BSAVA Manual of Exotic Pets

Fifth edition

A Foundation Manual

Editors:

Anna Meredith

MA VetMB CertLAS DZooMed MRCVS
RCVS Recognised Specialist in Zoo and Wildlife Medicine
Royal (Dick) School of Veterinary Studies, Hospital for Small Animals,
Easter Bush Veterinary Centre, Roslin, Midlothian EH25 9RG

and

Cathy Johnson-Delaney

DVM DipABVP(Avian)
Eastside Avian and Exotic Animal Medical Center, 13603
100th Avenue Northeast, Kirkland, WA 98034, USA

Published by:

British Small Animal Veterinary Association
Woodrow House, 1 Telford Way, Waterwells
Business Park, Quedgeley, Gloucester GL2 2AB

A Company Limited by Guarantee in England.
Registered Company No. 2837793.
Registered as a Charity.

Copyright © 2024 BSAVA
Third edition 1991
Fourth edition 2002
Fifth edition 2010
Reprinted 2014, 2015, 2017, 2018, 2020, 2021, 2022, 2023, 2024

Front cover images: sugar glider, courtesy of D. Johnson; snake, courtesy of P. Raiti; toucan, courtesy of M. Stanford; and koi, courtesy of HE Roberts. Back cover images: grey parrot, courtesy of M. Stanford; White's tree frog, courtesy of TD Bennett.

Illustrations 14.5b, 15.6 and 16.4 were drawn by S.J. Elmhurst BA Hons (www.livingart.org.uk) and are printed with her permission.

A catalogue record for this book is available from the British Library.

ISBN 978 1 905319 16 9

The publishers and contributors cannot take responsibility for information provided on dosages and methods of application of drugs mentioned in this publication. Details of this kind must be verified by individual users from the appropriate literature. Veterinary surgeons are reminded that they should follow appropriate national legislation and regulations, for example in the UK the prescribing cascade.

Printed in the UK by Hobbs the Printers Ltd, Totton SO40 3WX
Printed on ECF paper made from sustainable forests

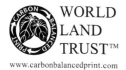

www.carbonbalancedprint.com
CBP2250

Carbon Balancing is delivered by World Land Trust, an international conservation charity, who protects the world's most biologically important and threatened habitats acre by acre. Their Carbon Balanced Programme offsets emissions through the purchase and preservation of high conservation value forests.

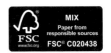

19589PUBS24

Other titles in the BSAVA Manuals series:

Contents

Contributors

Tracy D. Bennett DVM DipABVP(Avian)
Bird and Exotic Clinic of Seattle, 4019 Aurora Ave North, Seattle, WA 98103, USA

Michelle Campbell-Ward BSc BVSc (Hons I) DZooMed (Mammalian) MRCVS
RCVS Recognised Specialist in Zoo and Wildlife Medicine
Taronga Conservation Society Australia, Taronga Western Plains Zoo, Obley Road, Dubbo,
NSW 2830, Australia

John Chitty BVetMed CertZooMed MRCVS
Wombourne, Allington Track, Allington, Salisbury, Wilts SP4 0DD

Kevin Eatwell BVSc (Hons) DZooMed (Reptilian) Dip ECZM (Herp) MRCVS
RCVS Recognised Specialist in Zoo and Wildlife Medicine
ECVM Recognised Veterinary Specialist in Zoological Medicine (Herpetological)
Royal (Dick) School of Veterinary Studies, Hospital for Small Animals,
Easter Bush Veterinary Centre, Roslin, Midlothian EH25 9RG

Ruth Francis-Floyd DVM MS DipACZM
College of Veterinary Medicine, University of Florida, PO Box 100136, Gainesville, FL 32610, USA

Darryl Heard BSc BVMS PhD DipACZM
College of Veterinary Medicine, University of Florida, PO Box 100136, Gainesville, FL 32610, USA

Mike Jessop BVetMed MRCVS
Ash Veterinary Surgery, Aberdare Road, Georgetown, Merthyr Tydfil, Mid Glamorgan CF48 1AT

Dan Johnson DVM
Avian and Exotic Animal Care, 8711 Fidelity Boulevard, Raleigh, NC 27617 USA

Cathy Johnson-Delaney DVM DipABVP(Avian)
Eastside Avian and Exotic Animal Medical Center, 13603 100th Avenue Northeast, Kirkland,
WA 98034, USA

Nic Masters MA VetMB MSc MRCVS
International Zoo Veterinary Group, Keighley Business Centre, South Street, Keighley,
West Yorkshire BD21 1AG

Anna Meredith MA VetMB CertLAS DZooMed MRCVS
RCVS Recognised Specialist in Zoo and Wildlife Medicine
Royal (Dick) School of Veterinary Studies, Hospital for Small Animals,
Easter Bush Veterinary Centre, Roslin, Midlothian EH25 9RG

B. Denise Petty DVM
College of Veterinary Medicine, University of Florida, PO Box 100136, Gainesville, FL 32653, USA

Romain Pizzi BVSc MSc DZooMed FRES MACVSc(Surg) MRCVS
RCVS Recognised Specialist in Zoo and Wildlife Medicine
Inglis Veterinary Centre, 120 Halbeath Road, Dunfermline, Fife KY11 4LA
Royal Zoological Society of Scotland, Edinburgh Zoo, Corstorphine EH12 6TS

Paul Raiti DVM
Beverlie Animal Hospital, 17 West Grand Street, Mt Vernon, NY 10552, USA

Helen Roberts DVM
Aquatic Veterinary Services of WNY/5 Corners Animal Hospital, 2799 Southwestern Boulevard, Orchard Park, NY 14127, USA

Ian Sayers BVSc CertZooMed MRCVS
South Devon Referrals, c/o Abbotskerswell Veterinary Centre, The Old Cider Works, Abbotskerswell, Newton Abbot, Devon TQ12 5GH

Peter Scott MSc BVSc FRCVS
Vetark Professional, PO Box 60, Winchester SO23 9XN

Francis Scullion MVB PhD MRCVS
Royal (Dick) School of Veterinary Studies, Hospital for Small Animals,
Easter Bush Veterinary Centre, Roslin, Midlothian EH25 9RG

Geraldine Scullion MVB MRCVS
Veterinary Services, 16 Cranlome Road, Ballygawley, Co. Tyrone BT70 2HS

Nico Schoemaker DipECZM DipABVP(Avian)
Division of Zoological Medicine, Utrecht University, Yalelaan 108, 3584 CM Utrecht, The Netherlands

Stephen Smith BVetMed (Hons) CertZooMed MRCVS
Wendover Heights Veterinary Centre, 1 Tring Road, Halton, Aylesbury, Bucks HP22 5PN

Michael Stanford BVSc FRCVS
RCVS Recognised Specialist in Zoo and Wildlife Medicine (Avian)
Birch Heath Veterinary Centre, Birch Heath Road, Tarporley, Cheshire CW6 9UU

Thomas N. Tully Jr DVM MS DipABVP(Avian) ECZM(Avian)
Louisiana State University, School of Veterinary Medicine, Department of Veterinary Clinical Sciences, Skip Bertman Drive, Baton Rouge, LA 70803, USA

Foreword

It is an exciting time for exotic pet medicine as the past decade has seen tremendous growth and interest in exotic pets, which has concomitantly led to a greater demand for top quality veterinary care for these species. Small animal veterinary practitioners worldwide are now asked to provide care for these pets and are seeking additional training in exotic animal medicine at a greater rate than ever before. Veterinary schools are providing more coursework and rotations to help young veterinarians understand the needs of these patients, and internships, residencies and certifications in exotic pet medicine are providing advanced training in exotic pet medicine and surgery.

In order to provide excellent care for these animals, exotic pet practitioners must have: (1) solid foundations in the biology of each species in order to evaluate appropriate husbandry, abnormal behaviours and signs of disease; (2) the knowledge and skills to diagnose and treat the many different diseases of these pets; and (3) the ability to provide life-saving supportive and critical care to stabilize each patient. We must set the bar high in educating ourselves in all of these areas, and continue our education as exotic pet medicine advances in the future.

The *BSAVA Manual of Exotic Pets, fifth edition* is a well-organized reference that provides the foundations for care for the most commonly kept pet exotics. Each chapter addresses important biology, husbandry and handling/restraint for each species as well as the approach to differential diagnoses, specific diagnostic and therapeutic techniques, anaesthesia and analgesia, and supportive and critical care. Updated formularies are included throughout. Young veterinary graduates will find this Manual extremely useful for organizing their approach to the veterinary care of these pets. Established practitioners will find new approaches to the common diseases of these species and new, in-depth, information on less commonly presented species including primates and aquatic pets. The chapters on exotic pet legislation are especially timely as welfare of these pets is an integral component of their veterinary care and practitioners must be familiar with local, state, federal and international regulations pertaining to the exotic pet trade.

It is a true honour to be invited by the editors to write this foreword for the fifth edition of the *BSAVA Manual of Exotic Pets*. This is a Manual written by practitioners for practitioners, and I believe it should be included in the library of every pet veterinarian.

Michelle G. Hawkins VMD DipABVP(Avian)
Associate Professor, Companion Avian and Exotic Pet Medicine and Surgery
School of Veterinary Medicine, University of California Davis, Davis, CA 95616, USA
November 2009

Preface

The best-selling *BSAVA Manual of Exotic Pets* has been a 'must-have' text for so many clinicians since the first edition was published in 1991. Since then veterinary knowledge of, and exposure to, exotic pets has increased greatly, and this new updated edition reflects this. Looking back and comparing the first edition to this new one, the progress, expansion and development in the field has been vast. This fifth edition includes some new species (otters, skunks, marsupials, ratites) while other species now have expanded stand-alone chapters (e.g. African pygmy hedgehogs, axolotls and salamanders). One species (fancy pigs) has been moved entirely to the *BSAVA Manual of Farm Pets*.

The main aim of the Manual is to provide clinicians with easy access to necessary information in a standardized format for each chapter and species. The chapters are set out to lead the clinician from the natural history of a species, through the anatomy and physiology, husbandry, housing, dietary requirements, handling and restraint, diagnostic approach and major common conditions. Each chapter has tables of information providing quick access to biological data, bloodwork, common diseases and drug formularies so that a problem-oriented system approach can be carried out.

The authors and editors recognize that, as exotic pet medicine evolves, this Manual can no longer cover all species in sufficient depth, and so many chapters refer to the clinician to other BSAVA Manuals that provide more detailed information. This Foundation Manual can thus be seen as a starting point, designed to provide busy practitioners with a quick guide and the basic knowledge that enables them to deal professionally with a particular species even if it is unfamiliar.

The invited authors have done a fantastic job of providing the most up-to-date coverage of their subjects from a practical point of view, and we thank them sincerely for their time and effort. Several chapters combine expertise from both North America and the UK, as species typically seen by practitioners vary considerably between countries and continents. We hope this combination of material from North America as well as the UK and EU provides information that is applicable and useful worldwide. Many medications and even diagnostic techniques may not be available in every country and this is noted frequently. It is our hope that this will foster contact between readers and the authors, to try and bridge medical and therapeutic gaps to bring the level of veterinary practice in every country to the highest level.

As editors, one of us [CJD] for the first time for a BSAVA Manual, it has been a rewarding experience to work with so many authors, sharing their expertise about so many 'non-traditional' pets and captive species. It has been an incredible learning experience as well, as none of us can really know every species as well as the authors of the specific chapters do. We have also had a wonderful working relationship with each other, and with the BSAVA team (Marion, Nicola and Ben) and thank them sincerely for their guidance and patience. We have thoroughly enjoyed the experience and hope that you continue to find this new edition to be useful in daily practice and that it becomes an active part of your patient care.

Anna Meredith
Cathy Johnson-Delaney
November 2009

Mice, rats, hamsters and gerbils

Ian Sayers and Stephen Smith

Introduction

The order Rodentia contains over 2000 species. Those most commonly presented to veterinary surgeons are the domestic rat (*Rattus norvegicus*), domestic mouse (*Mus musculus*), Mongolian gerbil (*Meriones unguiculatus*) and Syrian, or golden, hamster (*Mesocricetus auratus*). Other species gaining in popularity are the Siberian, Russian, Djungarian or dwarf hamster (*Phodopus sungorus*), Chinese hamster (*Cricetulus griseus*), Roborovski hamster (*Phodopus roborovskii*), degu (*Octodon* spp.) and jerboa (*Jaculus* spp.). The term 'rodent' comes from the Latin *rodere,* meaning to gnaw or chew, and the Latin *dent,* for teeth.

Rodents have often been referred to as 'children's pets' but this term is no longer appropriate. There are many adults who care for rodents, and in the UK under the Animal Welfare Act 2006 there should always be a *responsible adult* supervising children caring for pet rodents. A lot of information is available about disease problems within laboratory rodents; not all of these are seen commonly in pet varieties but this does not mean that they are immune to such problems. Similarly, because a disease problem has not yet been reported in a species does not mean that it cannot occur.

It is important to approach cases in a similar manner to that used in more commonly seen patients. Signs of pain may be subtle and overlooked by the owner or clinician. Invariably the costs of investigation and treatment will exceed the purchase price but the authors wish to emphasize that we must not assume the owner's financial limits, and this should not prevent a full medical service being offered. Full clinical examination should be performed and appropriate diagnostic testing should be discussed with the owner to reach an appropriate action plan. Where necessary referral should be discussed and considered. Where cost is a problem, patient welfare should be paramount.

Rats and mice

Rats can make excellent pets as they rarely bite, especially if well socialized from an early age. They are also highly intelligent. Rats are less nocturnal than mice and are more easily trained. They benefit from companions, ideally same-sex littermates; otherwise, population control can quickly become an issue. Introduction of adult males is not recommended as fighting may ensue. It is easier to introduce older females of both species. Males tend to have a stronger scent than females and this is more noticeable in mice.

About 65 varieties of domestic rat are recognized by the National Fancy Rat Society in the UK, classified into five sections: Self Varieties; Marked Varieties; Any Other Varieties (AOV); Guide Standard Varieties; and New Varieties (see www.nfrs.org). Similarly, varieties of fancy mice are classified into five sections: Selfs; Tans; Marked; Satins and Any Other Variety (AOV) (see www.thenationalmouseclub.co.uk).

Hamsters

Hamsters are short-tailed stocky rodents of the family Muridae, subfamily Cricetinae and comprise 24 species in five genera, dispersed across Europe and Asia. The most common species kept in captivity is the Syrian, or golden, hamster *Mesocricetus auratus,* which is endangered in the wild. All golden hamsters in captivity originate from only 13 individuals captured in Syria in 1930. Golden hamsters are solitary and nocturnal but should rouse rapidly when disturbed. Most are the 'wild-type' colour which is a reddish-golden brown hair coat with a white ventrum (see Figure 1.5); other variations include cinnamon, dark brown, cream, white, piebald, albino and long-haired ('Teddy Bear').

Chinese hamsters (*Cricetulus griseus*) are smaller than golden hamsters and are also solitary and nocturnal, but more aggressive. Russian hamsters (*Phodopus sungorus*) are slightly larger than the Chinese hamsters and are relatively tame and placid compared with the other dwarf species. Russian hamsters are colonial and can be housed in groups (Figure 1.1), with the males tending to the young.

Gerbils

The Mongolian gerbil *Meriones unguiculatus* is one of 95 species and 14 genera in the order Rodentia, family Muridae, subfamily Gerbillinae – which are all correctly called gerbils. Gerbils are adapted to a desert environment and range from Africa, through the Middle East to Asia. In their natural environment they can produce most of their water requirement from metabolic processes; however, as pets, fresh water should be made available at all times. Gerbils are burrowing diurnal rodents with crepuscular tendencies (active at dusk and dawn). Gerbil pelage

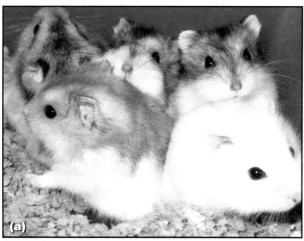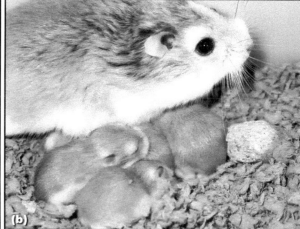

1.1   Dwarf varieties of hamster such as **(a)** Russian and **(b)** Roborowski are becoming more common. (Courtesy of C. Johnson-Delaney.)

colour can be black, grey, piebald, blue, Burmese, Himalayan, silver, white or the 'wild-type' agouti, which has dark pigmented skin with a light buff to white ventrum and mixed white, yellow and black hairs – giving a mixed brown appearance. Gerbils are highly sociable animals but appropriate management, i.e. single-sex groups, is required to prevent a surplus of unwanted pets. A total of 25 varieties are recognized, classified into Selfs, White Bellied, Any Other Variety (AOV) and Provisional (see www.gerbils.co.uk).

Biology

Biological data for small rodents are summarized in Figure 1.2.

Anatomy and physiology

Hamsters

Hamsters are renowned for their extensive cheek pouches that are used to carry food and, occasionally, young. The pouches are evaginations of the oral mucosa and can extend as far caudally as the scapula. They are emptied by squeezing the cheek contents forwards with the paws.

Hamsters are permissive hibernators, and at temperatures below 4°C will enter a deep sleep; some individuals will go into torpor between 4 and 10°C. This state of torpor should not be mistaken for death.

The stomach is demarcated from the oesophagus distinctly by a muscular sphincter, which prevents vomiting. The stomach is made up of the forestomach

	Mice	Rats	Hamsters	Gerbils
Lifespan (years)	1–2.5	2–3.5	1.5–2	2–3
Average weight (g) Males: Females:	20–40 20–60	270–500 225–325	87–130 95–130	46–131 50–55
Number of digits Front: Rear:	4 5	4 5	4 5	5 4
Heart rate (beats/min)	420–700	310–500	300–470	260–600
Respiratory rate (breaths/min)	100–250	70–150	40–110	85–160
Rectal temperature (°C)	~37.5	~38	36.2–37.5	37.4–39
Dentition	2 (I1/1 C0/0 P0/0 M3/3) Only incisors open-rooted			
Environmental temperature (°C)	24–25	21–24	21–24	18–22
Relative humidity (%)	45–55	45–55	40–60	45–50
Daily water intake	15 ml/100 g	10 ml/100 g	10 ml/100g	4–5 ml
Fluid therapy	100 ml/kg/24h			40–60 ml/kg/24h
Diet	Omnivorous			Largely granivorous
Food intake per day per animal (g)	3–5	15–20	10–15	5–7
Coprophagy/Caecotrophy?	Yes	Yes	Yes	Yes

1.2   Biological data for small rodents.

(pars cardiaca), which has a high pH and contains microorganisms for fermentation, and the glandular stomach (pars pylorica). Both sexes possess lateral flank glands (Figure 1.3) that are used to mark territory and stimulate mating behaviours. These brown patches are covered by fur and are more developed in the male than female. In the sexually aroused male they become easily visible as secretions cause matting of the overlying fur. Hamsters have acute hearing and olfaction so communication is achieved by sound, ultrasound and scent.

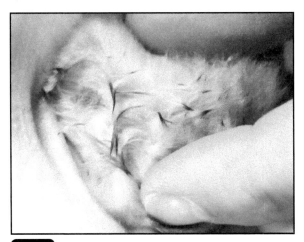

1.3 Lateral flank scent gland in a hamster.

Gerbils
The gerbil has a long furry tail, strong claws for burrowing and muscular back legs for jumping and standing. To help avoid predation they have a large middle ear to hear low-frequency sounds such as the beat of an owl's wing. Dorsal placement of their eyes gives a wider field of vision and their contrasting tail tip colour can distract predators. The tail will easily deglove if grasped to allow escape from a predator – an adaptation that should be borne in mind when handling.

Gerbils produce very concentrated urine, which is an adaptation to survival in dry environments. Both sexes possess an elliptical testosterone-responsive ventral scent gland; this enlarges in the pubescent male. Female gerbils have two pairs of thoracic and inguinal teats. The adrenal glands are normally large relative to bodyweight and lie at the cranial poles of both kidneys.

Dentition
The dental formula for mice, rats, hamsters and gerbils is similar (see Figure 1.2). Only the incisors are elodont (continually erupting), with the molars being brachydont (closed-rooted). It is important to recognize the normal lower to upper incisor crown ratio of 3:1, to avoid inappropriate teeth burring. The anterior surface of the incisor is enamel, whilst the caudal surface is softer dentine. During gnawing the cheeks are drawn into the diastema (gap between incisor and cheek teeth), which allows particles to be expelled easily from the mouth. Gnawing wears the teeth and maintains the sharp chisel-shaped tip. The yellow colour of the teeth is normal and is related to the deposition of iron pigments.

Sexing
Rodents possess open inguinal canals, allowing the testicles to be retracted into the abdominal cavity. Neutering of animals is becoming more common, and thus sexing via presence or absence of testicles is not reliable. The most reliable method of sexing is to assess the anogenital distance, which is shorter in females than in males (Figure 1.4).

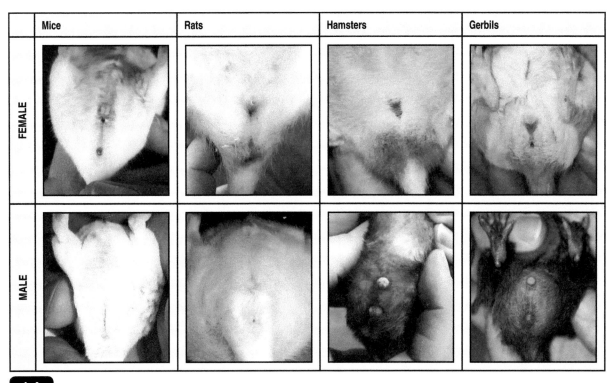

	Mice	Rats	Hamsters	Gerbils
FEMALE				
MALE				

1.4 Sexing by external genitalia.

Husbandry

Housing

Rats and mice

Rats and mice like to gnaw, so sufficient environmental enrichment and toys are needed to keep them active. Cages must be of material impervious to gnawing. Multi-level housing is beneficial to allow sufficient exercise and normal behaviour patterns. Mesh or wire flooring may cause feet problems.

Preferred humidity levels for rats are around 50%. Ventilation and cleanliness are important to prevent build-up of ammonia, which is highly irritating to the eyes and airways. There is a positive correlation between rising ammonia levels (25–250 ppm) and *Mycoplasma pulmonis* lung infections. Frequency of cleaning will depend on stocking density but it is stressful for the animal to have scent marks and olfactory clues removed by excessive cleaning. Supervised time out of the cage can be beneficial for rats, and their owners, but areas should be suitably 'rat-proofed'. A cage should have the following:

- Shelter or bolt-hole
- Absorbent substrate (wood shavings, shredded paper)
- Nesting material
- Sufficient substrate to scatter food to promote foraging
- Other environmental enrichment (gnawable items, empty boxes, sheets of paper, ladders).

Hamsters

Hamsters are inquisitive animals and will eagerly explore the perimeter of their housing, looking for ways to escape; thus cages need to be resistant to gnawing. Multi-floor caging with solid floors or plastic housing with interconnecting tubes can be used. Hamsters need plenty of exercise, and benefit from the provision of wheels and other toys. In the wild, hamsters can travel up to 10 km at night, so this should be re-created in captivity. Exercise wheels should be solid on the back and underfoot (Figure 1.5), to prevent damage to feet or tails. Hamsters usually urinate (cream colour) in one area of the cage

(latrine), and spot cleaning of this area should be done frequently. A nesting box containing nesting material (avoiding synthetic fibres) should be available, and it should be checked daily to prevent spoilage of hoarded food. A deep layer of substrate allows hamsters to engage in natural burrowing behaviour.

Gerbils

Gerbils are highly social animals and should be housed together as single-sex groups (introduced before sexual maturity), a breeding pair or in harems. Females are more likely to fight than males. Housing should have a tight-fitting lid with ventilation holes. Deep substrates (>15 cm) such as sawdust, shavings, peat and hay are recommended; sand should be avoided as it is too abrasive on the face during burrowing. Gerbils will create their own system of tunnels, which are constantly remodelled.

Gerbils should be kept in a dry environment. Relative humidity should be kept below 50%, otherwise an unkempt oily coat will result. A sand or dust bath should be provided, in a similar manner as for chinchillas, to allow dust bathing and promote a good coat quality. Playthings will prevent stereotypical behaviours, and items should be rotated to prevent boredom. Wood and cardboard will provide things to chew and ceramic pots or mugs provide good areas to hide in.

Gerbils produce scant amounts of urine, so enclosures often need less frequent cleaning than those of other rodents.

Diet

Rats and mice

Many mouse and rat owners think that rodents eat a seed-based diet, but this lacks a number of nutritional requirements to maintain health. Historically, 'muesli' diets have been fed, but care has to be taken to avoid selective feeding, particularly where high-fat seeds, such as sunflower seeds, are included, as obesity is not uncommon (Figure 1.6). Commercial pellets with >14% protein for mice and 20–27% protein for rats are recommended and are becoming more widely available. Items including commercial rodent-specific treats, fruit, nuts, vegetables, pasta and cheese should only be used in limited quantities to avoid imbalance or digestive upsets. However, these can help with training, especially for rats.

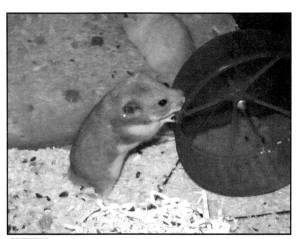

1.5 Exercise wheels for hamsters should be of solid construction.

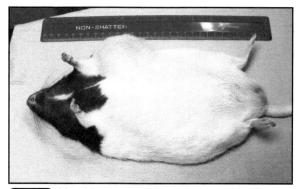

1.6 Morbidly obese rat. There is a mammary tumour in the left axilla.

Hamsters and gerbils

Hamsters and gerbils have similar dietary requirements in captivity and should be provided with a minimum of 16% protein (>20% for gerbils) and 4–5% fat. Again complete pellets are recommended to prevent selective feeding, and treats should be limited to items high in protein and low in fat. Hamsters fed exclusively on seed diets are prone to osteoporosis. Hamsters eat around 12 g of food per 100 g of bodyweight per day, and gerbils eat around 8 g of feed per day per 100 g bodyweight.

Water

Water bottles are recommended to prevent contamination – but water should be changed daily and the sipper cleaned and checked for debris or air locks. If bowls are used they should be heavy enough to prevent their being overturned, thus avoiding trauma. Gerbils are from very arid environments and only drink around 4 ml of water per gerbil per day compared with 10 ml of water/100 g bodyweight per day in hamsters.

Breeding

Reproductive parameters of small rodents are summarized in Figure 1.7.

Cannibalism can occur if litters are disturbed. Several factors can affect the incidence of cannibalism including low bodyweight, cold ambient temperatures and lean diets. Owners should provide ample food, water, nesting material and warm environmental temperatures and ideally leave the nest undisturbed for 1–2 weeks after parturition. Handling of litters can also increase cannibalism or desertion. A disturbed hamster mother may stuff the pups in her cheek pouches to move them to safety. If she is not allowed to hide quickly, the pups may suffocate.

	Mice	Rats	Hamsters	Gerbils
Oestrous type	Continuous polyoestrous	Continuous polyoestrous	Seasonal polyoestrous	Continuous polyoestrous
Post-partum oestrus?	Yes	Yes	No	Yes (resulting in delayed implantation)
Age at puberty (months)	1.5	1	Males: 2 Females: 1.5	Males: 2–4.5 Females: 2–3
Gestation length (days)	19–21	21–23	Syrian: 16–18 Russian: 18–21 Chinese: 21–23 Roborovski: 23–30	23–46
Oestrous cycle (days)	4–5	4–5	4–5	4–6
Oestrus duration (hours)	9–20	9–20	8–26	12–18
Litter size	7–12	6–13	5–10	3–8
Birth weight (g)	1–1.5	4–6	1.5–3	2.5–3.5
Altricial/Precocial	Altricial	Altricial	Altricial	Altricial
Eyes open (days)	12–14	12–15	12–14	16–21
Age at weaning (days)	18–21	21	19–21	21–28
Number of pairs of teats	5	6	6–7	4
Minimum breeding age (months)	2	2	2	2.5–3.5
Ratio for breeding (M:F)	1:1–6 If polygamous remove female before parturition	1:1–6 If polygamous remove female on day 16	1:1 Remove male after mating (except for Russian hamsters)	1:1 Form monogamous lifelong pairs in captivity. **Do not remove the male**
Comments	They will eat the litter if disturbed in the first 2–3 days	They will eat the litter if disturbed in the first 2–3 days	A vaginal discharge on day 2 of the oestrous cycle is normal and should not be confused with pyometra Cannibalism will occur if handled within 5 days of parturition Born with erupted incisors	Pseudopregnancy is common following infertile mating, lasting 14–16 days

1.7   Reproductive parameters of small rodents.

Handling and restraint

Conscientious interpatient hygiene is recommended for all animals. Particular attention should be paid to washing hands so that potential prey species are not stressed by the scent of a potential predator. Appropriate handling at all times can help reduce stress to an already ill animal.

Handling of rodents should be firm yet gentle and confident; the grip used will relate to the needs of the particular procedure. Restraint by 'scruffing' is often unnecessary for initial examination and should be reserved for appropriate procedures.

All small rodents should be handled close to a stable surface. This will minimize the risk of trauma if the animal jumps or is dropped and, on the rare occasion when a bite is inflicted, the animal can easily be placed on the solid surface where it will usually release its grip. It is common for rodents to pass urine and or faeces when restrained, which can be advantageous for sample collection.

Mice

Mice are quick and have a tendency to bite when in unfamiliar surroundings, so should be handled with care. They can be lifted by the base of the tail and placed on a surface that provides good grip (Figure 1.8ab). Palpation and auscultation may be performed in this manner, but when necessary the skin of the scruff can be grasped with the other hand, ensuring that there is sufficient amount to prevent the mouse turning its head and biting. The grip on the tail can then be transferred to the third and fourth fingers of the same hand (Figure 1.8c).

Rats

Rats bite less frequently than mice, even when startled, particularly if they have been well socialized. If a rat does bite during handling it may well be a pain response. Rats are nocturnal so it is important to ensure that a rat is awake before attempting to handle it. Rats can be grasped around the shoulders, with the other hand supporting the hind feet (Figure 1.9). For a painful procedure (e.g. injections), a thumb can be placed under the mandible to prevent biting. It is important not to grasp so firmly that respiration is impaired, especially if respiratory problems are suspected. If necessary the base of the tail can be grasped to lift the animal, but scruffing and overzealous restraint are usually resented and cause increased distress.

Hamsters

Hamsters have a reputation for biting, but if allowed to rouse from sleep and handled correctly they will only bite occasionally, especially if regularly handled in the home. They are best approached from the side, rather than from above, and cupped between the hands (Figure 1.10a). Subsequently they can be palmed or held around the shoulders and pelvic girdle with the head between the first and second fingers (Figure 1.10bc). As needed, gentle pressure can prevent the head turning to bite, and examination can be performed with the other hand. Handling in such a manner minimizes the risk of inadvertent ocular prolapse. Scruffing should be reserved for aggressive individuals or for administering medication.

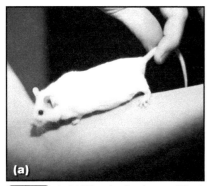 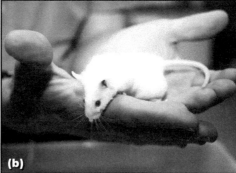 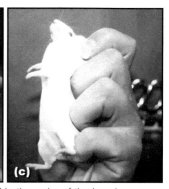

1.8   **(a)** Lifting by the base of the tail and front limbs supported once lifted. **(b)** Held in the palm of the hand. **(c)** Scruffing may occasionally be required.

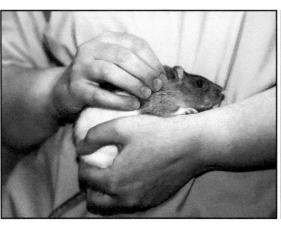 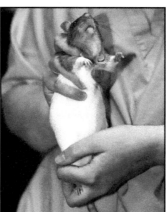

1.9

A rat can be grasped around the shoulders, with the other hand holding the hind feet.

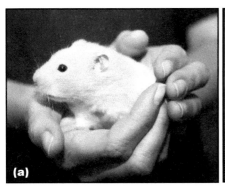 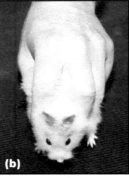 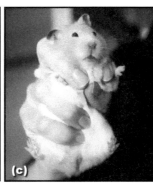

1.10
(a) A tame hamster can be held in cupped hands.
(b,c) Holding the shoulders and pelvic girdle, with the head between the first and second fingers.

Gerbils

Gerbils can be lifted in a similar manner to hamsters (Figure 1.11) They rarely bite, unless never handled at home. Gerbils should never be lifted by the tail. The skin on the tail is very thin and may tear off ('tail-slip'), exposing underlying connective tissue and bone (Figure 1.12) which will become necrotic. Analgesia and surgical amputation, to the level of healthy skin, will then be required.

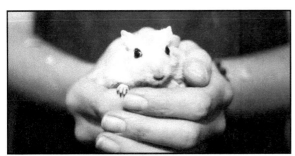

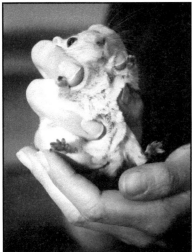

1.11
Gerbils can be lifted in a similar manner to hamsters.

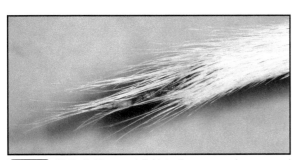

1.12 'Tail-slip' in a gerbil. Note the exposed coccygeal vertebrae and desiccated soft tissues.

Diagnostic approach

The principles of a thorough history-taking and clinical examination are similar to those applied to other patients, once the clinician is familiar with the species' husbandry, anatomy and biology. Animals should initially be viewed from a distance to assess demeanour, respiration rate and other parameters, whilst simultaneously taking a detailed history from the owner. Direct clinical examination should then be performed.

Rodents are primarily nocturnal but activity during daylight hours varies between the species. A large proportion of their time is spent grooming, to help keep coats in a good clean and shiny condition. They are generally inquisitive animals and if disturbed should rouse quickly. Signs of ill health may include reduced food and water intake, poor unkempt coat, reluctance to move, hunched posture, separation from cagemates, irrascibility and lack of interest in surroundings. Rodents are prey species, thus signs of disease may be concealed in the early stages. Since signs of pain and illness are not readily demonstrated, even apparently acute problems are likely to have been present for some time.

Accurate measurement of weight is critical for therapeutic dosing and patient monitoring. For small rodents, scales accurate to 0.1 g are recommended.

History

When obtaining the history, it is important that the correct person is asked about the patient. Although an adult is ultimately responsible, the majority of the care and attention may be given by a child.

Questions should address:

- Length of ownership
- Age
- Previous problems
- Current problem
- Diet
- Housing details
- Thirst
- Any other pertinent information.

Clinical examination

When performing a clinical examination, the clinician should be confident but careful. It is important that hands do not smell of food or predators. Particular attention should be paid to assessment of the oral cavity and to chest auscultation and abdominal palpation.

Imaging

Radiography
The approach to radiography should be similar to that in other species but, due to the small size of the patient, whole body views are often taken. Thought should be applied to correct positioning and optimal exposure setting for the area of interest. The use of high-quality film (e.g. mammography film) or newer higher definition digital systems is recommended to obtain images with superior detail.

The small size of the thoracic cavity, and superimposition of the triceps muscles, can make thoracic interpretation difficult. On occasion it may be beneficial to radiograph subjects through radiolucent boxes (e.g. induction chambers) to avoid the need for general anaesthesia, although correct positioning cannot be relied upon.

Ultrasonography
Ultrasound examination can be a useful aid to diagnosis of many disease problems of small rodents. High-frequency probes are recommended

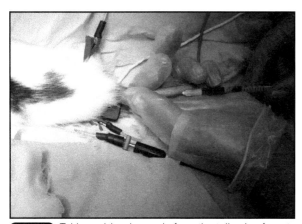

1.13 Taking a blood sample from the tail vein of a rat. Note also the presence of a rectal temperature probe and ECG leads.

and stand-offs may be beneficial. General anaesthesia may be required, and is essential for ultrasound-guided cystocentesis or other fluid removal.

Sample collection

Blood
Circulating blood volumes in rodents range from 5 to 8% of bodyweight, and approximately 10% of this can be safely taken from a healthy animal in a 3–4 week period. Sample volumes should be kept to the minimum required for testing, and the health status of the patient and subsequent potential blood loss (e.g. surgery, haematoma) must be considered. Sample sites depend upon species and sample size required. Sedation or anaesthesia is often required.

The lateral saphenous vein can be used in all these species. The vessel is punctured using a small-gauge needle and blood collected into a heparinized syringe or capillary tube. The use of small-volume syringes is recommended to minimize venous collapse.

Lateral tail veins can be used with proper restraint in mice, rats and gerbils (with care to avoid tail-slip), but sampling under anaesthesia is less stressful for the patient. Warming the animal or placing its tail in warm water or under a heat lamp will aid sampling. The vein is occluded at the tail base and sampling attempted one-third of the way down the tail (Figure 1.13), moving proximally if unsuccessful. Larger volumes can be obtained from the ventral tail artery in the rat or the anterior vena cava in the hamster.

The authors recommend contacting the commercial laboratory to ask about their ability to and experience of processing these small amounts of blood so that valuable information is not lost. A fresh blood smear should be made at the time of sampling to enable manual haematology if blood volumes are very small. Figure 1.14 gives average reference ranges for haematology and biochemical parameters for small rodents.

Parameter	Mice	Rats	Hamsters	Gerbils
Total blood volume (ml/kg)	70–80	50–65	65–80	60–85
Approximate recommended maximum blood collection volume (ml)	0.14	1.3	0.65	0.3
Haematology				
RBC (x10^{12}/l)	7.9–10.1	5.4–12	3.96–10.3	7–10
MCV (%)	46–62	46–68	no data	no data
HCT (%)	37–46	36–52	36.5–58	41–52
Hb (g/dl)	11.0–14.5	11.1–17.4	10.7–19.2	12.1–16.9
WBC (x10^9/l)	3.4–13.7	4.0–12.2	2.7–10.6	4.3–15
Neutrophils (%)	7–40	6–50	17–32	5–34
Lymphocytes (%)	55–95	50–88	50–95	60–95
Monocytes (%)	0.1–3.5	0–5	0–2.4	0–3

1.14 Average ranges from multiple sources for haematology and biochemistry parameters for adult rodents. It is recognized that differences occur according to strain, age, sex, fasted animals and site of venepuncture and these figures should therefore be viewed as a guide only. It is recommended that clinical parameters are interpreted using verified ranges from the laboratory producing the results. (continues) ▶

Parameter	Mice	Rats	Hamsters	Gerbils
Haematology continued				
Eosinophils (%)	0–4	0–6	0–3	0–4
Basophils (%)	0–1.5	0–2	0–3	0–1
Platelets (x10⁹/l)	600–1610	760–1120	300–570	400–600
Biochemistry				
Total protein (g/l)	56–103	59–84	55–72	43–147
Albumin (g/l)	25–48	32–46	20–42	18–58
Globulin (g/l)	60	22–48	25–49	8–100
Creatine kinase (IU/l)	155	111–334	366–776	–
AST (IU/l)	101–400	54–262	43–134	–
ALT (IU/l)	44–87	52–144	22–63	–
ALP (IU/l)	43–200	40–250	6–18	3.7–7
LDH (IU/l)	366	225–275	134–360	–
Sodium (mmol/l)	128–164	129–150	124–147	143–147
Potassium (mmol/l)	4.8–6.8	4.3–6.3	3.9–6.8	3.6–5.9
Chloride (mmol/l)	105–110	100–109	92–103	93–118
Glucose (mmol/l)	4.0–10.1	4.0–8.9	3.3–8.8	2.58–7.5
Cholesterol (mmol/l)	1.53–2.67	1.14–3.6	1.69–3.84	2.34–3.66
Urea (mmol/l)	6.42–11.06	4.28–7.85	4.99–9.63	6.1–10.7
Creatinine (μmol/l)	35–97	35–70	35–88	53–124
Total bilirubin (μmol/l)	5.13–13.68	4.0–8.2	4.1–12.31	13.68–27.36
Phosphate (mmol/l)	1.67–3.03	1.71–2.73	1.29–2.64	1.19–3.61
Calcium (mmol/l)	1.1–2.4	1.9–3.15	2.1–3.07	0.92–1.52

1.14 (continued) Average ranges from multiple sources for haematology and biochemistry parameters for adult rodents. It is recognized that differences occur according to strain, age, sex, fasted animals and site of venepuncture and these figures should therefore be viewed as a guide only. It is recommended that clinical parameters are interpreted using verified ranges from the laboratory producing the results.

Urine

Many rodents will urinate during handling, so handling them over a clean receptacle, or non-absorbent surface should be considered. Urethral catheterization and conscious cystocentesis are usually precluded by the small size of the patient. Sample size is also often small, so the clinician needs to be selective with their choice of tests.

Common conditions

Eye disease

The basic anatomy of rodent eyes is similar to that of other mammals, but there are notable differences. The smaller rodents have large globes in shallow orbits, resulting in prominent eyes. The rat and mouse have an intraorbital tear gland and an extraorbital tear gland. They also have a Harderian gland, which is in a similar position to the nictitans gland found in dogs, but has a slightly different function. The Mongolian Gerbil has both a Harderian and a nictitans gland. The Harderian gland produces lipid and porphyrin-rich secretions that appear to play a role in ocular lubrication and are groomed over the pelage. The retinal vascular supply is holangiotic.

Ocular infections

In rats and mice the most common causes of conjunctivitis are not associated with intraocular signs. Agents including *Corynebacterium* spp. and *Pasteurella* spp. may be involved in outbreaks where up to 50% of animals may be affected. Sialo-dacryoadenitis, caused by a coronavirus, is an important disease of adnexal tissue. It can be acute or chronic, causing conjunctivitis, periorbital swelling, photophobia and blepharospasm amongst other clinical signs (see Viral infections, below). Inappropriate substrate such as sand may result in a greater incidence of conjunctivitis or ocular foreign bodies in gerbils. Ocular infections, if unnoticed, can result in symblepharon formation or rupture of the globe (Figure 1.15). This can also be a common problem in hamsters where, due to their nocturnal nature, early signs are often overlooked by owners. Treatment of ocular infections is by appropriate topical and/or systemic antibiotics and analgesia. A ruptured globe should be enucleated.

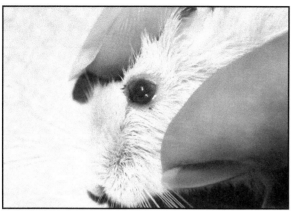

1.15 Ruptured globe subsequent to infection in a gerbil.

Other

Microphthalmos is a common problem and not all cases have a genetic basis. Cataracts may occur spontaneously or be congenital. Reversible cataract has been reported after the systemic use of xylazine. Glaucoma may be seen either due to inherited factors, or other causes, e.g. persistent pupillary membranes or anterior lens luxation. Entropion may also be seen, particularly in naked rats. Age-related corneal calcification, with production of central white plaques, is reported to occur in gerbils.

Corneal ulceration

Due to the prominence of the globe in these species, it is necessary to consider corneal lubrication during anaesthesia, otherwise exposure keratopathy corneal ulceration all too readily occurs. Application of appropriate paraffin products during the perianaesthetic period is recommended. If trauma is the suspected cause of ulceration it is necessary to check for signs of deeper injury.

Chromodacryorrhoea ('red tears')

As a response to stressors, production of porphyrin is increased, and often grooming is decreased with a resultant accumulation around the eyes and/or nose, either unilaterally (Figure 1.16) or bilaterally. These red crusts should not be mistaken for blood. Porphyrins are irritant, which can result in rubbing of the face, self-trauma and secondary infection. Porphyrins are reported to fluoresce under ultraviolet light, but the

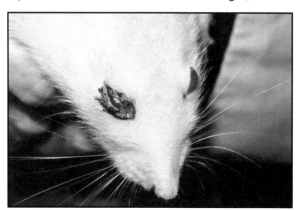

1.16 Unilateral chromodacryorrhoea in a rat.

authors have been unsuccessful in demonstrating this. The underlying cause should be investigated and treated appropriately.

Retinal atrophy

This is an age-related change seen in some albino rats and mice. It can be exacerbated by the level of lighting that occurs in most households. Some animals are seen to head-weave but it is unknown whether that is a behavioural or a neurological problem.

Ocular prolapse

The reputation of hamsters to bite readily when handled inappropriately means that, of the small rodents, ocular prolapse is most likely to occur in this species. When it is necessary for an individual to be scruffed, care should be taken to ensure that sufficient loose skin is restrained to avoid the animal being able to turn within the skin and deliver a bite, but also to make sure that excessive pressure is not applied around the eyes, which may potentially result in ocular prolapse.

Iatrogenic ocular prolapse is largely avoidable but should this occur it is necessary to lavage and replace the eye as soon as possible, ideally under anaesthesia. Analgesia should be administered and broad-spectrum topical antibiosis applied for 5–7 days.

Respiratory disease

Rats

Respiratory disease is one of the most frequent problems in rats and can be a complex multifactorial syndrome. *Mycoplasma pulmonis*, *Streptococcus pneumoniae*, cilia-associated respiratory (CAR) bacillus and Sendai virus are the most common aetiological agents, but infections are often mixed.

Sendai virus is a highly contagious paramyxo-virus contracted via aerosol from the respiratory tract. Transmission is possible over a distance of 6 feet. Infection with Sendai virus infection alone in rats is of little significance but it causes serious disease in mice.

M. pulmonis is a Gram-negative bacterium that causes serious disease in rats. Transmission can be intrauterine or via aerosol. The organism survives poorly outside the host and is susceptible to drying. It is thought that it is a normal commensal and only causes disease when there is concurrent Sendai virus infection or rising ammonia levels (> 19 μg/l) due to poor sanitation.

CAR bacillus is a Gram-negative bacillus that is a normal commensal in rats. The clinical picture is similar to that for *M. pulmonis*, with the addition of pulmonary abscesses and bronchiectasis in young rats. Disease due to CAR bacillus is always associated with *M. pulmonis* and occasionally Sendai virus infection.

Diagnosis is based on the presence of clinical signs, which can vary from mild dyspnoea to severe pneumonia and death. Rodents are obligate nasal breathers so open-mouth breathing is a poor sign. Clinical signs include nasal discharge, weight loss, 'rattling', dyspnoea, porphyrin-staining around the eyes, head tilt and a hunched stance. Radiography may aid diagnosis and show areas of abscessation or consolidation (Figure 1.17).

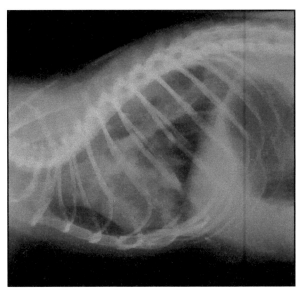

1.17 Right lateral thoracic radiograph of a rat, demonstrating lung lesions consistent with respiratory disease.

Initial aggressive treatment is rarely curative. Many cases will require lifelong therapy, or may never be well controlled. In-water medications are ineffective but most rat owners can give medication directly by mouth. Whilst not active against the viral component, antibiotics are very often useful in mixed infections. There are many choices (see Figure 1.36); combinations of fluoroquinolones with tetracylines or macrolides are often effective at reducing clinical signs and managing the disease. Pulse treatment is often required. Concurrent use of anti-inflammatories is beneficial; non-steroidal anti-inflammatory drugs (NSAIDs) should be tried initially, reserving steroids for non-responsive, chronic disease.

Bronchodilators and mucolytics can be used to open airways and increase mucociliary clearance. Nebulization should also be considered for delivering therapy (antibiotics, steroids) to the respiratory tract with minimal systemic effects. Commercial nebulizers or inhalers in a small chamber can be used to good effect. Importantly, environmental issues need to be addressed on the first presentation. This includes ensuring that: the substrate is dust-free; there is provision of good ventilation; and cages are cleaned regularly to prevent the build-up of ammonia.

Mice

As in rats, acute and chronic respiratory infections may be caused by Sendai virus or *Mycoplasma pulmonis*. Acute respiratory infections are usually associated with Sendai virus; adult mice survive but neonates often die. Chronic respiratory infections, with clinical signs of pneumonia, suppurative rhinitis and occasionally otitis media, may be the result of *M. pulmonis*. Both infections should be treated in a similar way to that described for rats.

Hamsters

In hamsters the true incidence of respiratory disease is unknown. Some reports state that it is uncommon, whereas other reports from laboratory colonies state that respiratory disease is second only to diarrhoea. Purulent rhinitis associated with pneumonia and ocular discharge ('sticky eyelids') carries a poor prognosis, but other clinical signs can include head tilt and dyspnoea. *Mycoplasma* has been isolated from hamsters but its pathogenicity is unclear; more common pathogens include *Pasteurella* spp. and *Streptococcus* spp. (which can be transmitted *from* children to the hamster). Other organisms isolated include *Klebsiella* spp., *Bordetella* spp. and *Staphylococcus* spp. Ideally, antibiotic therapy should be based on culture and sensitivity results, or broad-spectrum antibiotics can be used empirically.

Gerbils

Respiratory disease is rarely reported in gerbils, although they are susceptible to various pathogens, and clinical disease is seen in practice. *M. pulmonis*, *Pasteurella pneumotropica*, *Streptococcus pneumoniae* and *Bordetella bronchiseptica* have all been reported. Gerbils can also be carriers of Sendai virus. Clinical signs can include poor coat quality, weight loss, anorexia, dyspnoea, porphyrin around the eyes and nose, sneezing, and cyanosis if the problem is severe. Radiography and culture and sensitivity testing can aid diagnosis and treatment. Therapeutic options include appropriate antibiotics, NSAIDs, mucolytics, bronchodilators, diuretics and oxygen therapy.

Gastrointestinal disease

Enteritis and diarrhoea are common signs of ill health in rodents. General supportive therapy should be employed alongside therapies for specific causes. Sudden dietary changes can result in diarrhoea, in which case the original diet should be reintroduced with appropriate supportive measures. Dietary changes should be gradual, as with other species.

Salmonellosis

Salmonella typhimurium or *S. enteritidis* can cause acute or chronic diarrhoea in rodents, though in some cases the faeces can be normal. Other signs shown by infected animals include septicaemia, chronic wasting and abortion. In pets the incidence is low. The zoonotic potential and likelihood of developing carrier status if treated means that euthanasia is recommended upon diagnosis.

Tyzzer's disease

This can affect all rodents and is caused by infection of the gastrointestinal tract with *Clostridium piliforme*. Gerbils, followed by hamsters, are most commonly affected and these suffer increased mortality compared with rats and mice. The disease is often triggered by underlying stressors such as rehoming, overcrowding, poor husbandry, high environmental temperatures and humidity, prior antibiotic use, heavy parasite burdens and other disease.

Clinical signs in hamsters and gerbils are often non-specific and can include watery diarrhoea, scruffy coat, dehydration, lethargy and death. Diagnosis is based on post-mortem findings (necrotic hepatic foci and sometimes intestinal lesions) and by silver, Giemsa or PAS staining of affected tissues.

Generalized supportive treatment is rarely successful, but oral tetracyclines for 30 days may decrease morbidity in groups alongside appropriate treatment for any concurrent infection present.

Viral enteritis
Mouse hepatitis virus, a coronavirus, can cause severe enteritis in neonates but is rarely seen in pet mice. Accepted means of control in colonies is to stop breeding for 6–8 weeks and prevent introduction of new animals.

Parasitic enteritis
Faecal examination may demonstrate the presence of parasites, but many are coincidental findings and considered non-pathogenic unless high numbers are seen. Figure 1.18 outlines the gastrointestinal parasites that may be found in rodents.

Cheek pouch problems
Hamster cheek pouches often become impacted with various materials, including food and bedding. Animals present with distension of the face, unilateral or bilateral, which can extend as far back as the scapulae. If present for a long time, rupture of the pouch in the subcutaneous space can occur, leading to infection. Treatment involves everting, emptying and flushing the pouches under general anaesthesia. Abrasions and infection should be treated with appropriate antibiosis (topical or systemic), and any rupture in the pouch can be sutured to prevent recurrence. Potential underlying causes such as dental malocclusion should be evaluated.

Occasionally the cheek pouch(es) can evert spontaneously. This is likely to recur if simply pushed back in, so inversion and placement of a full skin thickness, non-absorbable, tacking suture is recommended. Food need not be withheld, and following suture removal after 2 weeks the problem should not recur.

Proliferative ileitis ('wet tail')
This is caused by the intracellular bacterium *Lawsonia intracellularis*, and is a proliferative enteropathy affecting young hamsters 3–10 weeks of age. Underlying stress factors, such as weaning, are involved in development of the disease. Signs include anorexia, lethargy and poor coat appearance followed by diarrhoea (Figure 1.19). Aggressive supportive treatment with fluids and nutritional support is required, along with broad-spectrum antibiotics such as tetracycline, doxycycline, enrofloxacin, chloramphenicol, neomycin or trimethoprim. Prognosis is poor and those animals that do survive may subsequently develop obstruction, intussusception or rectal prolapse.

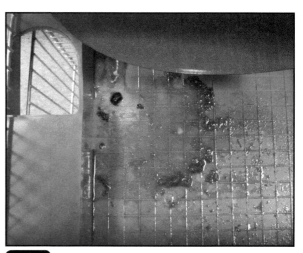

1.19 Diarrhoea characteristic of 'wet tail'.

Antibiotic-associated diarrhoea/enterotoxaemia
Selection of an appropriate and safe antibiotic is very important in rodents if adverse effects are to be avoided. Hamsters possess a predominantly Gram-positive gastrointestinal flora, which is susceptible to disruption by the administration of antibiotics. This disturbance in balance can allow proliferation of clostridial species (and suppression of normal *Lactobacillus* spp. and *Bacteroides* spp.), leading to a change in lumen pH and increased production of volatile fatty acids. The volatile fatty acids inhibit the normal bacteria further and cause production of iota toxin by the resident *Clostridium* species. These toxins destroy the mucosal epithelium and will cause

	Parasite	Disease	Diagnosis	Treatment (see Figure 1.36 for doses)
Protozoa	*Spironucleus muris, Giardia muris* (and other non-pathogenic commensals)	Mild enteritis in large numbers	Detection of oocytes in faeces	Metronidazole
Nematodes	*Syphacia* spp., *Aspicularis* spp., *Dentostomella translucida*	Mild enteritis in young animals. Large worm burdens can cause straining and rectal prolapse	Faecal flotation or adhesive tape strips around anal areas for *Syphacia* eggs	Ivermectin: three doses at 2-week intervals. Good sanitation
Tapeworms	*Rodentolepis* (formerly *Hymenolepis*) *nana* (dwarf tapeworm)	Found in lower small intestine. Infection is often asymptomatic but heavy burdens can cause severe gastroenteritis, weight loss and death. **ZOONOTIC**	Identification of segments on faecal flotation	Direct (15 days) and indirect lifecycle (via fleas and beetles). Frequent bedding changes and good hygiene. Praziquantel or niclosamide
	Rodentolepis (formerly *Hymenolepis*) *diminuta*	Affects upper small intestine. Low zoonotic risk	Identification of segments on faecal flotation	Frequent bedding changes and good hygiene. Praziquantel or niclosamide

1.18 Gastrointestinal parasites of small rodents.

diarrhoea and enterotoxaemia, which may lead to more severe disease and death.

The effects of antibiotics on individuals can vary widely, generating some confusion as to the safety of their use.

The use of narrow-spectrum antibiotics, with action against Gram-positive organisms, is more dangerous than using broad-spectrum agents.

Oral administration carries a higher risk than parenteral administration, due to direct action on the gastrointestinal tract flora.

Amoxicillin, amoxicillin/clavulanate, ampicillin, bacitracin, cephalosporins, clindamycin, erythromycin, lincomycin and other penicillins are capable of causing antibiotic-associated diarrhoea when given orally to small rodents (and rabbits, guinea pigs and chinchillas).

Treatment of antibiotic-associated diarrhoea and enterotoxaemia should start with aggressive supportive care aimed at cardiovascular support (fluid therapy), reducing production and effect of toxins, and support of normal flora. Colestyramine is an ion exchange resin capable of binding bacterial toxins and has been shown to prevent enterotoxaemia associated with clindamycin. Other general supportive treatment includes correction of hypothermia and supplemental feeding via syringe if there is not adequate voluntary intake of dietary fibre. Metronidazole or chloramphenicol have been suggested to reduce the levels of clostridial organisms. Transfaunation can be attempted from healthy animals and probiotics may be helpful. The incidence of clostridial enterotoxaemia is higher in intensive situations where the environment is contaminated with clostridial spores; therefore efforts should be made to keep the environment clean.

Urinary tract disease

Protein-related nephrotic syndrome
Nephrotic syndromes causing polyuria, polydipsia, chronic weight loss and proteinuria are seen in all the small rodent species and have various underlying aetiologies. High dietary protein levels have been implicated in the development and progression of these problems. There are no specific treatment regimens recommended, but general supportive care, fluid diuresis and potential use of anabolic steroids may be palliative. Decreasing levels of dietary protein has also been found to be beneficial. Using benazepril may be beneficial where there is renal protein loss (as in other species), though the hypotensive effects have been fatal in some rabbits when used at the higher end of the dose range. Starting at the low end of the dosage range and monitoring blood pressure is recommended with its use, even though this can be difficult.

Chronic progressive nephropathy
This is a common age-related problem in rats; the kidneys are enlarged and pale and have a pitted, mottled surface with pinpoint cysts. Clinical signs are

polydipsia and polyuria and the most marked change is proteinuria exceeding 10 mg/day. Glomerulosclerosis and interstitial fibrosis are seen histologically. The disease affects males at a younger age than females and is usually more severe. It is thought that high-calorie, high-protein diets are implicated in progression of the disease, and therefore calorie restriction and reduced protein levels (4–7%) are recommended to help limit the severity. Administration of anabolic steroids may be palliative.

Amyloidosis
Amyloidosis is caused by deposition of the almost insoluble proteinaceous matrix amyloid in the kidneys, spleen, adrenal glands or liver. The incidence is higher in females. Clinical signs are associated with organ failure and nephrotic syndrome if the kidneys are involved. Proteinuria, decreased serum albumin, oedema, ascites, hypercholesterolaemia, anorexia and increased total globulin are usually seen. Polyuria, polydipsia and haematuria are seen only occasionally. Prognosis is poor and palliative treatment is indicated, ensuring hydration and decreased protein intake.

Arteriolar nephrosclerosis
Hamsters fed high levels of dietary protein are prone to developing arteriolar nephrosclerosis. Signs exhibited include uraemia, proteinuria and polyuria. Amyloid deposition often occurs concurrently.

Gerbils
Little is reported with respect to urinary problems in gerbils. This may be related to this species' ability to produce only small amounts of concentrated urine, obtaining most of their fluid requirements from metabolic processes. However, chronic interstitial nephritis is considered to be common in older gerbils and may be associated with clinical signs of polydipsia, polyuria, weight loss and anorexia. Renal fibrosis, amyloidosis and glomerulosis have also been reported.

Reproductive system disease

Ejaculatory plugs
These are formed normally in rats and mice from epithelial cells and spermatozoa and are often seen in the bladder of males on post-mortem examination due to retro-ejaculation. It is important not to mistake them for uroliths causing obstruction of the urinary tract. Occasionally they can cause urethral obstructions, which can result in severe urinary tract infection and subsequent renal disease and/or death.

Pyometra
Pyometra is observed clinically in hamsters, gerbils and rats, but is not common. Diagnosis is by ultrasonography and cytology of vaginal discharge. Ovariohysterectomy is the treatment of choice (Figure 1.20). In hamsters it is important to differentiate pyometra from the normal creamy/white stringy postovulatory vaginal discharge.

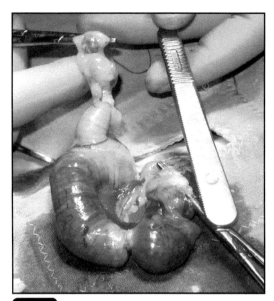

1.20 Ovariohysterectomy to treat pyometra in a rat.

Cystic ovarian disease

Cystic ovaries have been reported in all small rodents but are most often seen in hamsters (2% of females) and gerbils (up to 50% of animals <400 days of age). Clinical signs include poor coat quality, symmetrical alopecia, abdominal distension and dyspnoea. Nutritional intake may also be affected due to abdominal crowding. Diagnosis is made using radiography and ultrasonography. Ovariohysterectomy is the treatment of choice; medical options using human chorionic gonadotrophin and gonadotrophin-releasing hormone (GnRH) agonist implants have not yet been evaluated in rodents.

Neoplasia

Ovarian and mammary gland tumours have been reported (see Neoplasia, below).

Mastitis

Inflammation and infection of the mammary tissue has been reported in rats and may occur in other rodents. Clinical signs include swollen painful warm and/or lumpy mammary glands, poor appetite and hunched posture. The mother may have stopped allowing pups to nurse. Diagnosis is based on clinical signs; milk can be aspirated for culture and sensitivity testing. Treatment is with appropriate antibiotics, NSAIDs and warm compresses four times a day to promote drainage and decrease swelling.

Neurological disorders

Head tilt/vestibular signs

Torticollis and circling are seen more often in rats than in mice, and older individuals are more commonly affected. Central brain lesions can be the cause, but more often a head tilt is due to otitis interna, frequently caused by *Mycoplasma pulmonis* infection. Medical treatment is usually ineffective, but steroids and antibiotics in acute cases are reported to be useful.

A head tilt is also common in aged gerbils. It can be associated with a bacterial ear infection or may be secondary to respiratory infection, aural cholesteatoma (accumulation of keratinized epithelium), papilloma or polyp formation. Antibiotics may prevent worsening of the clinical signs but will rarely resolve the infection. There is no treatment for aural cholesteatomas, but papillomas and polyps require surgical excision.

Hydrocephalus

This can occur in rats due to a congenital malformation that causes CSF to accumulate in the ventricles of the brain, causing the cranium to become enlarged. The head is noticeably larger in the first few weeks of life, with seizures and poor motor coordination developing later. The disease is progressive, ultimately requiring euthanasia.

Hindlimb ataxia

This is a not uncommon presentation in aged rodents, particularly rats. It is seen as a progressive paralysis that can affect both hindlimbs. Aetiology is not fully understood but may be related to degenerative changes. It is important to rule out other causes such as trauma.

Toxicities

Streptomycin is toxic to gerbils and hamsters, causing a fatal ascending paralysis.

Lead toxicity is not uncommon in gerbils, due to their propensity to chew metal items, such as bars and bowls. Since gerbils produce very concentrated urine, they are susceptible to chronic lead accumulation. Clinical signs include weight loss, poor appetite, anaemia and neurological signs such as ataxia and seizures. Longer-term exposure will cause hepatic and renal failure, and typical microcytic hypochromic anaemia with basophilic stippling will be seen on haematology. Diagnosis can be made with radiography (if particulate lead is ingested) or by measuring blood lead levels. Treatment is by chelating agents (EDTA or D-penicillamine) and removal of the source.

Epilepsy

Twenty to forty percent of gerbils from certain strains develop spontaneous epilepsy starting at 2 months old and progressing to more severe disease up to 6 months of age. After this they seem to outgrow the problem. The inherited susceptibility is caused by a deficiency in the cerebral enzyme glutamine synthetase, and may have developed from a survival mechanism to deter predators. Episodes usually pass in a few minutes and can be triggered by handling or change of environment. Seizures may be mild or severe. Treatment is rarely indicated but phenytoin and primidone have been used. Epilepsy may be less likely to develop if gerbils are handled frequently within the first 3 weeks of life.

Skin disease

Ectoparasites

A wide range of ectoparasites occur on pet rodents (Figure 1.21). Clinical signs are largely associated with alopecia, scaling, ulceration and secondary bacterial infection associated with self-trauma. Skin scrapings,

	Parasites	Comments
Mice	*Myobia musculi, Radfordia affinis*	Fur mites. Low numbers rarely cause signs. Alopecia and ulceration in large infestations or immunosuppression
	Myocoptes musculinis, Trichoecius rombousti (rare)	Mange mites. Similar to fur mites but less severe
	Polyplax serrata	Sucking louse rarely seen on mice but zoonotic importance as vector of tularaemia
	Psorergates muricola	Burrowing mite that causes small white nodules on ear pinnae and body
	Liponyssoides sanguineus	House mouse fur mite. Asymptomatic unless very large numbers. Environmental control required
Rats	*Myobia musculi, Radfordia affinis, R. ensifera* (Figure 1.22)	Fur mites. Pruritus around head and shoulders, leading to self-inflicted ulcerative and scabbing lesions
	Notoedres muris	Watery papular lesions associated with yellow crust on the nose and ear flaps. Can also be erythematous and vesicular or papular lesions on tail, limbs and genitalia
	Polyplax spinulosa	Sucking louse of laboratory rats. Can cause pruritus, restlessness and anaemia and act as a vector for disease
	Demodex spp.	Incidental; unknown if associated with disease
Hamsters	*Demodex criceti* (in keratin and pits of epidermis), *D. aureti* (in hair follicles)	Alopecia, dry scaly skin, erythema and small haemorrhages. Not often pruritic unless infected and associated with immunosuppression or ageing (although small numbers can be found in healthy hamsters)
	Notoedres notoedres (ear mite), *N. cati* (cat mange mite)	Thick, yellow crust with associated alopecia and erythema on the pinnae, tail, genitalia, paws and muzzle
	Trixacarus caviae	May be pruritic
	Sarcoptes scabiei	Intense pruritus and alopecia. May be passed to humans/other animals
Gerbils	*Demodex meroni*	Associated with immunosuppression and underlying disease such as old age, poor diet and husbandry-related problems. Causes alopecia, scaling and focal ulcerative dermatitis with secondary infection
	Acarus farris (fur mite)	Alopecia, scaling and thickening of the skin over the tail, hindquarters and head
	Liponyssoides sanguineus	Asymptomatic unless very large numbers. Environmental control required
	Tyrophagus castellani	Copra itch mite. Asymptomatic
Any rodent	*Liponyssus bacoti*	Tropical rat mite. Lives in the environment and only comes on the host to feed
	Fleas	Seen where there are dogs and cats

1.21 Ectoparasites of small rodents.

coat brushing, hair plucks (trichograms) or adhesive tape strips (Figure 1.22) should be used to demonstrate the presence of adult mites and insects, nymphs or eggs. Examination of the coat with a hand lens may also reveal large parasites. In a single pet mouse that has signs of mites but scrapes are negative and there is no history of contact with others, biopsy for dermal hypersensitivity should be considered.

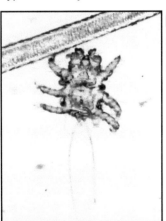

1.22

Radfordia ensifera found on tape strip sampling of a rat.

Treatment options are broadly similar for most of the parasites, and for specific details the reader should consult the Further reading. Reportedly effective treatments include ivermectin, selamectin, amitraz, benzoyl peroxide shampoo and lime sulphur dip. Regular bedding changes and good environmental hygiene and decontamination will help treatment of many infestations. Some sources recommend fragrant wood chips to control ectoparasites, but these can also be associated with skin hypersensitivity, so plain paper or recycled litter is preferable. Cedar should not be used as it contains oil that inhibits liver metabolism.

Bacterial infections

In rodents bacterial skin disease is usually due to opportunistic pathogens. *Staphylococcus aureus*, *Pasteurella pneumotropica* and *Streptococcus pyogenes* are common isolates. Abscesses often occur after bites or other trauma (Figure 1.23). Diagnosis can be based on demonstration of bacteria on impression cytology. Culture and sensitivity can be used to determine antibiotic therapy. Abscesses are best excised surgically leaving the abscess capsule intact

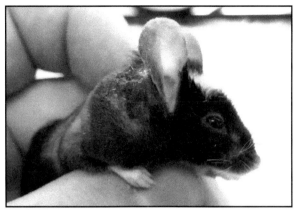

1.23 Cutaneous abscess associated with bacterial skin disease in a mouse.

but where this is not possible lancing and lavage under anaesthesia may be attempted. Treatment requires appropriate topical and/or systemic anti-biosis and analgesia. Recurrence is common if the underlying cause is not addressed or the abscess capsule is not removed. In gerbils, infection of the ventral scent gland may complicate diagnoses of scent gland neoplasia on initial presentation.

Dermatophytosis
Dermatophytosis is not uncommon in rodents but can often be asymptomatic. Where signs are present they are often dismissed as being due to mites. The most common causal agents are *Trichophyton ment-agrophytes*, *Microsporum canis* and *M. gypseum*. Secondary bacterial infection will often complicate the disease. Affected animals may be asymptomatic or may show typical dry circular lesions, alopecia, erythema and scaling. Toothbrushing of the entire animal is recommended for sampling for culture; or microscopy of hair samples can be used for diagnosis. *Trichophyton* spp. and 50% of *Microsporum* spp. do not fluoresce; thus, examination with a Wood's lamp can be unrewarding.

Treatment should be attempted, with topical therapy to remove spores from the hair shafts and systemic therapy to act at the hair follicles. Small lesions can be clipped, but with multiple lesions a whole-body clip may be beneficial. Systemic treatment with ketoconazole, itraconazole and terbinafine have all been reported. Under the prescribing cascade in the UK, itraconazole should be the first choice since it is authorized for use in cats. Topically, enilconazole can be applied daily or every other day with a toothbrush or cotton bud (although it can be toxic if ingested), or a miconazole/chlorhexidine shampoo used every other day may be helpful. Treatment should be continued until there have been two negative cultures 2–4 weeks apart. Removal of spores from the environment is essential to prevent reinfection.

Therapy in rodents is more challenging than in cats and dogs. Therapy usually lasts longer than in other patients due to the difficulty of preventing self-licking and scratching. Owner compliance can be variable when challenged with having to bathe and medicate a rodent daily for an extended period. Care should be exercised because of the potential for zoonosis.

Facial dermatitis
Facial (nasal) dermatitis, also known as facial eczema or 'sore nose', is a common condition in gerbils, especially in sexually mature, group-housed animals and incidence may be as high as 15%. The Harderian gland is located inside the orbit and secretes mucoprotein and lipids, which are released via the nasolacrimal duct at the external nares and then usually groomed away. Stress factors trigger hyper-secretion and accumulation in debilitated animals due to decreased grooming.

Initial signs include erythema around the nares (Figure 1.24) that can spread to include the face, paws and abdomen. Areas of alopecia develop and progress to extensive moist dermatitis. Diagnosis is based on clinical signs, bacterial culture and cytology of impression smears. Treatment for secondary infection is indicated, but improving husbandry, environmental temperature and reducing humidity (to <50%) are important. Provision of a sand bath will improve fur quality and promote grooming.

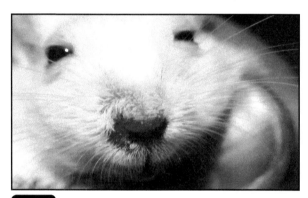

1.24 Early facial dermatitis in a gerbil.

Epitheliotropic lymphoma
Epitheliotropic lymphoma (see Figure 1.25) is the second most common tumour in hamsters (see Neoplasia, below).

Hamster scent gland inflammation
Syrian hamsters have scent glands over the hip area (see Figure 1.3), which are raised, pigmented structures that produce secretions during sexual activity. Occasionally these glands can become inflamed, swollen and crusted. Treatment is with clipping and topical antiseptics. These glands can also become neoplastic (see below).

Neoplasia
Neoplasia in small rodents is a common presentation in practice. For example, 25–40% of gerbils between 2 and 3 years old are reported to develop tumours. Scent gland carcinoma in males, and ovarian granulosa cell tumours in females, account for 80% of tumours in gerbils over 3 years of age. Mammary tumours are very common in rats.

Skin
Skin tumours, e.g. trichoepithelioma, are seen in rats and mice, but the majority of skin masses are abscesses. In hamsters the most commonly reported

cutaneous tumours are melanomas and melanocytomas, followed by epitheliotropic lymphoma. Subcutaneous masses in rats and mice are most commonly related to neoplasia of the extensive mammary tissue (see Mammary gland tumours, below). Old hamsters often present with clinical signs consistent with skin neoplasia, but failure to reach a diagnosis and report findings means the true aetiology of these signs can be unclear.

Epitheliotropic lymphoma: Epitheliotropic lymphoma is the second most common tumour in hamsters. There are three reported presentations of lymphoma in the hamster: a haemopoietic form; a cutaneous form (similar to mycosis fungoides in humans); and an epizootic form caused by hamster polyomavirus. For the cutaneous form, mean survival time from presentation to euthanasia has been reported as 9.6 weeks, but this was only a case series of six hamsters (Harvey *et al.*, 1992).

Epitheliotropic lymphoma can be confused with demodicosis or hyperadrenocorticism. Clinical signs vary depending on the extent and progression of the disease but include alopecia (Figure 1.25), pruritus, dry flaky skin, secondary infection, cutaneous plaques or nodules, cutaneous ulceration, and crusts. Diagnosis is based on biopsy and impression smears.

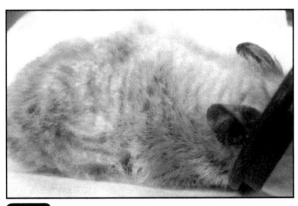

1.25 Epitheliotropic lymphoma in a hamster.

Treatment has not previously been recommended and euthanasia is carried out when the disease has progressed sufficiently to cause suffering. There is limited information about chemotherapy and survival times in hamsters with lymphoma, and much is anecdotal or incomplete. Protocols have been based on drugs that can be given subcutaneously and orally at dosages used in other animals. With venous access ports, intravenous protocols may also be of use. Prednisolone therapy has been used with good effect by the authors as a palliative measure.

Scent glands: Neoplasia of the scent glands occurs in both hamsters (flanks) and gerbils (ventrum), with or without secondary infection. It may be difficult to differentiate between simple infection of a normal gland and secondary infection of a neoplastic gland. Glands can appear matted and moist during normal glandular secretion. Cytological examination of impression smears and response to antibiosis can be useful.

Tumour growth is usually androgen-dependent; castration has therefore been recommended, but the authors do not routinely do this. If the scent gland is incompletely removed the tumour will recur unless the source of sex hormones is removed. Leuprolide acetate has been used with success anecdotally to block sex steroid production (C. Johnson-Delaney, personal communication). Benign adenoma, malignant adenocarcinoma and squamous cell carcinoma are seen. In the authors' experience neoplasia of the ventral scent gland is a common presentation in gerbils (Figure 1.26). Total gland excision is recommended, ideally in the early stages. Removal is usually achieved by a simple cutaneous incision and attention to haemostasis, which decreases the chances of local spread.

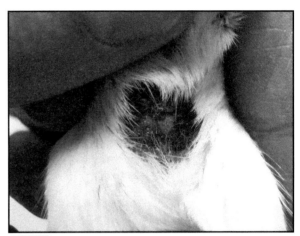

1.26 Advanced ventral scent gland neoplasia in a gerbil.

Gastrointestinal tract
Neoplasia affecting the stomach is reported in hamsters. Benign primary squamous papillomas in the glandular portion of the stomach are most common. Intestinal adenomas are also reported.

Reproductive tract
Ovarian tumours are reported in hamsters; they are usually unilateral, and metastasis is uncommon. Uterine endometrial adenocarcinoma has been reported in Chinese hamsters and results in vaginal haemorrhage.

Neoplasia of the reproductive tract in gerbils may present with vulval discharge and is often associated with secondary bacterial infection. Tumours reported include granulosa and thecal cell tumours, leiomyomas and adenocarcinoma of the uterus. Testicular teratomas and seminomas have been reported in the male gerbil.

Mammary gland tumours
These are the most common spontaneous neoplasms of mice and rats, but are rare in hamsters and gerbils. Most mammary tumours in rats and hamsters are benign, whereas in mice and gerbils they are more often malignant. In mice 90% of mammary tumours are malignant adenocarcinomas and fibrosarcomas. In rats 90% of mammary tumours are benign fibroadenomas; mammary tumours are uncommon in rats under 1 year old. The tumours are usually single

and firm, and unattached to deeper structures; they do not metastasize, but their size can be a problem if not treated early (Figure 1.27). In rats, ovario-hysterectomy at a young age reportedly reduces the incidence of mammary neoplasia.

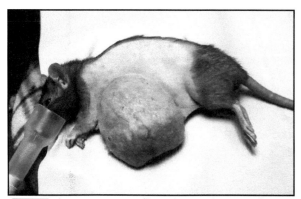

1.27 Large mammary fibroadenoma in a rat prior to surgery. This mass had been present for some time before the owner sought veterinary advice.

Surgical excision is indicated in the early stages. If surgery is not performed, continued growth of the mass can result in ulceration, ambulatory problems, self-trauma or other welfare issues. Mammary gland tissue is extensive in rats and mice, extending from the neck to the groin and as high as the flanks and shoulders. In hamsters and gerbils mammary tissue is confined to the ventral thorax and abdomen. During surgery there are generally several large blood vessels that should be identified and ligated; speed and accurate haemostasis have shown to be vital for a successful outcome. Histology is recommended, as further neoplasia at local or similar sites is not uncommon.

Behavioural and husbandry-related disorders

Barbering
Barbering is typically reported in groups, or pairs, of rats and mice where a hierarchy is established. The dominant animal nibbles the whiskers (Figure 1.28) and hair of subordinates; most commonly the face is

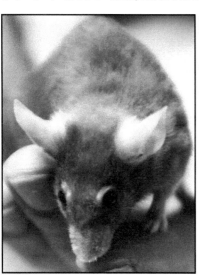

1.28 Barbering in a mouse. Notice the bare nose and shortened whiskers.

affected. The underlying skin appears normal and there are no signs of pruritus. Often only the dominant animal is unaffected. Removal of this individual can resolve the problem, but this may only be temporary, as subsequent dominant individuals may show the same behaviour. Barbering can also occur in other species. If it occurs in large groups of gerbils, bare areas are generally seen on the dorsal head and tailbase. Decreasing the stocking density is recommended.

Aggression
Aggression is seen, particularly in certain lines of rats and mice. Aggressive behaviour can sometimes be controlled by castration, but success depends on age of onset and how soon castration is performed. It may be beneficial in 'rescue' situations but cannot be relied upon. Adult Syrian hamsters should not be housed together as most will fight.

Ring tail
In rats aged 7–15 days, low environmental humidity (<20–40%) is associated with the development of annular constrictions of the tail, often near the base. The tail becomes oedematous, inflamed and then necrotic. Aetiology is unclear but factors involved may include fatty acid deficiency, low or high temperature, genetics, dehydration and trauma. Treatment requires increasing humidity to approximately 50% (e.g. by placing water bowls next to the cage or decreasing air flow). Attempts can be made to release the constriction surgically with small longitudinal incisions of the constricting band of tissue.

Cardiovascular disease
Atrial thrombosis is described in up to 73% of certain strains of aged laboratory hamsters. Cardiomyopathy, amyloidosis and vascular disease are all thought to contribute to heart failure and cardiac thrombus formation in the left atrium that, in turn, leads to a consumptive coagulopathy. Clinical signs of cardiomyopathy are usually present, including tachypnoea, cyanosis, lethargy, anorexia, cold extremities and ascites. Hamsters showing these signs typically die within a week. Diagnosis is based on clinical signs, radiography and echocardiography. Treatments reported include medications used in other species, such as diuretics, angiotensin-converting enzyme (ACE) inhibitors, prophylactic anticoagulants, digoxin and calcium-channel blockers.

Endocrine disease
While endocrine disease is possible in species of rodent, recognition and appropriate diagnostic sampling may not be available. Treatments follow guidelines for other species. Owners should be given the option to try treatment.

Hyperadrenocorticism
This can be primary (through neoplasia of the adrenal cortex), secondary (excess adrenocorticotropic hormone (ACTH) secretion due to a pituitary tumour) or iatrogenic (from glucocorticoid therapy). Hamsters demonstrating signs similar to hyperadrenocorticism

(HAC) in dogs do occur in practice, but only one case report has been published, with one animal possessing elevated serum cortisol levels. HAC has also been reported as a rare occurrence in aged gerbils and rats.

Clinical signs can include bilateral symmetrical flank alopecia, hyperpigmentation, comedones and thinning of the skin, polydipsia, polyuria and polyphagia. Differential diagnoses of dermatophytosis, lymphoma and demodicosis need to be ruled out, though the latter can often occur secondary to HAC. Diagnosis is normally based on clinical signs, as use of the ACTH stimulation or dexamethasone suppression test, although described for laboratory rodents, may not be possible for the pet animal. Urine cortisol:creatinine ratio may be easier to use to rule out HAC but reference ranges need to be established. Elevated serum cortisol (normal range 13.8–27.6 nmol/l) or alkaline phosphatase (normal range 6–18 IU/l) may be present, but can also be due to stress. The use of metyrapone was effective in one hamster but other medications have not been fully evaluated.

Diabetes mellitus

Diabetes is a spontaneous disease usually seen by 90 days of age in specific lines of Chinese hamster. Signs include polydipsia, polyuria, weight loss, hyperglycaemia, glucosuria and polyphagia. Blood glucose levels can be elevated above 16.65 mmol/l (normal range 3.3–8.8 mmol/l), although 'normal' values as high as 12.7 mmol/l are reported for mice, probably resulting from stress-induced hyperglycaemia. Treatment using neutral protamine Hagedorn (NPH) insulin (2 IU s.c. q24h) may be useful.

Diabetes can also be a sequel to obesity in aged gerbils, and obesity and high-calorie diets have been known to induce spontaneous diabetes mellitus in mice. Spontaneous diabetes has been reported in strains of rats that are used as models for juvenile diabetes in humans. One report indicates good response to twice-daily injections of medium duration insulin for rats using an initial dosage of 1 IU/kg rising to 10 IU/kg for final stabilization. In all species, urine glucose can be used for monitoring, to avoid the complications of repeated venepuncture.

Other

Other reported endocrine diseases include insulinoma, pituitary adenoma and hyperplasia, thyroid adenoma, hypothyroidism and parathyroid neoplasia. Some have been diagnosed *post mortem* so the clinical significance is unclear.

Viral infections

Lymphocytic choriomeningitis

Lymphocytic choriomeningitis virus (LCMV) is an RNA arenavirus that causes a chronic fatal wasting disease of young hamsters. Individuals are often asymptomatic, and clinical signs depend on age and immune status of infected individuals and the virulence of the viral strain. Reported signs include weight loss, photophobia, tremors and seizures. Wild mice are a common primary reservoir of infection (but hamsters and guinea pigs can also be a reservoir) and transmission occurs vertically *in utero* or horizontally via direct or indirect contact with infected urine, faeces or saliva. Diagnosis is via PCR, serological detection of anti-LCMV antibodies or virus isolation from tissue. **Treatment should not be attempted due to the zoonotic risk from LCMV.** Rodents suspected of having the disease should be euthanased and submitted for post-mortem examination. Housing and furniture should be disinfected or discarded. Humans may become infected by exposure to urine and faeces or from a bite, causing symptoms consistent with 'flu, malaise, headaches, fever, myalgia or arthritis. Fatal aseptic meningitis or meningoencephalitis is rare. Other primate species such as callitrichids (marmosets and tamarins) can also be affected (see Chapter 8). Strict hygiene and protective clothing will reduce the likelihood of exposure to those working with rodents.

Hamster polyomavirus (papovavirus)

Hamster polyomavirus (HaPV) causes cutaneous epitheliomas in Syrian hamsters, with up to 50% affected in laboratory colonies. The host-specific virus is also thought to be the cause of transmissible lymphoma (abdominal, thoracic or epitheliotropic) and other skin tumours (see Neoplasia, above). Wart-like lesions are seen in young (3–12 months) hamsters around the eyes, mouth (Figure 1.29) and perianal area. The virus is transmitted via urine and is highly contagious. There is a long incubation period (4–8 months) and the virus is very resistant in the environment. There is no spontaneous resolution. Individual tumours can be removed surgically.

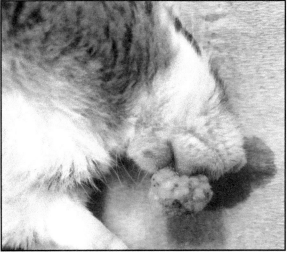

1.29 Hamster polyomavirus lesion on the lower lip of a young hamster.

Coronavirus

This has been identified as causing sialodacryoadenitis in rats. Clinical disease caused by this agent alone is self-limiting and is *highly* infectious. Sneezing, oculonasal discharge, cervical oedema, enlarged cervical lymph nodes, necrotic inflamed salivary glands, swelling or infection of the eyes or surrounding eye tissues, ulcers of the cornea and hyphaema can be seen. Signs may be present for several weeks in a colony, but each individual rat will only show signs for a week. Secondary infections will cause other associated clinical signs. There is no treatment other than supportive care and antibiosis for secondary infection.

Supportive care

Hospitalization
Small rodents are prey animals and as such they should be hospitalized away from the scent, sound and smell of predators. This will decrease stress levels and ultimately improve recovery from illness. It is often beneficial to hospitalize them with their normal cagemates and keep them within their usual housing to minimize stress. They should be offered familiar foods, even if the diet is not ideal, in the short term to encourage intake. Dietary changes can subsequently be implemented upon recovery. Provision of water in a familiar container is also essential. Signs of disease and discomfort are not overtly displayed, so attention to nursing time to allow observation is required. It should be remembered that whilst it is important to maintain temperature these animals are unable to sweat or pant, and signs of heat stress can occur when exposed to high temperatures (see Figure 1.2 for recommended ranges).

Drug administration
An accurate weight for each patient needs to be established to enable accurate drug dosing. Using average weights for the species is not appropriate.

Injection sites

- Subcutaneous injection is easy and poses the least risk to the animal. Small rodents can be held by the scruff and the injection given into the tent of skin between the thumb and forefinger.
- Intramuscular injections are less useful due to the small muscle mass. The anterior thigh muscles and triceps are the largest muscle masses for small-volume injection.
- The intraperitoneal route exposes drugs to first pass through the portal circulation, so there may be premature metabolism or biotransformation.
- Venous access for intravenous injections invariably requires anaesthesia, unless the animal is very depressed. Larger rodents may be amenable to intravenous injections while conscious.

Figure 1.30 gives general guidelines for routes and volumes for injections. Drug volumes calculated for administration can be impractically small. To give accurate doses and to avoid tissue irritation, drugs may have to be diluted. Ideally, diluents should be the same as the drug carriers but water for injection or 0.9% NaCl appear to be acceptable alternatives for aqueous preparations.

Oral medications
Medications given in food or water rarely achieve adequate therapeutic blood levels of the drug. Medication of drinking water for individual treatment is considered poor practice by the authors: when ill, rodents may drink and eat less than normal, and will reject unfamiliar-tasting food or water. However, medicated tasty treats can sometimes be useful.

When hospitalized, drugs can be administered with a gavage tube if necessary. The tube is premeasured from the nares to the last rib and lubricated with KY jelly. The animal is held with the neck extended and the tube passed through the oropharynx into the oesophagus. Smooth advancement and failure to aspirate air indicates correct placement, whereas struggling suggests incorrect placement (although a bulb-ended tube helps prevent entry into the trachea). If a soft tube is used, a mouth gag should be placed to prevent the animal biting through the tube. The suggested maximum volume for gavage is 5–10 ml/kg.

For oral medication at home, a solution of appropriate concentration needs to be used. To improve palatability and owner compliance drugs can be mixed (and diluted) with flavoured syrups or fruit juices. Other compounding systems such as Flavorx are also available. To administer oral medications, the rodent should be held as previously described and the tip of the syringe inserted into the mouth via the diastema. Alternatively, some rodents readily accept sweet-tasting medication. It is important to ensure that the client is competent at giving the oral medication. Slow and careful administration reduces the risk of aspiration pneumonia.

Nebulization
Nebulization can be beneficial for the administration of various drugs and solutions for respiratory problems. Machines are readily available but it is necessary to ensure appropriate particle size (between 2 and 10 μm). Efficacy of inhalation is also affected by the rate and depth of respiration and by tidal volume.

Route	Mice	Rats	Hamsters	Gerbils
Subcutaneous	Neck, back, abdomen (2–3 ml)	Neck, back, abdomen (5–10 ml)	Neck, back, abdomen (3–5 ml)	Neck, back (2–3 ml)
Intramuscular	Quadriceps (0.03 ml)	Quadriceps/gluteal (0.2–0.3 ml)	Quadriceps/gluteal (0.1 ml)	Quadriceps/gluteal (0.1 ml)
Intraperitoneal	Right caudal quadrant of abdomen (1–3 ml)	Right caudal quadrant of abdomen (10 ml)	Right caudal quadrant of abdomen (3–4 ml)	Right caudal quadrant of abdomen (2–3 ml)
Intravenous	Lateral tail vein (0.2–0.3 ml)	Lateral tail or saphenous vein (0.5 ml slowly)	Not described	Lateral tail vein (0.2–0.3 ml)

1.30 Injection volumes and sites for small mammals. These recommended volumes vary throughout the literature and are given as a guide only. Thought should be given to the effectiveness of uptake and amount of discomfort caused.

Fluid therapy

Fluid therapy should be used in situations of fluid deficit or anticipated fluid loss, i.e. anaesthesia and surgery. Generally 100 ml/kg/day is recommended for maintenance, although only 40–60 ml/kg/day is recommended for gerbils due to their adaptation to dry environments. Dehydration can be estimated subjectively based on bodyweight, mucous membrane dryness, skin tenting, sunken eyes and altered mentation.

Fluid deficit is calculated as:

% dehydration x bodyweight (g)
= fluid required (ml).

In the first 24 hours, 50–75% of the fluid deficit can be replaced, with the remainder replaced over the following 48–72 hours, alongside maintenance requirements and ongoing losses. Fluids should be warmed to body temperature, regardless of the route of administration; warming to 39°C will not affect the composition. The patient's weight should be closely monitored to assess efficacy of fluid therapy. Weighing urine-soaked bedding can be done to assess urinary output. Choice of fluid follows that in dogs and cats.

Routes of administration

Where dehydration is >5%, **intravenous** fluid therapy is recommended, but this can be problematical due to the nature and size of these species, and subsequent catheter maintenance can be difficult due to vessel fragility. The **intraosseous** route has the advantage that similar fluid rates to intravenous administration can be used and there is easier access if there is vascular collapse. Intraosseous administration is easier to maintain due to stability of the medullary cavity. Spinal needles or hypodermic needles (with homemade metal stylets) can be used. Sites include the femur (through the trochanteric fossa) and the tibia (through the tibial crest). Flushing with heparinized saline should be done immediately to prevent rapid clotting of the bone marrow. Intraosseous catheters can be used for short-term volume expansion prior to intravenous catheterization. Asepsis, anaesthesia (local or general) and analgesia are required for intravenous or intraosseous catheter placement.

Intraperitoneal delivery allows for relatively large volumes with more rapid uptake than the subcutaneous route, especially when the animal is dehydrated. However, this route should not be used if there is abdominal disease. **Subcutaneous** administration is easily performed in the space over the neck and back but is painful and absorption is delayed in debilitated patients due to vasoconstriction. The **oral** route is recommended if the patient is <5% dehydrated and stable. Access is easy and it helps maintain intestinal tract function, but administration of large volumes can be difficult and may result in aspiration.

Fluid resuscitation

Hypovolaemic shock is difficult to treat in rodents but treatment can be accomplished with a combination of crystalloids, colloids and rewarming procedures. Ideally, blood pressure needs to be monitored but this can be problematic in rodents due to their body size, so clinical judgement may be relied upon. In the collapsed patient, compensatory mechanisms are blunted due to hypovolaemia and hypothermia.

1. Initially deliver a bolus of isotonic crystalloid at 10–15 ml/kg and colloid at 5 ml/kg over 5–10 minutes (i.v. or intraosseous).
2. Continue to give crystalloids at maintenance levels whilst warming the patient to above 36.7°C, at which point the adrenoceptors respond to the fluid deficit.
3. Then continue crystalloid and colloid increments until the patient responds clinically.
4. Maintenance fluid therapy should be continued as necessary.

Nutritional support

Nutritional support is often required for rodents as food intake is reduced when they are unwell; supplemental feeding is an essential component of long-term critical care.

- Oesophagostomy tubes may be considered but the size of tubing will often limit their usefulness. Assisted feeding using proprietary products or ground-up food pellets is often well tolerated, especially if these have a sweet flavour.
- Administration via gavage tube may be necessary if syringe feeding is not well accepted. Feed volumes of 5–10 ml/kg are usually appropriate. Commercial, scientifically derived products (e.g. Critical Care Formula (Vetark Professional, Winchester, UK) or Oxbow Critical Care for Herbivores (Oxbow Animal Health, Murdock, USA)) are widely available, so the use of baby foods should be unnecessary. If baby foods must be used it is important to avoid milk-based products that can contribute to intestinal upsets.
- The use of probiotics may be a useful adjunct to therapy.
- Gut transfaunation from a known healthy individual can be helpful with gastrointestinal disease.

Anaesthesia and analgesia

Preoperative care and preparation

All small rodents can be safely and effectively anaesthetized. Anaesthetic risks are greatly reduced when patients are suitably prepared and stabilized prior to the procedure. Apparently acute conditions are likely to have a chronic component, thus food and fluid intake will probably have been reduced for a period prior to presentation. Although often overlooked in rodents, administration of appropriate analgesia improves patient welfare, and allows delivery of a reduced amount of anaesthetic agent, thereby improving safety. Appropriate nutritional support and fluid therapy are also required.

Small rodents are unable to vomit, and have high metabolic rates, so pre-anaesthetic fasting is not required; indeed, it is contraindicated. Where a patient has been inadvertently starved the procedure (unless urgent) should be postponed. Careful thoracic auscultation is essential to identify previously undetected underlying respiratory problems, which would have a major impact on anaesthesia.

Small rodents have a high surface area-to-volume ratio, and thus potential for heat loss is high. Heat loss can be reduced by minimal clipping, avoiding use of alcoholic skin preparations, and using prewarmed skin disinfectants. Cold anaesthetic gases and open body cavities further increase heat loss, and anaesthesia removes the patient's ability to thermoregulate. Provision of heat via protected heat mats, infra-red heaters, warm air and appropriate ambient temperature is essential to prevent hypothermia. Whilst avoiding *hypo*thermia is crucial it is equally important to avoid *hyper*thermia and prevent skin burns that can occur with some heat sources. Body temperature should be recorded before and after the procedure to assess the efficacy of the chosen method(s); the use of continuous display rectal temperature probes is recommended throughout the anaesthetic period.

The use of multimodal analgesia in the perioperative period is recommended; a combination of NSAIDs, opiate analgesics and local anaesthetics should be used routinely (Figure 1.31).

Induction and maintenance

Anaesthesia can be induced and maintained with volatile agents, such as sevoflurane and isoflurane, or with injectable agents.

Gaseous

Sevoflurane is less irritant to the respiratory tract and less soluble than isoflurane, providing smoother and quicker induction. Pre-oxygenation is recommended, as breath-holding is not uncommon with gaseous induction. The authors' preference is to induce anaesthesia with sevoflurane and then maintain with either sevoflurane or isoflurane.

Induction chambers should be of an appropriate size, with gas inflow at the bottom and scavenging outflow at the top, to enable rapid air changes and a swift induction. Alternatively, patients can be held in a towel and a mask placed over their head or nose for delivery of the anaesthetic gas. Anaesthesia should be induced with the maximum percentage of volatile agent (5% for isoflurane; 8% for sevoflurane) to reduce induction time and patient stress.

Maintenance of anaesthesia can be achieved by a well fitted facemask (commercially available or homemade modified syringe cases), using cotton wool to maintain a good seal to prevent the escape of anaesthetic gas. Recommendation of an appropriate maintenance gas percentage is not possible as there are many factors to consider, such as analgesia used, fit of the facemask, painful stimuli. Sevoflurane is less potent than isoflurane; therefore, higher maintenance percentages will be required. It is important to maintain hydration of the cornea with an ocular lubricant during anaesthesia to prevent exposure keratopathy.

Endotracheal intubation is difficult in rodents and usually requires anaesthesia with an injectable agent. This is more common in the laboratory situation and specialized equipment is required. (See Further reading for more information.)

Injection

Injectable anaesthetic combinations can be used in rodents (Figure 1.32). A prerequisite of injectable

Drug	Species	Dose	Effect
Acepromazine	Rats	2.5 mg/kg i.p./s.c.	Sedation, but still active
	Mice, gerbils, hamsters	3–5 mg/kg i.p./s.c.	
Diazepam	Rats	2.5 mg/kg i.p.	Sedation
	Mice, gerbils, hamsters	5 mg/kg i.p.	
Fentanyl/Fluanisone	Mice, rats, gerbils, hamsters	0.5 ml/kg i.p./s.c.	Sedation and analgesia; often sufficiently immobilized for minor surgical procedures
Medetomidine	Mice, hamsters, rats	30–100 µg/kg i.p./s.c.	Sedation and some analgesia; immobilized at higher dose rates
Midazolam	Rats	2.5 mg/kg i.p.	Sedation
	Mice, gerbils, hamsters	5 mg/kg i.p.	

1.31 Pre-anaesthetic agents for use in small rodents.

Drug	Mice	Rats	Hamsters	Gerbils
Atipamezole	1 mg/kg s.c./i.m./i.p./i.v.	1 mg/kg s.c./i.m./i.p./i.v.	1 mg/kg s.c./i.m./i.p./i.v.	1 mg/kg s.c./i.m./i.p./i.v.
Doxapram	5–10 mg/kg i.v./i.p.	5–10 mg/kg i.v./i.p.	5–10 mg/kg i.v./i.p.	5–10 mg/kg i.v./i.p.
Fentanyl/Fluanisone + Diazepam	0.3 ml/kg FF i.m. + 5 mg/kg D i.p.	0.3 ml/kg FF i.m + 2.5 mg/kg D i.p.	1 ml/kg FF i.m. + 5 mg/kg D i.p.	0.3 ml/kg FF i.m. + 5 mg/kg D i.p.
Ketamine + Medetomidine	75 mg/kg K + 1 mg/kg M i.p.	75 mg/kg K + 0.5 mg/kg M i.p.	100 mg/kg K + 0.25 mg/kg M i.p.	100 mg/kg K + 0.25 mg/kg M i.p.

1.32 Anaesthetic and related drugs for use in small rodents (due to wide variation in response between strains, doses are intended only as a guide).

anaesthesia is accurate measurement of bodyweight and careful calculation of drug doses; dilution is often required. Intramuscular injection causes pain and muscle damage, and should be avoided where possible as the available muscle mass is minimal. Once administered there is less control of anaesthetic depth than with volatile agents. It is not possible to administer drugs *to effect*, unless the intravenous route is used, and there is often a wide range of response to injectable agents with certain combinations resulting in prolonged sleep times. Oxygen should be provided even when injectable anaesthetics are used, to prevent hypoxia from hypoventilation.

Monitoring

Plane of anaesthetic depth is most reliably assessed by the pedal withdrawal or tail pinch reflex. Tail pinch reflex is usually lost at light to medium planes, while the pedal response is lost at medium to deep planes of anaesthesia. The palpebral reflex may still be present at surgical planes of anaesthesia. The use of clear sterile drapes can aid monitoring of respiratory rate and depth; typical respiratory rates of anaesthetized rodents will be 50–100 breaths per minute.

It is possible to use similar monitoring equipment to that used for other small animal species, but it must be capable of measurement in the range required and be sensitive enough to register accurately the low amplitude cardiac electrical activity of some species. For example, a number of heart rate monitors show error codes at rates of 600 beats/min, so higher rates cannot be read. Capnography has the same benefits as in other species. However, the sample volume of mainstream capnographs is greater than the tidal volume of many small rodents and introduces excessive dead space into the system; side-stream capnographs are therefore recommended.

Recovery

Providing a stress-free area away from the sight, scent and sounds of predators is as important for recovery from anaesthesia as it is for hospitalization in general. Monitoring of patients at frequent intervals until fully recovered is essential. Thermal support should be maintained until the animal has fully recovered. Postoperatively, environmental temperature should be in the region of 35°C until fully recovered and then reduced to more normal levels.

Common surgical procedures

Preparation, equipment and principles of surgery

Small rodents often have subclinical respiratory disease or other undetected problems prior to anaesthesia. Thorough clinical examination is important prior to surgery and other diagnostic testing (e.g. haematology, biochemistry, imaging) is useful. Preoperative fasting is generally contraindicated as rodents cannot vomit and have limited glycogen stores; exceptions may include where oral or gastric surgery is planned.

Instrumentation

Specific microsurgical instrumentation is recommended for all rodent surgery; these instruments are of standard size but are counterbalanced for more comfortable and precise use. Ophthalmic instruments are a reasonable compromise but they are shorter, making deeper abdominal manipulations more difficult.

Recommended surgical instruments and equipment include:

- Microsurgical needle-holder
- Microsurgical artery forceps
- Halsted ring-tipped forceps
- Fine rat-toothed forceps
- No. 15 and no. 11 scalpel blades
- Small (2 x 2 cm) gauze swabs
- Large- and small-tipped cotton buds
- Lone-star retractor
- Haemoclips
- Haemostatic powder/gauze.

Magnification using surgical loupes or a surgical microscope will facilitate small rodent procedures. Practice is required to ensure the surgeon is confident and adept at using them when required for delicate abdominal surgery or precision haemostasis. Good quality illumination is essential. The use of clear plastic drapes is recommended as they are lightweight and allow anaesthetic monitoring of the patient.

Accurate haemostasis must be ensured, since blood loss can rapidly exceed dangerous levels (e.g. >0.3 ml for a 30 g mouse). Careful use of diathermy or radiosurgery will help minimize blood loss and is invariably appropriate for the size of blood vessels encountered. It should be remembered that it takes the circulating volume of more than two mice to soak a standard gauze swab. Hands or surgical instruments should not be rested on the patient, restricting respiration.

Wound closure

It can be challenging to prevent rodents interfering with surgical wounds, and they are particularly averse to the placement of Elizabethan-type collars. Use of fine suture materials (e.g. 0.7 to 1 metric (5/0–6/0 USP)), accurate closure of dead space, gentle tissue handling, minimal wound tension, appropriate analgesia and, in some cases, local anaesthesia will reduce the chance of problems. Surgical glue may be better tolerated, but some rodents can remove the glue from the incision, especially if applied too liberally. Skin staples are generally tolerated by rats.

Surgical neutering

Neutering can be considered for the prevention of disease, unwanted litters and undesirable behaviours associated with sexual maturity (such as aggression and urine marking), and for the treatment of reproductive disease.

Castration

In small rodents the testicles should descend into the scrotal sac; open inguinal rings mean that they can be withdrawn into the abdomen. Castration is described using scrotal, prescrotal or abdominal techniques, but the latter is more likely to cause intra-abdominal adhesions and therefore is not recommended by the authors.

A 'closed' technique is recommended by many to prevent herniation through the inguinal ring post-operatively, although this has not been clearly documented.

1. The patient is placed in dorsal recumbency. If the testes have retracted, ensure that the plane of anaesthesia and analgesia is adequate and apply gentle caudal abdominal massage to return them to the scrotum.
2. Make a scrotal skin incision.
3. Carefully dissect the vaginal tunic away from the skin and clamp it proximal to the testes. Place an encircling or transfixing ligature using fine (e.g. 1 metric (5/0 USP)) absorbable suture material (Figure 1.33) and remove the testicle caudal to the ligature.
4. A suture incorporating the tunic can be placed to close the inguinal ring.
5. Close the scrotum with tissue adhesive (prescrotal skin can be closed with subcuticular sutures).

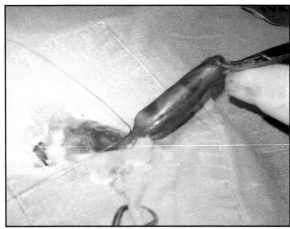

1.33 Ligation of the tunic and enclosed vasculature during closed castration in a rat.

If the initial incision penetrates the vaginal tunic this becomes an 'open' technique and the vas deferens and blood vessels are ligated directly. The tunic should be closed separately from the skin, although this can prove tricky in mice.

Males can remain fertile for up to 6 weeks after castration, although certain sexual behaviours may remain for many weeks.

Ovariohysterectomy

The technique is largely similar across the small rodents but is not commonly performed as an elective procedure.

1. With the patient in dorsal recumbency, make a 1–3 cm ventral midline incision between the umbilicus and pubis, into the abdominal cavity. If the ventral sebaceous gland interferes, divert the

incision around it and bluntly dissect back to the linea alba.
2. Identify the ovaries and the bicornate uterus, with its short uterine body and single cervix.
3. Clamp the ovarian pedicles and ligate with 1.5 metric (4/0 USP) or 1 metric (5/0 USP) absorbable monofilament suture material.
4. Bluntly dissect the broad ligament on each side to the level of the uterus.
5. Ligate the cervix with a transfixing suture and remove the reproductive tract. **Avoid handling the gastrointestinal tract as rodents are prone to developing adhesions.**
6. Close the abdominal wall incision with an interrupted or continuous pattern and then close the skin using a subcuticular continuous pattern or tissue adhesive.

Fracture management

When dealing with fractures in small rodents, patient stabilization and analgesia should be approached as diligently as in dogs and cats. Often euthanasia is considered, but other viable options are available for rodent fractures.

Fractures below the elbow and stifle (Figure 1.34) are commonly open, due to minimal soft tissue cover in these areas. When handling *open* fractures:

- Wear sterile gloves
- Use aseptic techniques
- Lavage the area after taking a swab for bacteriological culture
- Place a sterile bandage and temporary splint to prevent further soft tissue damage
- Maintain analgesia and perform radiography under anaesthesia when stable.

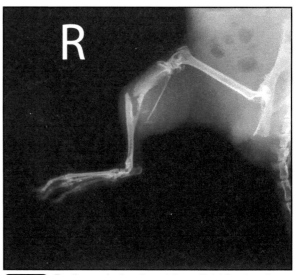

1.34 Radiograph showing oblique tibial fracture in a gerbil.

Whilst fixation maximizes patient comfort, improves bone blood supply and healing and reduces the chance of infection, small rodent fracture management may require a more imaginative approach than in dogs and cats. Confinement is easy, but rest is impossible to enforce. Rodents will often gnaw at splints and external fixators, and many of the implants available are too large. Techniques are described for external coaptation, intramedullary pinning, bone plating and external skeletal fixation.

External coaptation can be effective for closed simple interlocking fractures, but is poor for oblique fractures. However, the rapid callous formation in small rodents (7–10 days in hamsters) means that splinting can have a surprisingly effective outcome, even in poorly reduced fractures. When splinting a fractured limb, it is important to avoid further damage to the soft tissues and blood supply. Palpation will often establish whether the fracture is reduced but radiography is recommended to evaluate for misalignment. Standard splinting principles should be applied: keep the limb in normal position; immobilize the joint above and below the fracture; and achieve 50% cortical contact. Material used for splinting can include Vet-lite (Runlite SA, Belgium), crimped adhesive plasters for small limbs, and cocktail sticks or unfolded paper clips. Splints should be monitored to avoid soiling, pressure sores, infection and swelling. Application of bitter spray or superglue can be used to prevent chewing of the splint.

Rodents cope well with the loss of a limb, and amputation can be considered where there is a severe fracture, marked soft tissue damage or infection.

Dentistry

All the small rodent species can suffer from dental disease. It is important to remember the normal incisor crown length ratio of 3:1 lower to upper, and that only the incisors are elodont. Incisor malocclusion (Figure 1.35) can be an inherited condition or may be acquired through damage to the delicate periapical germinal layer from which the teeth grow, by trauma or chewing of unnaturally hard substances (cage bars). Treatment is with burring at regular intervals – on average every 4–5 weeks, but may be more frequent since the eruption rate increases when teeth are out of alignment. Clipping with nail clippers is not recommended as it **will** shatter the tooth; where or

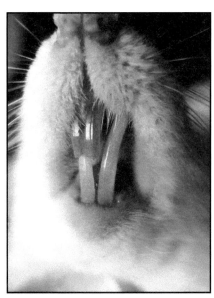

1.35

Incisor malocclusion and overgrowth in a rat.

how it shatters is purely down to chance, leaving sharp edges that further contribute to oral discomfort. Removal of the incisors has been described but is difficult because of the long reserve crown and fragility of the surrounding jaw bone; thus iatrogenic damage is likely, making it not a practical option. Provision of suitable objects to encourage gnawing, rather than cage bars, is recommended.

Euthanasia

It is recommended that small rodents should be anaesthetized prior to euthanasia to improve patient welfare and discomfort upon administration of irritant barbiturates. This enables safe and painless intravenous or intracardiac injection.

Drug formulary

Few drugs are authorized for use in small rodent medicine. In the UK, consideration should be given to adhering to the veterinary prescribing cascade. Where this is not possible informed consent for 'off-label' use must be obtained from the owner. It is worth remembering that in the UK the Small Animal Exemption Scheme does not fall within the cascade.

A drug formulary for small rodents is given in Figure 1.36. It is beyond the scope of this chapter to consider all possible drugs and doses reported. Many dosing regimens quoted in published texts have wide ranges, creating confusion when trying to select the correct dose. The reader is encouraged to make use of all the material available when considering choices of treatment and the doses listed in this formulary are intended only as a guide. An accurate weight for each patient needs to be established to enable accurate drug dosing. Using average weights for the species is not appropriate.

Antibiotics

Selection of an appropriate and safe antibiotic is very important in rodents if adverse effects are to be avoided (see Antibiotic-associated diarrhoea/enterotoxaemia, above). Antibiotics that are apparently safe in rodents include enrofloxacin, ciprofloxacin, marbofloxacin, trimethoprim/sulphonamide combinations and chloramphenicol. Doxycycline is used effectively in rats and mice for treatment of chronic respiratory disease.

WARNINGS
- **Gentamicin can cause renal problems, so care should be taken to prevent grooming and ingestion after topical application.**
- **Procaine is toxic to gerbils and mice (and rabbits and guinea pigs).**
- **Streptomycin can cause an ascending paralysis and death in gerbils, hamsters and mice.**
- **Nitrofurantoin causes neuropathological lesions in rats.**

Drug	Dose	Comments
Antimicrobial agents		
Amoxicillin/Clavulanate	Mice, rats: 100 mg/kg orally q12h	
Ampicillin	Mice, rats: 20–50 mg/kg orally/s.c./i.m. q12h Gerbils: 6–30 mg/kg orally s.c. q8h	**DO NOT USE IN HAMSTERS**
Azithromycin	Rats: 10–20 mg/kg orally q12h for 14 days then q24h for 14 days	For *Mycoplasma*
Cefalexin	Mice: 60 mg/kg orally or 30 mg/kg s.c. q12h Rats: 60 mg/kg orally or 15 mg/kg s.c. q12h	
Chloramphenicol	All species: 10–50 mg/kg orally/s.c./i.m./i.v. q6h–q12h	
Ciprofloxacin	All species: 7–20 mg/kg orally q12h	
Doxycycline	All species: 2.5–5 mg/kg orally q12h	Good for *Mycoplasma;* sometimes combined with enrofloxacin
Enrofloxacin	All species: 20–30 mg/kg orally q24h for 10–14 days	
Erythromycin	Mice, rats: 20 mg/kg orally q12h	Do not use in hamsters
Marbofloxacin	All species: 2 mg/kg orally/s.c./i.m. q24h	
Metronidazole	All species: 20 mg/kg orally q12h	
Neomycin	25 mg/kg orally q12h or 0.5 mg/ml in drinking water (group treatment)	For proliferative ileitis in hamsters
Oxytetracycline	All species: Tyzzer's disease: 10–20 mg/kg orally q8h All species: mycoplasmosis: 100 mg/kg s.c. q24h	
Trimethoprim/Sulphonamide	All species: 30–50 mg/kg orally/s.c./i.m. q12h	
Antifungal agents		
Enilconazole	Mice, hamsters, gerbils: dip in 0.2% solution weekly Mice, rats: 50 mg/m² topically twice weekly for 20 weeks	
Itraconazole	2.5–10 mg/kg orally q24h	For dermatophytosis
Ketoconazole	10–40 mg/kg orally q24h	For dermatophytosis
Terbinafine	8–20mg/kg orally q24h	For treatment of dermatophytosis
Antiparasitic agents		
Amitraz	Dilute 1.4 ml per litre and bathe weekly for 3–6 treatments	For *Demodex* – use with caution. Apply with cotton bud/brush. Can precede with benzoyl peroxide shampoo bath
Benzoyl peroxide shampoo	Topically, small amount, rinse well with warm water	Use prior to amitraz for mites
Fenbendazole	20–50 mg/kg orally q24h for 5 days	Use low end of dose range for *Giardia*
Fipronil	7.5 mg/kg topically every 30–60 days	For fleas
Ivermectin	0.2–0.4 mg/kg orally/s.c./topically every 7–14 days for a total of 3 treatments or 0.4 mg/kg q24h orally for 5–7 days	For demodicosis. Dissolve in 1:10 propylene glycol to improve topical absorption. If topical fails, repeat s.c. Large colonies: calculate 'total dose' based on group bodyweight; mix with propylene glycol; spray group evenly
Lime sulphur dip	All species: dip weekly for 4–6 treatments	For mites (*Demodex, Trixacarus*) and dermatophytosis
Metronidazole	All species: 10–40 mg/kg orally q24h	
Praziquantel	6–30 mg/kg orally/s.c. every 10–14 days	For cestodes
Selamectin	6–18 mg/kg topically every 14 days for 2–3 treatments	For mites
Analgesics		
Buprenorphine	Mice: 0.05–0.1 mg/kg s.c./orally q8h Rats, hamsters, gerbils: 0.01–0.05 mg/kg i.m./s.c. q6–12h	
Carprofen	All species: 5 mg/kg s.c. q24h	
Meloxicam	All species: 0.2–0.6 mg/kg orally/s.c. q24h	Some reports state doses of 1–2 mg/kg orally/s.c. q24h in mice and rats

1.36   Drug formulary for mice, rats, gerbils and hamsters. Doses are taken from multiple sources found in the references and further reading. (continues)   ▶

Drug	Dose	Comments
Miscellaneous		
Atropine	For bradycardia: 0.05–0.1 mg/kg s.c. For organophosphate toxicity: 10 mg/kg s.c. every 20 minutes	
Benazepril	0.05–0.1 mg/kg orally q24h	For protein-losing nephropathy; care, may cause hypotension
Diazepam	1–5 mg/kg i.m./ i.v./ i.p./intraosseously once	For seizures
Doxapram	5–10 mg/kg i.v./i.p. once or 1 drop orally	Respiratory stimulant
F10	1:250 dilution by nebulizer q8h	For nebulization (20 ml for 20–30 minutes) or for cleaning, delivered by spray bottle
Furosemide	All species: 5–10 mg/kg s.c./i.m. q12h or 1–4 mg/kg i.m. q4–6h	
Metyrapone	8 mg orally q24h for 1 month	Reported for treatment of hyperadrenocorticism in hamsters
Oxytocin	0.2–3.0 IU/kg s.c./i.m. once	
Phenytoin	Gerbils: 20–35 mg/kg orally q8–12h	For epilepsy
Prednisolone	1–2 mg/kg orally q12h	Palliative treatment for lymphoma
Primidone	Gerbils: 2.5–5 mg/kg orally/s.c./i.m. q12h	For epilepsy
Ranitidine	2–5 mg/kg orally q12h	Prokinetic and to reduce gastritis
Sucralfate	50 mg/kg orally q8h	Gastroprotectant
Verapamil	Hamsters: increasing from 0.25 to 0.5 mg s.c. q8h over a 4-week period	For cardiomyopathy

1.36 (continued) Drug formulary for mice, rats, gerbils and hamsters. Doses are taken from multiple sources found in the references and further reading.

References and further reading

Burgmann P (1997) Dermatology of rabbits, rodents and ferrets. In: *Practical Exotic Animal Medicine: The Compendium Collection*, ed. K Rosenthal, pp. 175–179, 184–185. Veterinary Learning Systems, Trenton, NJ

Carpenter JW (2005) *Exotic Animal Formulary, 3rd edn.* Elsevier Saunders, St Louis

Flecknell PA (2001) Analgesia of small mammals. *Veterinary Clinics of North America: Exotic Animal Practice* **4**(1), 47–56

Ellis C and Mori M (2007) Skin diseases of rodents and small exotic mammals. *Veterinary Clinics of North America: Exotic Animal Practice* **2**(4), 493–542

Hallowell Engineering and Manufacturing Corporation. *Intubation Techniques in Rats and Mice.* www.hallowell.com/index.php?pr=video_presentations

Harvey RG, Whitbread TJ, Ferrer L and Cooper JE (1992) Epidermotropic cutaneous T-cell lymphoma (mycosis fungoides) in Syrian hamsters (*Mesocricetus auratus*). A report of six cases and demonstration of T-cell specificity. *Veterinary Dermatology* **3**, 13–19

Hem A, Smith AJ and Solberg PL (1998) Saphenous vein puncture for blood sampling of the mouse, rat, hamster, gerbil, guinea pig, ferret and mink. *Laboratory Animals* **32**, 364–368

Keeble E (2001) Endocrine diseases in small mammals. *In Practice* **23**, 570–585

Keeble E and Meredith A (2009) *BSAVA Manual of Rodents and Ferrets.* BSAVA Publications, Gloucester

Krogstad AP, Franklin CL and Besch-Williford CL (2001) An epidemiological and diagnostic approach to murine skin lesions. *Proceedings, 52nd American Association for Laboratory Animal Science National Meeting, Baltimore* p.94 [abstract]

Lichtenberger MA (2007) Shock and cardiopulmonary-cerebral resuscitation in small mammals and birds. *Veterinary Clinics of North America: Exotic Animal Practice* **10**(2), 275–291

O'Malley B (2005) Clinical anatomy and physiology of exotic species. Elsevier, St Louis

Paterson S (2006) *Skin Disease of Exotic Pets.* Blackwell, Oxford

Quesenberry KE and Carpenter JW (2004) *Ferrets, Rabbits and Rodents: Clinical Medicine and Surgery, 2nd edn.* WB Saunders, Philadelphia

Renshaw HW, Van Hoosier GL Jr and Amend NK (1975) A survey of naturally occurring diseases of the Syrian hamster. *Laboratory Animals* **9**, 179–191

Schmidt RE, Eason RL and Hubbard GB (1983) *Pathology of Aging Syrian Hamsters.* CRC Press, Boca Raton, FL

Vincent AL, Rodrick GE and Sodeman WA Jr (1979) The pathology of the Mongolian gerbil (*Meriones unguiculatus*): a review. *Laboratory Animal Science* **29**, 645–651

2

Guinea pigs, chinchillas, degus and duprasi

Cathy Johnson-Delaney

Introduction

The hystricomorph rodents (literally meaning 'porcupine-like') include the guinea pig (*Cavia porcellus*), two species of chinchilla (*Chinchilla laniger* (long-tailed); *C. brevicaudata* (short-tailed)), and the degu (*Octodon degus*). Hystricomorph rodents are characterized by having relatively long gestation periods, precocial offspring and a membrane covering the vaginal opening, except at oestrus and during parturition. All teeth are open-rooted and grow continually. Guinea pigs, chinchillas and degus are hindgut fermenters and strict herbivores.

The duprasi (*Pachyuromys duprasi natronensis*) is a member of the subfamily Gerbillinae of the Muridae family of rodents, which have many characteristics typical of gerbils, rats and mice. Duprasi are also called fat-tailed gerbils or jirds. They are considered in this chapter as they are non-domesticated 'exotic' rodents.

Guinea pigs

Guinea pigs originated from the grasslands and Andes Mountains of South America. They were domesticated around AD 500–1000 and were raised for food and religious ceremonies. The Dutch brought the guinea pig (also called a cavy) to Europe in the sixteenth century. Although best known as pets or laboratory animals, they are still a staple food source in South America.

Guinea pig enthusiasts have bred a number of hair coats, patterns, markings and colours (Figure 2.1). Coat colours include white, red, tan, brown, chocolate, cream, golden beige, lilac and black.

Chinchillas

Chinchillas originated in the Andes Mountains of South America. There are two species, *Chinchilla laniger* and *C. brevicaudata*, although the latter is considered rare or possibly extinct in the wild. *C. laniger* has a longer tail and bigger ears than the larger *C. brevicaudata*. Chinchillas have been trapped to near extinction in their native habitat for their luxurious pelts.

The soft, dense fur has about 60 hairs per follicle. The tail is long and covered with short coarse hairs. They have long vibrissae (about 110 mm long) on either side of the upper lip, used as sensory organs to assist in nocturnal navigation. The natural coat colour is smoky blue-grey, but a number of colour

Breed	Hair coat
Abyssinian	Short, coarse hair in whorls or rosettes
Albino	No pigmentation; red eyes
American-crested	Short hair; single whorl of contrasting colour on forehead
Baldwin	Born with hair but becomes totally bald at weaning
English or American	Short, smooth, straight hair
Peruvian	Long, fine hair
Silkies (UK: shelties)	Long hair; doesn't cover face or part down the back
Skinny	Hairless except for head and lower legs
Teddy	Coarse, short, thick hair; kinked hair shafts; no ridges or rosettes
Texcel	Long hair in ringlets and curls all over body
Coat pattern	**Markings**
Agouti	Wild type colour; short, silky hair combination of black and brown on each hair
Bicolour	Blocks of two different coat colours
Brindle	Even mixture of black and white hairs
Dalmatian	White body interspersed with black spotting
Dutch	Self or agouti colouring on most of body; white 'saddle' across back; white 'blaze' running from forehead down to the nose; usually white cheeks; often white 'bib'
Himalayan	White, silky coat with black or chocolate ears, nose, feet
Roan	Similar to agouti, but body is black interspersed white hairs; solid black on head and feet
Self	Smooth-coated; coat all one colour
Silver	Dark-coloured coat interspersed with silver hairs
Tortoiseshell: • Bicolour • Tricolour	Red and black blocks of hair; similar to tortoiseshell cat Red, black and white blocks of hair Red, black, white and often tan or lilac coloured hair
Tricolour	Blocks of three different colours

2.1 Guinea pig breeds and coat patterns. (continues) ▶

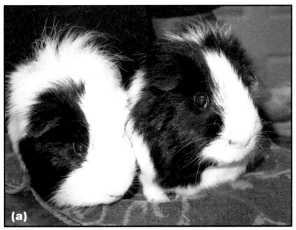

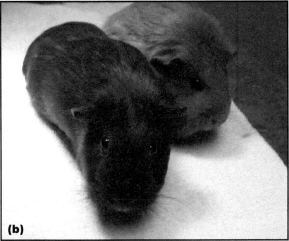

2.1 (continued) **(a)** Dutch colour pattern with typical white blaze down the nose. These are of mixed hair type (Peruvian long hair plus Abyssinian whorl pattern, plus English or Silkie straight hair). **(b)** Self colour pattern (i.e. coat is all one colour).

mutations have been developed including white, silver (Figure 2.2), beige, violet, charcoal, ebony and velvet. Eye colour may be black, or pink to red due to coat colour genes. Beige, white and ebony coat colours are transmitted as recessive genes. Homozygous white or black combinations are fatal.

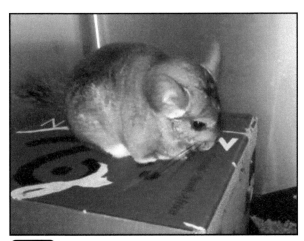

2.2 Silver coloured chinchilla.

Degus

The degu (Figure 2.3) is native to northern and central Chile on the West Andean slopes up to 1200 m. Degus are diurnal and active throughout the year. Vocalizations include soft chortles and whistles. Tooth chattering and hind foot thumping are warning sounds associated with agonistic behaviour. Alarm calls are sharp squeaks to alert conspecifics. Aroused but not frightened degus make a call that sounds like 'chuck-wee'. They also use urine and anogenital secretions to mark territory. Degus will use sand baths, but may saturate the sand or dust with urine and anal gland secretions. They live in colonies and construct burrows. Degus have a strong social organization based on group territories. The females rear their young in communal burrows.

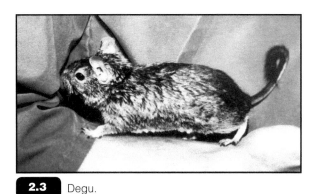

2.3 Degu.

Duprasi

Duprasi are native to the hamada (patches of vegetation) of the northern Sahara Desert from western Morocco to Egypt. They live in burrows up to 1 m deep. Wild duprasi are nocturnal with most activity at dusk. In captivity they are either diurnal or sleep and wake intermittently throughout the day and night. The coat is yellow-grey to buff brown, with white feet and underparts (Figure 2.4). There is a white spot behind each ear and a bicoloured club-shaped tail. They have well developed claws on the front feet. They are considered to be omnivorous, eating plants and at least two species of desert beetle (Felt *et al.*, 2008).

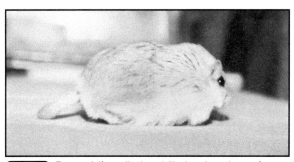

2.4 Duprasi (fat-tailed gerbil) showing signs of obesity.

Biology

Biological data for guinea pigs, chinchillas, degus and duprasi are summarized in Figure 2.5.

	Guinea pigs	Chinchillas	Degus	Duprasi
Lifespan (years)	5–6	Average 8–10 (maximum 18)	7–10	2–4
Adult bodyweight (g)	Males: 900–1200 Females: 700–900	Males: 450–600 Females: 550–800 (females are usually larger than males)	176–315	Males: 80.3–81.6 Females: 54.8–60.5
Dentition	2 [I 1/1, C0/0, P1/1, M3/3]	2 [I 1/1, C0/0, P1/1, M3/3]	2 [I 1/1, C0/0, P1/1, M3/3]	[I 1/1, C0/0, PM0/0, M3/3]
Body temperature (°C)	37.2–39.5	37–38	36.8–37.6	Not published
Heart rate (beats/min)	230–380	200–350	Not published	Not published
Respiratory rate (breaths/min)	90–150	40–80	Not published	Not published
Tidal volume (ml/kg)	5–10	Not found in the literature	Not found in the literature	Not found in the literature
Food consumption	6 g per 100 g bodyweight/day	21 g/day (adult); eat with fore feet	10.2–15.1 g/day (non-breeding adult)	5 g/day (adult)
Water consumption	10 ml per 100 g bodyweight/day	45–70 ml/day, depending on moisture content of food	10.3–40.4 ml/day, depending on moisture content of food	5 ml/day (adult)

2.5 Biological data for guinea pigs (Flecknell, 2002; Hrapkiewicz and Medina, 2007), chinchillas (Williams, 1976; Donnelly, 2002; Johnson-Delaney, 2002; Hrapkiewicz and Medina 2007), degus and duprasi.

Anatomy and physiology

Guinea pigs

Wild guinea pigs live in social groups of five to ten animals. Their vocalizations range from a chut or purr to loud squeals and shrieks when alarmed. Eleven different vocalizations have been recorded, some of which are inaudible to humans (Hrapkiewicz and Medina, 2007). Guinea pigs are active and tend to eat during the day. Although calm and docile normally, they can be easily excited or frightened by sudden noises or changes in the environment. Unfamiliar sounds or movements cause them to freeze and then run, characterized as stampeding, rapid circling of the cage or even jumping. Guinea pigs dislike change and develop rigid habits. Any change in food, water or habitat may cause the guinea pig to stop eating.

Guinea pigs have four digits on the forelimbs and three digits on the hindlimbs. They have large tympanic bullae. Hearing, olfaction and colour discrimination are well developed. The right lung has four lobes and the left has three lobes. The thymus surrounds the trachea rather than being located in the thoracic cavity as in other rodents. The adrenal glands are bilobed and large. The stomach is undivided and lined entirely with glandular epithelium. The small intestine lies primarily on the right side of the abdomen. The caecum takes up most of the central and left portion of the abdominal cavity (Figure 2.6), making up to 65% of the gastrointestinal capacity. Guinea pigs are caecotrophic and coprophagic and take pellets directly from the anus or cage floor. They have scent glands for marking, located circumanally as well as on the rump, and may walk or sit pressing the glands against surfaces. Guinea pigs lack L-gulonolactone oxidase, the enzyme required to synthesize vitamin C.

In comparison with other rodents, the packed cell volume (PCV), erythrocyte count and haemoglobin levels are relatively low in guinea pigs. Lymphocytes

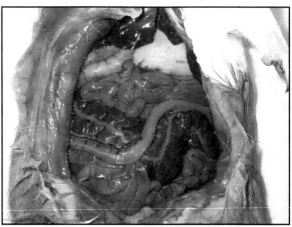

2.6 Normal presentation of the abdomen and large intestine in a guinea pig.

are the dominant leucocytes. Neutrophils have distinct eosinophilic cytoplasmic granules, similar to those of the rabbit. Sex chromatin drumsticks can be seen on the granulocytes in females (Hrapkiewicz and Medina, 2007). Guinea pigs have unique leucocytes called Kurloff cells. The Kurloff cell is a mononuclear lymphocyte with a large intracytoplasmic inclusion. It proliferates with oestrogenic stimulation. They are concentrated in the placenta and are thought to function as killer cells. They also appear to have a cytotoxic effect on leukaemic cells, which may explain why spontaneous tumours are uncommon in guinea pigs (Percy and Barthhold, 2007).

Chinchillas

Chinchillas are non-burrowing animals that in the wild are adapted to living in rock crevices or burrows at elevations above 4000 m (15,000 ft). The natural habitat is barren mountainous terrain. The thick fur protects them from cold temperatures. The footpads allow for agility on rocky surfaces. They are social animals that rarely fight. Although nocturnal, pet chinchillas adapt to owner schedules and are active during the day. They do not hibernate. They are clean, maintaining their coat with frequent dust baths. They are extremely active, quiet and even slightly shy animals that are more appropriate as pets for older children and adults.

Chinchillas have four toes on the front and rear feet, each with a small claw. The palms and soles of the feet are devoid of fur. The thymus gland is entirely intrathoracic. The gastrointestinal tract is long (approximately 2.5–3.0 m), with the jejunum filling nearly the entire abdomen. The caecum is large but holds less intestinal content than that of the rabbit or guinea pig. The proximal colon is highly sacculated. The terminal colon is smooth. Chinchillas cannot vomit and are caecotrophic and coprophagic.

Chinchillas have large ears with thin-walled pinnae and well developed auditory bullae. They have a shallow orbit, large cornea and densely pigmented iris with a vertical pupil.

Degus

Degus are semi-fossorial, diurnal rodents that live in colonies or families of up to 100 animals in the wild. Degus are similar anatomically to both guinea pigs and chinchillas. They have a grey/brown coat with creamy underparts. The tip of the tail is a black brush. The claw of the fifth digit is reduced and there are comb-like bristles over the claws of the hind feet. Degus are herbivorous with microbial fermentation of ingesta occurring in the large haustrated caecum. The stomach is simple and glandular. The intestine is the primary site of nutrient absorption. The colon lacks haustra. Colonic absorption of water from digesta results in very dry faeces. Degus are caecotrophic and coprophagic, with one study reporting that 38% of faeces produced within 24 hours were re-ingested; 87% of this activity occurred at night. Caecotrophy and coprophagy begins in juveniles as young as 3 days of age (Edwards, 2009).

Duprasi

Duprasi are similar in anatomy to domestic gerbils with the exception of the fleshy tail. The tail contains some fat stores, but does not seem to decrease in size in cases of starvation or emaciation. Adult males are approximately 25% heavier than adult non-gravid females (Felt *et al.*, 2008).

Dentition

Guinea pigs

The incisors are white and chisel-like, with the maxillary pair being shorter than the mandibular pair. The oral cavity is small, and the soft palate is continuous with the base of the tongue. The soft palate has a hole in it, the palatal ostium. This is the only opening from the oropharynx to the remainder of the pharynx, making intubation and stomach tubing (gavage) extremely difficult (Popesko *et al.*, 2002; Hrapkiewicz and Medina, 2007). All teeth grow continuously. There are deep longitudinal grooves on the buccal surface of the cheek teeth. Each mandibular cheek tooth occludes with one single opposing maxillary tooth. Mandibular and maxillary teeth of each arcade are aligned so that the occlusal plane is a 30 degree oblique that slopes

from buccal to lingual, dorsal to ventral. The diet must contain sufficient fibre for the proper wearing of the teeth otherwise severe malocclusion can occur, which often traps the tongue and prevents eating, which in turn causes less tooth wear, exacerbating the malocclusion and leading to starvation.

Chinchillas

Like the guinea pig, all teeth grow continuously. The incisors are yellowish in contrast to the molars which are cream. The cheek teeth (one premolar and three molars in each quadrant) are arranged in a straight line, so the arcades converge mesially (towards the front of the mouth). The cheek teeth are all similar in form, with multiple folded parts producing transverse ridges on the mandibular teeth. The difference in angulation of the ridging at the mandibular and maxillary occlusal surfaces allows the teeth to slide smoothly over each other without locking. Differential wear of the exposed enamel, dentine and cementum produces an effective surface for grinding fibrous plant material. Normal occlusion results in a horizontal occlusal surface that should be flush with the gingiva, except at the mesial surface of the mandibular premolar. The oral cavity is narrow. The palate is similar to that of the guinea pig.

Degus

The incisors are pale orange. The premolars and molars are flat-crowned and hypsodontic, with deep infolded margins in the mid-region of the tooth resembling a figure eight. This tooth characteristic led to its genus name Octodon. All teeth continually grow and must be worn by chewing fibrous material.

Duprasi

Duprasi have similar dental anatomy to gerbils (see Chapter 1) with open-root incisors. The maxillary incisors are slightly grooved. The cheek teeth do not grow continuously.

Sexing

Guinea pigs

Superficially, the external genitalia may appear similar in young male and female guinea pigs. In young boars, there is no obvious scrotum but the penis can be protruded by pressing gently on either side of the genital opening. The penis can also be palpated in the midline, just cranial to the genital opening. The penis has two prongs at the tip. Males have a slit-shaped anogenital opening.

Both males and females have an obvious pair of nipples in the inguinal region, and in the male the inguinal canal remains open. Males have several accessory sex glands that include large, transparent, smooth seminiferous vesicles that extend 10 cm into the abdomen from the pubis. These should not be interpreted as enlarged lymph nodes on abdominal palpation (O'Malley, 2005).

The sow has a shallow vaginal groove between the urethral orifice and the anus. The vagina is covered by a membrane except during oestrus (Figure 2.7) and parturition. The anogenital opening is Y-shaped.

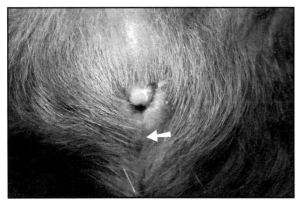

2.7 Female guinea pigs produce a mucoid discharge from the vagina during oestrus. The anus (barely visible) is arrowed.

Chinchillas

Male chinchillas do not have a true scrotal sac and the testes lie within the inguinal region (Figure 2.8). The inguinal canal remains open and requires surgical closure during castration.

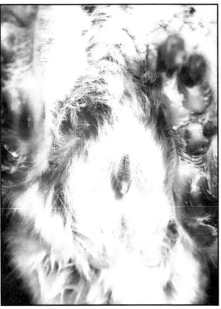

2.8 Male chinchilla genitalia. Note that the testes are not in a true scrotal sac.

Female chinchillas have a cone-shaped urogenital papilla. It almost resembles a penis; however, the urogenital distance is greater in males than in females. The urethral opening is seen within the papilla. The vagina is covered by a membrane except during oestrus (3–5 days) and parturition. The two uterine horns open separately into the cervix. There are three pairs of mammary glands.

Degus

Anatomically degus are most similar to chinchillas. Male degus do not have a true scrotal sac and the testes lie within the inguinal region. The inguinal canal remains open and requires surgical closure during castration. Female degus have two uterine horns, which open separately into the cervix. There are four pairs of mammary glands.

Duprasi

The genitalia and internal organs of duprasi appear similar to those of the domestic gerbil. In males there is a greater distance between the urogenital and anal openings than in females, and when held upright, the testicles descend into the scrotum. The inguinal canal remains open as in other rodents. There are four pairs of nipples in the female, which are visible by 16 days of age. Males do not have nipples.

Husbandry

Housing

Guinea pigs

Guinea pigs are social animals and best housed in pairs or small groups. These can be either single- or mixed-sex groups. Unless breeding is desired, males should be neutered. When group housed, guinea pigs tend to huddle next to a wall or in a tunnel or shelter, and walk along the periphery of the caging rather than cross into the middle. They will establish a social hierarchy, which is usually male dominated. Introduction of another male will destabilize the group. Although fighting is usually limited to intense vocalizations, nipping and prevention of subordinates from reaching food or water, the dominant animal may barber and chew the hair of subordinates. Barbering can also occur due to boredom or overcrowding. Adults may chew the ears of younger guinea pigs.

Guinea pigs are best kept in caging that has sufficient space for exercise and grazing (Figure 2.9). The minimum size should be 0.9 m² per adult. It should have an enclosed solid-sided nesting area or shelter for security. A large diameter polyvinyl chloride (PVC) or plastic drain pipe also works well for the guinea pig to run into for a quick hiding spot. Because they are a prey species, guinea pigs become frightened in large open spaces, and tend to stay at the edges of their enclosure. Caging should be constructed of wire mesh, stainless steel bars or a combination of both

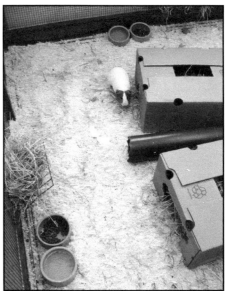

2.9 Typical guinea pig housing. (Reproduced from *BSAVA Manual of Rodents and Ferrets.*)

materials. Wood and some plastic may be gnawed through unless protected by wire mesh. The flooring should be smooth, and covered with either hardwood shavings, or shredded or pelleted recycled paper or hay. The substrate should be changed frequently to keep the environment dry and free of faeces.

Guinea pigs do not tolerate high heat or humidity. The preferred temperature range is 16–24°C, with humidity between 30 and 70%. Temperatures above 27–30°C may cause heat stroke. If the pen is placed outdoors in the summer, shade must be provided. The caging should also be secure to prevent attacks from predators such as dogs, cats, raccoons, coyotes and raptors. Wild bird access should be prevented as they may be sources of infections such as *Yersinia* and *Salmonella*. Most pet guinea pigs are housed indoors year-round.

Chinchillas

Chinchillas are not solitary animals. They should be housed in pairs, single-sex groups or polygamous groups of one male per up to five females. They are active animals and require both horizontal and vertical space, with a multi-level cage recommended. The cage should be made of wire mesh small enough to prevent foot and limb injury (15 x 15 mm). Part of the floor should be solid. A wooden nest box, which may need to be replaced frequently due to gnawing, is recommended for hiding and sleeping. Plastic boxes are not recommended as chinchillas quickly chew the plastic; accidental ingestion of foreign material is a potential problem, and can result in gastroenteritis.

Chinchillas require dust baths for grooming several times a week. Commercial dust products are available, usually composed of volcanic ash or a fine mixture of Fuller's earth (a type of kaolin) and silver sand (1:9 parts). A small amount of dust (2–3 cm deep) should be placed in a container large enough for the chinchilla to roll around in. Although totally enclosed dust bath containers are promoted by the pet trade as a way to keep the dust contained, they also increase the humidity, and the author has seen an increase in dermatophytosis with their use. An open container such as a large stainless steel dog feeding dish works well. The dust bath dish should be placed in a large, open-topped cardboard box or smaller cage in a location other than the home cage of the chinchilla. The baths should be kept clean, free of faeces and removed after use (usually <30 minutes). Overuse of dust, or bathing in contaminated dust, has been associated with conjunctivitis and dermatophytosis.

Chinchillas usually do well in normal home temperatures and humidity. They are prone to heat stroke if the ambient temperature rises above 28°C, especially if the humidity rises above 50–60%. Breeding facilities and commercial vendors prefer to keep the environmental temperature between 10 and 17°C with humidity <40% for optimal growth and production.

Degus

Caging for degus is similar to that for chinchillas. Many will use large rodent wheels. Deep bedding for digging and tunnelling should be provided. They will use burrows or nest boxes. Degus may stockpile food items, so routine changing of bedding should include 'dry' bedding as well as urine/faecal contaminated substrate. They should be offered a commercially available dust or sand for bathing several times a week. Degus normally do well at ambient temperatures <32°C, with humidity ≤50%. Artificial light cycles which provide 12–14 hours light have worked well in captive colonies.

Duprasi

Duprasi are often housed individually or in same-sex groups, depending on the temperament of the individuals. Mating pairs are often kept together for breeding for about 1 week, and then separated. Unlike domestic gerbils (*Meriones unguiculatus*), duprasi do not seem to form strong pair bonds and will successfully mate with unfamiliar conspecifics.

Caging for duprasi is similar to that used for hamsters (see Chapter 1). They will use rodent wheels for exercise and small nest boxes. Substrate should be provided for digging. In laboratory conditions, a 14-hour light, 10-hour dark cycle, with an ambient temperature of 24°C and 50% humidity tends to be used (Refinetti, 1998).

Diet

Guinea pigs

Many commercial diets are available but pelleted complete feeds are preferable to those based on seeds and grains. Guinea pigs are extremely fussy eaters, thus new bags of feed or an abrupt change in the type of feed may be rejected. A new supply of pellets should be mixed into the old bag to ease the transition. Timothy or grass hay should be available *ad libitum* as the fibre content is crucial for dental wear and gastrointestinal tract function. Fruit, seeds, candy-style treat foods and carbohydrate sources such as starchy vegetables are not recommended as the increased sugars may alter the gastrointestinal flora.

Heavy ceramic dishes work well as food bowls, but need to be emptied and washed frequently as guinea pigs often sit and defecate in them. Water is usually provided by dropper bottle with a metal drinking tube. These should be changed and the drinking tube cleaned daily as guinea pigs will spit back up into the tube. Any change to the flavour of the water or type of drinking tube used should be made gradually, as sudden change may result in the guinea pig refusing to drink.

Vitamin C: Vitamin C must be supplied in the diet. Adult non-breeding guinea pigs need 10 mg/kg of vitamin C per day. Breeding guinea pigs, and those stressed or ill, need 35–50 mg/kg of vitamin C per day. Clinical signs of deficiency can develop within 2–3 weeks due to defects in collagen synthesis. Signs include lameness, stilted or shuffling gait, swelling of joints and costochondral junctions, petechiation of mucous membranes, reluctance to move, pain upon touching or handling, depression, rough hair coat, ptyalism due to malocclusion, bruxism, anorexia and poor wound healing. The immune system is also depressed, leaving the guinea pig more susceptible to infections.

The diet must be corrected with the addition of fresh greens high in vitamin C such as kale, cabbage, dandelions and parsley; these will also serve as environmental enrichment for guinea pigs. In addition, attention must be paid to expiry dates on commercial pellets as vitamin C is perishable; some forms are unstable and oxidize readily. Stabilized forms of vitamin C are being used in several brands, although these still have a limited shelf-life. In severely deficient animals showing clinical signs, initial therapeutic doses of 100–125 mg/kg/day of vitamin C are given to promote rapid recovery.

Ascorbic acid can also be added to the drinking water at a rate of 250–500 mg/l. The drinking water should be changed every 12–24 hours to minimize vitamin C degradation by water, light and metal in the dropper bottle.

Chinchillas
The natural diet of chinchillas is high in fibre and low in energy content and consists of grasses, cactus fruit, leaves and the bark of small shrubs and bushes. To keep the teeth and gastrointestinal tract healthy, a high fibre intake and prolonged mastication for nutrient extraction, coupled with hindgut fermentation is required. In captivity, a diet of unlimited good quality grass hay (e.g. Timothy) along with a small amount (1–2 tablespoons) of commercial pellets is sufficient. A diet solely of pellets lacks sufficient fibre and is not adequate. Treats of fresh greens or cactus fruit (approximately 1 teaspoon per day) can be offered, although foods high in sugar should be avoided. Any change in the diet must be made gradually over several days with close attention paid to faecal output and consistency.

Degus
In the wild, the diet of the degu consists of herbaceous foliage (60% by volume), with young plants and new leaves preferred over mature plants. Seasonally, some seeds, grasses and even fresh cattle/horse droppings may be consumed. Grasses make up the remainder of the diet. Degus do not require the addition of ascorbic acid to the diet as they do have L-gulonolactone oxidase activity. In captivity the diet should include high-fibre herbivore rodent pellets (containing 15.9% crude protein, 3.3% crude fat and 28.3% acid detergent fibre), mixed grass and Timothy hay, and a small amount (20% of daily intake) of greens such as kale, collard, romaine lettuce, dandelion greens and roots such as beets, carrots, parsnips, sweet potatoes and turnips.

Duprasi
Duprasi are omnivorous and can be fed a combination of standard grain-based rodent pellets and insects (as suitable for African pygmy hedgehogs, see Chapter 7). In addition small amounts of fresh vegetables or greens can be offered. Quantities may need to be limited to prevent obesity.

Breeding
Reproductive data for guinea pigs, chinchillas, degus and duprasi are summarized in Figure 2.10.

Guinea pigs
The sow is usually bred at 2–3 months of age, corresponding to a bodyweight of 350–450 g. Sows should be bred before 6–7 months of age to prevent permanent fusion of the pelvic symphysis. The boar is bred at 3–4 months of age (600–700 g bodyweight). The

	Guinea pigs	Chinchillas	Degus	Duprasi
Sexual maturity (months)	Males: 3–4 (600–700 g) Females: 2–3 (350–450 g)	6–8	6 (range: 45 days to 20 months)	2.5–3.5
Oestrous cycle	15–17 days; breeding duration of 18–48 months	40 days; seasonally polyoestrous (November to May)	No regular oestrous cycle; presence of male may be needed to induce ovulation; breed all year in captivity	Breed all year in captivity
Duration of oestrus	1–16 hours	3–5 days	Receptive for several hours; multiple copulations	Likely similar to gerbils; copulatory plug is produced
Gestation length (days)	59–72 (varies inversely with litter size, longer for small litters)	111	90–93	20–22
Parturition	Early morning. Farrowing: approximately 30 minutes; 5–10 minutes between pups	Early morning; does not usually nest	Early morning; does not usually nest	Cup-shaped nest lined with nesting material
Post-partum oestrus	Yes	Yes	No	Unknown
Litter size	1–6 (average 3–4)	1–6 (average 2)	5–6 (1–10 per litter possible)	1–7 (average 3)
Birth weight (g)	60–100; precocial; fully furred; ears open; teeth present	30–50; precocial; fully furred; active	14.1–14.6 g; precocial; fully furred; active	2.4–2.6
Eyes open (days)	Open at birth	Open at birth	Open at birth	16
Eat solid food (days)	May begin day after birth to nibble solid foods	May begin day after birth to nibble solid foods	May begin day after birth to nibble solid foods	21; pellets

2.10 Reproductive data for guinea pigs, chinchillas, degus and duprasi. (continues)

	Guinea pigs	**Chinchillas**	**Degus**	**Duprasi**
Weaning (days)	14–21 (begin eating solid food and drinking water within 7 days)	42	28–42	28
Litters per year	Breeding colonies may have 3–4 litters to year	Produce 2 litters per year in captivity	More than 1 per year in captivity	Several per year, rest period of at least 30 days after weaning pups
Commercial breeding life	3–4 years	3 years, depending on culling rate	3–4 years	1–2 years
Chromosome number (diploid)	64	64	58	38

2.10 (continued) Reproductive data for guinea pigs, chinchillas, degus and duprasi.

sow is a non-seasonal, continuous polyoestrous breeder. Detection of oestrus is not necessary unless timed matings are needed. External signs of oestrus include a swollen congested vulva, and exhibition of lordosis upon stroking the back. The male will 'purr' and run around the sow, sniffing and licking her anogenital area prior to mounting. A vaginal plug confirms mating, but will fall out several hours after copulation. The plug is a solid mass formed from ejaculate fluids. Pregnancy can be confirmed with palpation or ultrasonography at 14–21 days gestation. Fetal skeletons are visible on radiographs at 6 weeks.

The sow will greatly increase in bodyweight during pregnancy, often doubling in weight by the end of the gestation period. During the last weeks of pregnancy, there is gradual relaxation of the pubic ligaments and spreading of the symphysis. If the sow is not bred until 9–12 months of age, the symphysis may not be able to separate, resulting in dystocia, and a Caesarean section will be required. Obese females and those with very large litters may become anorectic during the last 2–3 weeks of pregnancy. They may also become ketotic, dehydrated and develop hepatic lipidosis. Some guinea pigs also develop toxaemia due to the altered metabolism and enteric dysbiosis. Intervention to prevent stillbirths and death of the sow includes fluid therapy, assisted feeding, additional parenteral vitamin C and, in some cases, a Caesarean section.

Unless post-partum breeding is planned, the male can be separated from the female in late pregnancy. In addition, either pregnant females can be separated from other females in late pregnancy and housed with their young until weaning, or small groups of breeding females and their young can be housed together. Sufficient space and hiding shelters need to be provided to prevent inadvertent injury of the young if the group is startled. Sows housed together will 'cross-suckle' offspring, which helps survival of pups from sows that may have an inadequate milk supply. If the age of the litters differs by more than a few days, this may cause problems as the larger pups can prevent younger animals from reaching the teats. Although born precocial with fur, teeth, and open eyes and ears, the pups eat only small quantities of solid food in the first few weeks of life. Hay, pellets and a drinking tube for water should be positioned so that the pups can begin to chew and learn to drink. Care needs to be taken to ensure the pups do not become wet from the water bottle.

Chinchillas

Female chinchillas are seasonally polyoestrous (November to May in the northern hemisphere). The oestrous cycle is approximately 40 days. During oestrus the vaginal membrane disappears, making the opening slightly moist and easy to visualize. The female will expel a waxy plug from the vaginal opening during oestrus as well as after a successful mating. Females do not usually build a nest, although they may pile bedding in one corner of the cage. The precocial young are usually born early in the morning, fully furred, with open eyes and active. Although the pups can eat solid food from birth, they do nurse. Weaning takes place at about 6 weeks of age.

Degus

Female degus have no regular oestrous cycle; however, in wild animals a pattern of seasonal reproduction characterized by two peaks of parturition (early and late spring) with a non-reproductive period between summer and winter has been identified (Edwards, 2009). Captive degus breed throughout the year. The precocial young are born fully furred, with open eyes and are able to walk. The pups usually begin to eat solid food by day 7, although they should have access to the adult diet during the first week of life. Weaning normally takes place at 4–6 weeks, but young have been successfully weaned at 2–3 weeks of age.

Duprasi

Breeding in captivity follows guidelines used for gerbils (see Chapter 1). Sexual maturity is reached at 2.5–3.5 months of age. Gestation lasts 20–22 days with an average litter size of 3–6.

Handling and restraint

Guinea pigs

Guinea pigs are easy to handle and restrain, although they may run to avoid capture. The guinea pig should be grasped quickly and firmly around its shoulders and lifted out of its cage/pen. The hindquarters should be supported, and no pressure should be placed on the abdomen (Figure 2.11a). On the examination table, a towel or mat should be used to provide good footing and the guinea pig should be restrained at all times (Figure 2.11b). Guinea pigs object to being placed in dorsal recumbency, but if it is necessary for

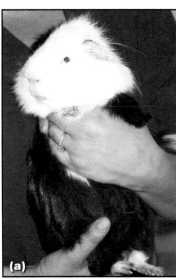

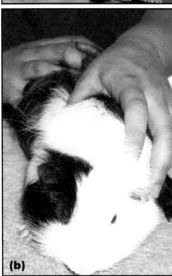

2.11

Handling and restraint of a guinea pig. **(a)** The shoulders and chest are held with one hand, whilst the rump is supported with the other hand. **(b)** Restraint of a guinea pig on a towel for examination. Note the hand placement used to prevent the guinea pig from scooting backwards.

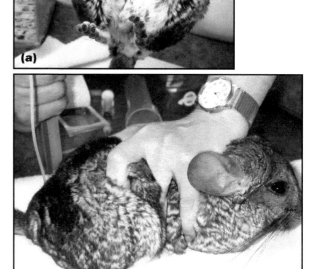

2.12 Handling and restraint of a chinchilla. **(a)** The chest is held with one hand, whilst the rump is supported with the other hand. **(b)** For examination, one hand can be used to approximate a harness and gently restrain the chinchilla over its back.

a brief examination, the thorax and shoulders should be elevated. If restraint for radiography or ultrasonography is required, midazolam at a rate of 0.4–0.5 mg/kg i.m. can be administered.

Chinchillas

Chinchillas can be shy and nervous, and wriggle when restrained. They rarely bite, but can quickly twist loose and jump, making recapture in the examination room very stressful. The chinchilla is best caught in its cage, and then held gently around the thorax with the hindquarters supported (Figure 2.12). Alternatively, the base of the tail can be grasped and the body supported with the other hand. Chinchilla fur is not tightly attached and the ability to 'slip' by dropping a patch of fur easily is a defence mechanism for escape. Rough handling during examination or procedures may result in loss of fur, and should be avoided.

Degus

Degus should be handled in a similar manner to chinchillas, although they are slightly more inclined to bite. Degus should be restrained on a towel or non-slip surface for examination. Degus should be weighed in a container, as all but the extremely ill will jump off the scales.

Duprasi

Duprasi are handled and restrained in a similar manner to hamsters, although they are less inclined to bite. They *should not* be handled by their tails.

Diagnostic approach

History and clinical examination

A detailed history is important to gather information on diet, husbandry, urination and defecation. A description of the number, character and consistency of the faecal pellets is important, particularly in cases of dental or gastrointestinal disease. However, many owners are not aware of changes until faecal material sticks to the perianal area, as substrate within the cage masks daily output. It is important to ascertain how often the substrate is changed, as moisture and faecal accumulation greatly affects health.

Changes in behaviour, including an increase or decrease in locomotion or vocalization, may also be an indicator of disease. The owner should be asked whether there have been any changes to the diet (including food dishes), water (including dropper or bowl), housing, ambient temperature/humidity (normal ranges should be ascertained), substrate, dust bath (type of dust, frequency and duration of bathing, type of container provided, how often the dust is replaced; normal information should also be noted) and routines at home, as well as whether there has been any addition/loss of conspecifics, pets or humans.

Prior to handling, general posture and coat condition can be assessed, along with the eyes and nose for evidence of discharge, and the mouth and perineal area for staining, wetness and odour. It is often useful to have an assistant gently restrain the patient, particularly during the oral examination, for injections or for toenail clipping. If guinea pigs, chinchillas or degus exhibit pain or are extremely frightened, butorphanol at a rate of 0.25–0.4 mg/kg s.c. or i.m. along with midazolam at a rate of 0.25–0.5 mg/kg i.m. may be administered. This will result in relaxation of the patient and allow a more thorough examination. A preliminary oral examination in guinea pigs, chinchillas and degus can be undertaken using an otoscope cone. A full oral examination in all patients requires sedation/anaesthesia.

Ill patients will sit hunched and be reluctant to move. If experiencing pain (e.g. associated with dental or gastrointestinal disease), they may exhibit bruxism and hypersalivation. They may also be tachypnoeic with shallow respirations and an elevated heart rate. The eyes may appear sunken or the nictitating membrane may be prominent. The fur may be matted, wet and have bedding stuck to it. Overgrown and curled toenails may be matted with faecal material, concealing ulceration. Gentle cleaning with warm water-soaked cotton wool removes the material, so the plantar surface of the feet can be examined (Figure 2.13). Thermometers should be of very small

diameter and well lubricated before insertion. Very ill, toxic or dehydrated animals may be hypothermic, and thus their temperature will not register on conventional thermometers. In these cases, an electronic probe thermometer capable of registering temperatures <37°C should be used. A paediatric stethoscope can be used for auscultation.

Imaging

While positioning for standard lateral (Figure 2.14a) and dorsoventral (DV) (Figure 2.14b) or ventrodorsal (VD) radiographs seems straightforward, most small rodents resist being restrained on the back or side, particularly with the limbs extended. Care must also be taken not to restrain the animal in dorsal recumbency for long, as it may compromise the thoracic cavity and respiration, particularly in guinea pigs and chinchillas. Frequently dental films are needed for chinchillas and guinea pigs. These require exact positioning so that cheek teeth roots are exposed. Sedation and/or full anaesthesia is necessary to accomplish good dental films and will usually facilitate positioning for standard lateral and DV/VD views. Dental and skull studies include oblique views (Figure 2.14c) as well as lateral, DV/VD and craniocaudal 'skyline' views to highlight the cheek teeth occlusion. Midazolam at 0.4–0.5 mg/kg i.m. once is usually adequate for most standard radiographs, but further anaesthesia with ketamine or isoflurane may be needed to achieve the necessary relaxation. Limbs can be held in place by household tape.

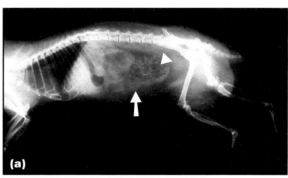

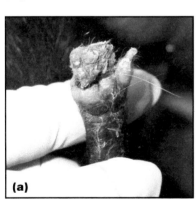

2.13 (a) Guinea pig presented with faeces and debris encrusted on its foot (can be considered a type of pododermatitis). (b) Foot following cleaning. Two toes were lost due to necrosis.

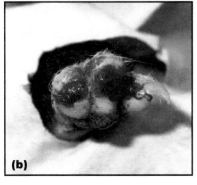

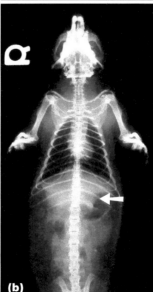

2.14 Radiographs of a guinea pig. (a) Lateral view. The pelvis is slightly rotated, which occurs if the dorsal leg is not propped square to the body. Note the apparent ingesta in the caecum (arrowed) and position of the bladder (arrowhead). (b) Dorsoventral view. This guinea pig was lightly sedated. Note the gas in the stomach (arrowed) and that the position of the head is not adequate to evaluate the teeth. (continues) ▶

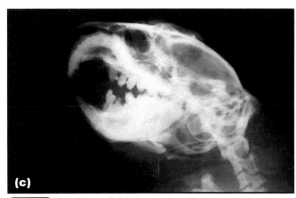

2.14 (continued) Radiographs of a guinea pig.
(c) Oblique view showing the occlusive surface and roots of the cheek teeth. This guinea pig had severe dental disease.

Ultrasonography is often used to examine the bladder, ovaries (Figure 2.15), kidneys, liver and heart. Due to the large hindgut, imaging from the ventral position (with the animal in dorsal recumbency)

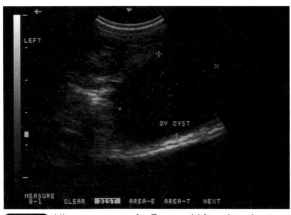

2.15 Ultrasonogram of a 7-year-old female guinea pig showing a large ovarian cyst, which caused abdominal distension and pain.

is non-productive, except for examination of the urinary bladder. The kidneys and ovaries can be approached from the paralumbar flank area. The heart is best viewed with the patient in a normal standing position. Hair must be clipped for guinea pigs, chinchillas and duprasi. The owner should be advised that chinchillas may not re-grow the hair until the next seasonal coat change. A 7.5–10 MHz probe should be used for imaging.

Sample collection

Blood

Blood samples should be collected from the following sites:

- Guinea pigs – cranial vena cava, jugular, femoral, cephalic or lateral saphenous vein. Sample volume for a healthy animal is equivalent to 1% bodyweight or 10% circulating blood volume (e.g. 0.5–3.0 ml)
- Chinchillas – cranial vena cava, jugular and lateral saphenous vein. Sample volume as per guinea pigs (e.g. 0.5–2.0 ml)
- Degus – cranial vena cava or jugular vein. Sample volume as per guinea pigs (e.g. 0.5–1.0 ml)
- Duprasi – jugular vein. Maximum sample volume is 0.3 ml.

Haematological parameters of note in chinchillas include a higher haemoglobin-oxygen affinity than other rodents and rabbits. There is also a seasonal effect with the red blood cell (RBC) count, white blood cell (WBC) count and haemoglobin level highest in winter. The higher WBC count continues into early spring as the reproductive season begins. Figure 2.16 gives average reference ranges for haematology and biochemical parameters in guinea pigs, chinchillas, degus and duprasi.

Parameter	Guinea pigs	Chinchillas	Degus	Duprasi (obtained under sedation)
Haematology				
RBC (10¹²/l)	4–7	5.6–8.4	Males: 8.69 ± 0.19 Females: 8.94 ± 0.16	–
PCV (%)	35–45	27–54	Males: 42.1 ± 0.59 Females: 40.0 ± 0.61	–
Hb (g/dl)	10.0–17.2	8–15.4	Males: 12.0 ± 0.15 Females: 11.7 ± 0.17	–
WBC (10⁹/l)	5.5–17.5 (average 11.2)	5.4–15.6	Males: 8.50 ± 0.39 Females: 8.20 ± 0.36	–
Neutrophils (%)	22–48	39–54	(Neutrophil:lymphocyte ratio is 40:60 in both males and females)	–
Banded neutrophils (%)	0–1	–	–	–
Lymphocytes (%)	29–72	45–60	–	–

2.16 Reference ranges for haematology and biochemical parameters in guinea pigs (Flecknell, 2002; Quesenberry and Carpenter, 2004; Wesche, 2009), chinchillas (Hoefer and Crossley, 2002; Johnson-Delaney, 2002; Wesche, 2009), degus (Murphy *et al.*, 1978) and duprasi (Felt *et al.*, 2009). Note that these values serve only as a general guide and laboratories/clinics should establish their own ranges. (continues) ▶

Parameter	Guinea pigs	Chinchillas	Degus	Duprasi (obtained under sedation)
Haematology continued				
Monocytes (%)	1–10	0–6	–	–
Eosinophils (%)	0–7	0–5	–	–
Basophils (%)	0.0–2.7	0–1	–	–
Reticulocytes (%)	2–3	0–2.8	–	–
Platelets (10^9/l)	260–740	200–482	–	–
Sedimentation rate (mm/h)	1.1–14.0	–	–	–
Biochemistry				
Total protein (g/dl)	4.7–6.4	38–56	Males: 5.70 ± 0.20 Females: 5.62 ± 0.18	4.9–6.2
Albumin (g/dl)	2.1–3.9	2.3–4.1	–	1.7–2.4
Globulin (g/l)	13.1–38.6	9–22	–	3.1–3.9
ALT (IU/l)	25–59	10–35	–	70.0–631.0
ALP (IU/l)	55–108	6–72	–	47–250
AST (IU/)	27–68	96	–	–
Bilirubin (µmol/l)	0–1.59	5.13–15.4	–	1.71–15.39
BUN (mmol/l)	3.34–10.33	6.06–16.06	–	4.64–13.2
Calcium (mmol/l)	2.4–3.1	1.4–3.02	–	2.25–2.63
Cholesterol (mmol/l)	0.31–1.67	1.3–7.85	–	–
Chloride (mmol/l)	90–115	108–129	–	–
Creatinine (µmol/l)	0–77	35.4–114.9	–	17.68–53.04
Glucose (mmol/l)	3.3–6.9	3.3–6.1	–	6.23–25.14
Phosphorus (mmol/l)	1.03–6.98	1.29–2.58	–	0.78–2.23
Potassium (mmol/l)	4.5–8.8	3.3–5.7	–	3.0–5.2
Sodium (mmol/l)	130–150	142–166	–	140–160

2.16   (continued) Reference ranges for haematology and biochemical parameters in guinea pigs (Flecknell, 2002; Quesenberry and Carpenter, 2004; Wesche, 2009), chinchillas (Hoefer and Crossley, 2002; Johnson-Delaney, 2002; Wesche, 2009), degus (Murphy *et al.*, 1978) and duprasi (Felt *et al.*, 2009). Note that these values serve only as a general guide and laboratories/clinics should establish their own ranges.

Urine

Samples for urinalysis should be obtained via cystocentesis under anaesthesia, preferably under ultrasound-guidance as the bladder may be small and the walls compromised from infection or inflammation. Free-catch urine samples are usually contaminated with faecal and bedding material. Figure 2.17 gives average reference ranges for urinary parameters in guinea pigs and chinchillas.

There is no published information for degus and duprasi.

Common conditions

Guinea pigs

Figure 2.18 details the common clinical conditions seen in guinea pigs.

Parameter	Guinea pigs	Chinchillas
Urine pH	8–9	8–9
Urine consistency	Creamy yellow; opaque; contains crystals	Yellow to slightly amber; cloudy
Urine specific gravity (SG)	Often >1.045	Often >1.045

2.17   Reference ranges for urinary parameters in guinea pigs (Flecknell, 2002; Quesenberry and Carpenter, 2004; Wesche, 2009) and chinchillas (Hoefer and Crossley, 2002; Johnson-Delaney, 2002; Wesche, 2009). Note that these values serve only as a general guide and laboratories/clinics should establish their own ranges.

Disease	Cause	Diagnostics	Treatment
Abdominal enlargement	Pregnancy; cystic ovaries; obesity; neoplasia; ascites; organomegaly (amyloidosis or cystic)	Radiography; ultrasonography; aspiration for cytology and culture	Resolution of pregnancy. Ovariohysterectomy for cystic ovaries. Diuretics/cardiac medication for ascites due to cardiomyopathy. Aspiration of cysts. Surgical removal of solid tumours. Slow weight loss for obesity. No treatment for amyloidosis
Alopecia:			
Bilaterally symmetrical	Cystic ovaries (hormone imbalance)	Palpation; ultrasonography; radiography	Ovariohysterectomy. GnRH analogue administration. Cyst drainage for temporary comfort. Pain management
Irregular	Barbering; stress; ectoparasites (mites, lice); wire/cage abrasions	History; cytology of skin scraping	Correct husbandry. For ectoparasites, ivermectin at 200–400 µg/kg s.c.
Anorexia/bruxism	Any illness; pain	History; physical examination, including dental (under sedation); radiography; CBC; serum biochemistry	Treat underlying condition. Analgesia. Supportive care. Fluid therapy. Nutrition
Cardiomyopathy (enlargement, arrhythmia, murmur)	Congenital defects; diet (vitamin E/selenium deficiency, high fat, high calcium); obesity	Radiography; echocardiography; electrocardiography; diet history	As per other species. Correct diet
Cataracts (Figure 2.19)	Hyperglycaemia (may be associated with diabetes mellitus)	Diet history; blood glucose levels; serum biochemistry; ophthalmic examination	Correct diet. Regular ophthalmic examinations
Cheilitis	Ulceration; discharge around mouth; abrasions; secondary bacterial infection; poxvirus	Culture	Gentle cleansing of face. Debridement of necrotic tissue. Antibiotics (topical, systemic). NSAIDs. Remove abrasive materials. Clean cage furnishings (especially water dropper)
Conjunctivitis	*Chlamydophila* conjunctivitis; corneal injury; bacterial conjunctivitis	Ophthalmic examination; fluorescein stain of cornea; conjunctival swab for PCR/culture	*Chlamydophila* infection may be self-limiting. Tetracycline topical ophthalmic preparations. Parenteral doxycycline. Appropriate antibiotics for bacterial conjunctivitis. Treat corneal injury as for other species. Topical ophthalmic and parenteral NSAIDs for comfort
Dermatitis:			
Wounds	Bites (self-inflicted or cage mates); secondary bacterial infection	Social history; culture; skin biopsy	Correct husbandry. Cleanse skin. Antibiotics. NSAIDs if skin appears irritated/painful
Hair loss (patchy, scaly, usually pruritic)	Dermatophytosis (*Trichophyton* spp., dermal cryptococcosis); *Trixacarus caviae*; immunosuppression as a result of stress, illness, overcrowding, introduction of new animals, increased ambient temperature/humidity with poor ventilation	Cytology of skin scraping; culture of fungal preparation; history	Griseofulvin at 15–25 mg/kg orally q14–28d. Topical antifungal cream if small area affected. Ivermectin at 200–400 µg/kg s.c. q14d, for 3 doses for *T. caviae*. May have both dermatophytes and mites. NSAIDs for inflammation/pruritus
Perianal (rump)	Urine scalding; inability to move; faecal accumulation; sebaceous scent gland impaction; spinal/orthopaedic problems; secondary bacterial infection; chronic pain; urolithiasis	Radiography	Gentle cleansing with antiseptic shampoo. Remove debris. Correct underlying condition
Pododermatitis (ulcerative foot lesions)	Swollen, ulcerated plantar surfaces of feet; obesity; poor sanitation; hypovitaminosis C; wire flooring	History of diet/husbandry; radiography for underlying osteomyelitis; culture	Removal of necrotic tissue. Systemic antibiotics. Topical antimicrobial cream/wound dressing (e.g. silver sulfadiazine). NSAIDs. Analgesia. Soft padded bedding. Correct vitamin C. Note: bandaging is difficult but can be done
Diarrhoea	Gastrointestinal dysbiosis (post-antibiotic therapy, diet change, motility change, caecal stasis); Clostridial overgrowth; enterotoxaemia; excessive fresh greens or fruits; Coccidia (*Eimeria caviae*); *Cryptosporidium*; *Paraspidodera uncinata*	Radiography (including contrast study); auscultation of the abdomen; faecal Gram stain; culture; faecal flotation; direct cytology; CBC; serum biochemistry	Analgesia. Parenteral fluid therapy. High-fibre diet. Antibiotics (may need metronidazole for *Clostridium* spp.). Cholestyramine. Motility enhancing drugs. Crypstosporidia may be self-limiting: supportive care. Antiparasitic agents

2.18   Common clinical conditions seen in guinea pigs (Data from Flecknell, 2002; Johnson-Delaney, 2002; Hrapkiewicz and Medina, 2007). GnRH = Gonadotrophin-releasing hormone. (continues) ▶

Disease	Cause	Diagnostics	Treatment
Masses: Cervical area	Cervical lymphadenitis; abscess (Figure 2.20); *Streptococcus*; *Staphylococcus*; *Yersinia pseudotuberculosis*; infected lymph nodes (may rupture)	Culture; history (with reference to bite wounds, sexual contact, coarse feed resulting in oral punctures); CBC; serum biochemistry for septicaemia	Surgically excise, flush and drain infected lymph nodes (may recur). Parenteral fluids. Separate affected animals. For breeding animals, remove from breeding colony, aggressive antibiotics, NSAIDs, surgery or euthanasia. For *Yersinia* infection, euthanasia (report if required)
Rump area	Trichofolliculoma (basal cell epitheliomas); sebaceous adenomas; impacted scent gland; secondary infection	Biopsy; culture	Surgical removal of the mass. NSAIDs. For scent gland impaction, cleansing area with antiseptic shampoo regularly may prevent recurrence
General	Neoplasia (lipomas, fibromas, fibrosarcomas); sebaceous cyst (Figure 2.21)	Biopsy	Surgical removal of the mass. Further treatment depends on histopathology
Otitis media/interna	Purulent exudate in tympanic bulla; head tilt; head shaking; ataxia; circling	Skull radiography; culture; ear canal flush (otitis media)	Appropriate systemic and topical antibiotics. NSAIDs for pain/inflammation. Surgical drainage of bulla. Prognosis guarded due to bulla involvement. [May be subclinical: infected bulla identified at necropsy]
Ptyalism (may be a chronic problem)	Heat stress; dental disease (malocclusion, abscess, fractured teeth)	History; dental examination (under sedation); dental/skull radiography	Correct ambient temperature/humidity. Parenteral fluids. Cool body temperature. For dental disease: correct occlusal surfaces within mouth using high-speed dental burrs; remove abscessed teeth. Antibiosis. Analgesia. NSAIDs. Fluid therapy and nutritional support.
Reluctance to move (lame, swollen joints, exhibiting pain)	Osteoarthritis; hypovitaminosis C; osteodystrophic fibrosa (Figure 2.22a); fractures due to trauma (Figure 2.22b); may have genetic component	History of diet and handling; radiography	Correct vitamin C deficiency. Long-term treatment plan for osteoarthritis includes NSAIDs and soft bedding. Fractures/luxations should be splinted, pinned or bandaged. If circulation compromised or severe fractures, consider amputation. For osteodystrophic fibrosa increase calcium in diet (decrease phosphorus). Pain management
Respiratory signs (dyspnoea, ocular/nasal discharge)	Pneumonia (hypovitaminosis C may contribute); *Bordetella bronchiseptica*; *Streptococcus pneumoniae*; *Klebsiella pneumoniae*; *Streptococcus zooepidemicus*; adenovirus; *Chlamydophila*; heat stress (if ambient temperature elevated, especially if humidity >70%; may have serous nasal discharge and ptyalism); overcrowding; stress	Housing and husbandry history; radiography; pulse oximetry or side-stream capnography to assess oxygen saturation; CBC; serum biochemistry; culture; cytology/PCR of conjunctival swabs (*Chlamydophila*)	Correct ambient temperature/humidity/oxygen provision. Appropriate antibiosis. Nebulization. Bronchodilators. NSAIDs. Midazolam (can be used to calm the guinea pig and encourage breathing deeply). Clean eyes/nose. Topical ophthalmic drugs
Urinary signs: Polyuria/glucosuria	Diabetes mellitus (may be associated with cataracts and polydipsia); diet high in carbohydrates and sugars; weight loss	Diet history; urinalysis; ophthalmic examination Note: hyperglycaemia may not be present or may be intermittent	Correct diet. Reports that insulin trials have not been successful as it is primarily a non-insulin-dependent form of diabetes mellitus (Quesenberry and Carpenter, 2004)
Stranguria/haematuria	Cystitis; urolithiasis; secondary bacterial infection	Urinalysis; radiography	Large stones may require cystotomy. Antibiosis. Fluid therapy. NSAIDs. Analgesia
Vulva enlargement/discharge/haemorrhage	Cystic ovaries; pyometra; pregnancy (with dead fetuses or dystocia); uterine neoplasia	History; radiography; ultrasonography; histopathology	Ovariohysterectomy. Antibiosis peri- and postoperatively for pyometra. Caesarean section

2.18 (continued) Common clinical conditions seen in guinea pigs (Data from Flecknell, 2002; Johnson-Delaney, 2002; Hrapkiewicz and Medina, 2007). GnRH = Gonadotrophin-releasing hormone.

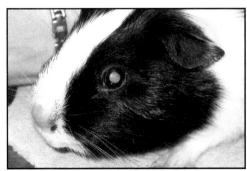
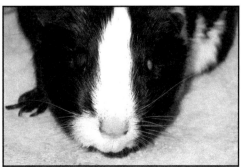

2.19 Cataracts in guinea pigs may be congenital or have a metabolic cause, such as diabetes mellitus. This guinea pig's cataracts were due to diabetes mellitus resulting from a diet high in carbohydrates and fruit.

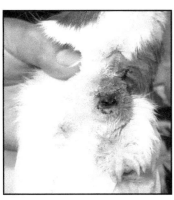

2.20

Cervical lymphadenitis in a guinea pig. The large abscesses (which may include numerous lymph nodes) need to be surgically removed. *Streptococcus* can usually be isolated from the abscesses, although other bacteria may also be involved.

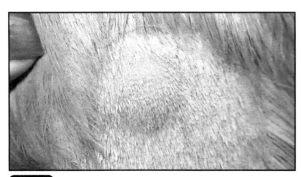

2.21   Sebaceous cyst in a guinea pig.

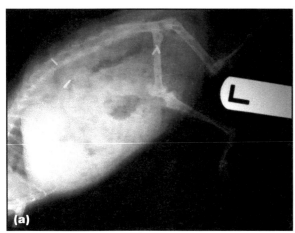

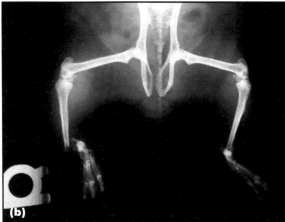

2.22   **(a)** Fibrous osteodystrophy in a neutered female guinea pig. Note the surgical clips placed at the ligature sites of the ovaries and uterus. Note also the moth-eaten appearance of the bones, primarily the legs. **(b)** Fractures frequently occur as a result of trauma. The guinea pig has a fractured distal tibia.

Dental disease

The teeth of the guinea pig grow continuously and depend on constant wear from chewing fibre and roughage. Overgrowth and malocclusion are relatively common and have many causes, including:

- Congenital defects (including conformation)
- Diet (hypovitaminosis C, inadequate fibre)
- Trauma (fractured teeth from falls, being dropped)
- Oral abscessation
- Systemic illness, causing anorexia (with secondary tooth overgrowth from lack of chewing)
- Osteoarthritis (temporomandibular joint, cervical vertebrae)
- Stress (including changes to the environment, diet and ambient noise levels, which alter eating habits).

The maxillary molars and premolars (cheek teeth) are angled outwards, whilst the mandibular cheek teeth are angled slightly inwards. Initially spurs can develop, which may lacerate the tongue or cheeks making chewing painful. The guinea pig then becomes anorectic, resulting in further tooth overgrowth. The mandibular cheek teeth may entrap the tongue, whilst the maxillary teeth may become embedded in the cheek (Figure 2.23). These guinea pigs are likely to experience pain, be anorectic and ptyalic, and begin to rapidly lose weight and condition. A full oral examination must be performed under general anaesthesia. Skull and/or dental radiographs are

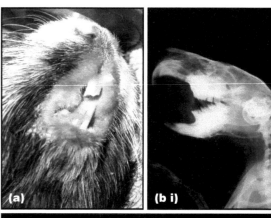

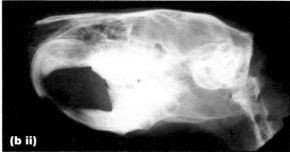

2.23   Malocclusion can involve the mandibular and maxillary incisors and cheek teeth. **(a)** Initial presentation. **(b)(i)** Open-mouth and **(ii)** closed-mouth dental radiographs prior to correction. Note the irregular occlusal surfaces of the cheek teeth. The closed-mouth view does not show the pinning of the tongue. The roots of the teeth on these views do not show abscessation, but additional views are required to fully delineate the roots. (continues)   ▶

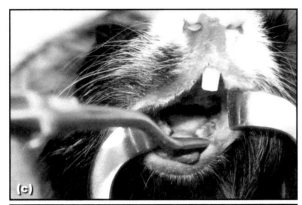

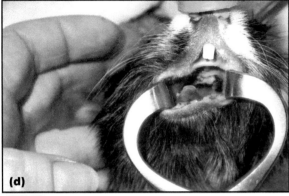

2.23 (continued) Malocclusion can involve the mandibular and maxillary incisors and cheek teeth. **(c)** The mandibular cheek teeth can be corrected by burring. The structure of these teeth is abnormal. Note that the mandibular incisors have also been burred, freeing the tongue. **(d)** The maxillary cheek teeth are irregular and in need of correction. No abscess material was found in the gingiva and the teeth appear solid.

recommended, as there may be tooth root abscessation requiring surgical debridement or tooth extraction. Analgesia and supportive care are critical in the postoperative period, while long-term diet correction may prevent recurrence (Capello and Gracis, 2005).

Gastrointestinal disease

Bacterial enteritis: Guinea pigs may develop diarrhoea from *Escherichia coli*, *Clostridium piliforme* (Tyzzer's disease) and *Campylobacter* spp. Stress and diet may alter normal gut flora, allowing pathogenic coliform bacteria to become dominant. Fluid therapy, antibiotics effective against anaerobic bacteria and supportive care may be successful.

Antibiotic-induced enterotoxaemia: The normal gut flora can be easily disrupted by antibiotics and allow enterotoxin-producing Clostridia to multiply. Acute ileus, gut pain, disruption of motility, and subsequent diarrhoea and death from enterotoxaemia can result. A wide range of antibiotics has been associated with this syndrome in guinea pigs. These include ampicillin, bacitracin, cephalosporins, clindamycin, erythromycin, gentamicin, lincomycin, penicillins, spiramycin and oral tetracyclines. In general, antibiotics considered 'safe' in guinea pigs are broad-spectrum and parenterally administered, rather than narrow-spectrum (particularly targeting

Gram-positive bacteria) and orally administered. Antibiotics considered 'safe' include chloramphenicol, trimethoprim/sulphonamides, and the fluoroquinolones such as enrofloxacin. Enrofloxacin has no anaerobic activity, and may be coupled with metronidazole if clostridial overgrowth is a possibility. Use of antibiotics in guinea pigs should be based on the results of bacterial culture and sensitivity testing.

Pseudotuberculosis: *Yersinia pseudotuberculosis* may be spread to pet guinea pigs via contaminated feed or bedding from wild rodents or birds. It is a zoonotic organism, which is reportable in many public health jurisdictions, and because of this euthanasia rather than treatment is advised. Guinea pigs infected with *Y. pseudotuberculosis* may have weight loss, diarrhoea and gradual loss of condition, resulting in death after several weeks of illness. Some animals die rapidly with septicaemia, whilst others develop a non-fatal infection restricted to the cervical lymph nodes. At necropsy, affected guinea pigs will have enlarged mesenteric lymph nodes, with necrotic foci in the liver and spleen. *Ante mortem* the organism can be cultured from lymph node aspirates and/or blood samples (if septicaemic).

Coccidiosis: This condition is caused by *Eimeria caviae*, which may result in watery diarrhoea in groups of younger animals, particularly with overcrowding, poor husbandry, and in the presence of other infections. Diagnosis is through faecal flotation and/or direct smear. Treatment includes sulfadimidine or sulfamethazine (2% in drinking water for 7–10 days) plus removal of all faecal material, improvement of husbandry and general sanitation, and alleviation of overcrowding.

Salmonellosis: In guinea pigs, salmonellosis results in septicaemia and sudden death, rather than enteritis and diarrhoea. Chronic infections can occur, characterized by progressive weight loss, poor general condition and abortion in pregnant sows. As the disease is zoonotic, affected animals should be euthanased. The disease may be reportable, depending on the public health jurisdiction requirements.

Candidiasis: *Candida* (*C. albicans*) in small numbers is part of the normal gastrointestinal flora in guinea pigs; however, overgrowth due to long-term antibiotic therapy and/or a diet high in sugars (fruits, processed carbohydrates, bakery goods) has been seen. Diarrhoea is the most common sign. Budding yeast can be identified on faecal Gram stain, and cultured. Treatment includes correction of the diet and, anecdotally, use of *Lactobacillus* probiotics.

Respiratory disease

Bacterial pneumonia: *Bordetella bronchiseptica* is the most common cause of respiratory disease in guinea pigs. Unfortunately, many guinea pigs in pet stores are housed with young rabbits and in close proximity to puppies that are likely to be carrying the bacteria. Many homes also have multiple pets, which may serve as the source of infection. *Streptococcus pneumoniae* may also cause pneumonia in guinea pigs, and presents with the same clinical signs as pneumonia caused by *Bordetella*.

Animals develop an ocular and nasal discharge, which progresses to signs of dyspnoea. There may be abnormal respiratory sounds, including audible wheezing, gurgling and sneezing. Ill animals become anorectic, depressed, lethargic and dehydrated, leading to weight loss. Many guinea pigs die soon after developing dyspnoea. Treatment consists of antibiotic therapy and supportive care, including vitamin C supplementation, fluid therapy, assisted feeding, bronchodilators and oxygen/nebulization for the most severely affected. Use of a non-steroidal anti-inflammatory drug (NSAID), such as meloxicam at a rate of 0.2 mg/kg s.c. q24h, seems to make the guinea pig more comfortable, as does keeping the eyes and nose free of discharge. The author may also use a benzodiazepine tranquillizer (midazolam, 0.3–0.5 mg/kg i.m.) at presentation for the severely ill, as it calms the guinea pig and seems to encourage deeper breathing.

Animals that recover may continue to carry the organism. Outbreaks have occurred in colonies, particularly associated with overcrowding, poor husbandry and diet. Both porcine and canine vaccines for *Bordetella* have been used in guinea pig breeding colonies to reduce clinical disease, but have not prevented the carrier state.

Viral pneumonia: Adenovirus has been reported in laboratory colonies during outbreaks of pneumonia. The incidence in pet guinea pigs is unknown. Serological testing is available and should be considered if a respiratory case is unresponsive to antibiotics.

Chlamydophilosis: This condition is most commonly caused by *Chlamydophila caviae* (although infection by *C. psittaci* has also been documented). While conjunctivitis is the primary clinical sign of chlamydophilosis (Figure 2.24), and in most cases in individual pet guinea pigs is self-limiting, it can progress to bronchitis and pneumonia, anorexia, weight loss and death. Stressed or breeding guinea pigs or those on suboptimal diets or with concurrent disease may require prolonged treatment and supportive care. Diagnosis is through cytology and/or PCR of conjunctival scrapings, or histopathology and immunohistochemistry of respiratory or conjunctival tissue retrieved at necropsy. Mild cases can be treated with tetracycline or fluoroquinolone ophthalmic ointments or drops, while more severe cases may require fluoroquinolones (enrofloxacin) orally or doxycycline parenterally. Supportive care includes keeping the eyes free of discharge. *C. psittaci* may be a reportable disease in some public health jurisdictions.

Urinary disease

Cystitis and urolithiasis: Cystitis is relatively common in pet guinea pigs but with fairly minor clinical signs. Owners may notice occasional stranguria or haematuria, although both may be overlooked.

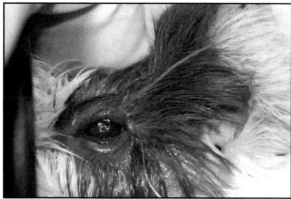

2.24 *Chlamydophila caviae* causes conjunctivitis and corneal ulceration in guinea pigs. The guinea pig may also experience pain and develop rhinitis, anorexia and bronchitis/pneumonia.

Severely affected animals may have abdominal pain, ill-health, and may scream during urination. Simple cystitis usually resolves with antibiotics (e.g. trimethoprim/sulphonamide). Recurrence is common. Palpation of the bladder may reveal thickening of the bladder wall, and in some cases identification of a urolith; however, radiographs should be taken to confirm the diagnosis. Recent stone analysis showed that most uroliths are composed of calcium carbonate and are radiopaque (Hawkins *et al.*, 2009). Large single and multiple small calculi can occur and be present in the ureters, bladder and/or urethra. The uroliths may cause partial or total urethral obstruction. Obstruction may lead to generalized depression, collapse and death if undetected. Cystotomy is indicated to remove the calculi. Antibiotics, NSAIDs and fluid therapy for the postoperative period are indicated. Recurrence of uroliths is common. Acidification of the urine is not possible.

Male guinea pigs may have an urethral obstruction due to plugs of material from the accessory sexual glands. Occasionally these plugs are visible at the end of the penis and can be removed with gentle traction.

Reproductive disease

Cystic ovarian disease: Intact females frequently develop ovarian cysts as they age (Figure 2.25). Many of these cysts can become quite large and fluid-filled, causing abdominal distension, pain, anorexia and gastrointestinal problems due to the mass effect of the ovary. If the ovary is hormonally active, the sow may present with bilateral endocrine alopecia. Ultrasonography is the most reliable diagnostic tool as it may highlight not only ovarian abnormalities but uterine (common) and/or bladder pathology as well. Both ovaries are usually affected, but to different degrees. For animals in severe pain, midazolam at a rate of 0.4–0.5 mg/kg i.m. along with buprenorphine at a rate of 0.05 mg/kg i.m. can be administered prior to extensive ultrasound examination. The skin can be surgically prepared for immediate ultrasound-guided fluid aspiration to relieve pressure and pain from the cyst. The guinea pig should be briefly anaethetized for the procedure. The long-term solution is usually ovariohysterectomy. The author has also used leuprolide acetate (30-day depot at 200 µg/guinea pig i.m.) to start regression of the ovarian follicles and decrease sex hormone production prior to surgery. Deslorelin implants (4.7 mg) may also be used as adjunctive therapy to suppress sex steroidogenesis and lessen the clinical signs. The guinea pig should be provided with nutritional support and analgesia until the ovariohysterectomy is performed.

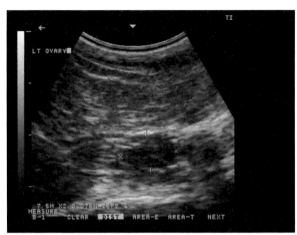

2.25 Ultrasonogram showing cystic ovaries in a sow. This condition is fairly common in guinea pigs.

Pregnancy toxaemia: This condition may occur in sows late in pregnancy or shortly after parturition. Obesity prior to pregnancy and large litters are predisposing factors. It can occur in non-pregnant obese animals that become anorectic for any reason. Animals become depressed, anorectic and dehydrated, and if left untreated, collapse, convulsions and death can occur. Animals are ketoacidotic, and urinalysis shows ketonuria, proteinuria and aciduria. At necropsy, hepatic lipidosis is present along with changes in abdominal fat (liquefied, necrotic or absent). In pregnant animals, it is not uncommon to find a gastrointestinal tract devoid of ingesta with virtually nothing in the caecum.

Treatment at the onset of clinical signs includes fluid therapy (warmed dextrose/saline s.c. or intraperitoneally) and oral feeding (e.g. Critical Care™ feed mixed with 50:50 water and unfiltered apple juice, and vitamin C at a rate of 35–50 mg/kg q24h). A Caesarean section may be performed, although aggressive supportive care of the sow should be continued. Owners of guinea pigs, particularly breeding females, should be advised to avoid overfeeding and ensure that the sow is eating and drinking regularly during the pregnancy.

Dystocia: Sows not bred until after 6–9 months of age, when the pubic symphysis has fused, as well as those with large litters or suffering from obesity prior to pregnancy may have difficulty delivering the pups. Straining, visible contractions, haemorrhage from the vulva, restlessness, anorexia and depression at or near the due date may signal dystocia. Ultrasonography and radiography can determine viability

of the fetuses. A Caesarean section should be performed, with the sow positioned with the head and thorax elevated. As recurrence of dystocia is common, ovariohysterectomy may be performed.

Mastitis: Poor husbandry and overcrowding may contribute to trauma to the mammary glands and the introduction of environmental and coliform bacteria. Treatment includes correcting the husbandry, antibiotics and NSAIDs to reduce pain and inflammation. The pups may need to be fostered with another sow. If the mammary glands are ulcerated or severely enlarged, topical treatment with wound cleaning cream may be necessary.

Skin disease

Ectoparasites: Dermatitis caused by the sarcoptic mite *Trixacarus caviae* is a common problem in guinea pigs. Infestation can result from direct or indirect contact, with active infestations causing severe pruritus. Self-trauma may result in secondary bacterial and/or fungal infection (Figure 2.26). Handling of severely pruritic guinea pigs may induce an apparent seizure. Prior to attempting skin scraping for cytology, midazolam or diazepam can be administered. Mites may be difficult to find in traumatized skin using superficial skin scrapings. In addition to ivermectin, NSAIDs and additional analgesics, antibiotics and/or antifungal medications may be needed.

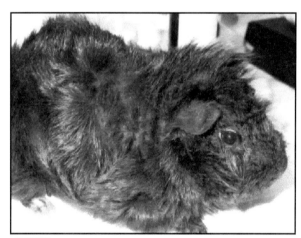

2.26 *Trixacarus caviae* infestation (mange). This guinea pig was so pruritic that it had scratched its eyes, causing a discharge and severe conjunctivitis. The lacrimal ducts were inflamed and not draining. It is recommended that the cornea is checked for laceration as a result of self-trauma in all cases of severe pruritic dermatitis.

Louse infestation with *Gliricola porcelli* or *Gyropus ovalis* is common, but rarely causes pruritus. Lice are usually easily seen and application of clear cellophane tape to the hair coat followed by microscopic examination of the hairs, nits and lice verifies the presence of the parasite. Transmission is by direct contact, and it is important to treat all exposed animals and clean all cages. Treatment with ivermectin is usually effective. Stress, inadequate diet and/or husbandry, overcrowding and concurrent disease may trigger a population explosion of lice.

Pododermatitis: Obese and sedentary guinea pigs may be predisposed to the development of ulceration on the plantar surfaces of the feet (Figure 2.27). Dirty bedding, wire cage flooring and vitamin C deficiency may also be contributing factors. Lesions can be mildly erythematous, hyperkeratotic and painful with progression to ulceration and osteomyelitis. Treatment of deep lesions is difficult, but mild lesions may resolve with: changing of the cage flooring to a smoother, softer bedding; removal of soiled/wet bedding; and vitamin C supplementation. Ulcerative lesions may require systemic antibiotics, NSAIDs, analgesics and topical antibiotic therapy. If osteomyelitis and necrotic tissue are present, surgical debridement and bandaging may be attempted. The prognosis is guarded to poor for full resolution of severe, deep lesions.

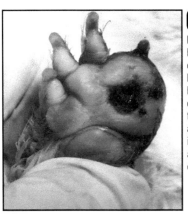

2.27
Pododermatitis can be caused by wire cage flooring, dirty bedding, sedentary behaviour and obesity. It should be treated aggressively as, in addition to the infection, there may also be secondary osteomyelitis.

Systemic disease

Hypovitaminosis C: Vitamin C must be supplied in the diet as guinea pigs lack L-gulonolactone oxidase, the enzyme required to produce vitamin C. Adult non-breeding guinea pigs need 10 mg/kg of vitamin C per day. Breeding guinea pigs, and those that are stressed or ill, need 35–50 mg/kg of vitamin C per day. Clinical signs of deficiency can develop within 2–3 weeks due to defects in collagen synthesis. Signs include lameness, stilted/shuffling gait, swelling of joints and costochondral junctions, osteoarthritis, petechiation of mucous membranes, reluctance to move, pain upon touching or handling, depression, rough hair coat, ptyalism due to malocclusion, bruxism, anorexia and poor wound healing. The immune system is also depressed, leaving the guinea pig more susceptible to infections. Dental disease and tooth growth irregularities have been linked to mild deficiencies, and additional sources of vitamin C should always be provided in cases of dental disease.

Chinchillas

Chinchillas are considered fairly hardy compared with guinea pigs, although dental disease (Figure 2.28), with or without gastrointestinal problems, is frequently seen in pet chinchillas. Dermatophytosis, trauma from falls, and geriatric conditions, including heart disease and arthritis, are commonly seen. Figure 2.29 details the common clinical conditions of chinchillas.

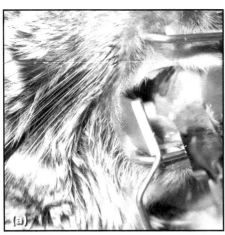

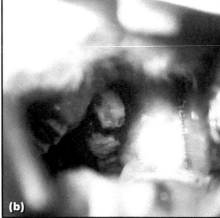

2.28 Matted fur around the mouth and under the chin in chinchillas occurs due to dental disease and malocclusion. **(a)** Oral ulceration due to lacerations from malocclusive teeth can contribute further to oral pain and anorexia. **(b)** Appearance of left maxillary cheek teeth following removal of necrotic debris and burring to approximate height of the right maxillary cheek teeth. Note the severe malformation of the teeth and the recession of surrounding tissue.

Disease	Cause	Diagnostics	Treatment
Abdominal enlargement	Gastrointestinal gas/fluid; pregnancy; obesity; neoplasia; ascites	Radiography (including contrast study); ultrasonography; fluid aspiration for cytology and culture	For ileus fluids, temperature regulation, anti-inflammatory drugs, analgesics and surgery for obstructions is indicated. Motility enhancement drugs (metoclopramide, cisapride) if no obstruction. Human paediatric anti-gas preparations containing simethicone may be helpful to decrease gas production, but efficacy in the caecum is questionable. Resolution of pregnancy. Diuretics/cardiac medication for ascites due to cardiomyopathy. Solid tumours (rare) may be surgically removed. Slow weight loss for obesity

2.29 Common clinical conditions seen in chinchillas (Data from Hoefer and Crossley, 2002; Johnson-Delaney, 2002). (continues) ▶

Disease	Cause	Diagnostics	Treatment
Alopecia (irregular patches)	Barbering; stress; possible dietary deficiencies; fur slip from inappropriate handling; dermatophytosis; ectoparasites (mites, lice); wire/cage abrasions	Behavioural assessment; history of husbandry; skin scraping for cytology; fungal culture if indicated	Correct husbandry. For ectoparasites, ivermectin at 200–400 µg/kg s.c. Dermatophytosis: topical antifungal creams if small area affected (do not use oil-based ointments; be sure cream is completely absorbed). Griseofulvin at 15–25 mg/kg orally q14–28d if widespread dermatophytic alopecia. Withhold dust bath until treated skin is dry. Change dust after every use. Use an open dish
Anorexia/bruxism	Any illness; pain	History; physical examination, including dental (under sedation); radiography; CBC; serum biochemistry	Treat underlying condition. Analgesia. Supportive care. Fluid therapy. Nutrition
Cardiomyopathy (enlargement, arrhythmia, murmur)	Congenital defects; diet (vitamin E/selenium deficiency, high fat, high calcium); obesity	Radiography; echocardiography; electrocardiography; diet history	As per other species. Correct diet
Conjunctivitis	Problems with dust bathing, ventilation and sanitation, resulting in irritation; secondary bacterial conjunctivitis	Ophthalmic examination; fluorescein stain of cornea; conjunctival swab for culture if exudate/discharge present	Correct dust bathing, ventilation, ambient temperature and humidity. Ophthalmic NSAIDs with appropriate topical antibiotics if secondary infection suspected. Treat corneal injury as for other species
Dermatitis: Wounds	Lacerations from sharp edges or wires in cage, on ramps or dishes; bites from cage mates	Skin examination; evaluation of housing and husbandry; culture (frequently *Streptococcus* or *Staphylococcus* isolated)	Correct husbandry. Cleanse skin and suture using subcuticular pattern if severe laceration. Inspissated exudates should be removed and abscesses excised and debrided. Parenteral antibiotics. NSAIDs if irritation or pain present. Avoid topical creams and ointments where possible. Dust baths should be withheld for a few days until open wound has formed a scab
Hair loss (patchy, scaly, may be pruritic)	Dermatophytosis; immunosuppression as a result of stress, illness, overcrowding, introduction of new animals, increased ambient temperature/humidity (particularly within dust bath container), dirty dust, wet substrate, poor ventilation	Cytology of skin scraping; culture of fungal preparation; history	Griseofulvin at 15–25 mg/kg orally q14–28d. Topical antifungal creams if small area affected (do not use oil-based ointments. Be sure cream is completely absorbed). Withhold dust bath until treated skin is dry. Change dust after every use. An open dish should be used for the dust bath. Correct husbandry. Parenteral NSAIDs for inflammation/discomfort/pruritus
Perianal or rump	Urine scalding; inability to move; faecal accumulation; poor hygiene; underlying condition; spinal/orthopaedic problems; urolithiasis; pain	Radiography; culture of skin lesions	Gentle cleansing with antiseptic shampoo. Remove debris. Dry fur thoroughly. Withhold dust bath until skin/fur dry. Correct underlying condition
Pododermatitis (ulcerative foot lesions)	Swollen, ulcerated plantar surfaces of feet; obesity; poor sanitation; wire flooring; pain	History of diet/husbandry; radiography for underlying osteomyelitis; culture	Removal of necrotic tissue. Systemic antibiotics. Topical antimicrobial cream/wound dressing (e.g. silver sulfadiazine). NSAIDs. Analgesia. Soft padded bedding. Note: bandaging is difficult but can be done
Diarrhoea	Gastrointestinal dysbiosis (post-antibiotic therapy, diet change, motility change, caecal stasis); Clostridial overgrowth; enterotoxaemia; excessive fresh greens or fruits; *Cryptosporidium*; *Giardia*	Radiography (including contrast study); auscultation of the abdomen; faecal Gram stain; culture; faecal flotation; direct cytology; CBC; serum biochemistry to assess metabolism; antigen assays and trichrome staining (*Giardia*)	Analgesics. Parenteral fluid therapy. Oral feeding with high-fibre diet. Antibiotics (may need metronidazole for *Clostridium* and *Giardia* infections). Cholestyramine to inhibit endotoxins. Motility enhancing drugs. *Cryptosporidium* infection is often self-limiting, just supportive care required
Heat stroke	Prolonged exposure to temperatures >28°C (80°F) (results in prostration, hyperthermia, panting); dehydration; secondary gastrointestinal stasis; bacterial shift; endotoxaemia followed by hypothermia/shock	History; temperature	Cool water baths. Intravenous fluids. Monitor and raise/lower blood pressure as needed. Treat Clostridial overgrowth prophylactically. Orally assisted feeding, antibiotics, gut motility enhancing drugs and cholestyramine for endotoxaemia

2.29 (continued) Common clinical conditions seen in chinchillas (Data from Hoefer and Crossley, 2002; Johnson-Delaney, 2002). (continues) ▶

Disease	Cause	Diagnostics	Treatment
Masses	Abscesses (often as a result of bites from cage mates); *Streptococcus*; *Staphylococcus*	History (with reference to bite wounds, sexual contact or coarse feed resulting in oral punctures); culture; CBC; serum biochemistry for septicaemia	Surgically excise, flush and drain site. Parenteral antibiotics. NSAIDs
Neurological signs (circling, tremors, convulsions, ataxia)	Vitamin B (thiamine) deficiency; calcium deficiency in young or pregnant adults; lymphocytic choriomeningitis (LCM; **zoonotic potential**); lead toxicosis (may also be blindness); listeriosis; cerebrospinal nematodiasis (due to exposure to raccoon faeces contaminated with *Baylisascaris procyonis*)	Assess diet; radiography; blood work; cerebrospinal (CSF) tap; cytology LCM: necropsy; serology Listeriosis: history of husbandry; serology; culture Lead: blood lead levels *Baylisascaris*: brain histopathology	Supportive care. Correct diet and husbandry. LCM: no treatment. Listeriosis: chloramphenicol 50 mg/kg orally q12h or oxytetracycline 10 mg/kg i.m. q12h; poor response once clinical signs present. Lead: calcium disodium versenate (EDTA at 30 mg/kg s.c. q12h)
Otitis media/interna/torticollis (purulent exudate in tympanic bulla, head tilt, shaking of head, ataxia, circling)	*Streptococcus*; subcutaneous abscesses; septic arthritis; chronic respiratory disease	Skull and chest radiography; culture; ear canal flush (otitis media) Surgical drainage of bulla (osteotomy)	Appropriate systemic and topical antibiotics. NSAIDs for pain/inflammation. Surgical drainage of bulla. Prognosis guarded due to bulla involvement.
Ptyalism (may be a chronic problem)	Heat stress; dental disease (malocclusion, abscess, fractured teeth)	History; dental examination under sedation; dental/skull radiography	Correct ambient temperature, humidity. Parenteral fluids. Cool body temperature. For dental disease: correct occlusal surfaces within mouth using a high-speed dental burr; remove abscessed teeth. Antibiosis. Analgesia. NSAIDs. Supportive fluid therapy and nutrition
Reluctance to move/fractures/luxations (lame, swollen joints, exhibiting pain)	Osteoarthritis; trauma (dropped, feet caught in caging); septic arthritis (spread from abscess elsewhere); age	Diet and handling history; radiography	Long-term plan for osteoarthritis, including NSAIDs and soft bedding. For fractures/luxations, splint/pin/bandage. Surgical repair may be difficult due to thin bones. External fixators (e.g. type II Kirschner–Ehmer) may work in some cases; padded bandages for distal forelimb fractures may be adequate if cage rest provided. Tape may irritate skin. If circulation compromised or fractures severe, consider amputation. Restrict exercise during healing
Respiratory signs (dyspnoea, ocular/nasal discharge)	Pneumonia; *Bordetella bronchiseptica*; *Streptococcus pneumoniae*; *Klebsiella pneumoniae*; *Streptococcus zooepidemicus*; heat stress (ambient temperature elevated, especially if humidity >70%; may have serous nasal discharge and ptyalism); overcrowding; stress	Housing and husbandry history; radiography; pulse oximetry or side-stream capnography to assess oxygen saturation; CBC; serum biochemistry; culture of discharge; conjunctival swabs; cytology	Correct ambient temperature/humidity and oxygen levels. Appropriate antibiosis/nebulization to aid breathing. (Nebulization may be best done with a mask rather than whole body in a chamber which may dampen the fur.) Bronchodilators. NSAIDs. Midazolam can be used initially, which helps to calm the chinchilla and get them breathing deeply. Clean eyes/nose; can use topical ophthalmics (antibiotic/NSAID) for further treatment
Urinary signs:			
Polyuria/glucosuria	Diabetes mellitus (may also see cataracts, polydipsia); diet high in carbohydrates and sugars; weight loss	Diet history; urinalysis; ophthalmic examination Note: hyperglycaemia may not be present or may be intermittent	Correct diet. Reports that insulin trials have not been successful as it is primarily a non-insulin dependent form of diabetes mellitus (Quesenberry and Carpenter, 2004)
Stranguria/haematuria	Cystitis; urolithiasis; secondary bacterial infection	Urinalysis; radiography	Large stones may require cystotomy. Antibiosis. Fluid therapy. NSAIDs. Analgesia
Stranguria/swollen prepuce	Paraphimosis in males (fur ring)	Examination of penis	Remove impacted fur ring
Vulvar enlargement/discharge/haemorrhage	Cystic ovaries; pyometra; pregnancy (with dead fetuses or dystocia); uterine neoplasia	History; radiography; ultrasonography; histopathology	Ovariohysterectomy. Antibiosis peri- and postoperatively for pyometra. Caesarean section

2.29 (continued) Common clinical conditions seen in chinchillas (Data from Hoefer and Crossley, 2002; Johnson-Delaney, 2002).

Degus

Degus typically do not drink much water, and with any amount of diarrhoea can easily become dehydrated. *Giardia* has been linked with fatal diarrhoea in both pups and adults. Other types of bacterial dysbiosis can occur, most likely due to dietary imbalances or poor sanitation. *Klebsiella pneumoniae* has been found in cases of acute suppurative bronchopneumonia. *Cryptococcus neoformans* was isolated from the faeces of a degu in a zoological collection, although no clinical signs were seen in the degu (Bauwens *et al.* 2004). Wild degus have been found infected with several helminth parasites, including the whipworm *Trichuris bradleyi* (Babero and Cattan, 1975). Most pet degus are free from intestinal parasites. Degus have also been found to carry *Trichophyton mentagrophytes*, usually subclinically, but may exhibit signs if the ambient humidity increases. As infection can be zoonotic, attention should be paid to any skin/fur abnormality, and the cleanliness of the caging and dust baths (Boralevi *et al.*, 2003).

Degus can develop spontaneous diabetes mellitus with islet amyloidosis. Guinea pig food or fresh fruit that elevate blood sugar levels, along with a cytomegalovirus-induced insulitis with the alpha-cell crystals showing the presence of a herpes-type virus have been implicated. Cataracts may develop within 4 weeks. Congenital cataracts were found in one colony of degus (Worgul and Rothstein, 1975).

Fractures and wounds from incorrect handling or attacks from other pets in the household have been reported. These are treated as for chinchillas and guinea pigs. Many types of neoplasia have been reported, including primary bronchoalveolar carcinoma with renal and hepatic metastases, reticulum cell sarcoma in a cervical lymph node causing tracheal compression, hepatocellular carcinoma, splenic haemangioma, lipoma and adrenal transitional cell carcinoma.

Figure 2.30 lists the common clinical conditions of degus.

Disease	Cause	Diagnostics	Treatment
Abdominal enlargement	Gastrointestinal gas/fluid; pregnancy; obesity; neoplasia; ascites	Radiography (including contrast study); ultrasonography; fluid aspiration for cytology and culture	For ileus fluids, temperature regulation, anti-inflammatory drugs, analgesics and surgery for obstructions is indicated. Motility enhancement drugs (metoclopramide, cisapride) if no obstruction. Human paediatric anti-gas preparations containing simethicone may be helpful to decrease gas production, but efficacy in the caecum is questionable. Resolution of pregnancy. Diuretics/cardiac medication for ascites due to cardiomyopathy. Solid tumours (rare) may be surgically removed. Slow weight loss for obesity
Alopecia (irregular patches)	Fur slip from inappropriate handling; stress; dermatophytosis; wire/cage abrasions	Behavioural assessment; history of husbandry; skin scraping for cytology; fungal culture if indicated	Correct housing and husbandry. Discuss appropriate handling with the owner. Dermatrophytosis: treat as for chinchillas and for hair loss (see below)
Anorexia/bruxism	Any illness; pain (including dental, skeletal, gastrointestinal, respiratory, ophthalmic)	History; physical examination including dental (under sedation); radiography; CBC; serum biochemistry	Treat underlying condition. Analgesia. Supportive care. Fluid therapy. Nutritional support
Cataracts	Diabetes mellitus; congenital; age	Diet history; blood glucose levels; full examination including blood work; ophthalmic examination	Correct diet to manage diabetes mellitus. If congenital, do not breed this animal (unknown if hereditary/genetic)
Conjunctivitis	Problems with dust bathing, ventilation and sanitation, resulting in irritation; secondary bacterial conjunctivitis; corneal abrasions	Ophthalmic examination; fluorescein stain of cornea; conjunctival swab for culture if exudates/discharge present	Correct dust bathing, ventilation, ambient temperature and humidity. Ophthalmic NSAIDs along with appropriate topical antibiotics if suspected secondary infection. Treat corneal injuries as in other species
Dermatitis: Wounds	Usually lacerations from sharp edges or wires in cage, ramps or dishes; bites from cage mates when in large groups	Skin examination; evaluation of cage and husbandry; culture (frequently *Streptococcus* or *Staphylococcus* isolated)	Correct husbandry. Cleanse skin and suture using a subcuticular pattern if severe laceration. Inspissated exudates should be removed and abscesses excised and debrided. Parenteral antibiotics. NSAIDs if irritation and pain present. Avoid using topical creams or ointments. Dust baths should be withheld for a few days until open wound has formed a scab
Hair loss (patchy, scaly, may be pruritic)	Dermatophytosis; immunosuppression as a result of stress, illness, overcrowding, introduction of new animals, increased ambient temperature/humidity (particularly within dust bath container), dirty dust, wet substrate, poor ventilation	Skin cytology; fungal preparation; culture; history	Griseofulvin at 15–25 mg/kg orally q14–28d. Topical antifungal creams if small area affected (do not use oil-based ointments. Be sure creams are completely absorbed). Withhold bath until treated skin is dry. Change dust after every use. Only use open dishes for dust bath. Correct husbandry. Parenteral NSAIDs for inflammation, discomfort and pruritus *Dermatitis continues*

2.30 Common clinical conditions seen in degus. (continues) ▶

Disease	Cause	Diagnostics	Treatment
Dermatitis: Perianal (rump)	Urine scalding; inability to move; faecal accumulation; poor hygiene; underlying condition; spinal/orthopaedic problems; urolithiasis; pain	Radiography; culture of skin if moist dermatitis; urinalysis if urinary tract infection/ urolithiasis	Gentle cleansing with antiseptic shampoo. Remove debris. Dry fur thoroughly. Withhold dust bath until skin/fur dry. Correct underlying condition
Pododermatitis (ulcerative foot lesions)	Swollen, ulcerated plantar surfaces of feet; obesity; poor sanitation; wire flooring; pain	Diet and husbandry history; radiography for underlying osteomyelitis; culture	Removal of necrotic tissue. Systemic antibiotics. Topical antimicrobial cream/wound dressing (e.g. silver sulfadiazine). NSAIDs. Analgesia. Soft padded bedding. Note: bandaging is difficult but can be done
Diarrhoea	Gastrointestinal dysbiosis (post-antibiotic therapy, diet change, motility change, caecal stasis); Clostridial overgrowth; enterotoxaemia; excessive fresh greens or fruits; *Giardia*	Radiography (including contrast study); abdominal auscultation; faecal Gram stain; culture; faecal flotation; direct cytology; CBC; serum biochemistry to assess metabolism; antigen assays and trichrome staining (*Giardia*)	Analgesics. Parenteral fluid therapy. Oral feeding with high-fibre diet. Antibiotics (may need metronidazole for *Clostridium* and *Giardia*). Cholestyramine to inhibit endotoxins. Motility enhancing drugs
Heat stroke	Prolonged exposure to temperatures >28°C (80°F) (results in prostration, hyperthermia and panting); dehydration; secondary gastrointestinal stasis; bacterial shift; endotoxaemia followed by hypothermia/shock	History; temperature	Cool water baths. Intravenous fluids. Monitor and raise/lower blood pressure as needed. Treat Clostridial overgrowth and toxaemia prophylactically. Oral assisted feeding. Antibiotics. Gut motility enhancing drugs. Cholestyramine to inhibit endotoxins
Masses	Abscesses (often from bite wounds from cage mates); *Streptococcus*; *Staphylococcus*	History (with reference to bite wounds, sexual contact or coarse feed resulting in oral punctures); culture; CBC; serum biochemistry (septicaemia)	Surgically excise, flush and drain abscess. Parenteral antibiotics. NSAIDs
Otitis media/interna/ torticollis (purulent exudate in tympanic bulla, head tilt, shaking of head, ataxia, circling)	*Streptococcus*; subcutaneous abscesses; septic arthritis; chronic respiratory disease	Skull/chest radiography; culture	Flush ear canal if primarily otitis externa. Surgical drainage of bulla (osteotomy). Appropriate systemic and topical antibiotics. NSAIDs for pain and inflammation. Prognosis guarded due to bulla involvement
Ptyalism (may be chronic problem)	Heat stress; dental disease (malocclusion, abscess, fractured teeth)	History; dental examination (under sedation); dental/skull radiography	Correct ambient temperature/humidity. Parenteral fluid therapy. Cool body temperature. For dental disease: correct occlusal surfaces within mouth using a high-speed dental burr; remove abscessed teeth. Antibiosis. Analgesia. NSAIDs. Supportive fluid therapy and nutrition
Reluctance to move/fractures/ luxations (lame, swollen joints, painful)	Osteoarthritis; trauma (dropped, feet caught in caging); septic arthritis (spread from abscess elsewhere); age	Diet and handling history; radiography	Long-term plan for osteoarthritis, including NSAIDs and soft bedding. For fractures/luxations, splint/pin/bandage. Surgical repair may be difficult due to thin bones. External fixators (e.g. type II Kirschner–Ehmer) may work in some cases; padded bandages for distal forelimb fractures may be adequate if cage rest provided. Tape may irritate skin. If circulation compromised or fractures severe, consider amputation. Restrict exercise during healing
Respiratory signs (dyspnoea, ocular/ nasal discharge)	Pneumonia; *Klebsiella pneumoniae*; other bacterial infections; heat stress (ambient temperature elevated, especially if humidity >70%; may have serous nasal discharge and ptyalism); overcrowding; stress	Husbandry history; radiography; pulse oximetry or side-stream capnography to assess oxygen saturation; CBC; serum biochemistry; culture of discharge; conjunctival swabs; cytology	Correct ambient temperature/humidity and oxygen levels. Appropriate antibiosis/nebulization to aid breathing. (Nebulization may be best done with a mask rather than whole body in a chamber which may dampen the fur.) Bronchodilators. NSAIDs. Midazolam can be used initially, which helps to calm the degu and get them breathing deeply. Clean eyes/nose; can use topical ophthalmics (antibiotic/NSAID) for further treatment
Urinary signs: Polyuria/glucosuria	Diabetes mellitus (may also see cataracts, polydipsia); diet high in carbohydrates and sugars; weight loss	Diet history; urinalysis; ophthalmic examination	Correct diet. Reports that insulin trials have not been successful as it is primarily a non-insulin dependent form of diabetes mellitus
Stranguria/ haematuria	Cystitis; urolithiasis; secondary bacterial infection	Urinalysis; radiography	Large stones may require cystotomy. Antibiosis. Fluid therapy. NSAIDs. Analgesia
Vulvar enlargement/ discharge/ haemorrhage	Cystic ovaries; pyometra; pregnancy (with dead fetuses or dystocia); uterine neoplasia	History; radiography; ultrasonography; histopathology	Ovariohysterectomy. Antibiosis peri- and postoperatively for pyometra. Caesarean section

2.30   (continued) Common clinical conditions seen in degus.

Duprasi

Pet duprasi can easily become obese if offered unlimited grain-based rodent pellets; however, rodent food containing 18% protein appears to meet other nutritional and dietary needs. Laboratory duprasi are usually screened and found to be free of common murine pathogens. *Escherichia coli* has been identified as a cause of septicaemia, suppurative metritis, caecocolitis and myocarditis. *Klebsiella pneumoniae* has been isolated from the blood, spleen and liver of a duprasi that died of hepatosplenomegaly (Felt *et al.*, 2008). *Serratia marcescens* has been isolated from the blood and muscle in a case of rhabdomyolysis affecting the distal hindlegs (Felt *et al.*, 2008). A single case of a novel *Bartonella* was reported as causing severe acute pulmonary haemorrhage and severe dyspnoea, although none of the cagemates were affected (Felt *et al.*, 2008). Wild-caught duprasi have been diagnosed with apparently non-pathogenic intestinal protozoa, although this is not common in captive animals. Wild-caught duprasi have also been diagnosed with *Rodentolepis* (formerly *Hymenolepis*) *diminuta*, as well as pinworms of undetermined genus. Eggs of *R. diminuta* and pinworms have been found on routine faecal flotation with zinc sulphate (Felt *et al.*, 2008). No clinical signs or pathology have been associated with either of these infections. *R. diminuta* has been eliminated with a single oral dose of niclosamide at a rate of 100 mg/kg bodyweight. Nematodes have been eliminated with weekly intraperitoneal doses of ivermectin at a rate of 0.2 mg/kg bodyweight for three treatments. Ova resembling *Strongyloides* have been found on direct smears of faeces from wild-caught animals. Wild-caught duprasi can be infested with mites (*Pyroglyphis moriani*) and camel ticks (*Hyalomma drommedarii*). These mites have been eliminated with two doses of ivermectin at a rate of 0.2 mg/kg bodyweight s.c. 14 days apart, along with frequent cage changes. The ticks are physically removed.

Excessive dental wear of the maxillary incisors with overgrowth of the mandibular incisors has been noted. This usually results in weight loss, and has been attributed to an excessive quantity of fruit and vegetables in the diet, which results in the improper wearing of the teeth. The teeth should be burred into the correct occlusion and the diet corrected to provide adequate fibre for tooth wear.

Chondrodysplasia (dwarfism) has been reported as a spontaneous mutation in one laboratory colony (Felt *et al.*, 2008). These duprasi only reached 25% of the normal adult bodyweight. They had visible skull and limb deformities, but were otherwise thriving until 5–10 months of age when they began to have problems walking.

Neoplasia has been reported in older duprasi. These include a trichofolliculoma and thoracic B-cell lymphoma. Trichofolliculomas can recur on the muzzle and nasal planum, despite repeated excisions. Figure 2.31 lists the common clinical conditions of duprasi.

Supportive care

Hospitalization

Hospitalization cages for guinea pigs and chinchillas are generally adapted from those for rabbits or ferrets. Depending on the severity of disease, and the need for oxygen or nebulization, the animal may be

Disease	Cause	Diagnostics	Treatment
Alopecia/pruritus	Mites (e.g. *Pyroglyphis moriani*)	Direct examination of skin; combing of fur; cellophane tape testing; skin scraping; microscopic examination	Change cage bedding and wash cage/furnishings. Ivermectin at 0.2 mg/kg s.c. 14 days apart for at least 2 treatments
Diarrhoea/enteropathy	Bacterial infection; ingestion of foreign body; stress; change or improper diet	Diet history; physical examination; faecal Gram stain; culture; sensitivity; radiography (including contrast study)	Correct diet. Appropriate antibiotics for dysbiosis. For foreign body, approach as with other animals
Malocclusion	Improper wear of incisors; dental abscess; fractured teeth	Full examination of mouth; skull radiography	Correct as for other rodents. Tooth extraction and debridement of abscess. Appropriate antibiotics. NSAIDs
Masses	Neoplasia; abscess	Physical examination; biopsy/fine needle aspiration; culture; sensitivity	Surgical excision of mass/abscess. Appropriate antibiotics for abscess. Postoperative NSAIDs and analgesia
Obesity/malnutrition	Improper diet; *ad libitum* grain-based diet; too many treat foods (fruit, carbohydrates); lack of exercise	History; physical examination; CBC; serum biochemistry; radiography	Correct diet and husbandry. Provide exercise. Limit food. Feed some live insects
Stunted growth/skeletal deformities/lameness	Chondrodysplasia (dwarfism)	Breeding history; radiography	No treatment. Do not breed
Trauma/ wounds/ fractures	Attacks from other pets; being dropped/mishandled; fights between cage mates (rare)	Physical examination; radiography; culture and sensitivity of wounds if infected	Appropriate antimicrobials. Wound care as for other animals. NSAIDs. Analgesia. Fracture repair similar to birds/small mammals. Correct husbandry
Weight loss	Malocclusion; systemic bacterial infection; neoplasia; pain; incompatible cage mates	History; physical examination; appropriate diagnostics for identified problem	Treat cause

2.31 Common clinical conditions seen in duprasi.

housed within an incubator/isolette constructed from a plastic storage container with ventilation holes, or a small wire cage. Towels can be used for bedding and a small amount of Timothy hay for burrowing can be provided. It is important for all prey species to be isolated from predators, and housed in a quiet area of the hospital, where ambient temperature and lighting can be controlled. Food and water consumption, and stool and urine output should be regularly monitored.

Drug administration

Injection sites

Injection sites and volumes are summarized in Figure 2.32.

- Subcutaneous injections can be given to guinea pigs, chinchillas and degus in the scruff or flank using similar restraint (Figure 2.32ab).
- For intramuscular and intraperitoneal injections, the animal can be restrained by an assistant as shown in Figure 2.11b. Intraperitoneal injections can be made into a posterior quadrant of the abdomen, along the line of the extended hindlimb. If there is abdominal distension or suspected abdominal disease, this route should not be used. Intramuscular injection is made into the quadriceps muscle; however, in general, intramuscular injections should be avoided as the muscle mass is small and iatrogenic damage and pain can be associated with this route.
- Intravenous injections can be made into the lateral saphenous vein using a 24–25-gauge needle. In anaesthetic emergencies in male guinea pigs, the penile vein is sufficiently large for injection. The brachiocephalic veins may be large enough in adult animals for small injections. Ear veins in pet animals are rarely used as the delicate vessels are easily damaged. If attempted, a local anaesthetic should be applied 20–30 minutes prior to venepuncture.
- For emergency fluid therapy, intraosseous catheters may be placed in either the tibia or the femur under anaesthesia, with an additional local anaesthetic infusion at the site of bone entry. Sterile preparation of the puncture site is needed. These catheters are usually removed within the first 12–24 hours as the rodent tends to chew any protective bandage material at the catheter site.

For duprasi, the routes of administration and volumes are essentially the same as for gerbils and hamsters (see Chapter 1).

Route	Guinea pigs	Chinchillas	Degus	Duprasi
Subcutaneous	Suprascapular, interscapular, dorsal back, flank (5–10 ml per site)	Suprascapular, interscapular, dorsal back, flank (5–10 ml per site)	Suprascapular, interscapular, dorsal back, flank (5–10 ml per site)	Suprascapular, interscapular, dorsal back, flank (3–4 ml per site)
Intramuscular	Anterior thigh (0.5 ml)	Anterior thigh (0.5 ml)	Anterior thigh (0.5 ml maximum)	Anterior thigh (0.1 ml)
Intraperitoneal	Posterior quadrant of the abdomen (5–8 ml)	Posterior quadrant of the abdomen (5–8 ml)	Posterior quadrant of the abdomen (5–8 ml)	Posterior quadrant of the abdomen (2–3 ml)
Intravenous/ intraosseous	Femur, tibia (8 ml)	Femur, tibia (5–8 ml slow bolus)	Femur, tibia (1–2 ml bolus)	Femur (up to 1 ml slow bolus)
Bolus	Saphenous, lateral metatarsal, penile, lingual or cephalic vein (1–2 ml slowly)	Saphenous or cephalic vein (1–2 ml slowly)	Saphenous or cephalic vein (1–2 ml slowly)	Jugular or saphenous vein (0.5 ml slowly, maximum)

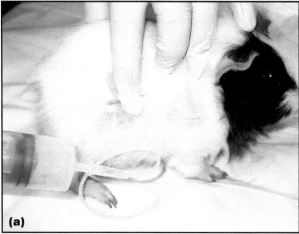
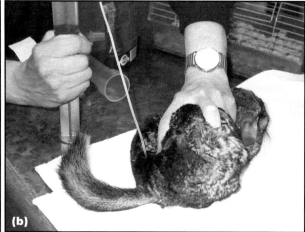

2.32 Injection sites and volumes (Data from Sirois, 2005; Johnson-Delaney, 2006). Subcutaneous fluids being administered to **(a)** a guinea pig and **(b)** a chinchilla via a butterfly catheter in the lose skin of the flank. Fluids should be warmed to body temperature.

Oral administration

Medications, oral liquids and assisted feeding with semi-liquid diets can be administered using a syringe placed in the diastema. Small amounts should be given and the animal coaxed to swallow. Passage of a stomach tube may be difficult due to the presence of the palatal ostium. Under anaesthesia, it may be possible to place a nasopharyngostomy tube; however, the small diameter makes adequate nutritional administration difficult. A pharyngeal feeding tube can be placed as for other species if longer term gavage feeding is required.

Fluid therapy

Intravenous, intraosseous, intraperitoneal and subcutaneous fluids should always be warmed to 37–38°C prior to administration. Fluids should be administered prior to anaesthesia and, if possible, during surgery for maintenance of blood pressure and perfusion. Fluid therapy should be continued in ill and hospitalized patients, particularly in cases of anorexia. Fluid supplementation is summarized in Figure 2.33.

Anaesthesia and analgesia

Preoperative preparation

Pre-existing illness, dehydration and anorexia may pose risks for anaesthesia and surgery. A careful clinical examination should be performed prior to induction of general anaesthesia or elective surgery. Anorexic patients may need additional nutritional and fluid support both before and following surgery.

It is not necessary to withhold food or water from any of these species as they cannot vomit. However, as they may hold food material at the back of the pharynx, removing food and water 1 hour prior to induction of anaesthesia may help to clear the mouth. During induction, the oral cavity should be swabbed out to remove any retained food. The anaesthetic gas itself may cause mucous membrane irritation, lacrimation and salivation, therefore pre-treatment with glycopyrrolate at a rate of 0.02 mg/kg s.c. and placement of eye lubricant ointment prior to induction is recommended.

Anaesthesia and intraoperative care

A balanced approach to anaesthesia and analgesia should be considered for each individual case, including:

- Pre-anaesthetic analgesics
- Anxiolytics
- Local/incisional anaesthetics
- General anaesthetics
- Post-anaesthesia analgesics.

The goal is to maintain the heart rate, blood pressure, oxygenation and body temperature as close as possible to that of the conscious animal. A thorough knowledge of the actions of the different drugs, physiology of the animal, and the duration and effect of surgery is necessary in choosing dosages and regimen. There are many published combinations. Injectable combinations may not allow much flexibility in controlling the depth of anaesthesia, but are useful for sedation or light anaesthesia. A surgical depth of anaesthesia can be achieved with the addition of inhalants such as isoflurane or sevoflurane.

Guinea pigs in particular become apnoeic with inhalant agents, and require careful monitoring and often the use of a respiratory stimulant (e.g. doxapram at a rate of 5–10 mg/kg i.v./i.m.) to keep respirations regular. Halothane has been shown to cause liver damage in some guinea pigs and should not be used. Use of an inhalant anaesthetic (via facemask) without prior administration of a sedative/anxiolytic (e.g. midazolam at a rate of 0.35–0.5 mg/kg i.m) should be avoided as it is stressful and can lead to a raised heart rate, blood pressure, and an increase in catecholamines and endogenous corticosteroids. These changes may alter the metabolism of the anaesthetic, making maintenance and a quick recovery difficult. A local or incisional anaesthetic utilizing a long-acting agent, such as bupivacaine (5%) diluted with sterile water to a volume appropriate for the area to be blocked, should be added to the regimen. Figure 2.34 details the various anaesthetic and analgesic agents and dosing regimens.

Fluid	Indication	Administration
Isotonic (normal) saline; isotonic dextrose (4%)/saline (0.18%); Lactated Ringer's solution (LRS); Normosol	Dehydration; electrolyte deficit (LRS, Normosol); toxaemia/septicaemia (isotonic dextrose/saline)	Severe dehydration (estimate >8–10%): 7–15 ml/kg/h i.v./i.o. via 24-gauge catheter Alternative: up to 30 ml/kg i.p. or up to 20 ml/kg s.c. Additional bolus administration q3–4h as needed to correct hydration Maintenance fluids: 50–100 ml/kg/day i.v./s.c.
Dextrose (5%) in water; glucose (20–50%, oral)	Pregnancy toxaemia; prolonged anorexia	Dextrose (5%): 7–15 ml/kg/h i.v. or up to 30 ml/kg i.p. Glucose (20–50%): 5 ml/adult orally every hour as needed
Colloids (e.g. Hetastarch)	Shock; hypotension; haemorrhage	Bolus at 3–5 ml/kg i.v./i.o. along with crystalloids at 5–10 ml/kg q30min until blood pressure and perfusion restored
Liquid diet (Critical Care for Herbivores, Oxbow Pet Products, Regular, Fine Grind); liquidized vegetables or pellets	Nutritional support	Hand/assisted feeding or via nasogastric, pharyngeal or oro/oesophageal tube (need to use a small mouth gag constructed from a 1 ml syringe barrel with hole drilled in it to pass premeasured feeding tube): 5–10 ml/adult per feeding. Feed 4–6 times a day for weight maintenance. For guinea pigs, add 10–30 mg vitamin C/kg/day

2.33 Fluid therapy and guidelines for use in guinea pigs, chinchillas, degus and duprasi.

Drug	Action	Guinea pigs	Chinchillas	Degus	Duprasi
Acepromazine	Pre-anaesthetic, light sedation, hypotensive	0.5–1.0 mg/kg i.m.	0.5–1.0 mg/kg i.m.	0.5–1.0 mg/kg i.m.	0.5–1.0 mg/kg i.m.
Acepromazine + Ketamine	45–60 minutes surgical anaesthesia; 2–6 hours recovery	5 mg/kg ACP + 100 mg/kg K i.p.	0.5 mg/kg ACP + 40 mg/kg K i.m.	Not published	Not published
Acepromazine + Ketamine + Xylazine	5–10 minutes sedation; sufficient for taking blood sample from jugular vein	Not published	Not published	Not published	1 mg/kg ACP + 30 mg/kg K + 6 mg/kg X i.p.
Acetylsalicylic acid (aspirin)	NSAID	80–85 mg/kg orally q4h	100–200 mg/kg orally q8h	100–200 mg/kg orally q8h	100–150 mg/kg orally q4h
Alfaxalone	Anaesthetic	40 mg/kg i.p.	Not published	Not published	Not published
Atipamezole	Reversal of dexmedetomidine	1 mg/kg s.c./i.m./i.p./i.v.	1 mg/kg s.c./i.m./i.p./i.v.	1 mg/kg s.c./i.m./i.p./i.v.	1 mg/kg s.c./i.m./i.p./i.v.
Atropine	Anticholinergic	0.05–0.1 mg/kg s.c./i.m.	0.05–0.1 mg/kg s.c./i.m.	0.05–0.1 mg/kg s.c./i.m.	0.1–0.4 mg/kg s.c./i.m.
Buprenorphine	Opioid analgesic	0.05 mg/kg s.c. q8–12h	0.05–0.10 mg/kg s.c. q8–12h	0.05–0.10 mg/kg s.c. q8–12h	0.05–0.10 mg/kg s.c. q12h
Butorphanol	Opioid analgesic	0.5–1.0 mg/kg i.m. q8h	0.5–2.0 mg/kg i.m. q8h	0.4–2.0 mg/kg i.m. q8h	1–5 mg/kg s.c. q4h
Carprofen	NSAID	5 mg/kg s.c. q24h	1–4 mg/kg orally q24h	4 mg/kg orally q24h	5 mg/kg orally q24h
Dexmedetomidine	Sedative; reverse with atipamezole	0.3 mg/kg s.c.; variable effects	Not published	Not published	0.1–0.2 mg/kg s.c.
Diazepam	Pre-anaesthetic, sedation	0.5–3 mg/kg i.m.	1–5 mg/kg i.m. (may irritate muscle) or 0.5–1.0 mg/kg i.v.	0.5–3 mg/kg i.m.	3–5 mg/kg i.m.
Fentanyl/ Fluanisone	Anaesthetic	0.5–1.0 ml/kg i.m.	Not published	Not published	Not published
Flumazenil	Reversal for benzodiazepines	0.1 mg/kg s.c.	0.1 mg/kg s.c.	0.1 mg/kg s.c.	Not published
Flunixin meglumine	NSAID; not recommended due to potential renal damage	1–2 mg/kg s.c. once	1–2 mg/kg s.c. once	1–2 mg/kg s.c. once	2.5 mg/kg s.c. q12–24h
Glycopyrrolate	Anticholinergic	0.01–0.02 mg/kg s.c./i.m.	0.01–0.02 mg/kg s.c./i.m.	0.01–0.02 mg/kg s.c./i.m.	0.01–0.02 mg/kg s.c./i.m.
Isoflurane	Inhalant anaesthetic	2–5% induction; 0.25–4% maintenance	1 mg/kg s.c./i.m./i.p./i.v.	1 mg/kg s.c./i.m./i.p./i.v.	1 mg/kg s.c./i.m./i.p./i.v.
Ketamine	Pre-anaesthetic, moderate sedation, little relaxation; usually a combination for short procedures	20–40 mg/kg i.m.	20–40 mg/kg i.m or 10–20 mg/kg i.v.	20–40 mg/kg i.m.	20–40 mg/kg i.m.
Ketamine + Dexmedetomidine	Pre-anaesthetic or heavy sedation; reverse dexmedetomidine with atipamezole	40 mg/kg K + 0.5 mg/kg D i.m./i.p.	Not published	Not published	50 mg/kg K + 0.5 mg/kg D i.p.
Ketamine + Diazepam	Sedation, relaxation	20–30 mg/kg K + 1–2 mg/kg D i.m.	20–40 mg/kg K + 3–5 mg/kg D i.m.	20–30 mg/kg K + 1–2 mg/kg D i.m.	Not published
Ketamine + Midazolam	Sedation, relaxation	5–10 mg/kg K + 0.5–1.0 mg/kg M i.m.	5–10 mg/kg K + 0.5–1.0 mg/kg M i.m.	5–10 mg/kg K + 0.5–1.0 mg/kg M i.m.	5–10 mg/kg K + 0.5–1.0 mg/kg M i.m.
Ketamine + Xylazine	Surgical anaesthesia; reversal with yohimbine (i.m.)	40 mg/kg K + 5 mg/ kg X i.p. or 20–40 mg/kg K + 2 mg/kg X i.m.	40 mg/kg K + 2–4 mg/kg X i.m.	40 mg/kg K + 2–4 mg/kg X i.m.	50 mg/kg K + 5 mg/ kg X i.p.
Meloxicam	NSAID	0.2–0.4 mg/kg s.c./ orally q24h	0.2–0.4 mg/kg s.c./ orally q24h	0.2–0.4 mg/kg s.c./ orally q24h	0.2–0.4 mg/kg s.c./ orally q24h

2.34 Anaesthetics, analgesics and sedatives used for guinea pigs, chinchillas, degus and duprasi. (continues) ▶

Drug	Action	Guinea pigs	Chinchillas	Degus	Duprasi
Meperidine	Analgesic	10–20 mg/kg s.c./i.m. q2–3h	20 mg/kg s.c./i.m.	10–20 mg/kg s.c./i.m.	20 mg/kg s.c./i.m. q2–3h
Midazolam	Better absorbed and less irritant i.m. than diazepam; benzodiazepine sedative, anxiolytic, amnesic	0.5–5.0 mg/kg i.m./i.p.	0.4–2.0 mg/kg i.m.	0.4–2.0 mg/kg i.m.	1–2 mg/kg i.m.
Morphine	Opioid analgesic	2–10 mg/kg i.m. q4h	2–5 mg/kg i.m. q4h	2–5 mg/kg i.m. q4h	2–5 mg/kg s.c. q2–4h
Naloxone	Narcotic reversal	0.01–0.1 mg/kg s.c./i.p.	0.01–0.1 mg/kg s.c./i.p.	0.01–0.1 mg/kg s.c./i.p.	0.01–0.1 mg/kg s.c./i.p.
Oxymorphone	Analgesic, opiate	0.2-0.5 mg/kg s.c. or i.m. bid or tid	0.2-0.5 mg/kg s.c. or i.m. bid or tid	0.2-0.5 mg/kg s.c. or i.m. bid or tid	0.2-0.5 mg/kg s.c. or i.m. bid or tid
Paracetamol	Analgesic	1–2 mg/ml in drinking water	1–2 mg/ml in drinking water	1–2 mg/ml in drinking water	1–2 mg/ml in drinking water
Tiletamine/ Zolazepam	Sedative; may have prolonged recovery	Not published	20–40 mg/kg i.m.	Not published	Not published
Xylazine	Sedative, hypotensive; use lower dose in combinations	Not used by itself	2–10 mg/kg i.m.	Not used by itself	Not used by itself
Yohimbine	Reversal of xylazine	0.5–1.0 mg/kg i.v. or 2.0 mg/kg i.m.	2.0 mg/kg i.m.	2.0 mg/kg i.m.	2.0 mg/kg i.m.

2.34 (continued) Anaesthetics, analgesics and sedatives used for guinea pigs, chinchillas, degus and duprasi.

Fentanyl/fluanisone combinations

Neuroleptanalgesic combinations, such as fentanyl/ fluanisone, when administered alone may produce sedation and sufficient analgesia for superficial surgery in most guinea pigs (Flecknell, 2002). There is poor muscle relaxation and marked respiratory depression at higher dosages. However, if it is administered in combination with a benzodiazepine (e.g. midazolam), surgical anaesthesia with good muscle relaxation and only moderate respiratory depression is produced. It can be partially reversed by butorphanol or other mixed agonist/antagonists. Benzodiazepine antagonists such as flumazenil can be used to speed recovery, but repeated doses are needed to avoid re-sedation. Even when reversal agents are used, recovery can be prolonged, particularly if a normal body temperature is not maintained (Flecknell, 2002).

Ketamine combinations

Ketamine alone has little analgesic effect, but will immobilize the animal. It can be combined with other agents for anaesthesia, but is often not as reliable in hystricomorphs as it is in other rodents or rabbits. Addition of an inhalant anaesthetic is frequently necessary to produce a surgical depth of anaesthesia. Medetomidine and xylazine produce glycosuria and polyuria. If a reversal agent for medetomidine or xylazine (atipamezole and yohimbine, respectively) is used, then an analgesic needs to be added to the regimen to provide postoperative analgesia.

Pentobarbital combinations

Pentobarbital is authorized for use in guinea pigs in the UK, but it has a very narrow margin of safety and variable effects. If it is used, a relatively low dose

(25 mg/kg i.p.) will immobilize and sedate the animal. The anaesthetic plane should be deepened using a low concentration of an inhalant anaesthetic such as isoflurane (at a rate of 0.5–1%). Close attention must be paid to maintaining normothermia during the procedure. Forced-air heating systems are preferable to warm water blankets, but care must be taken not to cause hyperthermia, particularly in chinchillas. Guinea pigs, chinchillas and degus are difficult to intubate, although using an endoscope it is possible to push past the ostium and place an uncuffed tube. Most inhalant anaesthetics are delivered via facemask. An induction chamber may be used initially, although there is the potential for the animal to injure itself as it passes through the excitation phase; it is advisable to remove the patient and continue induction with a facemask as soon as possible.

Monitoring

Due to their relatively small thoracic cavity and large abdomen, guinea pigs (and to a lesser extent chinchillas and degus) may be difficult to keep well ventilated during anaesthesia and surgery. If placed in dorsal recumbency, it is helpful to have the animal on a tilted surface with the head and thorax elevated above the abdomen. Monitoring during anaesthesia can be done using electrocardiography (ECG), a respiratory monitor, pulse oximetery and/or side-stream capnography, as well as via direct visualization of respiration, mucous membrane colour, capillary refill time, and auscultation or audio Doppler ultrasonography of the heart. Many electronic monitors designed for dogs/cats are not suitable for rodents as they do not record heart rates >250 beats per minute, and the clips/electrodes may be too large for these small animals. The author uses ECG and a respiratory monitor with 2 mm clips. An electronic thermometer probe can be fastened to the perineal area to continuously display the body temperature. Blood pressure measurements are difficult to obtain as the cuff size is usually larger than the limb, but the author has successfully measured blood pressure in the hindlimbs of guinea pigs, chinchillas and degus using a size 1 cuff with sphygmomanometer and audio Doppler ultrasonography, just above the medial tarsus. However, this may be difficult to do intraoperatively.

Postoperative care

As general anaesthesia can have adverse effects on both gut motility and flora, postoperative attention to gut health is important. Administration of gut motility enhancers such as metoclopramide, cisapride or ranitidine, as well as assisted feeding if the animal is not eating voluntarily, is recommended. Body temperature should be monitored and maintained by external heating if necessary until the animal is fully recovered. Ongoing fluid therapy may also be necessary until the animal is able to maintain hydration.

Analgesia

Pain is a major cause of postoperative inappetence and immobility. Suggested dosages and routes for analgesia are listed in Figure 2.34. An opioid analgesic such as buprenorphine, alone or in combination with an NSAID such as carprofen or meloxicam, will provide effective pain relief following major surgical procedures. Local anaesthetic infiltration of the incision site is a useful adjunct to systemic analgesics, and can be repeated if necessary postoperatively. An initial dose of the NSAID is given after blood pressure, heart rate and body temperature have returned to a pre-anaesthetic level, followed by an additional dose 12–24 hours later depending on the medication choice. In most circumstances, provision of analgesia for 24–48 hours post-surgery appears sufficient; however, if the animal shows reluctance to eat or move normally after analgesia is discontinued, it should be resumed and provided as necessary. There are no contraindications for administering pain medications.

Common surgical procedures

Guinea pigs

Orchidectomy

Guinea pigs have an open inguinal canal making a closed approach preferable. The scrotum is not readily visible; the testes can be palpated lateral to the penis.

1. Clip the hair and surgically prepare the incision sites. The guinea pig should be positioned on a slanted surface with the thorax and head slightly elevated above the abdomen.
2. Administer a testicular/cord local anaesthetic (e.g. 0.1 ml bupivacaine (5%) diluted to 0.3 ml with sterile water, injected into the cord at the level of the inguinal canal).
3. Make an incision over the proximal end of the testicle, through the skin and subcutis.
4. Dissect the testis and surrounding tunics free from the scrotum.
5. Apply gentle traction and double-clamp the cord and tunics.
6. Place a transfixing ligature proximal to the clamps.
7. Transect the cord between the two clamps and gently release.
8. Repeat the procedure with the other testis. If the tunic is damaged or opened, the incision should be lengthened so that the tunic can be repaired or the inguinal canal closed.
9. Close the skin with a subcuticular technique.

Ovariohysterectomy

The surgical approach is via a midline incision, and the ovaries and uterus are normally easily identifiable. In obese sows, the ovarian and uterine vessels may be embedded in adipose tissue and more difficult to identify and ligate.

1. Clip the hair on the abdomen from the pubis to the umbilicus, express the bladder, insert a rectal temperature probe and secure with tape to a hind foot, and attach ECG monitoring clips.
2. Surgically prepare the site using a non-alcohol based preparation (alcohol over such a wide site may reduce body temperature). The guinea pig should be positioned with the thorax slightly elevated above the abdomen on a slanted surface as is done for orchidectomy (see above).
3. Administer an incision site local anaesthetic (e.g. 0.1 ml bupivacaine (5%) diluted to 0.3 ml with sterile water).
4. Make a midline incision, starting approximately 1 cm anterior of the pubis and extending 1–2 cm for exposure of the uterus.
5. Elevate the cervix with the uterine horns. Transfix the cervix and ligate.
6. Follow the horns cranially to the ovaries, carefully reflecting the caecum and gastrointestinal tract. The uterine vessels are often embedded in fat and should be gently dissected and ligated. Ligate the ovarian pedicles. The ovarian pedicles, uterine body and associated vessels can then be removed.
7. Before closing, check the abdomen for haemorrhage, particularly in the area of the ovaries.
8. Close the peritoneum, incorporating it into the linea alba as the first layer. Close the abdominal muscle sheath as the second layer. Place a third layer subcuticularly to close the skin.
9. Use tissue glue to close any puckers or gaps in the skin.

Caesarean section

Supportive care for the sow is critical as this is often an 'emergency' procedure following prolonged dystocia. The sow may also be obese, have pregnancy toxaemia and a uterine infection. The surgical approach is via a midline incision (as for dogs or cats). If the young are dead, and the uterus is infected or has areas of necrosis, an ovariohysterectomy (see above) should be performed. If the dystocia is due to overly large but otherwise healthy fetuses, or the sow's symphysis has not separated, the decision may be to deliver the pups, and close the uterus. Generally this is not advised as subsequent pregnancies may also end in dystocia. Maternal mortality can be high if the pups are dead and there is a uterine infection. During the procedure, care must be taken to prevent exudates (if present) from the uterus entering the abdomen. The abdomen can be closed with two layers of simple interrupted sutures, and a subcuticular technique to close the skin. Postoperative antibiotics, fluid therapy and analgesia will be necessary. Orphaned pups can be fed on a mash of a commercial pellet diet diluted with cow's milk, using a dropper or syringe. Pups can be cross-fostered to other sows nursing pups.

Superficial abscesses
Guinea pigs may form thick, inspissated pus, often enclosed in a capsule (Figure 2.35). The skin should be shaved and disinfected. The abscess should be incised using a large cruciform incision. The contents should be thoroughly removed along with any capsule material. The cavity should be flushed with saline or a wound-cleansing fluid, then packed with a wound-cleaning cream. Systemic antibiotic therapy may be necessary if the animal is showing signs of generalized infection. The wound should be kept open for several days, and flushed and repacked with ointment daily as needed until healed. To prevent bedding from sticking to the wound, the guinea pig may need to be housed on towels or multiple layers of newspaper.

Chinchillas
The most commonly performed procedures in chinchillas are orchidectomy, ovariohysterectomy, dental abscess removal, with or without tooth extraction and occlusion adjustment, and orthopaedic surgery due to trauma. Caesarean sections are also performed due to dystocia. The techniques for orchidectomy, ovariohysterectomy and Caesarean section are the same as described for guinea pigs.

Correction of malocclusion from inside the oral cavity is complicated by the narrowness of the mouth, but as the normal occlusal surface of the cheek teeth is relatively straight, burring and polishing to obtain the horizontal bite can be easier than with the interdigitated occlusal surfaces of guinea pig or rabbit cheek teeth. Removal of teeth due to severe osteomyelitis or abscess is the same as in guinea pigs or rabbits.

Orthopaedic repair of fractures follows the principles for all bone repair; however, due to the likelihood of post-surgery splint or bandage chewing, internal fixation is often preferred. It is not uncommon for a chinchilla to self-amputate a limb due to either the fracture or the fracture repair. Prognosis for successful return to function *versus* post-corrective procedures must be evaluated. In many cases it is preferable to remove a limb distal to a fracture site to prevent self-mutilation. In all cases of fracture repair, strict cage rest without climbing or jumping for a minimum of 4 weeks is necessary. Non-union fractures are not uncommon in chinchillas due to their activity rates. Abscesses may arise secondarily from bite wounds. These should be surgically debrided and excised as they form inspissated pus, similar to those in guinea pigs.

Degus
Orchidectomy, ovariohysterectomy and all other surgical procedures are similar to those in chinchillas. There is a report of preputial damage with lateral penile displacement as a complication of castration, which caused bruising, swelling and severe oedema to the penis and prepuce (Powers *et al.*, 2008). Gentle tissue handling and fine surgical instruments should be used when working with small mammals.

Duprasi
Orchidectomy, ovariohysterectomy, abscess removal, dental repairs, wound repairs, orthopaedic procedures and mass removals are essentially the same as in the domestic gerbil. As with all rodents, postoperative pain management is essential to prevent self-mutilation of the surgery site.

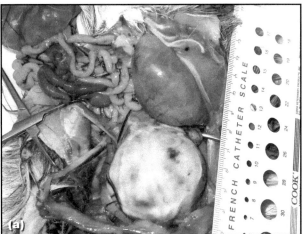 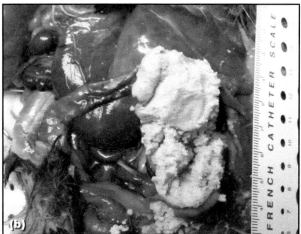

2.35 **(a)** Appearance of an abdominal abscess in a guinea pig at post-mortem examination. **(b)** The abscess has been opened to reveal the inspissated pus.

Euthanasia

Humane euthanasia of pets, particularly if owners wish to be present, must be done gently and efficiently. The author prefers to administer an intramuscular combination of midazolam (0.4 mg/kg), butorphanol (0.3 mg/kg) and low-dose ketamine (3 mg/kg). When the animal is fully sedated, a hindleg can be shaved and a vein located. An assistant then exerts proximal pressure to raise the vein. A euthanasia solution (pentobarbital preparation) is injected through a 25-gauge needle into the vein. If the owner is not present, euthanasia can be achieved following sedation with an intraperitoneal injection of the euthanasia solution.

Drug formulary

A drug formulary for guinea pigs, chinchillas, degus and duprasi is given in Figure 2.36. Doses for degus are adapted from those used for guinea pigs and chinchillas. Doses for duprasi are adapted from published dosages for domesticated gerbils (*Meriones* spp.). Antibiotics that have a primarily Gram-positive spectrum should not be used in guinea pigs, chinchillas and degus as they may cause a fatal dysbiosis.

Drug	Guinea pigs	Chinchillas	Degus	Duprasi	Comments
Antimicrobial agents					
Amikacin	10–15 mg/kg divided s.c./i.m./ i.v. q12h	10–15 mg/kg divided s.c./i.m./i.v. q12h	10–15 mg/kg divided s.c./i.m./i.v. q12h	10 mg/kg s.c./i.m. q12h	Antibiotic
Cefalexin	50 mg/kg i.m. divided q12h	50 mg/kg i.m. divided q12h	50 mg/kg i.m. divided q12h	Not used	Parenteral use only. May cause dysbiosis
Cefaloridine	10–25 mg/kg i.m. q8–12h	10–25 mg/kg i.m. q8–12h	10–25 mg/kg i.m. q8–12h	25 mg/kg s.c./i.m. q24h	Parenteral use only. May cause dysbiosis
Ceftiofur	1 mg/kg i.m. q24h	1 mg/kg i.m. q24h	1 mg/kg i.m. q24h	Not used	Parenteral use only. Pneumonia
Chloramphenicol	50 mg/kg orally q12h	50 mg/kg orally q12h	50 mg/kg orally q12h	50 mg/kg orally q12h	Antibiotic
Ophthalmic ointment or drops	1 drop topically q6–12h	1 drop topically q6–12	1 drop topically q6–12	1 drop topically q6–12	Topical antibiotic for eyes
Ciprofloxacin	10 mg/kg orally q12h	10 mg/kg orally q12h	10 mg/kg orally q12h	10 mg/kg orally q12h	Antibiotic
Doxycycline	2.5 mg/kg orally q12h	2.5 mg/kg orally q12h	2.5 mg/kg orally q12h	2.5 mg/kg orally q12h	Antibiotic. Use with caution in guinea pigs, chinchillas and degus as may cause dysbiosis
Enrofloxacin	10 mg/kg orally/s.c./i.m. q12h	10 mg/kg orally/s.c./i.m. q12h	10 mg/kg orally/s.c./i.m. q12h	10 mg/kg orally/s.c./i.m. q12h	Antibiotic
Gentamicin	5 mg/kg s.c./i.m. divided q12h	5 mg/kg s.c./i.m. divided q12h	5 mg/kg s.c./i.m. divided q12h	5 mg/kg s.c./i.m. divided q12h	Antibiotic
Ophthalmic ointment or drops	1 drop or small dab topically q12h	1 drop or small dab topically q12h	1 drop or small dab topically q12h	1 drop or small dab topically q12h	Topical antibiotic for eyes
Metronidazole	20 mg/kg orally q12h	10–20 mg/kg orally q12h	20 mg/kg orally q12h	20 mg/kg orally q12h	Anaerobes (also antiprotozoal)
Neomycin	15 mg/kg orally q12h	15 mg/kg orally q12h	15 mg/kg orally q12h	2.6 mg/ml drinking water	Antibiotic
Netilmicin	6–8 mg/kg s.c./i.m./i.v. divided q8–24h	6–8 mg/kg s.c./i.m./i.v. divided q8–24h	Usage not reported	Usage not reported	*Pseudomonas*
Oxytetracycline	5 mg/kg i.m. q12h	50 mg/kg orally q12h	Usage not reported	10 mg/kg orally q8h	Antibiotic. Toxicity reported in guinea pigs. Use with caution in chinchillas
Sulfadimethoxine	10–15 mg/kg orally q12h	10–15 mg/kg orally q12h	10–15 mg/kg orally q12h	10–15 mg/kg orally q12h	Antibiotic
Sulfamerazine	1 mg/ml drinking water	1 mg/ml drinking water	1 mg/ml drinking water	0.8 mg/ml drinking water	Antibiotic

2.36 Drug formulary for guinea pigs, chinchillas, degus and duprasi. (continues) ▶

Drug	Guinea pigs	Chinchillas	Degus	Duprasi	Comments
Antimicrobial agents continued					
Sulfaquinoxaline	1 mg/ml drinking water	1 mg/ml drinking water	1 mg/ml drinking water	1 mg/ml drinking water	Antibiotic
Tetracycline	10–20 mg/kg orally q12h	10–20 mg/kg orally q12h	Usage not reported	20 mg/kg i.m. q24h or 10–20 mg/kg orally q8–12h or 2–5 mg/ml drinking water	Antibiotic. Use with caution in guinea pigs and chinchillas as toxicity reported
Trimethoprim/ Sulphonamide	15–30 mg/kg orally/s.c.	15–30 mg/kg orally/s.c.	15–30 mg/kg orally/s.c.	15–30 mg/kg orally/s.c.	Antibiotic. Tissue necrosis can occur if given subcutaneously
Antifungal agents					
Captan powder	Not used	1 teaspoon per 2 cups of dust	1 teaspoon per 2 cups of dust	Not used	Fungicide to prevent dermatophytosis. Add to dust bath
Griseofulvin	15–25 mg/kg orally q24h for 14–28 days	25 mg/kg orally q24h for 14–28 days	15–25 mg/kg orally q24h for 14–28 days	15–25 mg/kg orally q24h for 14–28 days	Antifungal for dermatophytosis
Itraconazole	5 mg/kg orally q24h	5 mg/kg orally q24h for 6 weeks	Usage not reported	Usage not reported	Systemic candidiasis. Dermatophytosis in chinchillas
Ketoconazole	10–40 mg/kg orally q24h for 14 days	10–40 mg/kg orally q24h for 14 days	10-40 mg/kg orally q24h for 14 days	10–40 mg/kg orally q24h for 14 days	Systemic mycoses, candidiasis
Terbinafine	10–30 mg/kg orally q24h for 4–6 weeks	10–30 mg/kg orally q24h for 4–6 weeks	10–30 mg/kg orally q24h for 4–6 weeks	10–30 mg/kg orally q24h for 4–6 weeks	Antifungal
Antiparasitic agents					
Albendazole	Usage not reported	25 mg/kg orally q12h for 2 days	Usage not reported	Usage not reported	Giardiasis
Amitraz	0.3% solution topically q7d	Usage not reported	Usage not reported	1.4 ml of 0.3% solution/l topical q7–14d for 3–6 treatments	Anti-demodecosis
Carbaryl (5%) powder	Topical once a week for 3 treatments	Topical once a week for 3 treatments	Topical once a week for 3 treatments	Topical once a week for 3 treatments	Ectoparasites
Fenbendazole	20 mg/kg orally q24h for 5 days	20 mg/kg orally q24h for 5 days	20 mg/kg orally q24h for 5 days	20 mg/kg orally q24h for 5 days	Endoparasites. Some antiprotozoal activity
Ivermectin	0.2–0.4 mg/kg s.c. q7–14d	0.2–0.4 mg/kg s.c. q7–14d	0.2–0.4 mg/kg s.c. q7–14d	0.2–0.4 mg/kg s.c. q7–14d	Endoparasites and ectoparasites
Permethrin	0.25% dust in cage	0.25% dust in cage	0.25% dust in cage	0.25% dust in cage	Ectoparasites
Piperazine adipate	4–7 mg/ml drinking water for 3–10 days	500 mg/kg orally q24h	Usage not reported	200–600 mg/kg orally q24h for 7 days, off 7 days, repeat 7 days	Nematodiasis
Piperazine citrate	10 mg/ml drinking water for 7 days, off 7 days, repeat for 7 days	100 mg/kg orally q24h for 2 days	Usage not reported	2–5 mg/ml drinking water for 7 days, off 7 days, repeat 7 days	Nematodiasis
Praziquantel	6–10 mg/kg orally/s.c.; repeat in 10 days	6–10 mg/kg orally/s.c.; repeat in 10 days	Usage not reported	30 mg/kg orally q14d for 3 treatments	Cestodiasis
Pyrantel pamoate	50 mg/kg orally once	50 mg/kg orally once	50 mg/kg orally once	50 mg/kg orally once	Nematodiasis
Pyrethrin powder	Topical q7d for 3 treatments	Topical q7d for 3 treatments	Topical q7d for 3 treatments	Topical 3 times/ week for 3 weeks	Ectoparasites
Quinacrine	75 mg/kg orally q8h	75 mg/kg orally q8h	Usage not reported	Usage not reported	Giardiasis

2.36 (continued) Drug formulary for guinea pigs, chinchillas, degus and duprasi. (continues) ▶

Drug	Guinea pigs	Chinchillas	Degus	Duprasi	Comments
Antiparasitic agents continued					
Selamectin	6 mg/kg topically once per month	Usage not reported	Usage not reported	Usage not reported	Ectoparasites
Sulfadimethoxine	25–50 mg/kg orally q24h for 10 days	25–50 mg/kg orally q24h for 10 days	25–50 mg/kg orally q24h for 10 days	Usage not reported	Coccidiosis
Sulfamerazine	1 mg/ml drinking water	1 mg/ml drinking water	1 mg/ml drinking water	0.8 mg/ml drinking water	Coccidiosis
Sulfamethazine	1 mg/ml drinking water	1 mg/ml drinking water	1 mg/ml drinking water	0.8 mg/ml drinking water	Coccidiosis
Sulfaquinoxaline	0.1% in drinking water for 14–21 days	0.1% in drinking water for 14–21 days	0.1% in drinking water for 14–21 days	0.1% in drinking water for 14–21 days	Coccidiosis
Tiabendazole	100 mg/kg orally q24h for 5 days	50–100 mg/kg orally q24h for 5 days	100 mg/kg orally q24h for 5 days	100 mg/kg orally q24h for 5 days	Ascaridiasis
Miscellaneous					
Adrenaline	0.003 mg/kg i.v.	0.003 mg/kg i.v.	0.003 mg/kg i.v.	0.003 mg/kg i.v.	Cardiac arrest
Aluminium hydroxide	20–40 mg/animal orally as needed	20–40 mg/animal orally as needed	20–40 mg/animal orally as needed	20–40 mg/animal orally as needed	Hyperphosphataemia due to renal failure
Aminophylline	50 mg/kg i.m.; maintenance 10 mg/kg orally q8–12h	50 mg/kg i.m.; maintenance 10 mg/kg orally q8–12h	Usage not reported	Usage not reported	Bronchodilator
Atropine	10 mg/kg s.c. q20min	10 mg/kg s.c. q20min	10 mg/kg s.c. q20min	10 mg/kg s.c. q20min	Organophosphate toxicity
Benazepril	Usage not reported	0.10 mg/kg orally q24h	0.10 mg/kg orally q24h	Usage not reported	Dilated cardiomyopathy
Calcium gluconate	100 mg/kg i.m.	100 mg/kg i.p.	100 mg/kg i.p.	Usage not reported	Hypocalcaemic tetany, eclampsia, dystocia
Chlorphenamine	0.6 mg/kg orally q24h	Usage not reported	Usage not reported	Usage not reported	Antihistamine
Chorionic gonadotrophin	1000 IU/animal i.m.; repeat in 7–10 days	Usage not reported	Usage not reported	Usage not reported	Cystic ovaries
Cimetidine	5–10 mg/kg orally/s.c./i.m./i.v. q6–12h	5–10 mg/kg orally/s.c./i.m./i.v. q6–12h	5–10 mg/kg orally/s.c./i.m./i.v. q6–12h	5–10 mg/kg orally/s.c./i.m./i.v. q6–12h	Gastric antihistamine. Gastric and duodenal ulceration, oesophagitis
Cisapride	0.5 mg/kg orally q8–12h	0.5 mg/kg orally q8–12h	0.5 mg/kg orally q8–12h	0.1–0.5 mg/kg orally q12h	Gastrointestinal motility enhancer
Colestyramine	2 g in 20 ml of water orally q24h; can be divided into 3–4 doses	2 g in 20 ml of water orally q24h; can be divided into 3–4 doses	2 g in 20 ml of water orally q24h; can be divided into 3–4 doses	Usage not reported	Ion exchange resin that binds bacterial toxins. Useful for Clostridial toxaemias
Cyclophosphamide	300 mg/kg i.p. q24h	Usage not reported	Usage not reported	Usage not reported	Antineoplastic
Deslorelin	4.7 mg implant for cystic ovaries, may suppress hormones for at least 6 months	Usage not reported	Usage not reported	Usage not reported	Deslorelin (Suprelorin®) 4.7 mg impant is a GnRH analogue which may be adjunctive therapy for ovarian cysts. Duration of action is at least 6 months
Dexamethasone	Pregnancy toxaemia: 0.6 mg/kg i.m. Shock: 4–5 mg/kg s.c./i.m./i.p./i.v.	Shock: 4–5 mg/kg s.c./i.m./i.p./i.v. Anti-inflammatory: 0.5–2.0 mg/kg orally/s.c. then decrease dose q12h for 3–14 days	Shock: 4–5 mg/kg s.c./i.m./i.p./i.v. Anti-inflammatory: 0.5–2.0 mg/kg orally/s.c. then decrease dose q12h for 3–14 days	Shock: 4–5 mg/kg s.c./i.m./i.p./i.v. Anti-inflammatory: 0.5–2.0 mg/kg orally/s.c. then decrease dose q12h for 3–14 days	Corticosteroid. Anti-inflammatory. Shock, pregnancy toxaemia

2.36 (continued) Drug formulary for guinea pigs, chinchillas, degus and duprasi. (continues) ▶

Drug	Guinea pigs	Chinchillas	Degus	Duprasi	Comments
Miscellaneous continued					
Diazepam	1–2 mg/kg i.m.	Usage not reported	Usage not reported	Usage not reported	Calming, for intense pruritus
	1–5 mg/kg i.m./i.v./i.p./i.o.	1–5 mg/kg i.m./i.v./i.p./i.o.	1–5 mg/kg i.m./i.v./i.p./i.o.	1–5 mg/kg i.m./i.v./i.p./i.o.	Seizures
Diphenhydramine	5 mg/kg s.c. as needed or 7.5 mg/kg orally	1–2 mg/kg orally/s.c. q12h	1–2 mg/kg orally/s.c. q12h	1–2 mg/kg orally/s.c. q12h	Antihistamine. Anaphylaxis
Dopamine	0.08 mg/kg i.v.	Usage not reported	Usage not reported	Usage not reported	Hypotension
Doxapram	2–5 mg/kg i.v./i.p.	5–10 mg/kg i.v./i.p.	5–10 mg/kg i.v./i.p.	5–10 mg/kg i.v./i.p.	Respiratory stimulant
Edetate calcium disodium	30 mg/kg s.c. q12h	30 mg/kg s.c. q12h	Usage not reported	Usage not reported	Chelation of lead and zinc
Ephedrine	1 mg/kg i.v.	Usage not reported	Usage not reported	Usage not reported	Antihistamine, stimulant
Furosemide	1–4 mg/kg s.c./i.m. q6h or 5–10 mg/kg s.c./i.m. q12h	1–4 mg/kg s.c./i.m. q6h or 5–10 mg/kg s.c./i.m. q12h	1–4 mg/kg s.c./i.m. q6h or 5–10 mg/kg s.c./i.m. q12h	1–4 mg/kg s.c./i.m. q6h or 5–10 mg/kg s.c./i.m. q12h	Diuretic for oedema, pulmonary congestion, ascites
Glycopyrrolate	0.01–0.02 mg/kg s.c.	0.01–0.02 mg/kg s.c.	0.01–0.02 mg/kg s.c.	0.01–0.02 mg/kg s.c.	Bradycardia
Hydralazine	1 mg/kg i.v. as needed or 1–2 mg/kg orally q12h	Usage not reported	Usage not reported	Usage not reported	Antihistamine
Loperamide	0.1 mg/kg orally q8h for 3 days, then q24h for 2 days; give in 1 ml water	0.1 mg/kg orally q8h for 3 days, then q24h for 2 days; give in 1 ml water	0.1 mg/kg orally q8h for 3 days, then q24h for 2 days; give in 1 ml water	Usage not reported	Anti-diarrhoeal. Enteropathy
Leuprolide acetate depot (30-day formula)	0.2–0.3 mg/kg i.m. q30d	Usage not reported	Usage not reported	Usage not reported	Cystic ovaries
Metoclopramide	0.2–1.0 mg/kg orally/s.c./i.m. q12h	0.2–1.0 mg/kg orally/s.c./i.m. q12h	0.2–1.0 mg/kg orally/s.c./i.m. q12h	0.2–1.0 mg/kg orally/s.c./i.m. q12h	Gastrointestinal motility enhancer. Gastric stasis
Oxytocin	If pubic symphysis is not fused: 1.0–3.0 IU/kg s.c./i.m./i.v.	0.2–3.0 IU/kg s.c./i.m./i.v.	0.2–3.0 IU/kg s.c./i.m./i.v.	0.2–3.0 IU/kg s.c./i.m./i.v.	Unobstructed dystocia. If no young produced 15 minutes after at least 1 IU/kg, then Caesarean section is indicated
Phenobarbital	10–20 mg/kg i.v./i.p.	Usage not reported	Usage not reported	Usage not reported	Anti-seizure
Potassium citrate	10–30 mg/kg orally q12h	Usage not reported	Usage not reported	Usage not reported	Electrolyte
Pseudoephedrine	Usage not reported	1.2 mg/chinchilla orally q12h	Usage not reported	Usage not reported	Antihistamine
Sucralfate	25–50 mg/kg orally q8–24h	25–50 mg/kg orally q8–24h	25–50 mg/kg orally q8–24h	25–50 mg/kg orally q8–24h	Upper gastrointestinal protectant
Tropicamide (1%)	1 drop each eye	1 drop each eye	1 drop each eye	1 drop each eye	Mydriasis. Do not use in albino eyes
Vitamin A	50–500 IU/kg i.m. once	Usage not reported	Usage not reported	Usage not reported	Hypovitaminosis A
Vitamin B complex	0.02–0.2 ml/kg s.c./i.m.	0.02–0.2 ml/kg s.c./i.m.	0.02–0.2 ml/kg s.c./i.m.	0.02–0.2 ml/kg s.c./i.m.	Deficiency, haemorrhage, appetite stimulant
Vitamin C	Severe case: initial dose 125 mg/kg s.c./orally q24h Ill, stressed: 35–50 mg/kg s.c./i.m./orally q24h	Not a requirement	Not a requirement	Not a requirement	Ascorbic acid deficiency, arthritis, additional need in stressed/pregnant/ill guinea pigs. Supplementation should be provided to all hospitalized/surgical guinea pigs

2.36 (continued) Drug formulary for guinea pigs, chinchillas, degus and duprasi. (continues) ▶

Drug	Guinea pigs	Chinchillas	Degus	Duprasi	Comments
Miscellaneous continued					
Vitamin D2	200–400 IU/kg s.c./i.m. once	200–400 IU/kg s.c./i.m. once	200–400 IU/kg s.c./i.m. once	200–400 IU/kg s.c./i.m. once	Hypovitaminosis D, osteomalacia. Correction of the diet required
Vitamin E	Usage not reported	100–400 IU/chinchilla orally as needed	Usage not reported	Usage not reported	Myopathy
Vitamin K1	Warfarin poisoning: 1–10 mg/kg i.m. q24h for 4–6 days 2.5–5.0 mg/kg q24h for 21–28 days	Warfarin poisoning: 1–10 mg/kg i.m. q24h for 4–6 days 2.5–5.0 mg/kg q24h for 21–28 days	Warfarin poisoning: 1–10 mg/kg i.m. q24h for 4–6 days 2.5–5.0 mg/kg q24h for 21–28 days	Warfarin poisoning: 1–10 mg/kg i.m. q24h for 4–6 days 2.5–5.0 mg/kg q24h for 21–28 days	Warfarin poisoning, brodifacom poisoning

2.36 (continued) Drug formulary for guinea pigs, chinchillas, degus and duprasi.

References and further reading

Babero BB and Cattan PE (1975) Helmintofauna ndel Chile: III. Parasitos del roedor degu, *Octodon degus* Molina, 1782, con la descriptcion de tres nuevas especies. *Bolivan and Childean Parasitology* **30**, 68–76

Bauwens L, Vercammen F, Wuytack C, Van Looveren K and Swinne D (2004) Isolation of *Cryptococcus neoformans* in Antwerp Zoo's nocturnal house. *Mycoses* **47**(7), 202–206

Boralevi F, Leaute-Labreze C, Roul S, Couprie B and Taieb A (2003) Lupus-erythematosus-like eruption induced by *Trichophyton mentagrophytes* infection. *Dermatology* **206**(4), 303–306

Capello V and Gracis M (2005) Anatomy of the skull and teeth. In: *Rabbit and Rodent Dentistry Handbook*, ed. V Capello *et al.*, pp. 3–43. Zoological Education Network, Lake Worth, Florida

Donnelly TM and Quimby FW (2002) Biology and diseases of other rodents. In: *Laboratory Animal Medicine, 2nd edn*, ed. JG Fox *et al.*, pp. 247–307. Academic Press, San Diego, California

Edwards MS (2009) Nutrition and behavior of degus (*Octodon degus*). *Veterinary Clinics of North America: Exotic Animals* **12**(2), 237–253

Felt SA, Guirguis FI, Wasfy MO, Howard JS, Domingo NV and Hussein HI (2009) An effective venipuncture technique and normal serum biochemistry parameters of the captive fat-tailed jird (*Pachyuromys duprasi*). *Journal of the American Association for Laboratory Animal Science* **48**(1), 57–60

Felt SA, Hussein HI and Mohamed Helmy IH (2008) Biology, breeding, husbandry and diseases of the captive Egyptian fat-tailed jird (*Pachyuromys duprasi natronensis*). *Lab Animal* **37**(6), 256–261

Flecknell P (2002) Guinea pigs. In: *BSAVA Manual of Exotic Pets, 4th edn*, ed. AM Meredith and S Redrobe, pp. 52–64. BSAVA Publications, Gloucester

Hawkins MG, Ruby AL, Drazenovich TL and Westropp JL (2009) Composition and characteristics of urinary calculi from guinea pigs. *Journal of the American Veterinary Medical Association* **234**(2), 214–220

Hoefer HL and Crossley DA (2002) Chinchillas. In: *BSAVA Manual of Exotic Pets, 4th edn*, ed. AM Meredith and S Redrobe, pp. 65–75. BSAVA Publications, Gloucester

Hrapkiewicz K and Medina L (2007) *Clinical Laboratory Animal Medicine: an introduction, 3rd edn.* Blackwell Publishing, Ames, Iowa

Johnson-Delaney CA (2002) Other small mammals. In: *BSAVA Manual of Exotic Pets, 4th edn*, ed. AM Meredith and S Redrobe, pp. 102–115. BSAVA Publications, Gloucester

Johnson-Delaney CA (2006) Common procedures in hedgehogs, prairie dogs, exotic rodents and companion marsupials. *Veterinary Clinics of North America: Exotic Animal Practice* **9**(2), 415–435

Meredith AM and Redrobe S (2002) *BSAVA Manual of Exotic Pets, 4th edn.* BSAVA Publications, Gloucester

Murphy JC, Niemi SM, Hewes KM, Zink M and Fox JG (1978) Hematologic and serum protein reference values of the *Octodon degus. American Journal of Veterinary Research* **39**(4), 713–715

O'Malley B (2005) Guinea pigs. In: *Clinical Anatomy and Physiology of Exotic Species, Structure and Function of Mammals, Birds, Reptiles and Amphibians*, ed. B O'Malley, pp. 197–208. Elsevier Saunders, London

Percy DH and Barthold SW (2007) Guinea pigs. In: *Pathology of Laboratory Rodents and Rabbits, 3rd edn*, ed. DH Percy and SW Barthold, pp. 217–252. Blackwell Publishing, Ames, Iowa

Popesko P, Rajtova F and Horak J (2002) Cavia aperea f. porcellus. In: *A Colour Atlas of Anatomy of Small Laboratory Animals Volume One: rabbit, guinea pig* (*Octodon degus*), ed. P Popesko *et al.*, pp. 147–240. Saunders, St Louis, Missouri

Powers MY, Campbell BG and Finch NP (2008) Preputial damage and lateral penile displacement during castration in a degu. *Journal of the American Veterinary Medical Association* **232**(7), 1013–1015

Quesenberry KE and Carpenter JW (2004) *Ferrets, Rabbits and Rodents: Clinical Medicine and Surgery, 2nd edn.* Saunders, St Louis, Missouri

Refinetti R (1998) Homeostatic and circadian control of body temperature in the fat-tailed gerbil. *Comparative Biochemistry and Physiology Annals of Molecular Integrated Physiology* **119**(1), 295–300

Rush HG, Lee TM and Young AT (2000) Growth and reproductive performance of degus (*Octodon degus*) on commercial rodent diets. *Contemporary Topics* **39**, 104

Sirois M (2005) The guinea pig. In: Laboratory Animal Medicine: principles and procedures, ed. M Sirois, pp. 115–138. Elsevier Mosby, St Louis, Missouri

Williams CSF (1976) Practical Guide to Laboratory Animals. CV Mosby Company, St Louis, Missouri

Worgul BV and Rothstein H (1975) Congenital cataracts associated with disorganized meridional rows in a new laboratory animal the degu (*Octodon degus*). *Biomedical Express* **23**, 1–4

Wesche P (2009) Rodents: clinical pathology. In: *BSAVA Manual of Rodents and Ferrets*, ed. E Keeble and A Meredith, pp. 42–51. BSAVA Publications, Gloucester

3

Chipmunks and prairie dogs

Cathy Johnson-Delaney

Introduction

Chipmunks

Chipmunks occur in North America, Europe and Asia. The genus *Eutamias* consists of two subgenera and 24 species. The term *Eutamias* is often used as a synonym for *Tamias*, although *Walker's Mammals of the World* (Nowak, 1999) separates *Eutamias* from *Tamias* (single species *T. striatus,* the eastern American chipmunk found throughout the eastern USA and southeastern Canada, rarely kept as pets).

Most pet chipmunks in the USA and Europe are *Eutamias sibiricus* (Figure 3.1a). The original range of this species is Siberia, Mongolia, northern and central China, Korea and the Japanese island of Hokkaido. The information in this chapter refers to this species, but is applicable to most other chipmunks of the genus *Eutamias*.

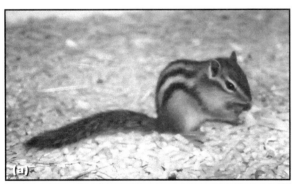

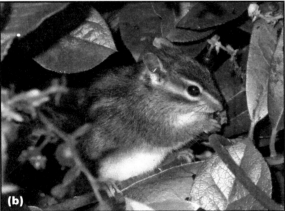

3.1 **(a)** Captive pet chipmunk (*Eutamias sibiricus*). (Courtesy of E. Keeble.) **(b)** *Eutamias townsendii* (wild Western American chipmunk), demonstrating coat coloration typical of all chipmunks. These are not kept as pets.

Chipmunks are typically distinguished by characteristic black and white stripes along the back, as well as through the eyes (Figure 3.1b). The wild-type colouring is brown to grey fur, with a white or yellowish ventrum. They have a long, bushy tail with dark guard hairs tipped with white. There are colour variations in captive-bred chipmunks, including all-cream, albino and piebald. In many of these colour variants, the striping is no longer visible.

Chipmunks are not domesticated rodents and retain much of their wild behaviour in captivity. Because of this, they do not make ideal pets. They are easily stressed and may exhibit stereotypical behaviours.

Prairie dogs

The black-tailed prairie dog *(Cynomys ludovicianus)* is native to North America (Figure 3.2). It is diurnal and does not truly hibernate. It may have dormant periods in inclement weather and tends to gain weight in the autumn as the light cycle and temperature decrease. Vocalizations include a 'bark' when excited, and various chatters and growls.

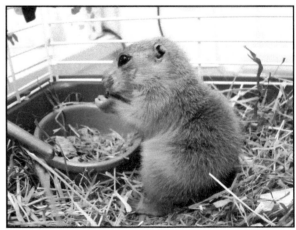

3.2 Black-tailed prairie dog (*Cynomys ludovicianus*). (Courtesy of D. Johnson.)

Until 2003 prairie dogs in the American pet trade were harvested from the wild, although a few captive-bred animals were available. In 2003 prairie dogs housed with imported exotic rodents, principally Gambian giant rats (*Cricetomys* spp.) from Africa, became infected with monkeypox. These prairie dogs developed systemic disease with lesions in numerous organs resembling monkeypox lesions in non-human

primates and smallpox lesions in humans. A number of humans became infected with monkeypox. The Centers for Disease Control and Prevention (CDC) and the Food and Drug Administration of the United States (FDA) brought about regulations that implemented an embargo on importation of all rodents from Africa. The regulations also prohibited transport, sale and distribution, including release into the environment, of prairie dogs and various African rodents. States were also empowered to enact measures to prohibit importation, sale, distribution or display of animals that could result in transmission of infectious agents. Because of this, the number of prairie dogs seen as pets has been decreasing as the owned animals age and die. In September 2008 the FDA lifted its restrictions as there had been no additional cases for 5 years but the CDC have not rescinded; so, at time of writing, the regulations are still in effect. In the UK prairie dogs may legally be kept as pets.

Biology

Chipmunks

Eutamias sibiricus primarily inhabit forests of evergreen trees, such as firs, pines and spruce, as well as woodlands of deciduous trees and brush. They reside in burrows and are active during the day. Nests may be in hollow logs, tree branches or, in the winter, in chambers in burrows underground. Wild chipmunks are omnivorous, with a diet of seeds, buds, leaves and flowers. They will climb trees to obtain food. They have cheek pouches to carry food back to the nest, and tend to hoard food items. They are coprophagic, allowing uptake of vitamins B and K. Biological data are summarized in Figure 3.3.

Lifespan in captivity (years)	Males: up to 8 Females: up to 12 Average: 4–6
Adult bodyweight (g)	70–142
Body temperature (°C)	38; during torpor, a few degrees above ambient
Heart rate (beats/min)	264–296; during torpor may drop to 3–6
Respiratory rate (breaths/min)	75; during torpor may drop to less than 1 per minute and is barely detectable
Food consumption	25–30 g/day
Fluid consumption	75–100 ml/kg/day
Activity	Diurnal
Dentition	Incisors open-rooted: I 1/1, C 0/0, PM 2/1; M 3/3 x 2 = 22 teeth
Mammary glands	4 pairs

3.3 Biological data for *Eutamias sibiricus*.

Chipmunks do not truly hibernate in cold weather but they will become torpid; they hoard food in their nest in preparation. In captivity, extra nest material should be supplied in the winter months but food stores should not be removed. Generally, pet chipmunks kept at indoor temperatures do not exhibit winter torpor episodes, although there is still a tendency to hoard more food in the autumn. Lifespan and health in pet chipmunks may be better if they are not allowed to follow a torpor episode pattern.

Prairie dogs

Biological data for the black-tailed prairie dog are summarized in Figure 3.4.

Lifespan in captivity (years)	6–10
Adult bodyweight (kg)	0.5–2.-2 (males larger than females, weight increases during autumn/winter)
Body temperature (°C)	35.3–39.0
Heart rate (beats/min)	83–318
Respiratory rate (breaths/min)	40–60
Food consumption	Calorie consumption varies throughout the year; diet should be modified to prevent obesity
Fluid consumption	Varies depending on diet; dry pelleted diet encourages more water intake. Water should always be available
Activity	Diurnal
Dentition	Incisors open-rooted: I 1/1, C 0/0, PM 1/1, M 3/3 x 2 = 20 teeth
Mammary glands	8–12 pairs

3.4 Biological data for the black-tailed prairie dog (*Cynomys ludovicianus*).

Prairie dogs will enter a state of torpor if the ambient temperature drops below 20.5°C for prolonged periods. Prairie dogs have a number of vocalizations, ranging from yips and excited barks when they recognize their owners or other prairie dogs, to chatters, growls, chirps and a loud 'yell' signifying alarm. Different postures are important in their social structure and for communication. A defensive posture (Figure 3.5) includes a stance with the tail raised, often with teeth bared. An excited or nervous prairie dog may sit up on its haunches frequently and flick its tail. A content pet prairie dog may put its head against its owner and cuddle close.

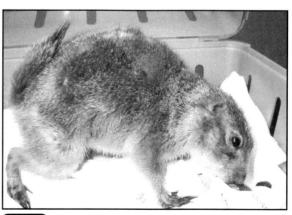

3.5 Prairie dog showing a typical defensive posture.

Prairie dogs are hindgut fermenters and require roughage in their diet. They are coprophagic and caecotrophs should be passed, although they are not fastidious about it. Prairie dogs possess a unique anatomical feature: trigonal anal sacs, ducts that appear as white papillae beside the anus (Figure 3.6).

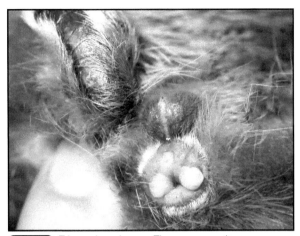

3.6 Trigonal anal sacs. These are a unique anatomical feature of prairie dogs.

Sexing

Chipmunks
Anogenital distance is greater in males than in females and the prepuce is obvious in males. Testes are obvious in mature males: seasonal enlargement begins in January, with the breeding season commencing in March (northern hemisphere); the testes stay enlarged until September.

Prairie dogs
The testicles in the male descend relatively late, and are more prominent during the breeding season (spring in the northern hemisphere). There is no distinct scrotal sac.

Husbandry

Housing

Chipmunks
Chipmunks can be housed singly, in pairs, or in harem groups comprising one male to two or three females. If there is sufficient space, same-sex groups may be compatible, but usually adult males fight.

Chipmunks require larger enclosures than domesticated rodents of a similar size. They are best kept outdoors or at least with some outdoor access. Outdoor housing should be sheltered from direct sun and prevailing weather. Indoor caging should be placed out of direct sunlight and away from human noise and disturbances. Good ventilation and air quality are essential in designing and placing housing.

Caging must be of strong metal mesh, no larger than 2.5 cm spacing, with a metal support structure (Figure 3.7). Minimal cage dimensions for one chipmunk are 1.2 m high and 3.5–4.5 m wide and deep; there is no upper limit on size. Double doors with secure locking mechanisms are recommended.

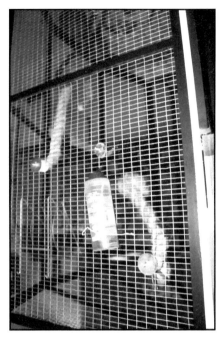

3.7 Typical chipmunk housing. (Courtesy of E. Keeble.)

Outdoor habitats may be similar to walk-in aviaries. Wood or heavy plastic can be used for furnishings, nest boxes and for exercise, although it will need to be replaced frequently as chipmunks gnaw incessantly. Non-toxic hardwood such as apple or other fruit trees, willow or maple branches work well for climbing and nest box construction. PVC pipes and fittings can be used for furnishings. Exercise wheels available for small pet rodents may also be utilized. Water should be provided by sipper tube and bottle and changed daily.

Chipmunks burrow and forage on the ground, so the base of the cage should be solid and impervious to gnawing or digging through. A deep layer (3–6 cm) of substrate such as paper pellets, shredded recycled paper substrate or hardwood chips will allow normal behaviour.

Nest boxes should have a flap door that can be closed when the chipmunk is asleep, securing the animal in the box. Nest material can be paper-based, dry hay or straw that cannot become impacted in the chipmunk's cheek pouches or entangle toenails. The nest box should be cleaned about once a month, except during the winter when the animal should be left undisturbed. Soiled bedding should be removed frequently so that faecal material, moisture and ammonia levels do not build up in the cage. This can be done in the evening or when the chipmunk is secure in the nest box to minimize disturbances. The cage can then be cleaned, and substrate and furnishings replaced with minimal disturbance.

Prairie dogs
Prairie dogs are social animals and live in large communities or 'towns' in the wild. They are housed in large social groupings in zoos but are frequently kept as solitary pets. They require companionship and when solitary may develop behavioural abnormalities, including self-mutilation and aggressiveness towards humans. They are not agile climbers but many try to climb in a household environment.

Caging must be of strong metal not wood (those used for rabbits and guinea pigs are suitable) and allow for a deep substrate of newspaper pellets or hardwood shavings for digging (Figure 3.8a). Nest boxes can be made from terracotta planters covered with cotton t-shirts (Figure 3.8b). Prairie dogs like to have walls around them for sleeping. Food dishes should be attached securely to the cage and water bottles should be fixed from the outside. Other cage furnishings can include aluminium baking dishes filled with hay, cotton rope and cardboard/PVC tubes for tunelling and chewing. The cardboard must be free of glues and varnishes, and the cotton rope should not contain any dyes or plastic tips that could be ingested. Commercial exercise wheels are available, although not all animals will use them. Prairie dogs prefer an environmental temperature range of 20.5–22°C.

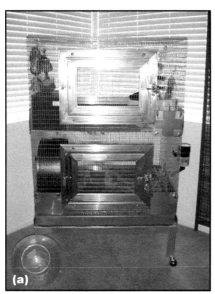

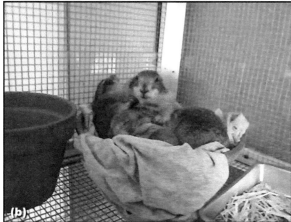

3.8 **(a)** Typical prairie dog housing. **(b)** Nest boxes can be made from terracotta planters and cotton t-shirts. (Courtesy of G. Seaberg.)

Diet

Chipmunks
The captive diet can be based on a general rodent pellet suitable for rats and mice. This can be supplemented with small amounts of vegetables, fruit, nuts and seeds. A seed-based rodent mix is inadequate as it is largely composed of sunflower seeds and peanuts, both of which are high in fat and low in calcium. Occasional treat foods can include mealworms, hard-boiled eggs, cooked meat, dog food, or day-old chicks from a reputable source that do not have an antibiotic or antiparasitic drug level. Pregnant or lactating females require extra protein. Uneaten or hoarded fresh foods need to be removed daily to prevent moulding, except in the winter (see above).

Prairie dogs
In the wild prairie dogs eat grasses, prairie herbs and weeds. In captivity they should be provided with an unlimited source of grass or hay, with small amounts of fresh greens given as treats. Juvenile animals should also be given a pelleted guinea pig or rodent chow and alfalfa hay. Adult animals should be given 1 or 2 rodent chow blocks per week but no alfalfa hay. Prairie dogs should not be fed peanuts, raisins, french fries, cereal, bread or dog biscuits.

Breeding

Chipmunks
Reproductive data are summarized in Figure 3.9. The breeding season in the northern hemisphere is from March to September in response to lengthening light cycle and increasing temperatures. Indoor housing with constant long light days can lead to infertility. Male testicular enlargement starts in January, prior to the onset of the female oestrous cycle in March. Ovulation is spontaneous. Chipmunks in oestrus vocalize repeatedly. Mating usually occurs on Day 2. In captivity, unless continuously housed as a pair, the female should be taken to the male for mating. Females are aggressive to non-paired males when not in oestrus.

Sexual maturity (years)	Approximately 1
Oestrous cycle (days)	Average: 13–14 (range: 11–21)
Oestrus length (days)	3
Post-partum oestrus	No
Gestation (days)	Average: 31–32 (range: 28–35)
Litter size	Average: 3–5 (range: 1–10)
Litters per year	Usually 1; if wean early, may have second smaller litter
Emergence from nest	Approximately Day 35 after birth
Weaning	Approximately 42 days old

3.9 Reproductive data for *Eutamias sibiricus*.

Hand-rearing: The young are altricial (naked, blind) at birth. Any stress, such as noise (television, radio, human disturbances) or proximity of predators (house cats, dogs particularly) may cause the female to abandon her young. Hand-rearing can be successful if the young are over 1 week old. Evaporated

milk diluted 1:2 with water can be fed by syringe every 4 hours during the first week. Baby cereal can then be added and feeding intervals extended to 6–8 hours. Probiotics can be added. Urination/defecation should be stimulated before and after each feeding by rubbing the anogenital area with warm moist cotton wool.

The volume to feed depends on overall health, stomach capacity and individual tolerances:

- Start at 5% of bodyweight and gradually increase, as long as there are no indications of gastrointestinal upset such as gas, bloat or diarrhoea. Example: 0.5 ml per 10 g bodyweight to start
- When bodyweight is >100 g, feed at 7% of bodyweight (7 ml/100 g) until weaning.

Prairie dogs

Reproductive data are summarized in Figure 3.10.

Sexual maturity (years)	2–3
Oestrous cycle	Monoestrus
Oestrus length (days)	5–6 hours on a single day; usually mate with only one male
Post-partum oestrus	No
Gestation (days)	30–37
Litter size	2–10 (average 5)
Litters per year	1
Weaning	6 weeks old
Breeding season	Spring in northern hemisphere; usually colony social situation necessary for successful captive breeding and rearing

3.10 Reproductive data for the black-tailed prairie dog (*Cynomys ludovicianus*).

Preventive healthcare

Digging is a primary activity for prairie dogs, which have long sharp toenails that need frequent trimming and blunting.

Handling and restraint

Chipmunks

Some hand-reared chipmunks will allow minimal handling by cupping in the hands (Figure 3.11a) or by the scruff of the neck, similar to handling a hamster. Most are not tame, however, and may inflict a powerful bite if handled, despite acceptance of food by hand. A lightweight net can be useful to catch the chipmunk; then it can be carefully grasped around the shoulders or scruffed. Chasing the animal should be avoided as it is very stressful. Heavy leather gloves for restraint do not allow the dexterity and sensitivity needed to safely restrain the chipmunk (Figure 3.11b). Double layers of latex gloves or surgical orthopaedic gloves will afford

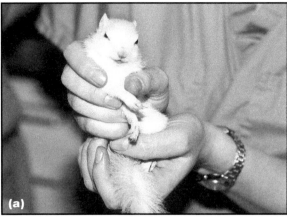

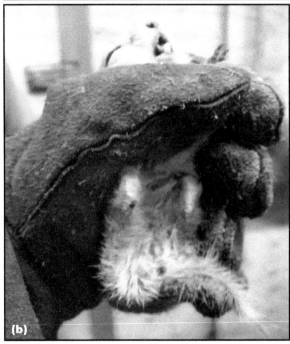

3.11 **(a)** Some hand-reared chipmunks will allow minimal handling by cupping in the hands. (Courtesy of A. Meredith.) **(b)** Most chipmunks resent handling. Leather gloves may be worn; however, they are cumbersome and do not always allow the dexterity and sensitivity needed to safely restrain chipmunks. (Courtesy of E. Keeble.)

some protection. The chipmunk should not be grasped by the tail as degloving injuries can occur similar to those in gerbils and degus (see Chapters 1 and 2).

For clinical examination, mild sedation with midazolam at 0.25–0.3 mg/kg i.m. is recommended. Full anaesthesia may be necessary for blood sampling or other diagnostic tests.

Prairie dogs

Most pet prairie dogs are used to some amount of handling (method should be ascertained from the owner), although they are likely to roll quickly and bite unfamiliar people; animals that have a strong bond with their owners or social group are likely to regard any other human as an intruder or competition. They may also squirt musk from the anal sacs. In addition, they have long, sharp nails designed for digging that can cause significant scratches.

To handle a prairie dog, a small towel can be placed over the head and, taking care to control the head to prevent biting, it can then be lifted in a similar manner to guinea pigs (see Chapter 2). Many prairie dogs have to be handled using gloves. Prairie dogs can also be wrapped in a towel 'burrito' (Figure 3.12) for examination or medication administration. Care must be taken to prevent inhibition of respiration or exacerbate stress during restraint.

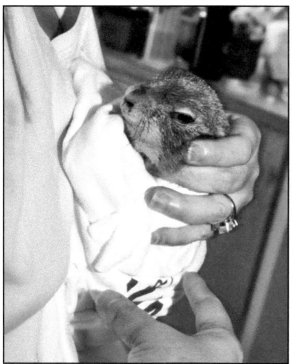

3.12 Restraint of a prairie dog using a t-shirt. The prairie dog can be wrapped in the t-shirt and held with the hindquarters supported. This position is excellent for syringe feeding and oral dosing of medication. (Courtesy of G. Seaberg.)

For clinical examination, mild sedation with midazolam at 0.5 mg/kg i.m. may be required. Full examination requires sedation or general anaesthesia (see below). A thorough check for ectoparasites (e.g. fleas and ticks) should be performed, particularly if the prairie dog is housed outdoors.

Diagnostic approach

Chipmunks

- If possible, the animal should first be observed in its home cage to assess activity level, locomotion, balance, behaviour and content of the latrine area. Confinement of the awake chipmunk in a clear plastic container will afford assessment of body condition, respiratory pattern or injury.
- General signs of illness, pain or distress in the chipmunk are similar to those seen in other rodents (see Chapter 1). Low body temperature must be interpreted with consideration of time of year and housing conditions.

- Full examination requires sedation or full anaesthesia (see below).
- Under anaesthesia, blood may be obtained from the jugular or saphenous vein. A safe volume to withdraw depends on the bodyweight and condition of the chipmunk, but 0.1–0.2 ml can usually be withdrawn from most adults.
- Serological testing for the presence of rodent pathogens is not usually done as the tests have not been validated for this species. However, many diagnostic laboratories may be able to screen wild-caught pet chipmunks for rodent-borne zoonotic infections such as lymphocytic choriomeningitis virus (LCMV), *Salmonella* spp., *Yersinia pestis* (plague), *Borrelia burgdorferi* (Lyme disease) and rabies (see Chapter 1).

Other diagnostic sampling techniques and imaging are the same as for similarly sized rats or hamsters (see Chapter 1).

Prairie dogs

- Normal stools are similar to those of a guinea pig, which are dry and oval in shape.
- Urine is normally alkaline (pH 8–9) and clear yellow.
- Radiographic positioning is essentially the same as that used for the guinea pig (see Chapter 2). Intraoral radiographs are useful to examine the roots of teeth and assess possible odontoma or osteomyelitis.
- Blood samples may be taken from the lateral or medial saphenous, cephalic or jugular vein, or the cranial vena cava (see Figure 3.19). Collection from the latter two sites needs to be performed under anaesthesia. Most adult prairie dogs weighing >300 g can safely have 0.25–0.5 ml of blood withdrawn; however, if the animal is ill or dehydrated, the lower value would be most appropriate. In severely ill or stressed prairie dogs, and for emergencies when obtaining sufficient volumes from a vein proves difficult, enough blood to fill several microhaematocrit tubes for doing a packed cell volume (PCV), slides for an estimated total and differential white blood cell count, and serum for determining total protein, glucose and blood urea nitrogen levels can be obtained from a clipped toenail. The toenail should be cleansed with chlorhexidine scrub and dried prior to clipping, and the bleeding stopped with a haemostatic powder upon completion. Whilst not ideal, the clinician may gain immediate valuable information with little stress to the animal.

Common conditions

Chipmunks
Common diseases of chipmunks are listed in Figure 3.13. Many of the disease conditions present in other rodents are found in captive chipmunks. Treatment regimens for chipmunks are based on successful treatments used in other rodents.

Disease	Cause	Clinical signs	Diagnostics	Treatment
Anorexia	Stress; overcrowding (subordinate animal); torpor; any systemic illness	Emaciation; poor coat condition; no faecal output; lethargy; porphyrin staining around the eyes	CBC; biochemistry; radiography/ultrasonography	Correct husbandry/social situation. Treat systemic illness. Supportive care: fluid therapy, gavage feed, vitamin B complex for appetite stimulation
Bacterial cystitis/urethritis	Ascending infections; concurrent urogenital infections; dehydration; calculi	Haematuria; dysuria (may vocalize); penile swelling/protrusion; anorexia	Urinalysis; culture; radiography/ultrasonography to rule out concurrent uroliths	Analgesia. Antibiosis. Anti-inflammatories. Be sure cage latrine area is kept clean
Bacterial enteritis	*Salmonella;* wild rodents may be source; faecal accumulation in habitat	Diarrhoea; dehydration; weight loss; anorexia; stained/wet perineum; death	Faecal culture	Appropriate antibiosis. Fluid therapy. Supportive care. Euthanasia if zoonosis (e.g. *Salmonella*)
Cage paralysis	Vitamin E deficiency (general dietary deficiencies including calcium may contribute)	Weakness; paresis; paralysis; weight loss and muscle atrophy if untreated	Review diet; elevated creatine phosphokinase (CPK)/cholesterol; radiography to rule out fractures	Dietary supplementation with Vitamin E. Other diet corrections. NSAIDs. Supportive care. Keep in smaller habitat until strength returns
Cataracts	Cause unknown; reported in older chipmunks, especially males	Partial/complete blindness; usually bilateral	Ocular examination	Surgical excision possible but captive chipmunks appear to 'learn' their environment and do not require treatment
Comatose, unresponsive	Torpor during winter or cold weather; end stage of any disease	Low body temperature/heart rate/respiratory rate; stays curled up; does not respond to touch	History and physical examination	Warm slowly with external heating. Subcutaneous fluids if torpor
Dental disease (including overgrowth, fracture, tooth root/gumline abscess)	Insufficient wear (usually diet-related); trauma; infection	Overgrown incisors; anorexia; salivation; facial soft tissue penetration; swelling; may cause rhinitis; may paw at mouth frequently	Oral examination; radiography	Burr teeth under sedation/anaesthesia (see Chapter 2). If abscess: drain, antibiosis. If non-viable cheek teeth: remove. Correct diet to include items for tooth wear: nuts in shell, dog biscuits, branches of hardwood
Dermatitis	Bacterial (may start with small bite wounds); fungal (particularly if wet environment, stressed animal); may be secondary to ectoparasites	Areas of scabbing, alopecia, erythema; may be pruritic	Skin scraping; fungal/bacterial culture	Antibiosis if bacterial. Antifungal medication if fungal. NSAIDs. Eleviate stress. Correct husbandry (see also Chapters 1 and 2)
Ectoparasites	Fleas; ticks; mange mites (may be indistinguishable from bacterial or fungal dermatitis without diagnostics)	Areas of alopecia, erythema ± pruritus; parasites may be visible	Visual examination under magnification; skin scrapings; hair plucks	Appropriate topical/systemic preparation as used in guinea pigs for similar ectoparasites (see Chapters 1 and 2). Correct husbandry: clean out caging, furnishings, substrates. Treat environment surrounding caging if appropriate. Remove ticks, may submit to laboratory as can be a vector for zoonotic diseases such as borreliosis (Lyme disease)
Fractures (limbs/spine/tail)	Usually history of fall, fight or mishandling	Lameness; paresis; paralysis; may chew affected area if there is pain	History; physical examination; radiography	Small cage confinement. Analgesia. NSAIDs. Amputate if severe limb fracture as splints/bandages not well tolerated. Euthanasia if spinal fracture with paralysis
Hypocalcaemia	Poor diet both sexes; may follow parturition, particularly if large litter; during lactation	Posterior paresis/paralysis; incoordination; tremors; collapse; semi-conscious state	Review diet/reproductive status; serum chemistry for calcium level	0.5 ml of 10% calcium gluconate s.c. (may dilute in 2–3 ml warm lactated Ringers solution). Calcium supplementation short-term. Diet correction to include calcium-rich foods
Hypothermia	Winter torpor; result of malnutrition; poor husbandry; systemic illness; shock following injury	Subnormal body temperature; slow to rouse; may stay curled up	Review diet/husbandry; history; physical examination; other diagnostic testing as appropriate	Warm slowly with external heating. Subcutaneous fluids. Correct underlying problems

3.13 Common diseases of chipmunks. (continues) ▶

Disease	Cause	Clinical signs	Diagnostics	Treatment
Mammary tumours	Usually benign fibroadenomas	Mammary mass ± ulceration	Clinical signs; FNA; biopsy; radiography to check metastasis	Surgical removal. Ovariohysterectomy/ castration and hormonal suppression (leuprolide acetate depot 30 day) may slow recurrence
Metritis/pyometra	Metritis: usually due to retained fetus; may progress to peritonitis/ toxaemia Pyometra: as for other species	Vaginal discharge; abdominal enlargement; pain; anorexia; unthriftiness; if lactating, may cease	Clinical signs; history; bacterial culture of discharge; abdominal ultrasonography/ radiography	Antibiosis. Supportive care. Ovariohysterectomy
Neurological signs	Hypocalcaemia; waking from torpor; general malnutrition with weakness; trauma (particularly skull); toxicosis (environmental); encephalitis (bacterial/viral)	Incoordination; paresis; paralysis; seizures; tremors; anisocoria; hypersalivation	Review history/diet/ husbandry; full work-up including blood; radiography; serology	Trauma: assess feasibility of recovery. Supportive care, NSAIDs, analgesics and antibiosis as determined by aetiology
Pneumonia	Predisposing stressors include overcrowding, poor ventilation, damp conditions, ammonia build-up from latrine area; assumed bacterial, although can contract human influenza viruses	Dyspnoea; tachypnoea; anorexia; unkempt coat; often fatal	Clinical signs; radiography; tracheal wash cytology and culture	Anti-anxiety relaxant such as midazolam. NSAIDs. Antibiosis. Bronchodilators. Consider nebulization. Supportive care: oxygen, heated environment, fluids, assisted feeding, rest and quiet (see also Chapters 1 and 2)
Rhinitis/upper respiratory infection	May occur in association with incisor overgrowth/ chronic suppurative periodontal disease; dusty or poorly ventilated environment (irritation)	Nasal discharge; upper respiratory tract stridor; epistaxis; face rubbing; conjunctivitis; may see matting of forearms from grooming	Clinical signs; oral examination; ocular examination; radiography of skull; culture and sensitivity	Antibiosis. Analgesia. NSAIDs. Consider nebulization. Supportive care: oxygen, heated environment, fluids, assisted feeding, rest and quiet. Correct dental disease if possible
Trauma (lacerations, bite wounds)	Fight wounds from cagemates (improper social combinations); predator attacks	Wounds; scabs; alopecia; pain; lameness; guarding a body area	Review social situation/ husbandry; clinical signs; culture and sensitivity	Antibiosis. Surgical correction if wounds severe. Analgesia. NSAIDs. Correct social situation/husbandry
Tumours (masses anywhere on body)	Ageing may be a factor	Lumps; bumps; lameness and pain (if bone tumour); may ulcerate on surface; self-mutilation if painful	Clinical signs; palpation; radiography; ultrasonography; FNA; biopsy	Surgical removal if possible. Analgesia. Antibiosis if infected surface. Supportive palliative care. Euthanasia if quality of life severely compromised.

3.13 (continued) Common diseases of chipmunks.

Zoonotic infections
Wild-caught chipmunks may be asymptomatic hosts for a number of infections, including:

- LCMV
- *Salmonella* spp.
- *Yersinia pestis* (plague)
- *Borrelia burgdorferi* (Lyme disease)
- Rabies
- *Cryptosporidium parvum*
- *Eimeria* spp.
- Sarcoptiform mites
- Dermatophytosis.

A chipmunk brought in as a rescued animal must be considered a potential vector for zoonotic disease, and appropriate precautions taken while handling the animal at the veterinary clinic.

Behavioural problems
Chipmunks are extremely susceptible to stress and may remain quiescent for up to a day following a stressful event. Continued stress may result in hyperactivity and stereotypical behaviours, such as circling or looping around the cage. Stressors can include: catching; handling; small caging; overcrowding; insufficient nest boxes; proximity of predators (other pets, dogs, cats); electronic devices emitting electromagnetic and/or ultrasonic radiation; and transportation. Stress may exacerbate aggression from incompatible cagemates, and aggression adds to the stress of the subordinate animals. Aggression may increase in the autumn when food-hoarding increases.

Prairie dogs
Common diseases of prairie dogs are listed in Figure 3.14.

Disease	Cause	Clinical signs	Diagnostics	Treatment
Dental disease	Fractures: falls; chewing inappropriate hard objects; trauma Abscesses: may be due to improper wear; punctures from food; foreign objects Neoplasia (odontomas): possible repeated mouth trauma	Fractured teeth; malocclusion; tooth root abscesses; oral swellings; neoplasia	Oral examination under sedation/anaesthesia; skull radiography; endoscopy of nasal cavity	Remove abscessed teeth. Burr malocclusive teeth. Surgical excision of neoplastic tissue. Correct diet for proper tooth wear. Appropriate antimicrobials, NSAIDs, analgesics for oral lesions as with guinea pigs (see Chapter 2)
Dyspnoea (± sinusitis)/rhinitis	*Pasteurella multocida*; pulmonary mites	Respiratory rales; open-mouth breathing; sneezing; coughing; nasal discharge	Culture and sensitivity; cytology of tracheal/sinus wash; radiography; CBC; biochemistry	Appropriate antibiotics (fluoroquinolones first choice). Ivermectin for mites. Supportive care: nebulization, bronchodilators, NSAIDs
Neurological signs	*Baylisascaris* spp. (animals wild-caught/housed outdoors with exposure to skunks/raccoons, North America); heavy metal toxicosis (lead, zinc); inner ear infection; brain abscess; encephalitis (bacterial/viral/parasitic)	Ataxia; torticollis; stumbling; seizures; circling; abnormal vocalizations; changes in behaviour from normal personality; anorexia	*Baylisascaris*: CT, MRI, necropsy Heavy metals: history of chewed objects, blood lead/zinc levels, metal particulates in gastrointestinal tract on radiography CBC; biochemistry; ear/oral examination	There is no treatment for *Baylisascaris* lesions. Infections: antibiotics, NSAIDs, supportive care. Heavy metal toxicity: chelation therapy (CaEDTA or D-penicillamine). Remove dangerous toys/objects
Obesity	Overfeeding/improper foods; initiation of winter dormancy; lack of exercise	Fatty liver; lethargy; obesity	Review diet/husbandry/ambient temperature/light cycle; CBC; biochemistry; radiography; ultrasonography of liver	Correct diet (hay-based). Decrease total quantity of food intake. Correct light cycle/temperature. Exercise. If liver disease, supportive care as appropriate. To rouse from dormant condition: warm subcutaneous fluids, heated environment
Open-mouth breathing	Oral/maxillary odontoma or other neoplasia; nasolacrimal duct infection/blockage from tooth root abscess; sinus infection; severe respiratory tract infection	Dyspnoea; nasal/ocular discharge	Radiography; ophthalmic examination including nasolacrimal flush; culture and sensitivity of exudates; thorough oral examination; nasal endoscopy	Surgical excision of tumour if possible. Appropriate antibiotics, NSAIDs, analgesics as needed. Treatment as for abscesses (see above)
Pododermatitis	Poor husbandry; dirty/wet bedding; obesity; inactivity	Lameness; bedding stuck to bottom of feet; swellings/scabs on plantar foot surfaces	Radiography to assess bone/joint involvement; culture and sensitivity of edges of lesions	Treat as in guinea pigs (see Chapter 2): remove exudates, debride. Appropriate antimicrobials. Can try soft bandaging but likely to remove quickly and eat the bandage material. Soft flooring. NSAIDs. Correct sanitation/husbandry
Self-injurious behaviour	Solitary animal; improper husbandry; lack of social stimulation; boredom; stereotypical behaviour; wounds may become secondarily infected, painful, pruritic	Self-inflicted wounds; self-amputation	Assess husbandry; radiography if severe/bone involved; culture and sensitivity of infected wounds	Provide companionship, social stimulation, enriched environment (large/ability to dig/tunnels). Wound treatment as in rabbits/guinea pigs. Benzodiazepines may be needed to control self-injurious behaviour
Trauma/fractures/torn nails	Falls; injuries from other pets; nails caught in home furnishings/carpets	Lameness; bleeding from toenails; reluctance to move	Radiography for fractures	Trim nails. Repair fractures with guidelines used for guinea pigs (see Chapter 2)

3.14 Common diseases of prairie dogs.

Zoonotic infections
Wild-caught prairie dogs may carry potentially zoonotic infections such as *Yersinia pestis* or *Francisella tularensis*.

Obesity and dormancy
Captive prairie dogs frequently present with obesity due to overfeeding and lack of exercise. They may also be presented in a torpid or dormant state if the temperature in the home has dropped well below 20.5°C for several days, coupled with decreasing daylength. The dormant prairie dog may have elevated blood urea nitrogen levels, be slightly dehydrated and slightly hypothermic, but will rouse with warming and administration of warmed subcutaneous fluids.

Dental disease

Dental disease is common and includes fractured teeth (Figure 3.15), root abscesses and malocclusions associated with tooth loss or overgrowth. A thorough dental examination with radiographs must be performed under anaesthesia. Geriatric prairie dogs (>6 years of age) may present with molars worn down to the gum line, often with just the necrotic roots visible. Radiographs may disclose root absorption or bone lysis due to abscess; such wear is often coupled with dental pain, leading to anorexia. Removal of the roots can be done as per other rodents.

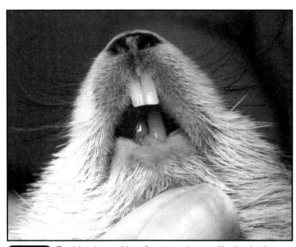

3.15 Prairie dog with a fractured mandibular incisor tooth. These injuries are commonly seen in pet animals.

Abscesses of the maxillary teeth may extend into the nasal cavities and sinuses, resulting in upper respiratory tract disease. Dental neoplasia (odontoma) has been associated with chronic dental disease or mouth trauma from chewing on inappropriate objects such as cage bars (Figure 3.16). With odontoma, the affected teeth must be removed and, if possible, a permanent opening into the nasal bones caudal to the tumour mass made to facilitate respiration. If possible, sections of the tumour may be resected, although it is often impossible to totally remove it. The condition is progressive. Symptomatic treatment includes non-steroidal anti-inflammatory drugs (NSAIDs), antibiotics and assisted feeding.

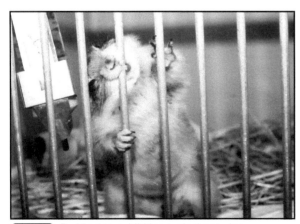

3.16 Prairie dog exhibiting typical gnawing behaviour.

Respiratory disease

Prairie dogs presented with open-mouthed breathing or dyspnoea must first be screened for odontoma blocking the nasal passages. Rhinitis can also be caused by maxillary teeth abscesses, neoplasia other than odontoma, pulmonary mites and bacterial infections. Wild-caught prairie dogs may carry pulmonary mites (*Pneumocoptes penrosei*); these can be diagnosed on cytology of a tracheal wash sample showing mites or eggs. Treatment is with ivermectin at 0.4 mg/kg s.c. q14d for three or four treatments.

Pasteurellosis

Pasteurella multocida infection has been associated with pneumonia, rhinitis and sinusitis. Bacterial culture and antibacterial sensitivity testing can be performed on nasal samples. Material for culturing can be obtained by instilling a few drops of sterile, non-bacteriostatic saline into the nasal cavity as a flush, and collecting the material sneezed or dripped out. Usually this is done under mild sedation and the prairie dog is briefly held with the head down just after the saline is instilled for collection. The prairie dog is then placed sternally, with the chest elevated, and given oxygen by facemask. It may continue to sneeze for a few minutes after the event. Material can be collected for cytology, staining and culture. The microbiology laboratory should be familiar with culturing *Pasteurella*.

Treatment of bacterial respiratory disease should be based on antibiotic sensitivity testing and follow guidelines for antibiotic choice used for treatments in guinea pigs and rabbits. Nebulization, bronchodilators such as aminophylline (10 mg/kg s.c. q12h), and NSAIDs such as meloxicam (0.2 mg/kg orally or s.c. q24h) can decrease the clinical signs of rhinitis, sinusitis and/or pneumonia, and make the prairie dog more comfortable. The author has also used ophthalmic NSAID drops placed in the eyes to reach nasal tissue and decrease inflammation, as in the rabbit: flurbiprofen ophthalmic drops, 0.03% solution, at one drop to each eye q12h.

Neurological disease

Neurological signs, including ataxia, torticollis, stumbling and seizures, have been reported in pet prairie dogs. *Baylisascaris* spp. has been implicated, particularly if the animal was wild-caught or housed outdoors and exposed to skunks or raccoons. This parasite is absent from the UK. Diagnosis may be aided by computed tomography (CT) or magnetic resonance imaging (MRI) for inflammatory lesions in the brain, but the definitive diagnosis is made at necropsy. There is no treatment.

Skin disease

Pododermatitis similar to that found in guinea pigs (see Chapter 2) has been seen. It is usually the result of poor husbandry, i.e. dirty wet bedding combined with obesity and inactivity. Treatment may be difficult as prairie dogs do not tolerate bandages well. Soft bedding and sanitation, along with systemic antibiotics and NSAIDs may be effective.

Trauma

Vertebral and long bone fractures (Figure 3.17), and fractured incisors are frequently seen due to trauma from falling in the home environment. Spinal or head trauma can also occur if a prairie dog falls or is dropped. Self-inflicted wounds including amputation and subsequent osteomyelitis, may be seen in solitary prairie dogs.

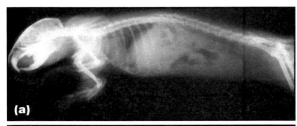

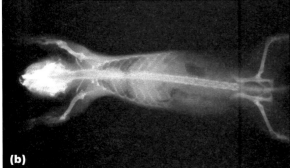

3.17 **(a)** Lateral and **(b)** dorsoventral radiographs of a prairie dog showing bilateral fractures of the radius and ulna sustained from a fall.

Toxicosis

Heavy metal toxicosis may present with vague neurological or gastrointestinal signs. Both zinc and lead toxicosis have been reported, usually due to chewing on cages or other household objects. Metal densities may or may not be present in the gastrointestinal tract on radiography. Generally, blood lead levels >10 µg/dl are considered diagnostic for lead toxicosis. Chelation is with edetate calcium disodium at 30 mg/kg s.c. q12h for 3–5 days or D-penicillamine at 30–55 mg/kg orally q12h for 1–2 weeks.

Supportive care

Chipmunks

An ill, hypothermic chipmunk needs to be slowly warmed and given warmed fluids to encourage revival from the torporous state. Fluids may be injected subcutaneously or intraperitoneally. If severe dehydration is present, intravenous or intraosseous administration of colloids and crystalloid fluids may be necessary. Supportive care and fluid therapy are similar to that for rats, hamsters and gerbils of a similar weight (see Chapter 1). Volumes for fluid and nutritional therapy are listed in Figure 3.18.

Prairie dogs

Injection sites and volumes are listed in Figure 3.19. Fluid therapy follows guidelines for guinea pigs (see Chapter 2).

Route	Volume	Fluid type and comments
Oral (gavage, syringe feeding)	2–5 ml per animal q6–8h and as needed, depending on hydration status	Oral rehydration solutions. Herbivore critical care formula (per bodyweight); human babyfood cereals; vegetable stews
Subcutaneous	Daily requirements 75–100 ml/kg divided over several sites (maximum of 3–8 ml per site) Example: If bodyweight is 300 g, then 30 ml/day fluid required; usually 15 ml q12h in a couple of sites (more sites for antibiotic distribution)	Isotonic crystalloids
Intramuscular (quadriceps)	Maximum of 0.1 ml	Medications suitable for intramuscular injection
Intraosseous (femur, tibia)	50–70 ml/kg bolus for shock Daily requirements 75–100 ml/kg	Crystalloids; colloids
Intraperitoneal	Maximum of 5–10 ml	Crystalloids; colloids. Contraindicated in presence of abdominal mass effect or fluid pressure
Intravenous (saphenous, jugular)	Up to 75–100 ml/kg/day (slow i.v. or bolus)	Medications suitable for intravenous administration (bolus form injection). Crystalloids, colloids (catheter for drip)

3.18 Fluid therapy, assisted feeding and medication routes in chipmunks.

Route	Site	Volume
Oral	Insert tip of syringe behind incisors into the diastema; placement of a gavage/stomach tube requires sedation to pass the tube through the palatial ostium	Estimate size of stomach based on bodyweight (approximately 10 ml per 150–200 g bodyweight)
Subcutaneous	Supra/intrascapular; dorsal back	10–15 ml/site
Intramuscular	Anterior thigh	0.5 ml
Intraperitoneal (do not administer if abdominal disease present)		5–10 ml
Intraosseous	Femur; tibia	1–2 ml bolus or slow infusion if catheter placed
Intravenous	Saphenous; cephalic	3–10 ml slow bolus
Venepuncture	Cranial vena cava (under anaesthesia)	0.3–0.5 ml/kg
	Saphenous; cephalic	0.1–0.2 ml

3.19 Fluid therapy, medication routes and venepuncture sites in prairie dogs.

Assisted feeding

Prairie dogs cannot easily be gavage-fed, due to the presence of the palatial ostium, similar to that in the guinea pig. If the prairie dog will not accept food through a syringe orally (Figure 3.20), then gavage feeding through a softened (in a cup of hot water) red rubber catheter, size 12 or 14 French or a similar gauge long feeding needle can be used. The prairie dog will need mild sedation (midazolam at 0.5 mg/kg i.m.) in order to pass the gavage tube. A herbivore formulation such as Critical Care or Critical Care Fine Grind (Oxbow Pet Products, Murdoch, NE, USA) or vegetable baby food can be used.

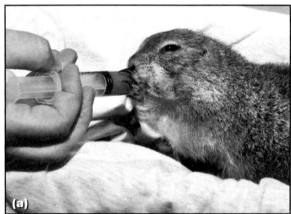

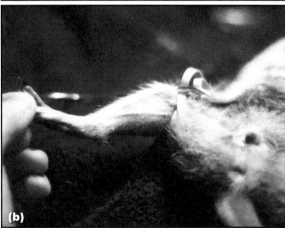

3.20 **(a)** Syringe feeding a prairie dog. (Courtesy of G. Seaberg.) **(b)** Preparation of saphenous vein for venepuncture in a prairie dog.

The tube should be pre-measured and the tip lubricated with a small amount of lubricating jelly. An oral speculum with a hole in the middle to pass a catheter through can be made from a 3 ml syringe casing. It is placed in the mouth behind the incisors in the diastema space and the pre-measured tube passed into the stomach. Gavage volume can be between 5 and 10 ml up to three times daily to maintain weight or until the prairie dog is eating on its own.

An alternative if prolonged assisted feeding is needed would be to place a nasogastric tube; however, the author has found that a 5 French tube is the maximum size for passage and this has been inadequate to deliver enough food for weight maintenance and fibre for digestive tract function.

Anaesthesia and analgesia

Chipmunks

Anaesthesia

Inhalational anaesthetic agents, such as isoflurane or sevoflurane, can be delivered without handling the chipmunk if it is confined in a container or in a large canine facemask. Administration of a sedative (e.g. midazolam at 0.25–0.3 mg/kg i.m.) prior to the administration of the anaesthetic gas decreases the anxiety produced during induction, but it does require handling of the chipmunk first. Doses of anaesthetic and analgesic agents used in rats and mice appear to be effective (see Chapter 1). Coaxial scavenging systems designed for laboratory rodents are clinically useful in this and other small rodent species. Once the chipmunk is anaesthetized in the chamber it can be removed, and anaesthesia maintained with a small facemask. It may be helpful to swab out the oral cavity and cheek areas to prevent aspiration of retained food.

Analgesia

The principles of pre-emptive analgesia as used in rats can be extrapolated to chipmunks. Buprenorphine at 0.02–0.1 mg/kg s.c. q6–12h has been used effectively for analgesia.

Prairie dogs

Anaesthesia

Pre-anaesthetic drugs used by the author for prairie dogs include glycopyrrolate at 0.02 mg/kg s.c., midazolam at 0.5 mg/kg i.m., and either butorphanol at 0.3–0.4 mg/kg i.m. or buprenorphine at 0.03–0.05 mg/kg i.m. Further induction can be achieved via masked delivery of isoflurane, or intravenous delivery of etomidate at a rate of 1 mg/kg. Prairie dogs can be intubated with a 2.0 or 2.5 mm uncuffed endotracheal tube, using a 'blind' technique or with the aid of a laryngoscope or endoscope.

For dental surgery, when the presence of an endotracheal tube would make oral access difficult, the author uses ketamine at a rate of 5–10 mg/kg along with midazolam at 0.5–1.0 mg/kg i.m. The ketamine dosage can be boosted at half the original dose after 20–30 minutes as needed. Local anaesthetic combinations of lidocaine (2%) plus bupivacaine (5%) can be used in a 50:50 ratio, diluted with an equal volume of sterile saline to infiltrate surgical sites or for dental blocks. Volume is based on bodyweight and area to be blocked, and should not exceed 1–3 mg/kg. For most procedures (e.g. single tooth blocks), the author uses 0.05 ml of lidocaine and 0.05 ml of bupivacaine with 0.1 ml sterile water.

The patient should be monitored throughout surgery, with particular attention paid to body temperature, heart rate and respiration. With a balanced anaesthesia approach, it is possible to maintain the animal at heart and respiratory rates, oxygenation and body temperature similar to that when it is awake. Blood pressure is difficult to measure in the prairie dog due to the size of the forelimbs *versus* the smallest cuffs available.

Analgesia

Analgesics used in prairie dogs are similar to those used in other rodents. The clinician should be aware that there is a possibility of gastrointestinal motility inhibition with prolonged use of opiates. Butorphanol seems effective at a rate of 0.2–0.5 mg/kg s.c. q2–6h, while buprenorphine at a rate of 0.03–0.05 mg/kg s.c. appears to provide analgesia for 8–12 hours. These drugs can be used in addition to an NSAID such as meloxicam (0.1–0.2 mg/kg s.c. or orally q24h). As with other animals, the clinician should address the type of pain relief required and modify dosages and combinations as needed. A prairie dog experiencing pain will sit hunched or be unresponsive to the usual social stimulation. It may also refuse to eat, or sleep with its nose and head curled under the body. It may also scream when touched. Many relaxed, healthy prairie dogs will sleep on their backs or sides and not be tightly curled.

Common surgical procedures

Chipmunks

Procedures for castration and ovariohysterectomy are similar to those in rats (see Chapter 1); closed castration is preferable, to prevent abdominal herniation. Wound repair, amputations and fracture repair are problematic, as the chipmunk may have already chewed the affected area: antibiotic therapy is required, as well as analgesia, in addition to the repair of the traumatic condition.

Intraoperative monitoring is as for other small rodents and includes electrocardiography (ECG), pulse oximetry, capnography and thermography. Monitors need to accommodate high heart rates and small body size. Several brands developed for laboratory rodent monitoring are available. Heat should be provided to maintain body temperature. As chipmunks will chew exposed sutures, all suture materials should be buried.

Prairie dogs

Ovariohysterectomy and castration are common procedures. It is preferable to perform these types of surgery in the first year of life as there is less body fat. Postoperative analgesia is necessary to prevent the prairie dog from chewing on and picking at the incision site.

Castration

Castration is easier in spring or early summer as the testicles are 'descended'. The testicles are lateral to the penis. The spermatic cord and vessels are best clamped and ligated using a closed technique because of the open inguinal rings. A local anaesthetic block consisting of 0.05 ml lidocaine (2%), 0.05 ml bupivacaine (5%) and 0.1 ml sterile water can be injected into each testicle prior to the incision. This allows for a lower systemic anaesthetic dosage to be used.

1. Make a separate skin incision over each testicle. If the testicles have not descended, perform a caudal coeliotomy.
2. The spermatic cords are located between the colon and bladder in a location analogous to the uterus of the female.
3. Retract the spermatic cord and exteriorize the testicle.
4. Ligate and transect the vas deferens and vessels.
5. Use intradermal or subcuticular sutures to close incisions.

Drug formulary

As there are no published formularies for chipmunks, the author refers to dosages used in rats (see Chapter 1). Therapeutic agents that seem to be efficacious and non-toxic in prairie dogs are those used for guinea pigs or chinchillas (see Chapter 2).

References and further reading

Avashia SB, Petersen JM, Lindley CM, *et al.* (2004) First reported prairie dog-to-human tularemia transmission: Texas, 2002. *Emerging Infectious Diseases* **10**, 483–486

CDC, Wilson P, Grahn B, *et al.* (2003) Multistate outbreak of monkeypox: Illinois, Indiana and Wisconsin, 2003. *Morbidity and Mortality Weekly Report* **52**: 537–540

Funk RS (2004) Medical management of prairie dogs. In: *Ferrets, Rabbits and Rodents: Clinical Medicine and Surgery, 2nd edn,* ed. KE Quesenberry and JW Carpenter, pp. 266–273. Saunders/Elsevier, St Louis

Johnson-Delaney CA (1997) Special rodents: prairie dogs. In: *Exotic Companion Medicine Handbook for Veterinarians,* ed. CA Johnson-Delaney, pp. 18–25. Wingers Publishing/ZEN Publications, Florida

Johnson-Delaney CA (2006) Common procedures in hedgehogs, prairie dogs, exotic rodents, and companion marsupials. *Veterinary Clinics of North America: Exotic Animal Practice* **9**, 415–435

Jones DL and Wang LCH (1976) Metabolic and cardiovascular adaptations in the western chipmunks, genus *Eutamias. Journal of Comparative Physiology B: Biochemical, Systemic and Environmental Physiology* **105**, 219–231

Langohr IM, Stevenson GW, Thacker HL and Regnery RL (2004) Extensive lesions of monkeypox in a prairie dog (*Cynomys* sp.). *Veterinary Pathology* **41**, 702–707

Lightfoot TL (2000) Therapeutics of African pygmy hedgehogs and prairie dogs. *Veterinary Clinics of North America: Exotic Animal Practice* **3**, 155–172

Mannelli A, Kitron U, Jones CJ, *et al.* (1993) Role of the eastern chipmunk as a host for immature *Ixodes dammini* in northwestern Illinois. *Journal of Medical Entomology* **30**, 87–93

Morera N (2004) Osteosarcoma in a Siberian chipmunk. *Exotic DVM* **6**(1), 11–12

Nowak RM (1991) Order Rodentia: Sciuridae. In: *Walker's Mammals of the World, 5th edn, Vol. I,* pp. 561–642. Johns Hopkins University Press, Baltimore

Perz JF and Le Blancq SM (2001) *Cryptosporidium parvum* infection involving novel genotypes in wildlife from lower New York State. *Applied Environmental Microbiology* **67**(3), 1154–1162

Seville RS and Patrick MJ (2001) *Eimeria* spp. from the eastern chipmunk (*Tamias striatus*) in Pennsylvania with a description of one new species. *Journal of Parasitology* **87**, 165–168

Slacherjt T, Ktron UD, Jones CJ, *et al.* (1997) Role of the eastern chipmunk (*Tamias striatus)* in the epizootiology of Lyme borrelliosis in northwestern Illinois, USA. *Journal of Wildlife Diseases* **33**, 40–46

Vourc'h G, Marmet J, Chassagne M, *et al.* (2007) *Borrelia burgdorferi* Sensu Lato in Siberian chipmunks (*Tamias sibiricus*) introduced in suburban forests in France. *Vector-borne and Zoonotic Diseases* **7**, 637–642

Wagner RA, Garman RH and Collins BM (1999) Diagnosing odontomas in prairie dogs. *Exotic DVM* **1**, 7–10

4

Rabbits

Michelle Campbell-Ward and Anna Meredith

Introduction

The species *Oryctolagus cuniculus* includes all breeds of domestic rabbit as well as the European wild rabbit from which the domesticated type originated. *O. cuniculus* is a member of the mammalian order Lagomorpha, which includes pikas, hares, cottontails and other species of wild rabbit. Over the centuries, the rabbit has been used for food, sport and clothing, as a scientific model, and as a hobby (the rabbit 'fancy'). In the UK, the keeping of rabbits as pets developed in Victorian times and since then their popularity has grown enormously. Rabbits are now well established as the UK's third most popular mammalian pet (Figure 4.1). Their popularity as a companion species in other countries has shown a similar trend in recent times.

As is the case with other domestic animals, the pet rabbit population is constantly evolving by selective breeding and mutation. A wide variety of different breeds and coat colours exist, although many pet rabbits are cross-breeds and owners are often unaware of their pet's breed lineage.

Advantages and disadvantages

Advantages of rabbits as pets include:

- Generally docile and responsive
- Good house pets
- Can be house-trained to use litter tray
- Relatively long-lived (up to 10 or more years).

Disadvantages of rabbits as pets include:

- Can become aggressive or nervous and difficult to handle
- Can be destructive in the house
- Can exhibit territorial marking (if not neutered)
- Can be easily injured by incorrect handling
- Larger breeds are difficult for young children to handle.

Biology

Rabbits are highly social, burrowing herbivores that are natural prey for a wide variety of carnivores. As a prey species, rabbits have evolved to be constantly vigilant, lightweight and fast-moving, with a highly

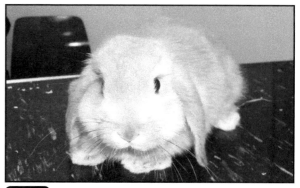

4.1 A Dwarf lop rabbit, a popular pet breed.

efficient digestive system that enables them to spend the minimum time possible above ground and in danger of capture. In the wild, feeding takes place mainly in the early morning and evening. To avoid attracting predator attention, rabbit behaviour is not overt and relies heavily on scent. Pet rabbits have retained many of the prey-based behavioural traits of their wild relatives (e.g. they do not elicit obvious signs of pain).

In the wild, rabbits live in warrens of 70 or more individuals, divided into small groups of two to eight. They spend a lot of time engaged in mutual grooming and lying together. Thumping with the hindleg is used as an alarm call. Fear elicits either complete immobility or a flight response, often with frantic attempts to escape and screaming. Rabbits are obligate nasal breathers. Biological data are summarized in Figure 4.2.

Lifespan (years)	5–12 (can be greater in some individuals)
Average weight (kg)	1–10 (breed-dependent)
Heart rate (beats/min)	180–300
Respiratory rate (breaths/min)	30–60 (higher if stressed)
Blood volume (ml/kg)	Approximately 60
Rectal temperature (°C)	38.5–40.0
Dentition	I2/1 C0/0 P3/2 M3/3
Daily water intake (ml/kg)	50–150
Daily urine production (ml/kg)	10–35
Food intake per day (g/kg)	50

4.2 Biological data for the rabbit.

Anatomy and physiology of the digestive tract

Rabbits are highly specialized hindgut fermenters, adapted to digest a low-quality, high-fibre diet consisting mainly of grass. Unlike other hindgut fermenters (e.g. the horse), the rabbit has a very rapid gut transit time and eliminates indigestible fibre from the digestive tract as soon as possible, whilst selectively retaining digestible dietary elements. This permits body size and weight to remain low, which is advantageous in a prey species. For further details on rabbit anatomy and physiology see *BSAVA Manual of Rabbit Medicine and Surgery, 2nd edition*.

Stomach

The stomach is large, J-shaped and located to the left of the midline in the cranial abdomen. There is a well developed cardiac sphincter, which prevents vomiting. The pH varies diurnally, but can be as low as 1–2. The stomach usually contains hair, food and fluid even after 24 hours or more of fasting/anorexia.

Small intestine

The small intestine is the primary site of nutrient absorption. The bile duct and a separate single pancreatic duct open into the duodenum. The terminal ileum enlarges into a dilatation known as the *sacculus rotundus* (a structure unique to the rabbit) at the ileocaecocolic junction. Retrograde movement of ingesta from the large intestine back into the ileum is inhibited by a valve-type mechanism.

Large intestine

The large intestine is highly developed in the rabbit. The caecum is the largest organ in the abdominal cavity and functions as a fermentation vat. It is located on the right side, is very thin-walled and coiled. The blind-ending vermiform appendix, which is rich in lymphatic tissue, is located at the distal caecum. The caecal contents are semi-fluid and rich in microorganisms.

The colon is functionally divided into 2 parts:

- The proximal colon, which features grossly distinct haustra (small pouches caused by sacculation)
- The distal colon, which is unhaustrated.

The proximal colon is the site of separation of particles (based on length) into the digestible fraction (which settles near the mucosa and is propelled in a retrograde fashion back into the caecum via coordinated contractions) and the indigestible fraction (which is passed in the centre of the lumen through to the distal colon for expulsion as hard faecal pellets). Normal function relies on a highly coordinated pattern of intestinal motility, which is itself promoted by indigestible dietary fibre. In this way, dietary fibre has a protective effect against enteritis. At the junction between the proximal and distal colon is the *fusus coli* (an area of thickened circular muscle unique to lagomorphs), which acts as the 'intestinal pacemaker' controlling colonic motility and faecal/caecotroph output.

The well established indigenous population of microorganisms in the caecum and, to a lesser extent, the colon, produce the volatile fatty acids acetate, butyrate and propionate. These products of fermentation provide up to 40% of the maintenance energy requirement of the rabbit, and may be absorbed directly through the caecal wall but, importantly, are also expelled and re-ingested as caecotrophs. The strict anaerobes of the genus *Bacteroides* are the predominant organisms within the caecum but many others are present also. Coliform bacteria and *Clostridium* spp. are present only in low numbers, if at all.

Caecotrophy: Rabbits produce two types of faeces: hard faeces and caecotrophs (also termed 'night faeces', although they are not only passed at night), which differ markedly in composition (Figure 4.3 and 4.4).

	Dry matter	Crude protein	Crude fibre
Faeces	53%	15%	30%
Caecotrophs	39%	34%	18%

4.3 Composition of hard faeces and caecotrophs.

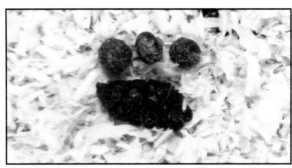

4.4 Rabbits produce two types of faeces: caecotrophs which are small, soft, mucus-coated balls of caecal contents arranged in grape-like clusters (bottom); and hard faeces which are larger and dry (top).

Caecotrophy (the ingestion of small packets of caecal contents) is an integral part of the rabbit's digestive physiology, the function of which is to improve feed utilization by maximizing the absorption of nutrients and bacterial fermentation products (amino acids, volatile fatty acids and vitamins B and K). In the normal rabbit, caecotrophs and hard faeces are not excreted at the same time. Caecotrophs are covered by a mucus 'envelope' secreted in the proximal colon and are passed as pellets of approximately 5 mm diameter arranged in clusters. Arrival of such clusters at the anus triggers a reflex licking of the area and ingestion of the caecotrophs, which are swallowed whole. Following consumption, caecotrophs remain in the stomach of the rabbit for 6–8 hours. They are preserved in an intact state due to the protective mucus coating, allowing the microorganisms within the caecotrophs to continue the fermentation process.

Pancreas

The pancreas is diffuse and located in a pocket formed by the transverse colon, stomach and duodenum. A gallbladder is present, and rabbits secrete mainly biliverdin in the bile rather than bilirubin.

Liver

The liver has four lobes. Overweight rabbits often have significant lipid stores in the liver, which predisposes them to hepatic lipidosis if they undergo periods of fasting or anorexia.

Dentition

The dental formula for rabbits is 2/1 0/0 3/2 3/3. All teeth are open-rooted, long-crowned and grow continuously. The part of the tooth embedded in the alveolus is referred to as the 'reserve crown' as it is not a true anatomical root. The visible part of the tooth is correctly described as the 'exposed crown'.

The unpigmented incisors have an enamel layer only on the anterior surface, which wears more slowly than the posterior surface, thereby maintaining a chisel shape for cutting herbage. Incisor wear, growth and eruption are generally balanced over time, at a rate of approximately 3 mm per week. The vestigial second pair of upper incisors are located directly behind the first pair and are known as 'peg teeth'. There is a long diastema between the incisors and premolar teeth. The term 'cheek teeth' refers to both the premolars and molars, which are functionally identical. They are wider apart on the maxilla than on the mandible, so only one side of the cheek teeth can be in occlusion at any one time. The mandibular cheek teeth grow faster than the maxillary ones. The temporomandibular articulation is positioned dorsal to the occlusal line.

The oral commissure is small and the oral cavity is long and curved. Cheek folds across the diastema make visualization of the cheek teeth difficult in the conscious animal. The tongue is large and has a mobile rostral portion and a relatively fixed thicker caudal portion (the torus). Prehension is achieved largely by the lips, whilst the incisors are used for slicing vegetation. Food is passed to the back of the mouth for grinding. When grinding fibrous natural foods, the mandible has a wide lateral chewing action, concentrating on one side at a time. This wears the whole cheek tooth occlusal surface. Grass is highly abrasive as it contains a high content of silicate phytoliths, so there is rapid wear of the teeth (around 3 mm per month) with equally rapid tooth growth and eruption to compensate for this.

Sexing

The anogenital distance is greater in the male (buck), which has a round preputial opening. The female (doe) has an elliptical vulval opening. Within a breed, does tend to be slightly larger than bucks, but bucks have broader heads.

Husbandry

Housing

- Rabbits are social animals and should be provided with a companion wherever possible.
- Litter mates can be kept together but should be neutered if of different sexes.
- Unrelated females will usually tolerate each other if there is sufficient space provided, but can fight.

- Intact bucks will fight and inflict severe injuries.
- All introductions should be supervised and gradual.
- Neutering minimizes the risk of conflict.
- The most stable pairing is a neutered buck and a neutered doe.
- Rabbits should not be housed with guinea pigs as bullying by either species can occur, particularly by the rabbit. Rabbits can also harbour *Bordetella bronchiseptica*, which is pathogenic to guinea pigs.

Outdoor housing

- Rabbits are generally hardy but need protection from extremes of weather.
- Direct sunlight should be avoided, as heat stress occurs easily.
- The hutch should be raised off the ground.
- Good ventilation is essential to prevent respiratory disease.
- For protection against bad weather, a waterproof roof and louvered panel to cover mesh-fronted areas should be provided, but it is important that these features do not compromise ventilation.
- The hutch should at least be big enough for the rabbit to stretch out fully, stand upright on its hindlegs and, if confined to the hutch for long periods, be able to take at least three 'hops' from one end to the other.
- A solid-fronted nesting area and a mesh-fronted living area should be provided, bedded with wood shavings and hay or straw.
- A hutch should never be considered adequate for permanent housing. Rabbits need daily exercise and should be permitted to graze whenever possible; the hutch can be placed within a grassed area, or if this is not possible, a separate ark, run or enclosure should be provided (Figure 4.5). Raised shelves or platforms can be readily used.
- Rabbits will burrow, so precautions should be taken to prevent escape.
- Rabbits can jump well and covering the run or pen with a mesh top will prevent escape, as well as provide protection from predators.
- Rabbits should always be provided with appropriate 'bolt-holes', such as empty cardboard boxes or drain-pipes, which they can retreat to if alarmed or to escape unwanted attention from other rabbits.

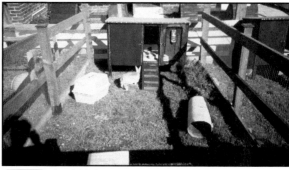

4.5 A rabbit in a run on grass, with bolt holes for shelter. (Reproduced from the *BSAVA Manual of Rabbit Medicine and Surgery, 2nd edition.*)

- Contact with wild rabbits should be prevented to minimize the risk of disease transmission by direct contact (e.g. viral haemorrhagic disease) or by vectors such as the rabbit flea (e.g. myxomatosis).
- Fly and mosquito control should be considered in summer months.

Indoor housing

- House rabbits should have a secure caged area where they can be placed when the owner is not present. Wire cages with plastic bases are suitable.
- Exercise around the house (and garden where available) should be encouraged.
- Rabbits will readily learn to use cat-flaps to gain indoor/outdoor access.
- Rabbits are easily trained to use a litter tray by repeatedly placing them in it (it may be necessary initially to place some droppings in the tray) or by allowing the rabbit to select a corner of the enclosure as a latrine and then placing a litter tray at that site. Wood- or paper-based litter should be used, as Fuller's earth products can be harmful if ingested.
- Electrical cables must be protected from chewing, and poisonous house plants such as *Dieffenbachia* (dumb cane) avoided.
- Rabbits enjoy chewable toys, such as cardboard boxes, telephone directories, straw baskets and commercial bird toys.

Diet

The best diet for a rabbit is *ad libitum* grass and/or good quality grass hay (e.g. Timothy or meadow) supplemented with fresh vegetables such as kale, cabbage, spinach, spring greens, watercress and the leaves of root vegetables as well as wild plants if available (e.g. bramble, groundsel, chickweed, dandelion). Hay can be fed from racks or nets to increase time spent feeding and thereby reduce boredom. Alfalfa hay can also be given to growing rabbits as a secondary fibre source, but the calcium and protein content is too high for it to be considered a useful dietary component for adults.

Restricted amounts (<30 g/kg bodyweight/day) of a pelleted/extruded concentrate diet may also be given, but should only be viewed as a minor component of the diet. Grass, the staple food of the wild rabbit, has a nutritional composition of approximately 20–25% crude fibre, 15% crude protein and 2–3% fat, and pellets with a nutritional composition as close to this as possible should be offered. Unfortunately, many commercially available rabbit diets are too low in fibre and too high in protein, fat and carbohydrate. In addition, many commercial foods come in the form of a mixed ration, consisting of pulses, grains, cereal flakes, grass pellets and biscuits. These products should be avoided as many rabbits are selective eaters and will leave the grass pellet and biscuit component of the ration, in favour of the grains, cereals and pulses. This results in poor nutrition due to low calcium and inadequate fibre levels as well as excessive carbohydrate intake.

Inappropriate feeding of concentrate rations (type and/or quantity) predisposes rabbits to caecocolic hypomotility, prolonged retention of digesta, increased volatile fatty acid production, and adverse alterations in caecal pH and microflora, leading to ileus, which can be life-threatening. Weanlings are particularly susceptible to gastroenteropathies, especially when dietary provision is suboptimal. Due to the energy content, nutritional inadequacies and ease with which they are eaten, consumption of excessive amounts of concentrate rations frequently also leads to obesity, dental disease due to lack of wear (Crossley, 1995) and/or metabolic issues (Harcourt-Brown, 2007), and boredom-associated problems such as stereotypical behaviour and aggression.

Treat items such as carrots or other root vegetables and small pieces of fruit can be used as a source of environmental enrichment, e.g. suspending them from the cage roof to act as edible toys. In this way, occasional items can be used to increase the time spent feeding without significantly increasing the calorie content of the diet. Sudden changes in diet, frosted or mouldy foods, and lawnmower clippings should be avoided. Rabbits enjoy sweet foods but sugar-rich treats should not be fed. Water intake is approximately 10% of bodyweight daily. Drinking bottles are easier to keep clean than water bowls and avoid wetting the dewlap, which can lead to a moist dermatitis.

Breeding

Rabbits become sexually mature at 4–8 months of age depending on sex and breed (does generally earlier than bucks; smaller breeds earlier than larger ones). Reproductive data are summarized in Figure 4.6.

Sexual maturity	4–8 months (does earlier than bucks)
Oestrous cycle	Induced (reflex) ovulation; oestrus January–October
Length of gestation	28–32 days
Litter size	4–12
Birth weight	30–80 g
Weaning age	6 weeks

4.6 Reproductive parameters for the rabbit.

Bucks

Bucks have two hairless scrotal sacs on either side of the penis (cranially). The testes descend at approximately 10 weeks of age, along with a large epididymal fat pad, and the inguinal canals remain open throughout life. There is no os penis. The accessory sex glands include seminal vesicles, small paired bulbourethral glands and the prostate gland.

Does

The ovaries are elongated and located more caudally in the doe than in the dog. Does have no uterine body, two separate uterine horns (long and coiled) and two cervices (opening into the vagina). The vagina is large and flaccid. The mesometrium is a major site of fat deposition, which can complicate ovariohysterectomy in older overweight individuals.

Does are induced ovulators and, although there is no definitive oestrous cycle, they have a variable receptive period (up to 14 days) followed by 2–4 days of non-receptivity during the breeding season (January to October in the UK). A receptive doe is very active, rubbing her chin on objects and exhibiting lordosis. The vulva becomes congested and reddish-purple in colour. Does may mount each other and this, or an infertile mating, can induce ovulation, leading to a pseudopregnancy of approximately 18 days. Does tend to be more territorial than bucks, and so the doe should be taken to the buck or to neutral territory for breeding in order to avoid aggression. Sexually mature bucks will mate at any time.

Nest building behaviour involves burrowing and pulling of fur from the dewlap, flanks and belly to line the nest and expose the nipples. Pregnancy can be detected by palpation at 12 days; gestation is 28–32 days. Parturition usually occurs in the early morning. The kits are altricial (i.e. hairless with ears and eyes closed). The placenta is haemochorial. Parturition is usually rapid (30 minutes) but will occasionally last several hours. The dam suckles the kits for only 3–5 minutes once (occasionally twice) a day. As such, the milk is very rich in protein and fat. Maternal transfer of immunity occurs before birth.

Kits

Kits emerge from the nest at about 2–3 weeks of age, when they start to show an interest in solid food; hay should be available at all times. Caecotrophy starts at about 3 weeks and weaning can take place at 4–6 weeks. If concentrate pellets are to be offered, they should be introduced gradually and only once the young are established on hay.

Preventive healthcare

Routine health checks

Regular health checks for rabbits are recommended every 6 months and can be combined with vaccination visits. Dietary factors as well as the physical and social environment of the rabbit can be discussed. By encouraging high husbandry standards, veterinary surgeons can actively play a role in reducing the incidence of preventable disease in the pet rabbit population.

Vaccination

Indoor housing does not protect rabbits from the risk of contracting myxomatosis or viral haemorrhagic disease (VHD). Both are highly infectious viruses that carry a very poor prognosis. Myxomatosis commonly presents as oedema and inflammation of the face and external genitalia, along with pyrexia, respiratory signs and debilitation, and is transmitted via insect vectors. VHD commonly presents as sudden death or collapse due to acute internal haemorrhage and anaemia, and is transmitted by fomites. As such all rabbits, regardless of proximity to wild rabbits, should be vaccinated.

Myxomatosis vaccines available in the UK are derived from the closely related Shope fibroma virus. The first inoculation is given from 6 weeks of age and repeated every 6 months throughout life. To ensure adequate immunity develops 0.1 ml of the reconstituted vaccine must be given intradermally; the remainder, subcutaneously. If heavily challenged, a vaccinated rabbit may develop a less severe form of myxomatosis characterized by localized cutaneous lumps; prognosis for this form of the disease is good.

VHD vaccination is provided annually throughout life and is administered subcutaneously. The first inoculation can be given from 12 weeks of age. Particular care must be taken when administering this vaccine as severe localized reactions in humans have been reported following accidental inoculation. Myxomatosis and VHD vaccination should not be carried out at the same time: 14 days should be allowed between inoculations. However, in some countries combined vaccines are available.

Neutering

Neutering of all non-breeding does (>6 months of age) is strongly recommended to prevent uterine adenocarcinoma. This neoplasm is alarmingly common, affecting 50–80% of intact does >3 years of age. Bucks (>4 months of age) are often also neutered for behavioural reasons and to prevent breeding. They have an open inguinal canal throughout life and so a closed castration technique is recommended (see Orchiectomy, below).

Parasiticides

Routine worming of pet rabbits is not necessary. In the summer months, cyromazine can be applied topically to the skin along the back of outdoor rabbits to prevent fly strike. Each application lasts 10 weeks and is especially important for rabbits with perineal soiling.

In the UK, imidacloprid is authorized for the treatment of fleas in rabbits. It is applied topically to the skin at the back of the neck. Environmental treatment (e.g. carpets) and treatment of in-contact animals is also required to control flea infestation.

Handling and restraint

As a prey species, rabbits are flighty animals and may react to threatening situations with little warning. Twisting and kicking out by the powerful hindlegs must be prevented, as serious back injury (e.g. lumbar fracture) can result. The risk of injury to the patient and handler can be minimized by following a few simple rules:

- Rabbits should always be approached in a quiet, calm and confident manner
- Sudden or rapid movements should be avoided
- The minimum effective level of restraint according to the animal's demeanour, health status and the procedure to be carried out should be used
- Slippery surfaces should be avoided (Figure 4.7)

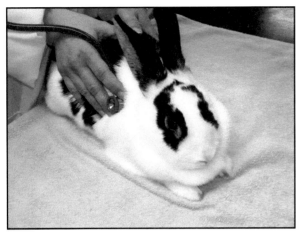

4.7 Examining rabbits on slippery surfaces should be avoided; covering the examination table with a towel makes the patient feel more secure, facilitating examination. Note that a paediatric stethoscope is being used to auscultate the thorax.

- The rabbit's back and hindquarters must be supported at all times during handling. Placing one hand over the rabbit's eyes and the other on the rump provides good restraint
- If the head is restrained, it should be ensured that the nares are not occluded
- On the rare occasion that a rabbit appears particularly aggressive, throwing a large towel over the animal and approaching from above will facilitate safe handling. Appropriately sized cat restraint bags can also be utilized for handling difficult rabbits
- Handling may be facilitated by wrapping the rabbit securely in a towel
- A rabbit should never be left unattended on a table (even if wrapped in a towel)
- Many rabbits require some form of chemical restraint to be placed in lateral recumbency safely
- If dealing with a particularly aggressive, nervous or stressed individual some form of chemical restraint should be considered
- Adequate analgesia (local or systemic) should be used if a potentially painful procedure is being undertaken.

Most rabbits can be effectively handled by grasping the scruff with one hand and placing the other hand on the rump supporting the back and hindlimbs. Docile individuals or heavy giant-breed rabbits can be picked up by placing one arm under the thorax and supporting the hindquarters as described for the 'scruff' method. Rabbits should never be picked up by their ears (as some older texts suggest).

Tonic immobility

A trance-like state (tonic immobility or 'hypnotization') can be induced in many rabbits by placing them in dorsal recumbency with the neck flexed and hindlimbs extended. Once positioned, covering the eyes or gently stroking the face or ventral body may help incite the reflex. The tonic immobility response is exhibited by wild rabbits that have been caught by a predator. During the trance, the rabbit's muscles relax, the righting reflex is lost and there is minimal response to external stimuli. Some veterinary surgeons and owners find the technique helpful to carry out brief minor non-painful procedures, e.g. nail clipping.

It is important to be aware that during tonic immobility a rabbit is neither truly hypnotized nor asleep, but is actually in a heightened state of awareness and undergoing physiological changes associated with a stressful situation. Whilst it is a useful restraint technique, some owners are under the impression that it is pleasurable to the rabbit and use it to enhance the pet–owner bond; this is highly unlikely and the technique should only be used when necessary. There appears to be considerable individual susceptibility to inducing tonic immobility; in some rabbits the response cannot be reliably invoked, whilst others can remain in an immobile state for over half an hour. Research indicates that animals that succumb easily to tonic immobility exhibit higher stress levels than those that resist it, perpetuating the mistaken belief that it is useful for calming or taming very nervous individuals.

Diagnostic approach

For information on history-taking, see *BSAVA Manual of Rabbit Medicine and Surgery, 2nd edition.*

Clinical examination

A methodical approach to the physical examination is essential as rabbits rarely show overt signs of disease, especially in the case of chronic illness.

Vital parameters

Respiratory rate and rhythm should be assessed prior to handling. It is also useful to obtain a resting heart rate, pulse rate (via the femoral or central auricular artery) and rectal temperature early in the examination process as all will tend to rise with the stress of handling. These parameters may already be elevated due to the stress associated with transport to the surgery or a prolonged wait in a noisy waiting room. If the animal is tachycardic, the heart rate may be too fast to measure accurately.

Condition and hydration status

The overall body condition of the rabbit should be assessed and an accurate bodyweight recorded. Visual assessment and palpation along the length of the body, concentrating on the soft tissues overlying the ribs, the dorsal spinous processes and the limb musculature is used to assess body condition. A basic body condition scoring system is as follows:

1. Emaciated.
2. Underweight.
3. Normal.
4. Overweight.
5. Obese.

Dehydration results in sunken eyes and a loss of skin elasticity. Rapid alterations in bodyweight may also provide some indication as to the degree of dehydration.

Integument

An initial assessment of coat quality is often made during the visual inspection, bearing in mind breed differences (e.g. Angora *versus* Rex rabbits). This is followed by a systematic inspection of the entire surface of the rabbit. The fur should be soft, dense, clean, dry and free of matts. Areas frequently associated with dermatoses in rabbits, which should be inspected during any physical examination, include the:

- Dorsum
- Face
- Ventral neck and dewlap (where present)
- Perineum
- Plantar surfaces of the feet
- Hocks (Figure 4.8).

Urine scald (Figure 4.9) or an accumulation of soft faeces in the perineal region (Figure 4.10) is always significant. Myiasis ('fly strike') should be considered an emergency.

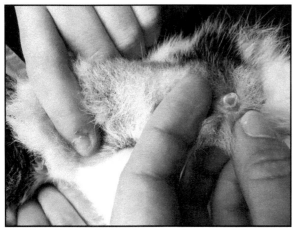

4.8 Rabbits lack footpads and as a result the plantar surfaces of the hind feet are a common site for focal skin disease to develop. This rabbit is showing signs of early plantar pododermatitis with mild alopecia and erythema of the hock area.

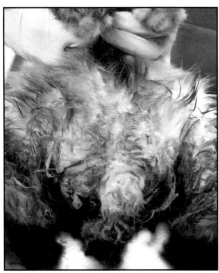

4.9 Perineal urine soiling has a variety of causes. Regardless of the underlying cause, it frequently leads to scalding of the perineal skin, resulting in pain and secondary bacterial dermatitis.

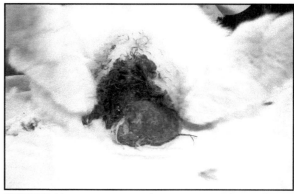

4.10 Uneaten caecotrophs may accumulate at the anus and in the perineal region, predisposing the rabbit to myiasis, urine scalding and perineal dermatitis.

Respiratory and cardiovascular systems

Following the initial respiratory rate and rhythm check, any sneezing, upper respiratory stertor or dyspnoea should be noted. The nares are then examined and should be equally patent and free of any discharge. Auscultation of the thorax and trachea is best performed with a human infant or paediatric stethoscope (see Figure 4.7). In the normal rabbit, short, regular and rapid inspiratory sounds are heard in all lung fields. Pulse rate and quality should be assessed.

Mucous membrane colour is assessed by inspection of the oral or conjunctival mucosa. The normal colour is light pink, slightly paler than that of a normal dog or cat. To improve efficiency and minimize handling, this assessment can be combined with the oral and/or ophthalmic components of the examination. Capillary refill time (CRT) is assessed via the gingival mucous membranes.

Gastrointestinal system

Inspection of the oral cavity in the conscious rabbit is limited. The rabbit is positioned in dorsal or sternal recumbency, depending on the patient's demeanour and clinician preference. The incisor teeth and oral mucosa are inspected by gently parting the upper lips at the philtrum. The cheek teeth and tongue are initially examined using an otoscope with a large plastic or metal cone attached, but sedation or anaesthesia is required to examine the mouth properly. Abnormalities that may be visualized include crown elongation, malocclusion, spike formation, tooth loss, infection, soft tissue trauma and haemorrhage. The face should be palpated along the maxillae, zygomatic arches and ventral mandible for asymmetry or foci of pain.

Abdominal palpation is performed with the hands held flat against each lateral body wall; it is important to be gentle as many of the rabbit's abdominal viscera are thin-walled. Abnormal, very firm or irregular structures should be noted as well as any regions of consistent discomfort. Abdominal auscultation and percussion are useful ancillary tests. The anus should be examined for evidence of diarrhoea or accumulated caecotrophs or the presence of a recto-anal papilloma.

Urogenital system

The kidneys are palpable, mobile and located slightly more cranially than those of dogs and cats. The bladder is usually palpable in the caudal abdomen; it should be handled carefully as it is very thin-walled.

Musculoskeletal system

Placing the rabbit on a non-slip floor surface and encouraging ambulation allows assessment of gait, degree of lameness (if appropriate) and limb position in relation to the trunk. The bones and joints can be palpated noting any swellings, pain or irregularities.

Ears

The pinnae are examined as for the rest of the skin, and both ear canals are inspected visually on either side of the tragus with an otoscope. A small amount of wax is a normal finding but should not be associated with any inflammation of the epithelium. The tympanic membrane should be white and translucent.

Eyes

Evidence of ocular discharge should be noted including wetness, alopecia or crusting of the periocular skin. Aberrations in eye position, nystagmus, exophthalmos or a sunken position of one or both eyes are significant findings. The opening to the lacrimal duct is examined by gently lifting the lower eyelid away from the globe near the medial canthus. At the same time, gentle pressure is applied to the face ventromedial to the eye to observe for discharge from the punctum. The eyelids, cornea and the remainder of the ocular structures are examined for abnormalities. The optic nerve is located above the horizontal midline of the eye, and the retinal vessels spread outwards from the optic disc. Rabbits have no tapetum lucidum.

Group examination

When dealing with large groups of rabbits (e.g. breeding establishments, commercial production units) key husbandry issues (e.g. diet, housing, hygiene), record-keeping, quarantine facilities and vaccination protocols (if appropriate) are critical to the evaluation of group health problems. Information regarding the source of new rabbits and the breeding programme utilized may also be useful.

Imaging

Radiography

Plain radiography can be used to evaluate the skull (Figure 4.11), thorax, abdomen, spine and limbs. Complete radiographic assessment of the skull (predominantly used to evaluate dental structures) includes 5 standard views:

- Left or right lateral
- Left lateral oblique
- Right lateral oblique
- Dorsoventral (DV) or ventrodorsal (VD)
- Rostrocaudal.

Features to note include incisor occlusion, cheek teeth occlusal plane, orientation, length and degree of curvature of all teeth, the radiodensity of the

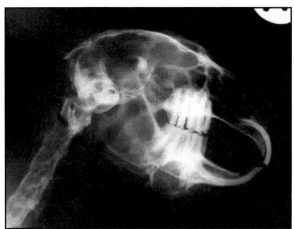

4.11 Lateral skull radiograph of a rabbit with a facial mass. The mass proved to be a *Pasteurella multocida* abscess that had developed at the apex of one of the mandibular premolars. Radiography was vital in this case to identify which tooth was involved. The tooth was subsequently extracted during surgery to debride the abscess.

surrounding bone and the symmetry of structures such as the tympanic bullae.

Thoracic radiography is best achieved in an anaesthetized, intubated rabbit to ensure that the lungs are inflated during exposure. Ideally left and right lateral and VD views should be taken. Intrathoracic fat and the presence of the thymus can complicate interpretation.

Abdominal radiography is useful for evaluation of the gastrointestinal tract, liver, urinary tract and occasionally the reproductive tract. It is an important tool for the evaluation of any rabbit with a distended abdomen. Gaseous distension of bowel loops indicative of ileus (Figure 4.12) and urinary calculi or 'sludge' (Figure 4.13) are common findings. Two views (lateral and DV) should be taken.

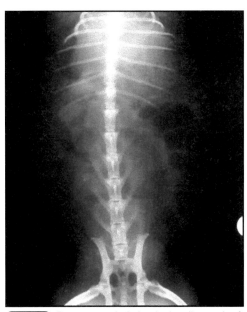

4.12 Dorsoventral abdominal radiograph of a rabbit revealing gaseous distension of the caecum suggestive of ileus. Aggressive medical therapy was instituted immediately and the rabbit made a full recovery.

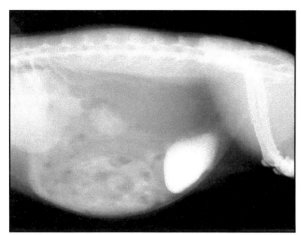

4.13 Lateral radiograph of a rabbit presented with non-specific signs of lethargy and inappetence. A large volume of radiopaque 'sludge' is present in the bladder warranting sedation, catheterization and lavage.

Once stabilized, trauma patients or those with a history of lameness, paresis or paralysis can undergo radiography to assess skeletal elements. Whole body views should be avoided and the aim should be to collimate accurately to the area of concern. Contrast agents are useful in the evaluation of the nasolacrimal duct, the gastrointestinal tract and the urinary tract.

Ultrasonography

Ultrasonographic evaluation of the abdominal viscera, intrathoracic masses/fluid, retrobulbar space and heart may be helpful in certain clinical situations. In rabbits with primary or secondary gastrointestinal hypomotility, the accumulation of gas within the intestines may impair the evaluation of abdominal structures via this imaging method. Ultrasound-guided needle biopsy or aspiration may be performed under sedation.

Computed tomography and magnetic resonance imaging

Computed tomography (CT) and magnetic resonance imaging (MRI) are advanced imaging modalities that are available at a limited number of referral practices. CT provides unparalleled information about bony and air-filled tissues (e.g. dental structures and the lungs), whereas MRI is most useful for evaluating soft tissues (e.g. brain; Figure 4.14).

Sample collection

Blood

Indications:

- Collection of blood.
- Administration of intravenous medication, including fluids.

Principles:

- Adequate lighting must be available to visualize the small veins of rabbits.
- The blood volume of a rabbit is 55–78 ml/kg and up to 10% of this can be removed safely in a normal animal (approximately 6.5 ml/kg); thus, sample volume is rarely a limiting factor.

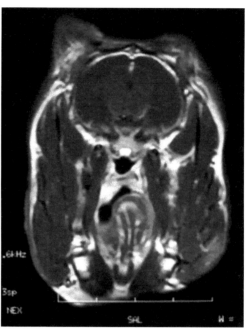

4.14 MRI is an incredibly powerful tool for evaluating a variety of soft tissue structures. It is particularly useful for the investigation of neurological disease. This MRI brain scan of a rabbit presented with severe, sudden onset torticollis shows no gross lesions (e.g. neoplasms, abscesses).

Sites: Marginal ear vein (Figure 4.15), jugular vein, lateral saphenous vein and cephalic vein.

Normal haematological and biochemical values are summarized in Figure 4.16.

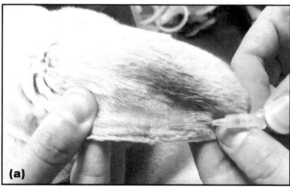

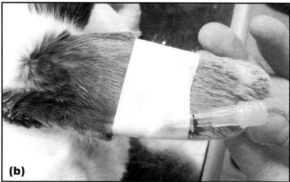

4.15 Venepuncture from the marginal ear vein. **(a)** An assistant raises the marginal ear vein by applying pressure at the base of the ear. **(b)** Intravenous catheterization of the marginal ear vein. (Reproduced from the *BSAVA Manual of Rabbit Medicine and Surgery, 2nd edition.*)

Parameter	Reference range
Haematology	
RBC (erythrocytes) (x 10^{12}/l)	4–7
HCT/PCV	0.31–0.45
Hb (g/l)	100–150
MCV (fl)	60–69
MCH (pg)	19–22
MCHC (%)	33–48
WBC (leucocytes) (x 10^9/l)	5.2–10.0
Lymphocytes (%)	30–60
Neutrophils (%)	30–50
Eosinophils (%)	0–4
Basophils (%)	0–7
Monocytes (%)	0–4
Platelets (x 10^9/l)	250–600
Biochemistry	
ALT (IU/l)	27.4–72.2
AST (IU/l)	10.0–78.0
Creatine kinase (IU/l)	58.6–175.0
LDH (IU/l)	27.8–101.5
GGT (IU/l)	0–5
Bilirubin (µmol/l)	2.6–17.1
Blood urea nitrogen (mmol/l)	6.14–8.38
Total protein (g/l)	49–71
Albumin (g/l)	27–50
Globulin (g/l)	15–33
Creatinine (µmol/l)	44.2–229
Glucose (mmol/l)	4.2–7.8
Calcium (total) (mmol/l)	3.0–4.2
Inorganic phosphate (mmol/l)	1.0–1.92
Sodium (mmol/l)	138–150
Chloride (mmol/l)	92–120
Potassium (mmol/l)	3.3–5.7

4.16 Normal haematological and blood biochemical findings in the rabbit.

Nasal

Nasolacrimal cannulation:

Indications:

- Flushing of the nasolacrimal duct in cases with suspected obstruction or infection.
- To instil topical medication into the nasolacrimal duct.
- To perform contrast dacryocystography.

Technique:

1. Sedate the rabbit and apply local anaesthetic drops to the eye (recommended in most cases).
2. Select a suitable cannula: 20–27-gauge plastic irrigating cannulae or intravenous catheters with the stylet removed are suitable; alternatively, a commercially available metal cannula can be used.
3. Gently pull out or evert the lower eyelid to expose the slit-like ventral punctum of the nasolacrimal duct in the lower conjunctiva medial to the lid margin.
4. Insert the cannula into the duct in a ventromedial direction (there should be little resistance if positioning is correct).
5. Attach a syringe filled with sterile saline, medication or contrast agent (as required) to the cannula and flush the duct (Figure 4.17). The instilled material and duct contents will be present at the ipsilateral nostril if the duct is patent. If the instillation of fluid leads to bulging of the globe, the duct has ruptured and the procedure should be abandoned immediately.

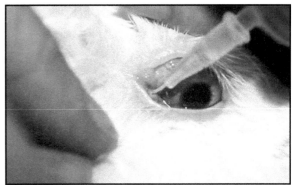

4.17 Cannulation of the nasolacrimal duct for flushing.

Deep nasal swab:

Indications:

- Collection of samples for bacterial/fungal culture and cytology in order to investigate nasal discharges or upper respiratory signs of unknown origin.

Technique:

1. Sedate or anaesthetize the rabbit to reduce the risk of iatrogenic damage to the turbinates and nasal mucosa.
2. Introduce a fine sterile microculturette/swab into the ventral aspect of the nasal cavity and advance to the level of the medial canthus of the eye (pre-measuring the distance is recommended) (Figure 4.18).

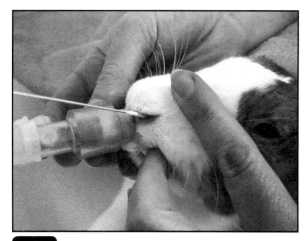

4.18 Deep nasal swab collection.

Urine

Urinalysis is an important diagnostic tool in the evaluation of many rabbit illnesses. Rabbit urine is alkaline, contains albumin, calcium carbonate and ammonium magnesium phosphate crystals, and is often pigmented (Figure 4.19).

Voided samples: These are easy to collect, especially from litter-trained rabbits, but are often contaminated. If possible collection by manual expression of the bladder, cystocentesis or catheterization is preferred.

Manual expression of the bladder: This is a relatively simple procedure.

1. Gradually increase the pressure applied to either side of the bladder via abdominal palpation until urine voided.

2. Collect the voided urine directly into a sterile universal container.

Excessive force should be avoided as the bladder is relatively thin-walled. Many rabbits who fail to void urine during this procedure will urinate soon after being replaced in their cage or on the floor, thereby providing a sample.

Cystocentesis:

1. Restrain the rabbit in dorsal or lateral recumbency.
2. Assess the degree of fill of the bladder prior to collection.
3. Clip and aseptically prepare a small window in the ventral midline, immediately cranial to the pubis.
4. Use one hand to isolate the bladder and the other hand to direct a 22–25-gauge 1 inch needle attached to a 5 ml or 10 ml syringe through the abdominal wall in the midline and into the bladder.
5. Slowly retract the syringe plunger to collect urine. If blood enters the needle, a second attempt should be made with a fresh needle and syringe.

Urinary catheterization:

Indications:

- To collect an uncontaminated urine sample.
- To treat a urinary obstruction.
- To therapeutically flush sludge from the bladder (Figure 4.20).
- To facilitate contrast radiography of the urinary tract.

Parameter	Normal findings	Comments/abnormalities
Appearance	Wide variation in colour from clear to pale yellow, orange/red to brown Often turbid or chalky	
Urine specific gravity (SG)	1.003–1.036	Urine SG >1.036 suggestive of haemoconcentration. Useful for assessing hydration status/renal function and monitoring response to fluid therapy in dehydrated patients
pH	Alkaline (>8.0, as with other herbivores)	pH <7.0 suggestive of metabolic acidosis and the need for immediate supportive therapy whilst investigating cause
Protein	None to trace	Moderate to large amounts suggestive of renal dysfunction
Ketones	None	Important for assessment of anorexia. Presence indicates ketosis. Often present in cases with hepatic lipidosis. Moderate to large amounts associated with poor prognosis and requirement for immediate intensive supportive care whilst investigating underlying cause
Glucose	None to trace	Higher amounts most often associated with stress hyperglycaemia
Blood	None	Important to differentiate false haematuria (presence of plant porphyrin pigments in urine) from true haematuria
Cytology	Calcium carbonate, calcium oxalate and struvite crystals; small number of red or white blood cells	Bacteria. Large numbers of inflammatory and/or red blood cells. Granular casts are observed in the advanced stages of renal failure. *Encephalitozoon cuniculi* spores may be seen as oval, strong Gram-positive structures with a coiled filament

4.19 Interpretation of urinalysis results in the rabbit.

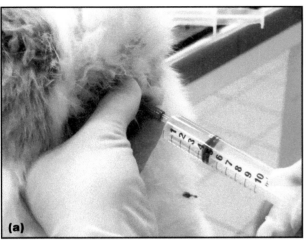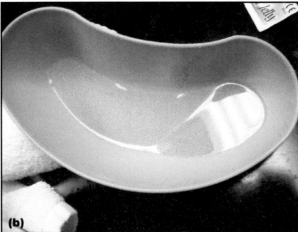

4.20 **(a)** Flushing the bladder of an anaesthetized rabbit suffering from sludgy bladder syndrome. **(b)** Urinary sludge (a thick accumulation of calcium crystals) removed from the bladder of the rabbit by catheterization and lavage.

Technique:

1. Sedate or anaesthetize the patient (preferably using a benzodiazepine in the premedication or sedation protocol).
2. Gently wash the vulva/prepuce with warm, dilute antiseptic solution and rinse.
3. Select a suitable catheter (usually 3–4 French). Cut open the package containing the sterile urinary catheter to expose the distal 3 cm of catheter and apply sterile, water-soluble lubricant to the catheter tip. Ensure an aseptic technique is used by wearing sterile gloves or insisting that the catheter remains wrapped in its packaging until immediately before use.

- *Bucks*: catheterization is a simple procedure. The patient is placed in dorsal or lateral recumbency, the prepuce is retracted to expose the penis, and the catheter introduced.
- *Does*: catheterization is more challenging but feasible in most does with practice. The patient is placed in sternal recumbency, the vulva is gently pulled caudally, and the catheter is introduced into the vagina and advanced along the floor. The urethral opening lies ventrally and the catheter should slide in without resistance.

Common conditions

Selected common diseases are summarized in Figure 4.21. Differential diagnoses based on clinical signs and the recommended diagnostic approaches are summarized in Figure 4.22.

Disease	Cause	Clinical signs	Diagnostics	Treatment
Abscess	*Pasteurella multocida, Staphylococcus aureus, Pseudomonas, Proteus, Streptococcus, Corynebacterium, Bacteroides* and other anaerobes; located on the face frequently as a result of acquired dental disease; abscesses may occur at wound sites or following haematogenous spread	Subcutaneous or facial swelling; draining tracts; may be dull, anorexic or pyrexic if bacteraemic; dyspnoea (if pulmonary or other respiratory tract abscess); neurological signs (if cerebral or spinal abscess); if not treated early, abscesses tend to behave as expansile masses; dental-related abscesses can displace teeth over time and tooth roots may adapt, growing to follow the capsule	Clinical signs; FNA; cytology/ bacterial culture; radiography (especially if dental-related); ultrasonography; CBC; biochemistry	*En bloc* surgical removal, including the capsule, is the treatment of choice. Marsupialization is an alternative approach if abscess is difficult to remove. Systemic and local antibiosis: injection of gentamicin into capsule (empirically 0.5–1 ml); placement of antibiotic-impregnated methylmethacrylate beads. Removal of associated teeth if abscess is dental-related to minimize risk of recurrence. Lance, drain and flush is very rarely successful and not an appropriate treatment
Allergic/irritant rhinitis/bronchitis	Environmental allergens or irritants	Sneezing; dyspnoea; nasal discharge	Exclusion of other causes; response to elimination of suspected allergen(s) and/or empirical treatment	Avoidance of allergen. Antihistamines (corticosteroids should be used with caution, especially if rabbit has concurrent *Pasteurella* or other bacterial infection)

4.21 Selected common diseases of the pet rabbit. (continues) ▶

Disease	Cause	Clinical signs	Diagnostics	Treatment
Antibiotic toxicity/ enterotoxaemia (clostridial overgrowth)	All antibiotics except fluoroquinolones and potentiated sulphonamides: especially oral penicillins, ampicillin, amoxicillin, clindamycin, lincomycin, cephalosporins, erythromycin	Diarrhoea (brown, watery, foetid, bloody); depression; dehydration; hypothermia; abdominal distension; collapse; death	History of antibiotic usage; faecal culture and toxin detection (rarely performed)	Aggressive fluid therapy. Cholestyramine. Metronidazole. High-fibre nutritional support (assisted feeding). Probiotics
'Blue fur' disease	Secondary dermatitis; *Pseudomonas aeruginosa*	Moist dermatitis; blue coloration of fur in moist areas (dewlap, skin folds)	Blue coloration pathognomonic; bacterial culture	Clip fur. Ensure affected area remains dry. Topical antibiotics/antiseptic. Address underlying cause
Clostridial overgrowth (see Antibiotic toxicity)				
Coccidiosis	*Eimeria* spp. (intestinal coccidiosis); *E. steidae* (hepatic coccidiosis); outbreaks frequently associated with suboptimal husbandry (e.g. overcrowding, low-fibre diet, stress, poor hygiene)	Diarrhoea; weight loss; anorexia; jaundice; dehydration; ascites; can cause high morbidity and mortality in weanlings	Faecal microscopy to detect oocysts; post-mortem examination	Toltrazuril or sulpha drugs. Disinfection; good hygiene. Reduce stress. Increase fibre content of diet
Conjunctivitis	Bacterial infection (usually *Pasteurella multocida*) or secondary to irritation (e.g. ammonia, dust, trauma); can occur secondary to dacryocystitis	Blepharospasm; chemosis; ocular discharge; photophobia	Conjunctival cytology; bacterial culture	Topical and subconjunctival antibiotics. Topical anti-inflammatory drugs may be considered with care if the underlying cause is irritation (ensure no corneal ulceration present before use)
Cystitis	Primary or secondary bacterial infection; may be associated with urolithiasis or sludgy bladder syndrome	Perineal urine soiling and scalding; dysuria; haematuria; urinary incontinence	Urinalysis including urine culture and cytology; radiography	Fluid therapy. Analgesia. Systemic antibiotic chosen on basis of culture results. Ensure calcium content of diet not excessive
Dacryocystitis (inflammation/ infection of nasolacrimal duct)	May be primary but more frequently occurs secondary to cheek tooth pathology; various bacteria may be involved	Epiphora; purulent ocular discharge; secondary conjunctivitis	Bacterial culture of nasolacrimal duct contents (collected from lacrimal punctum or from nares following duct flush); skull radiography and oral examination under sedation to evaluate dentition	Nasolacrimal duct flush: may need repeated treatments over days/weeks to clear. Topical antibiotic instillation. Systemic antibiotics. Treat any dental abnormalities. Clean and dry periocular skin daily
Dental disease (congenital)	Mandibular prognathism (especially common in dwarf breeds); primary incisor malocclusion	Incisor wear abnormalities; dysphagia or anorexia; weight loss	Physical examination; age of rabbit is important to differentiate between congenital and acquired incisor malocclusion	Incisor extraction is the treatment of choice. Alternatively, regular trimming (not clipping) of incisors with a low-speed burr. Clipping frequently results in tooth fracture, sharp edges and damage to the pulp and periodontal tissues, which in turn leads to infection
Dental disease (acquired, very common)	Mostly due to insufficient dental wear (diet-related) – causes cheek tooth elongation and malocclusion; overgrowth of both the crowns and apices ('roots') of affected teeth results in pathological bending of the teeth and deformation of surrounding bone; secondary incisor malocclusion may develop; low dietary calcium may be a factor in some rabbits	Dysphagia or anorexia; weight loss; ptyalism; dehydration; lack of grooming; lack of caecotrophy; palpable swellings on ventral border of the mandible; facial/retrobulbar abscesses; ocular discharge; dacryocystitis; incisor wear abnormalities; development of dental spikes with associated ulceration/laceration/scarring of oral mucosa, tongue, cheek, palate and lip; oral pain; food impaction between or around the teeth; missing teeth; secondary incisor malocclusion	Dental examination under sedation/ anaesthesia; skull radiography or CT (should be repeated periodically for monitoring purposes)	If detected in early stages, uncomplicated tooth elongation can be corrected simply by dietary change (i.e. reduction then elimination of concentrate rations and replacement with fresh and dried natural herbage). However, by the time clinical signs become apparent, tooth and jaw deformity are usually permanent. Regular (long-term) burring of cheek teeth to correct crown height and shape and removal of spikes is required – inter-procedure interval varies from 4 weeks to 6 months depending on severity of disease, rate of tooth growth, diet, etc. Extraction of severely diseased teeth or those associated with abscesses (including secondarily maloccluded incisors). Analgesia may be required long term, e.g. oral meloxicam. Antibiosis if infection present. Euthanasia if severe disease

4.21 (continued) Selected common diseases of the pet rabbit. (continues) ▶

Disease	Cause	Clinical signs	Diagnostics	Treatment
Dermatophytosis	Usually *Trichophyton mentagrophytes*	Alopecia; scaling; crusting; ± pruritus	Fungal culture; skin biopsy	Clip surrounding hair. Topical antifungal agents (e.g. miconazole, clotrimazole) for small areas. Systemic griseofulvin for widespread lesions
Dysautonomia (degeneration of autonomic ganglia, leading to gut stasis)	Unknown	Mucoid diarrhoea; gut stasis; caecal impaction; dehydration; anorexia; weight loss; abdominal pain and distension; death	Post-mortem examination; histology of mesenteric autonomic ganglia	For suspected cases: fluid therapy; metoclopramide, cisapride or ranitidine; analgesia; high-fibre nutritional support. Treatment usually ineffective
Ear mites	*Psoroptes cuniculi* (non-burrowing)	Thick crusts in external ear canal(s); head-shaking; pruritus; self-trauma to pinnae; lesions can spread to face and neck	Microscopy of ear crusts	Ivermectin. Selamectin. Analgesia in severe cases
Encephalito-zoonosis	*Encephalitozoon cuniculi* (an intracellular microsporidian parasite); potential zoonosis; spores shed in urine and ingested or inhaled	Kidney and CNS are target organs; infection often asymptomatic but can cause neurological signs (ataxia, torticollis, posterior paresis/paralysis, urinary incontinence, seizures); chronic weight loss and polyuria/polydipsia; ocular (lens) lesions	Clinical signs; serology; urine (PCR); post-mortem examination	Fenbendazole. Albendazole. Supportive care. Use of short-term corticosteroids in acute, severe cases may be considered but is controversial. Anticholinergics, antihistamines and benzodiazepines (short-term use) may be considered as adjunctive therapies. Treatment often ineffective if severe neurological signs. Cleaning and disinfection of the environment; quaternary ammonium compounds inactivate spores
Endometrial hyperplasia (common in unmated does)	Age-related; continuum of change from hyperplasia to adenocarcinoma	Haematuria; haemorrhagic vaginal discharge; palpably enlarged uterus	Ultrasonography; exploratory surgery and histopathology	Ovariohysterectomy
Endometrial venous aneurysm	Unknown	Haematuria; haemorrhagic vaginal discharge	Exclusion of other causes of haematuria; ultrasonography; exploratory surgery	Blood transfusion if severe haemorrhage. Ovariohysterectomy
Enteritis (bacterial – not related to antibiotic use)	*Escherichia coli*; Tyzzer's disease (*Clostridium piliforme*); *Salmonella*	Diarrhoea; depression; weight loss; hypothermia; abdominal distension; collapse; death; high morbidity and mortality in weanlings	Faecal culture; post-mortem histopathology for Tyzzer's disease	Fluid therapy. Appropriate antibiosis. High-fibre nutritional support (assisted feeding). Probiotics
Enteritis (viral)	Rotavirus; coronavirus	Diarrhoea; depression; anorexia; death; high morbidity and mortality in weanlings	Viral isolation	None other than supportive care
Fleas	Rabbit flea *Spillopsylla cuniculi* (important vector for myxomatosis); *Cediopsylla multispinosus* in USA; cat flea *Ctenocephalides felis*	Often none; pruritus	Physical examination (identification of fleas or flea faeces)	Imidacloprid. Feline/canine pyrethrum products. All in-contact animals and the environment should be treated. Fipronil spray should be **avoided** as adverse reactions have been reported
Fur mites	*Cheyletiella parasitovorax* (zoonotic); *Listrophorus gibbus* (not pathogenic or zoonotic); *Demodex cuniculi* (rarely reported)	Alopecia; scaling; crusting; minimal/no pruritus	Identification of mite by microscopy of skin crusts, hair plucks or cellotape preparations	Ivermectin. Selamectin. All in-contact animals and the environment should be treated (can use canine/feline environmental flea products)
Gastrointestinal hypomotility/impaction/ileus	Dietary (e.g. low-fibre diet); may occur secondary to stress, lack of exercise, anorexia or pain (e.g. concurrent disease); may occur after abdominal surgery	Reduced faecal output; anorexia; dehydration; depression; weight loss (if chronic); palpable impaction or gas accumulation in stomach or intestines; can be life-threatening	Physical examination; abdominal radiography; CBC, biochemistry and urinalysis to evaluate general health	Fluid therapy. Prokinetics (e.g. metoclopramide, cisapride, ranitidine). High-fibre nutritional support. If gastric bloating present, sedate and pass stomach tube to alleviate gas. Oral simethicone for mild bloating. Analgesia. Surgical exploration is frequently unrewarding and should only be considered if the rabbit fails to respond to medical therapy after 3–5 days

4.21 (continued) Selected common diseases of the pet rabbit. (continues) ▶

Disease	Cause	Clinical signs	Diagnostics	Treatment
Hepatic lipidosis/ pregnancy toxaemia	Overweight rabbits that have become anorexic (for any reason); pregnancy; pseudopregnancy; post-parturition	Anorexia; depression; collapse; neurological signs; dyspnoea; death	History and clinical signs; urinalysis (often aciduria, ketonuria); abdominal ultrasonography; liver FNA or biopsy	Intravenous fluid therapy (e.g. lactated Ringer's solution and 5% glucose). Nutritional support. Liver support. Lactulose. *S*-adenosylmethionine
Lice	*Haemodipsus ventricosus*	Pruritus; anaemia	Identification of louse/ eggs on microscopy of hair/skin samples	Ivermectin. Selamectin. Feline/canine louse powders or ectoparasitic shampoos
Mastitis	Bacterial (often *Pasteurella multocida*, *Staphylococcus aureus* or *Steptococcus* spp.) during lactation or pseudopregnancy; may be aseptic (in intact does >3 years of age)	Bacterial: depression, pyrexia, anorexia, polydipsia, swollen painful abscessated mammary glands; septicaemia; death. Aseptic: non-painful, may exude brown fluid	Bacterial: clinical signs, culture. Aseptic: clinical signs, biopsy	Bacterial: systemic antibiotics; supportive care; analgesia; drainage of abscesses; surgical excision for severe infections; wean young. Aseptic: benign; ovariohysterectomy will resolve
Myiasis (fly strike)	Occurs rapidly in hot weather, especially with perineal soiling with urine or caecotrophs	Malodour; perineal wounds; depression; shock; collapse; death	Physical examination, especially of perineal skin	Fluid therapy, analgesia and other supportive measures. Sedate and remove maggots. Flush wounds. Systemic antibiotics. Ivermectin. Address underlying cause. Severe cases require euthanasia, especially if larvae have penetrated and damaged the gastrointestinal, urinary or reproductive tracts. Fly control for outdoor rabbits. Prevent by cyromazine application in summer for susceptible rabbits
Myxomatosis	Poxvirus spread by the rabbit flea and other insect vectors	Facial and genital oedema/ swelling; blepharitis; conjunctivitis; ocular and nasal discharge; pyrexia; subcutaneous masses; nasal scabbing only in some mild cases; depression; death	Clinical signs	Supportive care in mild cases. Euthanasia. Prevention by vaccination
Otitis externa (bacterial)	Secondary to otitis media (following rupture of tympanic membrane); secondary to *Psoroptes cuniculi*; primary otitis externa	Purulent aural exudate; head-shaking; pruritus; head tilt	Bacterial culture	Systemic and/or local antibiotics. Flushing of external ear canal(s). Treatment of any underlying conditions (if secondary)
Otitis media/ interna	Usually ascending bacterial infection via eustacian tube from nasopharynx; *Pasteurella multocida* common but other bacteria also involved	Head tilt/torticollis	Skull radiography, CT, MRI; bacterial culture of material collected from middle ear (via tympanic membrane or bulla osteotomy)	Long course of antibiotics (based on culture and sensitivity results). Bulla osteotomy or aural resection if refractory. **Corticosteroids are contraindicated**
Pasteurellosis (*Pasteurella multocida* extremely common inhabitant of nasal cavity and tympanic bullae)	Overt disease usually follows injury or stressor (e.g. overcrowding, concurrent disease); spread by direct/ venereal contact, aerosol (slow), fomites, vertical/perinatal transmission	Nasal discharge; sneezing; conjunctivitis; dacryocystitis; bronchopneumonia; head tilt/ torticollis; abscesses; pyometra; mastitis; orchitis; epididymitis; depression; anorexia; pyrexia; death	Bacterial culture (e.g. deep nasal swabs or bronchoalveolar lavage); serology; thoracic radiography	Antibiotics (based on culture and sensitivity results): systemic and/or by nebulization. If respiratory congestion present, nebulization with mucolytics (e.g. bromhexine, *N*-acetylcysteine) to break up nasal secretions may be useful adjunct measure
Perineal soiling (with uneaten caecotrophs)	Reduced caecotrophy (overfeeding; physical problems, e.g. spinal pain, arthritis, obesity); abnormal caecotroph production (e.g. due to low-fibre/ high-protein and carbohydrate diet, ingestion of novel food item or recent abrupt diet change)	Caking of caecotrophs around perineum; often mistaken for diarrhoea, but hard faecal output is often unaffected; perineal dermatopathy; secondary myiasis	Clinical signs; history, physical examination, oral examination and radiography (skull, spine, limbs) to identify underlying cause	Treat underlying cause. Dietary reform to high-fibre content, including reduced or no concentrate ration. Analgesia (short- or long-term depending on the underlying problem). Probiotics. Clipping and cleaning of soiled fur. Increased exercise. Regular grooming or clipping of perineal hair. Meticulous cage hygiene. May take several months to resolve

4.21 (continued) Selected common diseases of the pet rabbit. (continues) ▶

Disease	Cause	Clinical signs	Diagnostics	Treatment
Pinworm	*Passalurus ambiguus*	Usually non-pathogenic	Identification of adult worm/ova in faeces or tape test from perineum; can be seen within gut during abdominal surgery	Fenbendazole
Plantar pododermatitis ('sore hocks')	Secondary to poor husbandry (e.g. wet, soiled bedding), obesity, inactivity and genetic factors (e.g. Rex rabbits lack guard hairs so fur covering plantar foot surface more delicate); various bacteria may be involved (e.g. *Staphylococcus aureus*, *Streptococcus* spp.)	Alopecia, erythema and ulceration of plantar surface of hind feet; lameness; abscessation	Clinical signs; bacterial culture of exudates; radiography to check for osteomyelitis	Topical and systemic antibiosis (based on culture and sensitivity results). Analgesia (NSAIDs). Bandaging. Surgical debridement. Treat any underlying condition that may result in inactivity. Ensure clean, dry bedding at all times. Ensure plenty of room available for exercise. Improved husbandry. Weight reduction
Pregnancy toxaemia (see Hepatic lipidosis)				
Rabbit syphilis/ venereal spirochaetosis	*Treponema cuniculi*; direct contact/venereal spread; kits can be infected at birth; not zoonotic; symptomless carrier state; overt disease precipitated by stress	Ulcerative, crusting lesions around genitalia and face/legs from autoinoculation; sometimes localized oedema; secondary bacterial infection and eosinophilic granuloma formation	Detection of organism in direct smear (dark field background) or biopsy (silver stain)	Injectable penicillin. Treat in-contact rabbits. May resolve spontaneously
Renolith (see Urolithiasis)				
Sludgy bladder syndrome/ hypercalciuria	Retention of urine in the bladder leading to calcium crystals forming sediment (calcium sand), resulting in mucosal irritation and secondary cystitis; predisposing factors: obesity, inactivity (any cause), prolonged periods in hutch, dehydration/poor water intake and high-calcium diet	Dysuria; perineal urine scald; haematuria; abdominal pain; non-specific illness (dullness, anorexia)	Radiography; urinalysis; urine culture	Fluid therapy. Analgesia (NSAIDs). Bladder lavage with sterile saline via catheter. Assisted urination (regular expression of bladder). Antibiosis (if secondary infection present). Dietary correction if required. If urine scald present, clip and clean the perineum, apply topical antibiotics and provide clean, dry bedding and sufficient room to exercise
Spinal fracture/ luxation	Usually traumatic; pathological	Paresis/paralysis	History; clinical signs; radiography; myelography; serology (to rule out encephalitozoonosis)	Cage rest. NSAIDs. Supportive care. Hydrotherapy/physiotherapy. In trauma patients, absence of deep pain >4 hours after the injury occurred indicates a grave prognosis
Splay leg	Inherited disease, several genes involved	1–4 legs adducted; subluxation of hip in some cases	Signalment (generally young); clinical signs; radiography	None
Trichobezoar (large concretion of food and hair in the stomach)	Secondary to gastric hypomotility	Non-specific; anorexia; lethargy; reduced faecal output	Characteristic 'radiolucent gastric halo' can be seen on plain radiography of the cranial abdomen	Despite size, rarely cause obstruction and usually respond to medical therapy for gastrointestinal hypomotility (fluids, prokinetics, analgesics, nutritional support)
Tyzzer's disease (Clostridium piliforme; see Enteritis, bacterial)				
Urolithiasis (kidney, ureter, bladder or urethra)	May be associated with high dietary calcium intake and sludgy bladder syndrome	Haematuria; dysuria; abdominal pain; non-specific illness (anorexia, depression)	Radiography; ultrasonography; urinalysis; urolith analysis	Surgical removal generally required (e.g. cystotomy). Supportive care. Antibiosis if secondary infection present/suspected. Not possible to acidify rabbit urine. Correct any dietary imbalances. Ensure adequate fluid intake. Provide opportunity to urinate freely in clean, dry enclosure
Uterine adenocarcinoma (extremely common in older unmated does)	Progressive changes from hyperplasia to neoplasia; rapidly metastasize locally and to the lungs	Haematuria; vulval discharge; weight loss; palpable abdominal mass	Radiography (thorax for metastases and abdomen to assess primary mass); ultrasonography; exploratory surgery	Ovariohysterectomy. Euthanasia if metastases detected

4.21   (continued) Selected common diseases of the pet rabbit. (continues)   ▶

Disease	Cause	Clinical signs	Diagnostics	Treatment
Vertebral spondylosis/ spondylitis/ ankylosis/ osteomyelitis	Congenital; degenerative; infection, usually by haematogenous spread (e.g. *Pasteurella*)	Reluctance to move; paresis; inability to practise caecotrophy	Radiography	Analgesia (NSAIDs). Antibiotics (if osteomyelitis present). Euthanasia if clinical signs severe
Viral haemorrhagic disease	Calicivirus; spread by direct or indirect contact (fomites)	Usually sudden death; pyrexia; depression; haemorrhagic discharge from nose and mouth	Post-mortem examination; virus isolation	None; prevention by vaccination

4.21 (continued) Selected common diseases of the pet rabbit.

Clinical sign	Differential diagnoses	Further investigations
Abdominal distension	Gastric dilatation; ileus and gaseous distension of bowel; ascites (e.g. liver or cardiac disease); abdominal mass; pregnancy; obesity	Radiography (plain, contrast); ultrasonography; blood biochemistry; faecal analysis (e.g. to check for coccidial oocysts); ultrasound-guided peritoneal tap or liver FNA if indicated; ECG; exploratory surgery
Abdominal mass	Impaction (e.g. caecal); neoplasia (e.g. uterine adenocarcinoma); abscess; non-neoplastic uterine pathology (e.g. pyometra, hyperplasia/metritis); abdominal fat; fetus(es); foreign body; trichobezoar	Radiography (plain, contrast); ultrasonography; exploratory surgery
Alopecia	Cheyletiellosis (zoonotic); *Listrophorus*; barbering; normal moult; dermatophytosis	Microscopy of tape preparation, hair and skin scrape; fungal culture; skin biopsy
Anorexia	Any disease (acquired dental disease and gastroenteropathies most common); pain	CBC; blood biochemistry; urinalysis; dental examination under sedation; radiography (e.g. skull, abdomen, thorax); ultrasonography
Ataxia/seizures	Encephalitozoonosis; bacterial meningitis (e.g. *Pasteurella*, *Toxoplasma, Listeria*); heat stroke; trauma; toxoplasmosis; listeriosis; baylisascariasis (USA); pregnancy toxaemia	Neurological examination; CBC; blood biochemistry; urinalysis; faecal analysis; serology/PCR (*Encephalitozoon cuniculi*); radiography; skull CT or MRI; CSF tap
Dermatitis	Ectoparasites; rabbit syphilis; urine scald; 'Blue fur' disease; eosinophilic granuloma; dermatophytosis; self-trauma; viral infection (e.g. cutaneous myxomatosis); injection site reaction (e.g. following viral haemorrhagic disease (VHD) vaccination)	Microscopy of tape preparation or skin scrape; bacterial and fungal culture; skin biopsy; if perineal dermatitis, investigate urinary tract and gastrointestinal tract disease
Dyspnoea	Any respiratory disease (e.g. bacterial pneumonia/rhinitis, pulmonary abscess, pulmonary neoplasia); thoracic trauma (e.g. pneumothorax); cardiac disease; thymoma; pregnancy toxaemia/ hepatic lipidosis; metabolic acidosis; severe pain; acquired dental disease; stress; heat stroke; foreign body inhalation; allergies	Immediate therapy includes the provision of a warm, dark, quiet environment with 100% oxygen; once stabilized, diagnostic tests include: complete physical examination, skull and thoracic radiography, collection of deep nasal swabs under sedation for bacterial/fungal culture, CBC, blood biochemistry and cardiac assessment (e.g. ECG); urinalysis; handle minimally to avoid stress
Facial swelling	Facial/dental abscess; neoplasia; myxomatosis; cellulitis	Vaccination/contact history; skull radiography; skull CT; dental examination under sedation; biopsy
Haematuria	False haematuria (red/brown porphyrin pigments in urine); bacterial cystitis; urolithiasis; sludgy bladder syndrome; uterine hyperplasia; uterine adenocarcinoma; uterine venous aneurysm; urinary or reproductive polyps; renal infarcts; DIC or other coagulopathy	Husbandry; physical examination; urinalysis: dipstick, urine culture and cytology, use of a Wood's lamp to detect plant porphyrin pigments (fluorescent); CBC; blood biochemistry; abdominal radiography (plain, contrast); ultrasonography of urinary and reproductive tracts
Head tilt (torticollis)	Otitis media/interna; encephalitozoonosis; CNS neoplasia; trauma; meningitis; cerebral abscess; baylisascariasis (USA); listeriosis; toxoplasmosis	Aural examination; neurological examination (using the criteria for defining central *versus* peripheral vestibular disease in dogs/cats); pharyngeal examination under sedation; skull radiography; skull CT or MRI; serology and/or PCR (*Encephalitozoon cuniculi*); CBC; blood biochemistry; bacterial culture of material collected from middle ear (via tympanic membrane or bulla osteotomy); CSF tap
Nasal discharge/ upper respiratory stertor ('snuffles')	Pasteurellosis; other bacterial URT disease; fungal URT infection; nasal foreign body; allergic/irritant rhinitis (e.g. high environmental ammonia levels); acquired dental disease (cheek tooth impingement on URT); myxomatosis	Bacterial and fungal culture of deep nasal swabs; skull radiography; skull CT; environmental history
Ocular discharge	Dacryocystitis (nasolacrimal duct obstruction or infection); conjunctivitis (secondary to poor air quality or the presence of a foreign body); traumatic corneal injuries	Ophthalmic examination including fluoroscein stain; plain (± contrast) skull radiography; bacterial/fungal culture and/or cytology of conjunctival swabs; nasolacrimal duct flush

4.22 Differential diagnoses and diagnostic options based on common clinical signs. (continues) ▶

Clinical sign	Differential diagnoses	Further investigations
Pale mucous membranes (anaemia)	Uterine adenocarcinoma; uterine venous aneurysm; VHD; renal disease; any chronic disease; lead toxicosis	Signalment and history; CBC; blood biochemistry; radiography; ultrasonography; exploratory surgery (following stabilization)
Paresis/paralysis	Spinal trauma (fracture/luxation, e.g. secondary to incorrect handling, struggling or kicking); encephalitozoonosis; spondylosis/spondylitis; spinal abscess; intervertebral disc disease; toxoplasmosis	History; plain spinal radiography; serology and/or PCR (*Encephalitozoon cuniculi*); myelography; spinal MRI
Subcutaneous mass	Abscess; neoplasia; cyst; granuloma; haematoma; myxomatosis	FNA; excisional biopsy and bacterial culture/histopathology; vaccination/contact history
Testicular swelling	Orchitis; epididymitis; testicular neoplasia; haematoma; myxomatosis; rabbit syphilis	FNA; bacterial culture of aspirated material; testicular ultrasonography; biopsy/orchiectomy and histopathology
Urinary incontinence/urine scald	Cystitis; urolithiasis; sludgy bladder syndrome; spinal disease; obesity; renal failure; encephalitozoonosis; conditions that prevent normal positioning during urination (pododermatitis, obesity, arthritis, inadequate space); conditions that prevent normal grooming (dental disease, systemic illness); hormone-responsive incontinence (spayed does); poor husbandry (urine-soaked bedding); perineal dermatopathy (e.g. secondary to accumulation of uneaten caecotrophs)	Evaluation of husbandry; physical examination; urinalysis; urine culture; radiography (abdomen, spinal, skull); serology and/or PCR (*Encephalitozoon cuniculi*); CBC; blood biochemistry; response to hormone therapy
Vaginal discharge	Pyometra; metritis; uterine hyperplasia/adenocarcinoma; dystocia	Cytology and bacterial culture of discharge; radiography; ultrasonography; exploratory surgery
Weight loss	Acquired dental disease; renal failure; any infectious or metabolic disease; neoplasia; bullying	Dental examination under sedation; radiography (skull, thorax, abdomen); ultrasonography; urinalysis; CBC; blood biochemistry; serology; faecal analysis/culture

4.22 (continued) Differential diagnoses and diagnostic options based on common clinical signs.

Non-specific illness

Non-specific signs such as anorexia, lethargy and weight loss are the most frequent presenting complaints in rabbit practice. Pain is very difficult to assess in this species and rabbits with painful conditions often present with these non-specific signs, as well as a hunched posture, grinding their teeth or showing increased aggression. Careful history-taking, patient evaluation and selection of diagnostic tests will aid in the identification of the underlying problem. Monitoring of appetite, urine and faecal production, and observation of behaviour from a distance may provide vital clues. The prevalence of dental disease warrants a complete oral examination under sedation in any patient with non-specific signs.

Behavioural problems

Rabbits have not been bred for positive behaviour traits and as a result behavioural problems are common. Individual rabbits have distinct 'personalities', from timid to bold to aggressive. In general, smaller breeds tend to be more flighty.

Aggression is generally learned (the owner leaves the rabbit alone if it behaves aggressively). Other causes include territorial behaviour, boredom, pain, improper socialization and negative association (a previous aversive or traumatic situation). Behavioural aggression can be treated successfully in many cases with techniques similar to those used for dogs.

Does are more territorial than bucks, and as they reach sexual maturity they may become aggressive towards other animals (and owners). Does may also bite, dig and chew flooring and household items,

spray urine and mount other rabbits. If housed outdoors on soil, the doe may excavate deep tunnels.

Socialization of young rabbits is often overlooked. A well socialized pet rabbit will beg for treats, 'hum' and circle the owner, stand on its hindlegs and lick the owner's hands and arms. Rabbits are inquisitive and enjoy exploring. Picking up objects with the teeth and throwing them is common, as is exploratory chewing.

Supportive care

Drug administration

Parenteral
The most common methods for administering parenteral medication include subcutaneous, intradermal, intramuscular, intraperitoneal, intraosseous and intravenous. The route used will depend on the drug, the condition of the patient and clinician preference. In all cases, the smallest gauge needle should be selected that is practical given the viscosity of the material to be injected, the route to be used and the size of the patient. Parenteral administration of drugs and fluids is summarized in Figure 4.23.

Intraosseous catheterization

Indications:

- Administration of fluids or drugs in situations where intravenous access is limited or non-existent (e.g. rabbits in cardiogenic shock, juvenile rabbits).

Route	Sites	Comments
Subcutaneous	Theoretically any part of the body; generally the medication is instilled under the skin at the base of the neck or along the dorsum	Well tolerated in most rabbits. Relatively slow absorption. Large volumes (up to 100 ml in 4–5 kg rabbits) can be given but may need to be administered at several sites
Intradermal	Skin at base of ears, flanks, back	Most often used for administration of 1/10 of myxomatosis vaccine. A 25–27-gauge needle should be used. A 'bleb' in the skin indicates successful administration
Intramuscular	Dorsal lumbar muscles that lie on either side of the vertebral column, quadriceps muscles, semimembranosus muscle, semitendinosus muscle	The needle should be introduced at right angles to the centre of the muscle mass. Only suitable for volumes <1 ml. Can be painful
Intraperitoneal	Caudal to umbilicus, paramedian	Can give volumes up to 20 ml/kg. Care is required to minimize risk of abdominal organ puncture
Intraosseous	Proximal humerus, proximal tibia, proximal femur	Second only to intravenous administration if rapid absorption required
Intravenous	Marginal ear vein, cephalic vein, lateral saphenous vein	Most medications that are administered intravenously should be given slowly. If administering intravenous fluids via a giving set, all tubing should be secured away from the rabbit's mouth to prevent chewing
Subconjunctival	Into the bulbar conjunctiva	The use of local anaesthesia is recommended. The volume administered varies from 0.25–0.5 ml

4.23 Routes of administration for parenteral drugs and fluids.

Contraindications:

- Metabolic bone disease.
- Fractured bones.

Sites: Proximal femur, proximal tibia and proximal humerus.

Technique:

1. Clip and aseptically prepare the skin overlying the selected bone.
2. Infiltrate lidocaine into the local tissues and periosteum (unless the rabbit is under general anaesthesia).
3. Select an appropriate needle based on the size of the bone to be catheterized and materials available: a spinal needle, a standard hypodermic needle (with a piece of sterile wire or a smaller gauge needle acting as a stylet) or a commercially available intraosseous needle can be used.
4. Position the selected needle over the appropriate site and ensuring that the needle is straight and aligned in the direction of the bone, use it to bore a hole through the cortex of the bone (a sudden lack of resistance will be felt as the marrow cavity is penetrated) (Figure 4.24a).
5. Remove the stylet (if present) and flush with heparinized saline to ensure patency (Figure 4.24b).
6. Confirm the position using radiography.
7. Bandage the site.

Maintenance:

- An aseptic technique should always be used when administering fluid or medication via the intraosseous catheter.

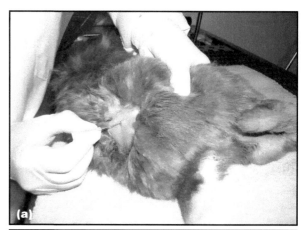

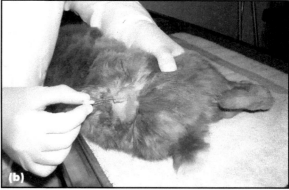

4.24 Intraosseous catheterization. **(a)** An intraosseous catheter (spinal needle) is placed in the proximal femur of a collapsed rabbit. **(b)** Removing the stylet. (Reproduced from *BSAVA Manual of Rabbit Medicine and Surgery, 2nd edition.*)

Other routes

Topical medication may be appropriate for certain ophthalmic, aural or dermatological conditions. Nebulization is a very useful therapeutic tool in the management of respiratory disease in rabbits.

Fluid therapy

Fluid therapy (most commonly with crystalloids) is frequently indicated in critically ill rabbits. Indications for colloidal fluids (including blood transfusion) are as for other species (i.e. shock, severe blood loss). Ideally, fluids should be given intravenously and warmed to body temperature. Alternative routes include oral, subcutaneous and intraosseous.

- Maintenance fluid requirements are 75–100 ml/kg/day.
- Estimates for dehydration include:
  - 5% for rabbits with mild gastrointestinal hypomotility
  - 5–8% if mucous membranes are dry and skin turgor increased
  - 10–12% if the eyes are sunken, CRT is slow, the rabbit is depressed and pulse is rapid and weak.

Nutritional support

The importance of nutritional therapy in the care of the ill rabbit cannot be overstated. Rabbits require a regular intake of high-fibre food to ensure gut motility is maintained, to facilitate rehydration, to support hepatic function, to provide a calorie intake sufficient to support recovery, and to maintain the population of gut microbes that are essential for normal physiological function. Fresh, quality food must be available at all times to hospitalized rabbits. Syringe feeding of commercially available high-fibre products or mashed pellets/vegetables is required if the animal is anorexic, and is well tolerated by most rabbits if carried out correctly with patience. For rabbits unable or unwilling to swallow, the placement of a nasogastric or oesophagostomy tube may be considered to facilitate life-saving nutritional therapy.

Syringe feeding

1. Restrain the patient in a suitable manner (on an examination table, on the floor or wrapped in a towel).
2. Gently insert the nozzle of a syringe into the mouth behind the incisor teeth on either side and direct towards the caudal mouth.
3. Administer a small volume of liquid (0.5–3 ml), remove the syringe, and wait for the rabbit to swallow before administering more. If the rabbit will not swallow the material, an alternative method of administration must be considered.

Nasogastric tube placement

Indications:

- To facilitate administration of oral fluids, nutrition and medication to critically ill rabbits in situations where syringe feeding is not possible (e.g. patients with swallowing disorders, following extensive oral surgery, or anorexic rabbits that do not tolerate frequent handling).

Technique:

1. Premeasure a 5–8 French catheter (depending on size of the rabbit) from the external nares to the caudal end of the sternum.
2. Instil a few drops of topical local anaesthetic into the nostril.
3. Apply a small amount of lubricant to the tip of the catheter.
4. Elevate the head and insert the catheter into the ventral nasal meatus, advancing ventromedially.
5. Keep the neck partially flexed as the catheter enters the oesophagus and advance the catheter to the predetermined level.
6. Radiography is recommended to ensure correct placement of the catheter before administration of fluids/food.
7. Secure the catheter to the rabbit's head using a flap of tape and tissue glue or a suture. The placement of an Elizabethan-style collar should be considered (Figure 4.25).

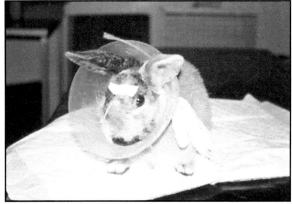

4.25 Nasogastric tube *in situ*. Note that the catheter has been secured to the rabbit's head using tape.

Anaesthesia and analgesia

Rabbits have an unnecessary reputation for being difficult to anaesthetize. With the correct techniques, there is no reason why rabbits can not be safely and successfully anaesthetized. The main problems relate to the high susceptibility of rabbits to stress, and underlying respiratory disease.

Preoperative care

It is not necessary to fast rabbits before anaesthesia as they are unable to vomit. Systemically ill rabbits are often dehydrated (if anorexic for any reason) and may be hypoglycaemic; these conditions must be corrected prior to anaesthesia to reduce complications. Rabbits with overt respiratory disease are considered high-risk patients, and ideally this should be treated or controlled before anaesthesia is attempted.

Anaesthesia

Premedication is an important consideration in rabbits as they are easily stressed. A high percentage of rabbits have serum atropinesterase, so glycopyrrolate at 0.01 mg/kg s.c. can be used as an alternative anticholinergic to atropine if desired. Suitable premedicants include:

- Fentanyl/fluanisone
- Medetomidine
- Xylazine
- Acepromazine
- Diazepam
- Midazolam.

Facemask or chamber induction without premedication should be avoided as rabbits breath-hold when exposed to all volatile agents, even at low concentrations, for periods up to 2 minutes. In addition, stress causes the release of catecholamines which can produce serious systemic effects under anaesthesia. Fentanyl/fluanisone or another premedicant, followed by mask induction results in the smooth onset of anaesthesia. Alternatively, an injectable combination can be used (Figure 4.26).

- Fentanyl/fluanisone plus midazolam, gives 30–40 minutes of surgical anaesthesia. Partial reversal with retention of analgesia can be achieved with buprenorphine or butorphanol.
- Alternatively, medetomidine plus ketamine is a good combination, to which butorphanol or buprenorphine can also be added. The addition of butorphanol prolongs anaesthetic time from approximately 30 minutes to about 80 minutes. This combination can be partially reversed with atipamezole.

When using an injectable regime, especially one containing an alpha-2 agonist, it is prudent to administer oxygen concurrently by facemask. Alternative anaesthetic agents include propofol and alfaxalone, which can be used alone or in combination with other drugs. An Ayres T-piece circuit or Bain circuit should be used.

Intubation

Rabbits are intubated either by direct visualization or using a blind technique; both methods rely on correct positioning of the rabbit's head and neck for success. Following induction, the rabbit is placed in sternal recumbency with head and neck extended vertically and the nose pointing toward the ceiling. The rabbit should be allowed to breathe 100% oxygen for 3–4 minutes before intubation is attempted. Severe, life-threatening laryngospasm can occur if the glottis is even moderately irritated during intubation, so use of local anaesthetic spray is recommended. The tube should never be forced into the larynx as this causes haemorrhage and oedema. Holding the tongue to one side is often useful. Endotracheal tubes with a 2–3 mm diameter are most commonly used for average-sized rabbits.

Direct visualization:

1. Visualize the larynx using a laryngoscope, otoscope or endoscope.
2. Insert the endotracheal tube (with the aid of an introducer if required).

Drug	Dose	Comments
Fentanyl/Fluanisone	0.2–0.5 ml/kg i.m. initially then incremental doses of 0.1 ml/kg i.m. may be administered every 30–40 minutes	Well tolerated by systemically unwell rabbits. Will produce sedation (not anaesthesia) within 10–20 minutes, provides analgesia without muscle relaxation. Can be reversed with buprenorphine at 0.01–0.05 mg/kg or butorphanol at 0.1–0.5 mg/kg s.c./i.m./i.v.
Midazolam or Diazepam + Buprenorphine	0.25–1.0 mg/kg Mi or D i.m./i.v. + 0.03 mg/kg Bp s.c.	Sedation
Ketamine + Acepromazine	25–40 mg/kg K + 0.25–0.5 mg/kg ACP i.m./i.v.	Sedation
Ketamine + Diazepam	25–40 mg/kg K + 0.5–2.0 mg/kg D i.m./i.v.	Sedation
Fentanyl/Fluanisone (Hypnorm®) + Diazepam or Midazolam	0.2–0.5 ml/kg FF i.m. + 0.5–2.0 mg/kg D or Mi i.v.	Full recovery may take 4–6 hours without reversal; if high-dose benzodiazepine used may have prolonged recovery. Reverse FF with butorphanol or buprenorphine (as above)
Propofol + Isoflurane	5–10 mg/kg P slow i.v. + 2–3% I	Intubation recommended as apnoea may occur. Rapid induction and recovery
Medetomidine + Ketamine ± Butorphanol	0.1–0.25 mg/kg Me + 5–10 mg/kg K ± 0.5mg/kg Bt i.m.	Good combination for healthy rabbits undergoing routine procedures. Will provide anaesthesia for 20–40 minutes. Can be reversed (at least 10–45 minutes after medetomidine administration to avoid risk of re-sedation) with atipamezole (same volume as medetomidine, i.e. 5 x medetomidine dose in mg). Rapid recovery
Medetomidine + Alfaxalone ± Isoflurane	0.25 mg/kg Me s.c. + 5 mg/kg Al i.m. ± 0.5–3% I	Reverse medetomidine with atipamezole (as above)
Alfaxalone	5 mg/kg Al i.v. then top-up slow i.v. or continuous infusion to effect for maintenance	Preoxygenate. Slow injection over 60 seconds minimizes risk of apnoea
Xylazine + Ketamine	3–5 mg/kg X + 35 mg/kg K i.m.	Results in 20–30 minutes anaesthesia, with recovery in 1–2 hours

4.26 Selected sedative and anaesthetic combinations. Note that individual variations in response occur with all these drugs.

Blind technique:

1. Pass the endotracheal tube over the tongue and advance whilst listening or (if using a clear tube) watching at the end of the tube for the presence of condensation at each breath.
2. Advance tube gently as the rabbit inhales, passing it into the trachea.

Intraoperative care

Depth of anaesthesia should be monitored by use of the ear pinch or the hindlimb toe pinch, both of which should be just absent for surgical anaesthesia. Standard monitoring equipment (electrocardiogram, pulse oximeter, capnograph, blood pressure measurement) should be used wherever possible. Eye position is not useful in the rabbit, and the palpebral reflex is not lost until the anaesthetic depth is dangerously deep. Heat loss should be minimized given the rabbit's relatively large surface area to bodyweight ratio. Clipping large areas should be avoided as should the overuse of cooling antiseptic solutions. In addition, an external heat source should be provided (e.g. heated surgical table, heat mat).

Postoperative care

Rabbits should be kept warm but not too hot, and excessive handling should be avoided in the postoperative period. Fluid therapy may be necessary and the rabbit should be monitored closely until eating again. Where possible, rabbits should be hospitalized to monitor appetite and faecal output, and to ensure adequate levels of analgesia are provided. Prokinetic medication (metoclopramide, cisapride and/or ranitidine) and syringe feeding of high-fibre gruels or mashes should be given at regular intervals until the rabbit's appetite has returned and faecal output is approaching normal. Rabbits should also be monitored for postoperative wound swelling, chewing of sutures and haemorrhage, depending on the procedure.

Analgesia

Pre-emptive analgesia in the pre- and perioperative period, and the alleviation of postoperative pain are essential components of rabbit anaesthesia and surgery. Insufficient analgesia will depress appetite, slow gut motility and hamper recovery. Buprenorphine and butorphanol are useful opioid agents, and reverse the respiratory and cardiovascular depressant effects of fentanyl whilst maintaining analgesia. The non-steroidal anti-inflammatory drugs (NSAIDs) meloxicam and carprofen are also highly effective and can be used alone or in combination with opioids (mixed or pure agonist opioids). Local anaesthetic agents may be indicated in some cases.

Common surgical procedures

The basic principles of veterinary surgery described for other domestic species are applicable to rabbits. However, surgical techniques and considerations may need to be modified to account for the unique anatomy, physiology and behaviour of rabbits. Rabbits can be challenging surgical patients but the chance of a successful outcome can be maximized by ensuring:

- Good knowledge of regional anatomy
- Adequate patient preparation
- Suitable instrumentation
- Steps are taken to minimize pain, fear and stress experienced by the patient.

Rabbits differ greatly from other species in response to pain, stress and surgical procedures. They may become anorexic following surgery with post-anaesthetic ileus a relatively common sequel.

General considerations

- During preparation of the surgical site, care must be taken to avoid tearing the thin skin with clippers. Tensing the skin minimizes the risk of trauma.
- Blood loss of 20–30% of total blood volume is critical; 10% of total blood volume may be lost without undue concern in healthy rabbits.
- Intra-abdominal adhesions are common in rabbits following surgery and the use of calcium-channel blockers has been advocated to counteract this (e.g. verapamil can be given postoperatively to patients who have suffered trauma to the abdominal organs). More importantly, organs must be handled gently to avoid adhesions.
- Suture material reactions are more common in rabbits due to the immune response to foreign material (the production of caseous pus) and the tendency to form adhesions. Fine-gauge, synthetic, absorbable, monofilament suture materials are recommended and haemostatic clips can be extremely useful.
- Intradermal suture patterns are preferred to close skin wounds in rabbits since they are fastidious at grooming and will commonly chew sutures. Similarly, rabbits are skilled at removing dressings.

Ovariohysterectomy

Ovariohysterectomy (spay) is recommended for all non-breeding does as a preventive measure against uterine adenocarcinoma. Additional indications may include aggressive and/or hypersexual behaviour, nest building and fur pulling. Generally rabbits are spayed at 5–6 months of age.

- Ovariohysterectomy is achieved via a standard ventral midline approach, with the incision made half way between the umbilicus and pubis.
- The abdominal musculature is extremely thin and care should be taken when entering the abdominal cavity. The caecum and bladder lie directly under the incision and iatrogenic damage is common.
- Reproductive anatomy is very different to that of the dog and cat. Does often has a large amount of periovarian and periuterine fat, the mesometrium being a primary site of fat storage. This makes identification of blood vessels difficult. The vagina in rabbits is very large and flaccid. The urethra enters the caudal vaginal vestibule and

retrograde filling with urine is common. The uterus is turgid and bright pink and is easily identified.

- Each uterine horn is followed carefully to locate the ovary. The ovarian vessels are small and haemorrhage is rare.
- Ligatures are placed around the ovarian vessels using a synthetic absorbable suture material. Vessels within the broad ligament may also need to be ligated if they are well developed.
- The uterine vessels lie several millimetres lateral to the uterus and should be ligated separately, followed by a transfixing ligature around the cranial vagina, just caudal to the cervices.
- Oversewing the vaginal stump is often performed to prevent urine contamination of the abdomen.
- Stump uterine adenocarcinomas can occur in rabbits that have been spayed with ligation proximal to the cervices.
- Abdominal and skin closure is routine.

Orchiectomy

Routine orchiectomy (castration) in bucks is recommended from 4–5 months of age. The indications include reduction of aggressive or hypersexual behaviour, cessation of breeding and cessation of urine spraying.

- Bucks have an open inguinal ring; therefore, a closed castration technique should be used, or an open technique followed by closure of the tunic. In the intact buck, large inguinal fat pads associated with the epididymis prevent herniation and intestinal strangulation. These lie in the inguinal canal when the testes are in the scrotum.
- The buck is placed in dorsal recumbency, and the scrotum and prescrotal area surgically prepared. Great care should be taken not to cut the skin in this area, which is extremely thin. There are two methods of castration commonly used:
  - *Closed technique:*
    - An incision is made over the scrotum on each side, taking care not to cut through the vaginal tunic.
    - The testis is removed from the scrotum and a ligature placed around the cord (following double clamping) (Figure 4.27) prior to removal of the testis.
    - The subcutaneous tissue and skin can be sutured as this tends to be more aesthetically pleasing to the client, but is not always necessary.
  - *Open technique:*
    - A scrotal or prescrotal incision is made on either side. The tunic is also incised and an open castration performed with a ligature again placed around the vas deferens and the vascular structures using a double clamp method. Following removal of the testis the tunic is closed with a continuous suture pattern and the skin closed routinely.

Bucks should be kept separate from entire does for 6 weeks postoperatively.

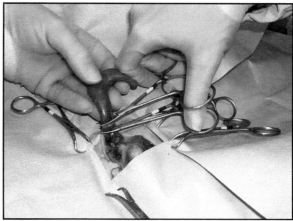

4.27 Castration of a buck using a closed technique. Following a scrotal incision, each testis is exteriorized without incising through the tunic. Double clamps have been applied to the cord prior to ligature placement.

Other procedures

Exploratory laparotomy

1. Midline approach.
2. Inspect all organs in sequence.
3. Take samples as required (e.g. liver biopsy).
4. Routine 2–3 layer closure.

Cystotomy

1. Midline incision.
2. Exteriorize the bladder and pack adequately to prevent contamination.
3. Place stay sutures (Figure 4.28).
4. Incise in an avascular location; urethral catheterization may be helpful.
5. Closure of bladder wall using a 2 layer inverting technique.
6. Routine closure of laparotomy site.

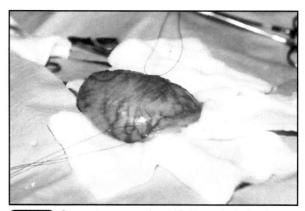

4.28 Stay sutures are placed in the exteriorized bladder of this rabbit undergoing cystotomy for removal of a urolith.

Gastrotomy

1. Midline incision.
2. Exteriorize the stomach and pack adequately to prevent contamination.

3. Incise in an avascular site along the greater curvature or between the greater and lesser curvatures.
4. Closure in 2 layers; as with any enteric surgery, gloves and surgical instruments should be changed prior to abdominal closure.

Abscess removal

Complete excision of the abscess and its capsule is recommended. In addition, any associated teeth should be removed if the abscess is of dental origin (Figure 4.29). If complete excision is not possible, marsupialization and daily flushing or instilment of an antibiotic preparation, or placement of antibiotic-impregnated gel/polymethylmethacrylate (PMMA) beads and closure should be considered.

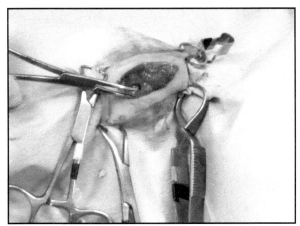

4.29 Surgical debridement of a mandibular abscess of dental origin. Associated teeth and tooth fragments must be removed to limit the risk of recurrence.

Enucleation

Enucleation can be achieved by either a trans-conjunctival (Figure 4.30) or transpalpebral technique. It should be noted that in the rabbit there is a large venous sinus behind the eye and, if damaged, the area should be packed for a minimum of 5 minutes; use of haemostatic aids is helpful. The Harderian and lacrimal glands and eyelid margins should be removed at the time of surgery.

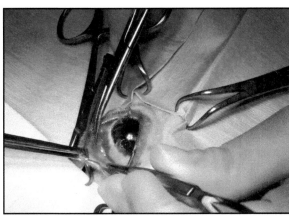

4.30 Transconjunctival approach to enucleation. This patient had a large retrobulbar abscess that had caused severe unilateral exophthalmos and subsequent refractory keratitis.

Orthopaedic repair

Normal rabbit bones have thin cortices compared with those of dogs and cats and are therefore more prone to splintering and shattering. Depending on the type and location of the fracture, fixation may be achieved with:

- External coaptation
- Internal fixation (e.g. intramedullary pin or bone screws)
- External fixation: Type I or Type 2 external fixators.

Limb amputation

Rabbits tend to cope well on three limbs following surgery, provided that they are not obese and that they do not have pre-existing arthritis.

- Forelimb: amputate at the level of the mid-humerus or at the scapula.
- Hindlimb: amputate at the level of the proximal third of the femur or at the coxofemoral joint.

Dental correction and extraction

Incisor coronal reduction

Incisor trimming can be performed without difficulty in conscious rabbits, using either high- or low-speed dental equipment (Figure 4.31). Clippers should not be used as they leave sharp edges and longitudinal cracks in the teeth and will often expose the pulp. Clipping also releases a considerable amount of energy into the tooth, concussing the pulp, and damaging the periodontal and periapical tissues.

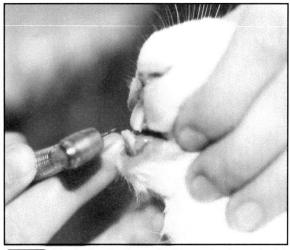

4.31 The incisor teeth can be trimmed using a dental burr.

Incisor extraction

Incisor extraction (Figure 4.32) is indicated in cases of primary and secondary incisor malocclusion. Cheek teeth should be evaluated at the time and any abnormalities corrected.

- Dental nerve blocks can be placed to improve analgesia as part of a multimodel strategy.
  - Upper incisors: infraorbital nerve – infiltrate local anaesthetic at the infraorbital foramen

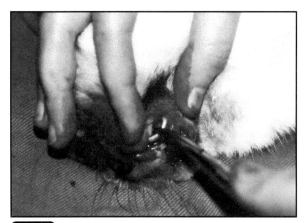

4.32 Incisor extraction.

on the lateral aspect of the skull, adjacent to the upper first premolar. The facial tuber can be palpated laterally as a bony protuberance and the infraorbital foramen lies 4–10 mm dorsal to this.
- – Lower incisors: metal nerve – the foramen is 2–4 mm rostral to the lower first premolar and located two-thirds of the way up the body of the mandible at this point.
- – Mix lidocaine (2%) with bupivacaine (0.5%) in a syringe and use 0.05 ml lidocaine and 0.18 ml bupivacaine per kg bodyweight as the total dose given, diluted with water to allow the total volume to be divided into the number of sites to block.
- The gingival attachment around the tooth should be cut using a proprietary elevator, a hypodermic needle or a No. 11 scalpel blade.
- The periodontal ligament should be elevated all around the tooth. It should be ensured that the elevator follows the line of the tooth, taking into account its natural curvature. The ligament is strongest on the medial and lateral sides of the tooth.
- Before the tooth is removed it should be gently rotated and pressed back into the socket to destroy germinal tissue and prevent re-growth.
- The tooth can then be extracted using gentle traction. Excessive traction may result in fracture of the tooth, especially if it is of poor quality. If a tooth breaks, the rabbit must be re-presented a few weeks later when the crown has re-erupted for completion of the extraction. If the periapical tissues have been damaged, re-growth may not occur and surgery may be required to retrieve the stump before it serves as a nidus for infection or progresses to tooth root abscessation.
- Analgesia must be provided in the postoperative period and food items should be prepared in bite-sized particles (e.g. vegetables may be chopped or grated).

The normal rabbit uses the incisors for grooming. An incisorless rabbit should therefore be groomed regularly by the owner to prevent matting of the coat.

Cheek teeth coronal reduction
Burring of the cheek teeth requires sedation/anaesthesia, a rabbit mouth gag and cheek dilators. A straight slow-speed dental handpiece with a long-shanked burr is recommended. Simply removing sharp edges or 'points' is not effective as this leaves the primary problem, tooth elongation, untreated. By reducing the exposed crowns to a normal height, the spikes will be removed in the process and, providing there are minimal apical changes, the teeth will start erupting again following treatment, allowing for more normal wear patterns. Rasps are unsuitable as they apply too much force, often tearing the periodontal ligament and on occasion causing tooth fracture. Burring removes the normal transverse occlusal ridging so chewing efficiency is greatly reduced until this re-forms. Chewing efficiency is also reduced for a few days as the jaw muscles recover following stretching associated with gag placement for exposure of the oral cavity.

Cheek teeth extraction
Some abnormal cheek teeth may be extracted intraorally by simple traction if the periodontal ligament is weak or root pathology is such that the tooth is loose.

- The curvature of the tooth should be taken into account when attempting to perform an extraction.
- If the periodontal ligament is still intact, it may be broken down using a modified elevator. The small size of the oral cavity relative to the instrument makes intraoral manipulation of the tooth difficult.
- Once loosened the tooth should be intruded into its alveolus and manipulated to help destroy any remaining germinal tissue prior to removal. The pulp should remain in the extracted tooth. If the pulp does not remain in the extracted tooth, the germinal tissues are probably intact and should be actively curetted using a sterile instrument.
- If the germinal tissues are left intact the tooth will re-grow, possibly as a normal tooth, but more likely with gross deformity.
- An extraoral approach must be considered if extraction is indicated but the periodontal ligament is intact.

Euthanasia

Euthanasia of rabbits is usually performed by intravenous injection of pentobarbital. The marginal ear vein is a useful site and the application of local anaesthetic cream will often prevent any discomfort associated with venepuncture. Nervous rabbits can be sedated (e.g. with a benzodiazepine or fentanyl/fluanisone) to aid restraint for the procedure. If intravenous access cannot be achieved, the rabbit can be anaesthetized (by injectable and/or inhalational methods) and the pentobarbital injection given into a well perfused organ (e.g. kidney or liver) or directly into the heart. Intraosseous administration is also effective.

Drug formulary

Given that the availability of authorized products for the treatment of disease in rabbits is limited, informed client consent should be obtained before proceeding with 'off-label' use of drugs.

- Ampicillin, clindamycin and lincomycin must not be administered to rabbits as they may induce a fatal gastrointestinal dysbiosis.
- Similarly, oral cephalosporins and oral penicillins should be avoided. If given parenterally (e.g. subcutaneously), cephalosporins and pencillins appear to be safe and effective choices for anaerobic infections.
- Fipronil is not recommended as an ectoparasiticide as adverse reactions (some fatal) have been reported with the use of both the spot-on and spray formulations in rabbits.
- Care should be taken with the use of corticosteroids in rabbits (both topical and systemic) as they are very sensitive to the adverse effects of these drugs. However, if considered clinically relevant, low doses of a short-acting formulation may be used with caution. In situations where longer term use is warranted, clients must be informed of the risks and close monitoring of the patient is recommended.

A basic drug formulary is presented in Figure 4.33.

Drug	Dose	Comments
Antimicrobial agents		
Cefalexin	15–20 mg/kg s.c. q12h	**DO NOT GIVE ORALLY**
Enrofloxacin	10 mg/kg s.c./orally q12h or 20 mg/kg s.c./orally q24h	Limited anaerobic activity. Baytril® authorized for use in rabbits
Fusidic acid	Ophthalmic preparation: apply to affected eye(s) q12–24h Dermatological preparation: apply to affected skin q24h for at least 3 days	Fucithalmic Vet® (ophthalmic preparation) authorized for use in rabbits
Gentamicin	Systemic preparation: 1.5–2.5 mg/kg s.c./i.m./i.v. q8h Topical preparation: 1–2 drops q8h for 5–7 days	Tiacil® (topical) authorized for use in rabbits
Metronidazole	20 mg/kg orally q12h	Good anaerobic spectrum
Oxytetracycline	15 mg/kg s.c./i.m. q24h	
Procaine benzylpenicillin	60,000 IU/kg s.c. q2–7d	**DO NOT GIVE ORALLY**
Trimethoprim/Sulphonamide	30–40 mg/kg orally q12h	
Antiparasitic agents		
Albendazole	15–20 mg/kg orally q24h for 2–4 weeks	For *Encephalitozoon cuniculi* infection
Fenbendazole	For gastrointestinal nematodes: 10–20 mg/kg orally; repeat in 14 days For *E. cuniculi*: 20 mg/kg orally q24h for 28 days	Lapizole® and Panacur Rabbit® available as oral formulations of fenbendazole for rabbits
Fipronil	**DO NOT USE**	Serious adverse reactions reported
Imidacloprid	40 mg for rabbits <4 kg 80 mg for rabbits >4 kg Apply topically to skin at back of neck once weekly as required	For flea treatment and prevention; Advantage® authorized for use in rabbits
Toltrazuril	25 mg/kg orally q24h for 2 days; repeat after 5 days	
Analgesics		
Buprenorphine	0.01–0.05 mg/kg s.c./i.m./i.v. q6–12h	
Butorphanol	0.1–0.5 mg/kg s.c./i.m./i.v. q4h	
Carprofen	2–4 mg/kg s.c. q24h	
Meloxicam	0.3–0.6 mg/kg s.c./orally q24h	Can be used long term
Miscellaneous		
Cisapride	0.5 mg/kg orally q8–12h	Prokinetic
Critical Care for Herbivores® (Oxbow)	Minimum of 50 ml/kg/day by syringe; divide into 4–5 doses throughout day	Nutritional therapy for anorexia
Dexamethasone	0.3–0.6 mg/kg s.c./i.m./i.v. q24h	**USE WITH EXTREME CAUTION.** Rabbits are highly sensitive to the adverse effects of systemic and topical corticosteroids
Furosemide	0.3–2 mg/kg i.v./i.m./s.c. q12h	Diuretic

4.33 Drug formulary for rabbits. (continues) ▶

Drug	Dose	Comments
Miscellaneous continued		
Lactated Ringer's Solution	Maintenance 75–100 mg/kg/day i.v./s.c.	Fluid therapy
Metoclopramide	0.5 mg/kg s.c./orally q6–8h	Prokinetic
Pentobarbital	20–45 mg/kg i.v./i.p.	Euthanasia
Ranitidine	2 mg/kg i.v. q24h or 2–5 mg/kg orally q12h	Prokinetic

4.33 (continued) Drug formulary for rabbits.

References and further reading

Crossley DA (1995) Clinical aspects of lagomorph dental anatomy: the rabbit (*Oryctolagus cuniculus*). *Journal of Veterinary Dentistry* **4**, 131–135

Harcourt-Brown FM (2007) The progressive syndrome of acquired dental disease in rabbits. *Journal of Exotic Pet Medicine* **16(3)**, 146–157

Meredith A and Flecknell P (2006) *BSAVA Manual of Rabbit Medicine and Surgery 2nd edn.* BSAVA Publications, Gloucester

O'Malley B (2005) *Clinical Anatomy and Physiology of Exotic Species*. Elsevier Saunders, Edinburgh

Paul-Murphy J and Ramer JC (1998) Urgent care of the pet rabbit. *Veterinary Clinics of North America: Exotic Animal Practice* **1(1)**, 127–152

Quesenberry KE and Carpenter JW (2004) *Ferrets, Rabbits and Rodents: Clinical Medicine and Surgery, 2nd edn.* Saunders, St Louis

Suter C, Muller-Doblies UU, Hatt J-M, *et al.* (2001) Prevention and treatment of *Encephalitozoon cuniculi* infection in rabbits with fenbendazole. *Veterinary Record* **148**, 478–480

Wiggs RB and Lobprise HB (1995) Dentistry in pet lagomorphs and rodents. In: *BSAVA Manual of Small Animal Dentistry, 2nd edn*, ed. DA Crossley and S Penman, pp. 68–92. BSAVA Publications, Cheltenham

5

Marsupials

Cathy Johnson-Delaney

Introduction

There are several types of marsupial, including:

- Petauridae – gliders (they do not have ossa marsupiala)
- Monodelphidae
  – South American opossums (e.g. the short-tailed opossum, *Monodelphis domestica*, is seen in the pet trade)
- Didelphidae – North American opossums (e.g. Virginia opossum, *Didelphis virginiana*)
- Phalangerids – include the Brushtail possum (*Trichosurus vulpecula*)
- Macropodidae ('large foot') – kangaroos, wallabies and wallaroos
- Dasyurids – carnivorous marsupials, which are not kept as pets (e.g. Tasmanian devil, *Sarcophilus harrisii*).

Possum or opossum?
Although the terms are used interchangeably, the correct nomenclature is as follows:

- **Old World possums (such as the Brushtail) are *possums***
- **New World 'possums' (such as the Virginia) are *opossums*.**

Companion marsupials commonly seen in exotic pet practice include the sugar glider, the short-tailed opossum, the Virginia opossum and wallabies (Figure 5.1). In addition, the Brushtail possum (*Trichosurus vulpecula*) is occasionally found as a pet; although it is banned from importation from New Zealand into the USA due to the high infection rate with *Mycobacterium bovis,* a number are still found, called 'phalangers' to avoid confiscation. It should be noted

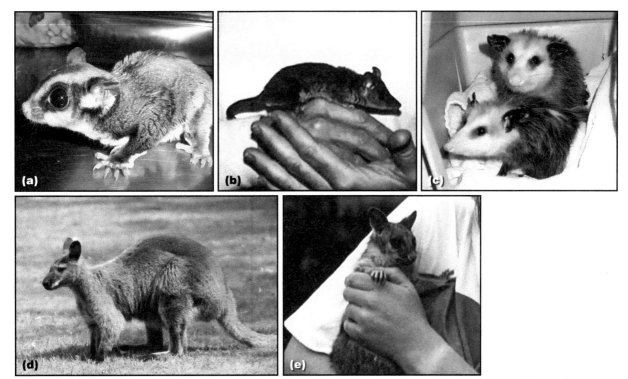

5.1 Marsupials seen in practice. **(a)** Sugar glider (*Petaurus breviceps*). (Courtesy of D. Johnson.) **(b)** South American short-tailed opossum (*Monodelphis domestica*). **(c)** Two 6-month-old Virginia opossums (*Didelphis virginiana*). **(d)** Bennett's wallaby (*Macropus rufogriseus rufogriseus*). (Courtesy of I. Sayers.) **(e)** A 6-month-old Brushtail possum (*Trichosurus vulpecula*).

that not all marsupials have pouches or the ossa marsupiala (i.e. the marsupial bones and pelvic ribs). One common feature of marsupials is that they all give birth to a fetus which develops outside the uterus. The general practitioner is encouraged to search the literature and build a reference collection concerning diet, husbandry, medical and surgical care.

Biology

Australian marsupials fill all the environmental niches that placental (eutherian) mammals fill on other continents. Kangaroos graze in a similar manner to wild cervids (e.g. deer, elk); possums, gliders and koala bears are primarily arboreal and utilize trees, fruit and bark in a similar manner to non-human primates and squirrels; and some marsupials are primarily carnivorous or insectivorous in a similar manner to wild canids, felids, procyonids (raccoons) and mustelids (pine martins, fishers, polecats). Many land-dwelling marsupials (such as the wombat) dig tunnels and utilize plants and insects in a similar manner to rodents and rabbits. Although, large carnivorous marsupials are now extinct, there existed one animal known as the Tasmanian tiger or wolf (*Thylacinus cynocephalus*), which hunted herbivorous mammals. Today the largest carnivorous marsupial is the Tasmanian devil, confined to the island of Tasmania, although smaller carnivores such as the quoll (*Dasyrurus* spp.) and other dasyurids exist throughout the rest of Australia.

Marsupials generally have woolly fur (i.e. the fur does not appear to lie in a particular direction). Their olfactory and tactile senses and hearing are well developed. Heart rates are usually about half those seen in equivalent-sized eutherian mammals.

Sugar gliders

The sugar glider (*Petaurus breviceps*; see Figure 5.1a) is native to New Guinea and Australia, with at least seven recognized subspecies. Their habitats are primarily open forest – either tropical or coastal, or dry inland sclerophyll tropical. Sugar gliders are nocturnal and arboreal, nesting in leaf-lined tree holes with up to six other adults and young. Gliding distance can be up to 50 metres. The gliding membrane (patagium) extends from the fifth digit of the forepaws to the ankles (Figure 5.2). The first and second digits of the hind feet are partially fused (syndactylous). The tail is well furred and weakly prehensile. Males have scent glands on the forehead, chest and cloaca (paracloacal glands); the female's scent glands are within the pouch. Sugar gliders are quite vocal, with a whole series of alarm yaps and screams. Biological data are summarized in Figure 5.3.

South American (Brazilian) short-tailed opossums

The short-tailed opossum (*Monodelphis domestica*; see Figure 5.1b) comes from eastern and central Brazil, Bolivia and Paraguay. It has been used extensively as a laboratory animal.

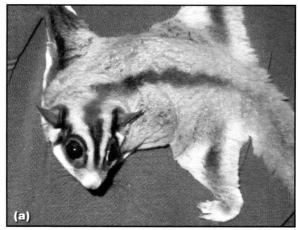

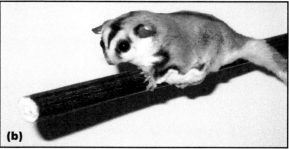

5.2 **(a)** The gliding membrane of the sugar glider extends from the neck to the tail, incorporating both the forelimbs and the hindlimbs. Note the lack of nail on the first digit on both the front and back legs. **(b)** The gliding membrane also gathers on the ventrum.

Lifespan (years)	In the wild: 4–5 (up to 9 recorded) In captivity: 12–14 (optimum diet and husbandry)
Bodyweight (g)	Varies with subspecies. Larger: males 115–160; females 95–135
Length (mm)	Head plus body: 120–132 Tail: 15–480
Body temperature (°C)	Average 32
Heart rate (beats/min)	Awake: 200–300
Respiration rate (breaths/min)	Awake: 16–40

5.3 Biological data for the sugar glider.

Short-tailed opossums usually dwell on the ground but they can climb. Nests are usually built in hollow logs. The animals are basically nocturnal but, as pets, they do spend time interacting with owners during the day. They will use rat wheels for exercise. In South America they live in human dwellings, where they are welcome, as they destroy rodents, insects, and arachnids such as scorpions. Individuals are highly intolerant of each other, though conflicts rarely result in serious injury. The tail is about half as long as the head and body, but always shorter than the body alone, and is sparsely haired. It is prehensile and is used to carry bedding and other items back to the nest. Dentition is closed rooted. Biological data are summarized in Figure 5.4.

Lifespan (years)	2–4 (up to 6 in captivity)
Bodyweight (g)	Males: 90–150 Females: 80–100
Length (cm)	Head: 11–20 Body: 7–16 Tail: 4.5–8
Food consumption (adults)	5 g per day
Water consumption (adults)	5 ml per day
Figures for body temperature, heart rate and respiration rate have not been published; however, in the author's experience they are comparable to those for the sugar glider	

5.4 Biological data for the short-tailed opossum.

Virginia opposums

The Virginia opposum (*Didelphis virginiana*; see Figure 5.1c) is the only marsupial that is native to North America. If hand-raised from a rescued infant (mother is usually road-kill) they make wonderful pets but, as they are considered wildlife, there may be local regulations preventing ownership. Many rescued opossums become too habituated to humans to be released; permits may be required to keep them.

Wild Virginia opossums are generally solitary, with males roaming in the spring seeking mates. They have a scaly, prehensile tail. Young may hang from trees using their tails but adults are too heavy to do this, although the tail does assist in balance and climbing. Adults may use their tails to carry bundles of leaves or bedding material. Opossums can run, climb trees, and dig under fences. They are nocturnal, but may adjust somewhat to a human schedule, particularly if fed during daylight. Human-socialized opossums appear to enjoy being carried and cuddled. They are curious, and highly motivated by food. They can learn their names and will come when called. As latrine animals, they easily adapt to using a litter box or newspaper for toileting. They also keep themselves clean by washing, in a similar way to a cat.

Virginia opossums have both a pouch and marsupial pelvic bones. Their fur can range in colour from black to white and in some regions has a cinnamon colour; cinnamon opossums have shorter fur. Ears can be all black or black with white tips. True albinos exist in nature, and another mutant has been found with white fur but normally pigmented skin.

They have 5 digits on each foot, including an opposable thumb on both front and hind feet. The dental formula is I 5/4; C 1/1; PM 3/3; M 4/4. Their brains are a quarter of the size (volume and weight) of a cat of comparable weight, and have large olfactory lobes. Both sexes have paracloacal (anal) scent gland that secrete a greenish fluid. Biological data are summarized in Figure 5.5.

The Virginia opossum makes four distinct vocalizations: hissing, clicking, growling and screeching. All may be used in aggressive actions or in fear. When threatened, the opossum may hiss, and then freeze in the position with its mouth slightly open, showing the teeth with excessive saliva dripping out.

Lifespan	2 winters in the wild; pets 3–5 years on average
Bodyweight (kg)	Males: 4–5 Females: 2–2.5
Length (cm)	Approximately 91 (including tail)
Cloacal body temperature (°C)	32.2–35
Blood volume	5.7% of bodyweight
Heart rate (beats/min)	70–100
Respiration rate (breaths/min)	25–40

5.5 Biological data for the Virginia opossum.

It can also go limp and feign death. This is the classic 'playing possum'.

Wallabies

All living macropods are members of the subfamily Macropodinae. Wallabies in general are social animals and get along well with humans, rabbits, and other herbivores. The author has seen red and grey kangaroos, common wallaroos, and Tammar, Bennett's and swamp wallabies kept as pets.

Tammar wallaby

The Tammar or 'Dama' wallaby (*Macropus eugenii*) originates in the southwest coastal area of Western Australia (south of Perth). It is one of the smaller wallabies and is often kept as a house pet, although it requires supervision when loose as it will dig in carpets, houseplants and furnishings, and may chew on furniture and doorframes. Cats and dogs may be perceived as predators, although many pets learn to live within the same household. Figure 5.6 lists biological data for the Tammar wallaby.

	Tammar wallaby	Bennett's wallaby
Lifespan (years)	10–15	12–15
Bodyweight (kg)	3.5–5.5	Males: 15–26.8 Females: 11–15.5
Cloacal temperature (°C)	35–36	35–36
Heart rate (beats/min)	125–150	120–150

5.6 Biological data for the Tammar and Bennett's wallaby.

Bennett's wallaby

Bennett's wallaby (*Macropus rufogriseus rufogriseus*; see Figure 5.1d) is a subspecies of wide-ranging red-necked wallaby and is found in Tasmania. It is mainly crepuscular and nocturnal. Groups may be seen at feeding areas and water holes, but these are not cohesive social groups. Adolescent males stay with their mothers beyond weaning and into the following year; females wean earlier than males. Related females form 'clans' with common feeding areas. Large dominant males reserve certain areas of their territory for their own use and have exclusive mating rights in those areas. Figure 5.6 lists biological data for the Bennett's wallaby.

Anatomy and physiology

Musculoskeletal system

Marsupials get their name from the presence of the marsupial bones (ossa marsupiala), which serve as attachment surfaces for several abdominal muscles, resting on and articulating with the pelvic and pubic bones (Figure 5.7). Generally boot-shaped and flattened, and varying in size, they have been referred to as 'eupubic bones' and may be considered comparable to abdominal ribs in reptiles. Once thought to support the pouch, this has generally been found not to be true, as they are present in males (no pouch) and are atrophied or absent in marsupial moles and sugar gliders.

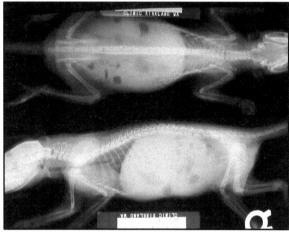

5.7 Radiograph showing marsupial bones extending from the pelvis in a Virginia opossum.

The forelimbs are often foreshortened and the hindlimbs elongated, with the best examples exhibited in the macropods. In several families, the second and third toes of the hind feet have grown out into grooming claws (Figure 5.8). The first toe is always clawless (except in the shrew opossum and marsupial mole).

The marsupial skull has palatal windows and foramina; these are important landmarks for dental anaesthetic blocks and oral surgery.

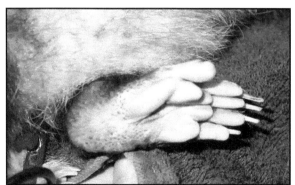

5.8 Virginia opossum. Note the lack of a claw on the first digit of the hind foot.

Urinary and reproductive systems

The kidneys of desert-adapted animals have enlarged medullas and an increased ability to concentrate urine.

The urogenital tract of marsupials is significantly different to that of placental mammals. In all marsupials the urinary ducts pass mesially to the genital ducts, whereas in eutherians they pass laterally. Thus, in male eutherians the vas deferens loops around the inside of the ureter to reach the testes, whereas in male marsupials this loop is absent.

In female eutherians the two oviducts fuse together in the midline to form a single vagina and uterus; in female marsupials this fusion cannot occur because of the presence of the ureters. The two lateral vaginas become united anterior to the ureters, where a median vagina is formed. At parturition, a birth canal is formed in the connective tissue between the median vagina and the urogenital sinus, through which the fetus passes. In most marsupials, this birth canal is transient and reforms at each birth, but in most kangaroos and wallabies it becomes lined with epithelium and remains patent after the first birth.

The cloaca is a common terminal opening for the rectum, urinary ducts and genital ducts.

The marsupium (pouch) is found with a variety of degrees of enclosure. It is well developed and forward-facing in the macropods, backward-facing in koalas and wombats, and absent in the short-tailed opossum, which is considered to be a more primitive marsupial. The pouch has evolved from annular skin creasing around each teat (primal pouch), to a common marsupial wall surrounding all teats, to a closed marsupium.

Endocrine system

The adrenal glands of females are twice the size of those in males, on the basis of weight (mg) per kilogram bodyweight. During lactation this discrepancy increases because of an enlargement in the 'X' zone of the cortex, and an increase in a testosterone-like steroid has been detected. Cortisol is the most abundant corticosteroid.

Body temperature

Marsupials are born without the ability to regulate their body temperature. During the first half of pouch life, the body temperature of the young will closely approximate ambient temperature if they are removed from the pouch. At about halfway through pouch life, young marsupials begin to regulate body temperature. This timing coincides with the start of thyroid function. Species from humid tropical climates, such as some of the *Phalanger* species, are not capable of compensating for evaporative water loss and cannot survive dry heat. Macropods exposed to high temperatures seek the shade of trees or cool caves. Most marsupials avoid activity in the heat of the day.

Cloacal temperatures are lower than actual body temperature; therefore, ear (tympanic) temperature readings are more likely to be accurate for core body temperature, but may be difficult to obtain in the very small marsupials.

Husbandry

Housing

Sugar gliders

Sugar gliders are highly social animals and should not be kept as a solitary pet: they become depressed when housed singly, and self-mutilation is not uncommon. Sugar gliders without proper socialization or exercise and territorial space may become aggressive. Both sexes scent-mark territory with secretions from their scent glands and, in addition, the female uses urine to mark territory. Males will fight if there is not enough distance between nest boxes. Males without adequate stimulation may also become aggressive towards humans. Neutering may help, but they will continue to scent-mark and will not be 'human-socialized' like a domesticated animal.

Sugar gliders live in groups with one adult male, one adult female, last year's joeys and the current pouch joeys. By the time the pouch joeys are ready to be weaned, usually last year's joeys are sexually mature and ready to leave their parents and establish their own territory and family. In captivity, females generally have two litters per year, and the joeys are removed as soon as they are observed to be eating solid food and spending little time in the pouch (from 4–8 weeks 'out of pouch').

Enclosures should be a minimum of 2 m wide x 2 m long and at least 1.8 m high (Figure 5.9). Bird cages are not suitable. Supplemental heating is usually necessary as temperatures in human homes are at the lower end of the glider's metabolic tolerance and comfort zone. Sugar gliders become almost torpid during the day (their night) or if they are too cold, and can be extremely difficult to rouse.

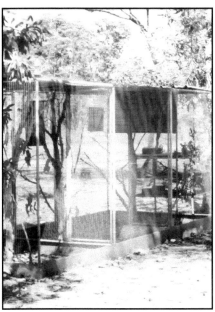

5.9 Outdoor enclosure for sugar gliders. The nest box is positioned in the upper part of the cage and substitute trees have been provided for the animals to glide between. The food and nectar feeders are elevated off the ground.

The animals need large areas for activity and exercise – ideally the freedom of a whole room, fitted with vertical 'trees'. This may be impractical in a typical home and many owners are reluctant to allow such freedom because gliders scent-mark and are active at night.

Hospital caging: In hospital, sugar gliders can be housed in a small animal incubator or plastic bin with ventilation holes in the lid ('isolette') as used for small rodents, kittens and ferrets. The temperature should be maintained between 27 and 32°C with 60–80% humidity. A cloth towel can be provided as bedding.

South American (Brazilian) short-tailed opossums

Large bird or rodent cages can be adapted for these opossums (Figure 5.10). The bars should be closely spaced together so that the animal cannot escape. Branches should be provided for climbing along with a large exercise wheel (such as that for rats). A small box can be used as a nest box. This can be placed near a radiant heat source as temperatures in human homes are at the lower end of the opossum's wild habitat temperature range. Ceramic heat emitters can be used to provide supplemental heating; they should be placed far enough from the cage so that the animal cannot be burned. These raise the ambient temperature but do not heat the cage bars. Recycled newspaper pellets or shreds can be used as bedding; opossums will also shred paper towels and transport the material back to the nest box, using the tail.

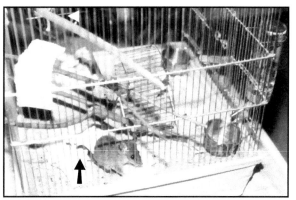

5.10 Housing for a short-tailed opossum. This female has gathered pieces of shredded paper towel by her tail (arrowed) ready to transport them back to the nest box. Note the paper towel deposited on a branch. A dish has been placed beneath the water bottle to catch drips and prevent the bedding from becoming soaked. Branches and an exercise wheel have been provided. The ceramic heat emitter (arrowhead) is just visible attached to the cage.

Short-tailed opossums are housed singly, and are only brought together for short periods to allow breeding: the male and female's cages can be connected via a tunnel, or a separate neutral cage can be provided. Fighting between opossums rarely results in death, but can result in wounds that require medical treatment.

Virginia opossums

Immature opossums as pairs or individuals can be accommodated in cages 45 x 75 cm; a sloping roof 80 cm at the highest point and 35 cm at the lowest allows for some climbing. Standard coated wire cages for rabbits or ferrets may also be used, although it should be multi-level (Figure 5.11). Adults

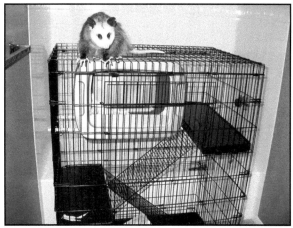

5.11 A large ferret cage adapted for a Virginia opossum. A nest box has been made from a plastic storage container and secured to the cage. The bottom of the cage is lined with newspaper, although opossums generally choose a latrine away from the sleeping area.

may fight in limited quarters. Large groups of neutered males and females can be kept in gang yards 30 x 40 m, either indoors or outdoors, provided the individuals are compatible or were raised together.

Substrate such as shredded or pelleted newspaper allows digging and can be dragged around. Wet or wire floors may lead to sore feet. A nest box should be provided and can be attached to the outside of the cage. Human house temperatures are ideal, but opossums can tolerate a wide range as long as they have shelter. Temperature ranges of 10–30°C, with humidity >58% are considered appropriate.

Wallabies

Wallabies require a large area (minimum of 900 x 900 cm, enclosure must be large enough to allow the animal to run) without obstacles or escape routes but with shade. Group housing is possible with several males and multiple females per group. A group of marcopods is called a mob. Some adult males may fight, but generally they are peaceful, social animals. Wallabies will dig, so fencing should extend at least 30–60 cm below the ground, and should be at least 244 cm (8 feet) high. Chain link fencing is suitable for outdoor enclosures, provided the link spacing is too small for the wallaby to get a foot or leg caught it in when attempting to jump over the fence. Solid wall fencing may be preferred by some owners to prevent such injuries, although the wallaby may try to chew the wood. Hay can be used as bedding.

Tammar wallabies require a temperature above 16°C, with a dry bedding area sheltered from wind and rain. Bennett's wallabies are more tolerant of a temperate climate, including brief exposure to snow and rain but still need shelter from precipitation and wind. If temperature drops below freezing at night, heat should be provided to keep the shelter above 15–16°C.

Hospital caging: When housed in the veterinary clinic, a very large dog cage or kennel can be used. The cage should be large enough to allow the animal

to sit upright and lie down with the legs extended. Most owners will have a small stall or pen for confinement indoors during inclement weather; this can be used for home confinement during convalescence. Bedding of newspaper covered with a deep layer of hay should be provided, which must be changed daily to prevent the build up of faeces and moisture. Water and food should also be replaced daily.

Diet and metabolism

Marsupials have a lower basal metabolic rate than placental mammals – generally considered to be about two-thirds that of placental mammals of equivalent size. However, marsupials can increase their metabolism in response to high rates of heat loss or reproductive needs. These adaptations allow energy reserves to last longer in adverse conditions, so that the animals have lower food requirements and greater environmental tolerance.

In captivity, energy requirements are lower than in the wild. Dietary-related disease is frequently seen and obesity is common. Appropriate diets and quantity must be stressed to owners.

- Heterothermy (difference in body temperature when awake/active *versus* asleep/torporous) is common in insectivorous animals. Insects are consumed in different quantities throughout the year and are the main source of proteins, carbohydrates, fats, fibre, vitamins and minerals. Nectar, gum and sugary exudates from plants are metabolized quickly, while insects take longer to digest. Since a constant supply of insects is unlikely in the wild, and insect food cannot be cached, insectivores may enter a state of torpor to conserve energy. The Didelphids, Monodelphids, Australian Petaurids and the Tarsipedidae (honey possum) can have torporous states lasting up to 11 hours (longer than this puts the animal into a negative calorie balance). During torpor, body temperature, heart rate, respiration rate and overall metabolism decrease; the same state may occur during anaesthesia if care is not taken to maintain normal awake levels. If torpor is induced during anaesthesia, it can complicate postoperative recovery (e.g. haemorrhage can occur due to the increase in blood pressure, which occurs as the body temperature and metabolism return to normal awake levels).
- Sugar gliders have a basal metabolic rate similar to that of macropods. Part of their endogenous nitrogen is retained and recycled to the digestive tract to increase protein availability. Sugar gliders have a larger caecum than most omnivores to ferment ingested gums.
- Herbivorous marsupials recycle urea and have resident flora to degrade and resynthesize protein.

The bottom line for clinicians is that there is enough information available from captive and field studies of the major species of marsupials (metabolic rates, effects of food habits, activity levels) to develop appropriate diets. Micronutrient components still need to be studied in many but little should be left to guesswork, and diets should not be fed simply because the animal prefers certain food items. It is easy to overfeed captive marsupials.

Sugar gliders

The natural diet in the wet season (winter) is primarily the sugary sap or gum of eucalypts and acacias, and nectar from the flowers of eucalypts, banksias, acacias and several types of native apple. For the rest of the year, sugar gliders are mainly insectivorous, the diet including a range of insects plus arachnids and small vertebrates.

Sugar gliders have specialized incisors for gouging the bark of trees. Small insects trapped in wattle or acacia gum (a carbohydrate-rich sap) are consumed. Favourite trees include the Australian 'bloodwood', the red sap of which crystallizes, mixes with the decaying pulp of the trees, and attracts insect activity. Other trees produce 'manna', a deposit of white encrusting sugars from wounds made by sap-sucking insects, birds, other gliders or possums. The sugar glider has also been observed to eat honeydew, secreted by sap-sucking insects. Despite published advice, sugar gliders do not rely on nuts, grains, seeds or table fruit. The diet for a captive glider should contain a variety of foods appropriate for insectivores – at least 50% of total intake, particularly if they are active breeders. Most of the remaining 50% should be sources of fruit sugars, preferably in the form of a sap or nectar. Gum arabic (acacia) can be purchased as a powder, mixed into a thick paste, and used to simulate native gums; it can be used in holes in branches and on surfaces, with insects or bits of fruit stuck to it for enrichment and foraging. The diet should be offered in fresh portions in the evening.

Commercially available adult insects should be fed a calcium-rich insect diet for several days prior to being offered. Larval forms should be kept to a minimum. In the absence of a large variety of insects, a zoo-formula insectivore food can be used. Portion size for one glider is roughly 15 g of insects or insectivore diet, 15 ml of nectar, and 2.5 g of fruits, other insects, etc. Some suggested diets are given in Figure 5.12.

South American (Brazilian) short-tailed opossums

In laboratory facilities short-tailed opossums are fed a pelleted fox diet, insects and 'pinky' mice. They are fed in the evening. Live foods are let loose in the cage, and fruit can be placed on branches to encourage foraging and exercise. Some suggested daily diets are given in Figure 5.13.

Diet 1 (Johnson-Delaney and Ness, in press)

For one sugar glider portion, fed in the evening:
- 15 ml Leadbeater's mix (approximately 45–50% of diet):
    - 150 ml warm water
    - 150 ml honey
    - 1 shelled, boiled egg
    - 15 g baby cereal (flakes, rice-based)
    - 5 g powdered avian vitamin/mineral supplement.
    - Mix warm water and honey. In a separate container, blend egg until homogenized. Gradually add water/honey, then vitamin powder, then baby cereal, blending after each addition until smooth. Divide into 15 ml portions (ice cube tray), freeze unused portions. Thaw and keep refrigerated until served
- 15 g insectivore/carnivore diet (approximately 45–50% of diet)
- Treat foods: various fruits (chopped), may add bee pollen, vitamin/mineral supplement, enriched diet-fed adult insects (2 adult crickets/serving). Total treat intake should be maximum 10% of daily intake.

Fresh water should always be available.

Diet 2 (Booth, 1999)

Offer a total of 15–20% of bodyweight daily. Select one diet (a or b) from each of the following groups (1, 2 and 3) every day. Rotation between the diets is recommended but not necessary. Animals will benefit from a regular supply of vitamin/mineral-enriched insects.

Group 1
    a. Insects: 75% moths, crickets, beetles; 25% fly pupae, mealworms.
    b. Meat mix: commercial small carnivore or insectivore mix.

Group 2
    a. Nectar mix: 337.5 g fructose, 337.5 g sucrose (brown sugar), 112.5 g glucose made up to 2 litres with warm water; commercially available mixes have some vitamin/mineral additives and may be used.
    b. Dry lorikeet mix: 900 g rolled oats, 225 g wheat germ, 225 g brown sugar, 112.5 g glucose, 112.5 g raisins or sultanas.

Group 3
    a. Fruit and vegetables: select from diced apple, nectarine, melon, grapes, raisins, sultanas, figs, tomato, sweet corn kernels, sweet potato, beans, shredded carrot, butternut pumpkin.
    b. Greens: mixed sprouts, leaf/romaine lettuce, broccoli, parsley; with a vitamin/mineral supplement at the manufacturer's directions.

5.12 Two suggested diets for sugar gliders.

Diet 1 (adapted from the National Zoo, Washington DC, USA)

5 g of a blended meat mixture comprising:
   225 g chopped, cooked lean meat (horse or beef)
   1 hard-boiled egg
   15 g wheat germ flakes
   10 g powdered milk
   2.5 g powdered multivitamin/mineral supplement.
 	
This mixture is supplemented daily with:
   1 cm cube of fresh fruit (kiwi, orange, apple, grape, banana)
   1 cm cube of commercial marmoset diet
   1or 2 calcium gut-loaded crickets, 6 small mealworms OR two king mealworms OR 10 small mealworms. Note: adult insects are more nutritious than larval forms.

Diet 2 (Johnson-Delaney and Ness, in press)
5 g commercial insectivore diet (hedgehog dry kibble or semi-moist zoo insectivore diet) 2.5 g cooked meat (turkey, chicken, beef, deboned fish) sprinkled with powdered multivitamin/mineral supplement 1 cm cube of fresh fruit (kiwi, orange, apple, grape, banana) sprinkled with powdered multivitamin/mineral supplement 1 or 2 calcium gut-loaded crickets 1 large mealworm and 6 small mealworms OR 2 large mealworms OR 10 small mealworms. Note: adult insects are more nutritious than larval forms In addition, 3–5 times a week: 1.25 g hard-boiled egg (chop white and yolk together, sprinkle with vitamin/mineral supplement) 1.25 g cottage cheese or skim-milk cheese.

5.13 Two suggested diets for short-tailed opossums.

Virginia opossums

The diet in the wild is truly omnivorous: green and yellow vegetables; grass; fruits; carrion; snails and slugs; earthworms; flies, earwigs, cockroaches and other insects; rats and mice; snakes; amphibians; eggs; crayfish; and fish. They may eat birds, but will rarely eat the entire carcass. In captivity, adults can be fed a varied diet, which should include a good dry cat food or zoo insectivore or omnivore pelleted diet, various vegetables, fruits, occasional egg, supplemental calcium, vitamin A, live foods (such as commercially raised crickets, slugs or mealworms) and yoghurt (Figure 5.14).

Food consumption required is 150–200 g per day. To prevent obesity, dry food may need to be limited and fed as meals rather than *ad libitum*. Commercial dry hedgehog diet is being used in place of dry dog/cat food. No feeding trials have been done, but the hedgehog diets are generally lower in fat than the dog and cat foods, which may be advantageous for controlling weight. The faeces resemble large, soft cat faeces; with usually one defecation per 24 hours. Water consumption is 100–150 ml per day. Both food and water should be provided in heavy crockery bowls (Figure 5.15).

Wallabies

Diets should be based on Timothy or grass hay, with a mix of rabbit and horse pelleted feed used as approximately 25% of the daily intake. Many fairly sedentary captive macropods are fed strictly mixed grass hays to decrease obesity. Small amounts of

Diet 1

Evening:
   112.5 g chopped mixed vegetables (not corn, peas)
   15 g mixed chopped fruits (not citrus)
   15 ml non-fat yoghurt
   56 g insectivore or omnivore zoo pelleted diet (pet hedgehog diet has been used).
 	
   3–4 times a week:
   0.25 hard cooked egg OR 15 g canned salmon OR 56 g cooked tofu
   50 mg pharmaceutical grade calcium carbonate or calcium gluconate powder can be mixed into the vegetables/fruit at least 3 times a week
   Children's multiple vitamin can be given 1–2 times a week as a treat.
 	
   Other treats: 1 king mealworm OR 1–2 calcium loaded crickets OR 3–4 mealworms – 2–4 times a week
 	
Morning:
56 g dry cat food.

Diet 2

Evening:
   56 g dry dog food, insectivore, omnivore or hedgehog kibble
   56 g meat-based canned dog or cat food mixed into kibble
   56 g mixed fruit
   56 g mixed vegetables
   Calcium carbonate should be sprinkled on fruits/vegetables and mixed in.
 	
Morning:
   56 g dry cat, insectivore, omnivore or hedgehog kibble.
 	
Treats:
   5 ml non-fat fruit yoghurt OR 1 children's multiple vitamin OR 1 king mealworm OR 1–2 calcium loaded crickets OR 3–4 mealworms – offer ONE of these daily.

5.14 Two suggested diets for Virginia opossums. These amounts are for one adult female; males may require slightly more.

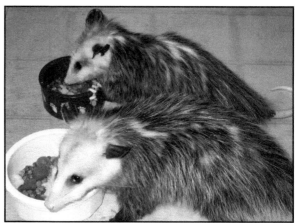

5.15 Virginia opossums eating out of heavy crockery-type dishes. Water should also be provided in this type of dish. Opossums are messy eaters, often spitting out food bits they do not like (e.g. apple skin). After eating, they will wash the face and forelegs in a similar manner to cats.

dark leafy greens are enjoyed. Starches, processed carbohydrates and fruits, although liked should not be fed as these may have detrimental effects on gastrointestinal flora.

Breeding

Reproductive data for sugar gliders, short-tailed opossums, Virginia opossums and wallabies are summarized in Figure 5.16.

Sugar gliders

Male sugar gliders have a bifurcated penis. Intact males also have a pendulous sac in the mid-ventral abdomen containing the paired testicles (Figure 5.17).

	Sugar gliders	Short-tailed opossums	Virginia opossums	Tammar wallaby	Bennett's wallaby
Age at sexual maturity	Males: 12–14 months Females: 8–12 months	4–5 months Males: reproductive life of 39 months Females: reproductive life of 28 months	12 months (puberty occurs at 6–8 months)	Males: >14 months Females: 11–16 months Earlier in captivity than in the wild	Males: 19 months Females: 14 months
Oestrous cycle	Polyoestrous; may have 2 litters per year	Up to 4 litters per year; breed all year round in captivity	Polyoestrous; 23–28 days	30 days	Seasonal
				Post-partum oestrus and embryonic diapause: wallabies will mate within a few hours of birth. The embryo remains quiescent during lactation. It will reactive when the young leave the pouch (usually 8–9 months following fertilization). If the nursing pouch is lost, the female is still affected by the inhibitory influence of day length/season and will not reactivate the embryo until the optimum time of year for survival/weaning of joeys	
Length of oestrus	29 days	3–12 days (up to 1 month)	1–2 days		
Gestation	16 days	14–15 days	12–13 days	25–28 days	30 days
Birth weight (fetus)	<1 g; by the time it emerges from the pouch the joey weighs 5–8 g and is furred	Approximately 1 g	2 g	<1 g	<1 g
Litter size	1–2	5–14	8–20 embryonic young (average 13)		
Milk composition			86% water 4.7% fat 4.5% protein 4.5% sugar		
Development of young (inside pouch)			34 days: vibrissae developed 43 days: hair on back 56–64 days: eyes open		
Weaning age	Joeys leave the pouch at about 70 days; independent at 17 weeks but may remain in parental nest	50 days	Joeys leave the pouch at about 60 days; weaned at 10–12 weeks	Joeys leave the pouch at about 250 days; weaned at 10–11 months	Joeys leave the pouch at about 7–8 months; weaned at 12–17 months

5.16 Reproductive data for marsupials.

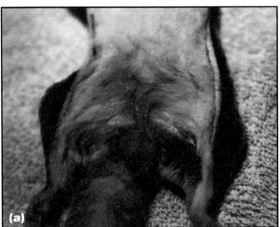

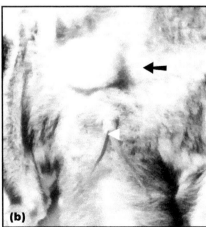

5.17
(a) Normal reproductive anatomy of a male sugar glider. **(b)** Extension of the penis (under anaesthesia) showing the bifurcation. The urethra terminates proximally to where the penis exits the cloaca (arrowhead). Note the large testicular sac proximal to the penis (arrowed).

Courtship begins with the male rubbing his scent glands on the female, although this activity continues to a lesser extent year round in mated pairs. The male also marks his territory using the various scent glands.

The female has the typical marsupial bilobed uterus with lateral vaginas and central birth canal. The pouch contains four teats, although two offspring per litter is most common. The allows the previous litter's joeys to wean during the beginning of the next litter's pouch development. The teats can secrete milk of different composition, related to the age of the joey (Figure 5.18). Females increase marking from pouch scent glands to indicate breeding readiness to the male. The female may rub her ventrum over branches as part of the scent marking.

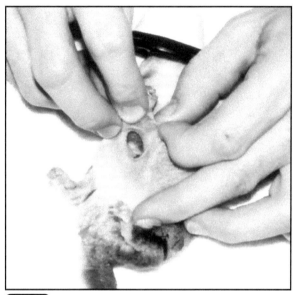

5.18 Female sugar glider with a joey in the pouch.

Both sexes may fight and become irritable at the beginning of breeding. In captivity, sugar gliders will breed throughout the year and produce, on average, two litters per year.

South American (Brazilian) short-tailed opossums

Male short-tailed opossums have a mid-abdominal testicular sac (as for other marsupials). In the female the pouch is not developed (see Figure 5.20), and the mammae (8–14) are arranged in a circle on the abdomen. Neonates cling to the nipples of the mother; later they ride on her back and flanks. Breeding occurs throughout the year in tropical ranges. Short-tailed opossums may have up to four litters annually.

Virginia opossums

There are two distinct breeding periods for Virginia opossums: a short period of high breeding activity, covering 6–7 weeks in the early spring; and a longer, less intense period, beginning 2–4 weeks later and lasting for 2 months into early summer. Females may have a second litter in the same season. Virginia opossums have two lateral and one central vaginal canal and two separate uterine horns. Ovulation is spontaneous.

There are no behavioural/external outward signs of oestrus except excessive drooling and washing of objects to mark locations; males will 'click' when females are in oestrus. A female may kill a male if she is not receptive to breeding and he persists. Copulation lasts 20–40 minutes, with the animals lying on their sides. After mating, they each go their separate ways and remain solitary.

The pouch has a variable number of nipples. After emerging from the pouch, youngsters are carried on the back of the mother until they are independent.

Wallabies

Male wallabies have a testicular sac hanging ventrally from the abdomen. Females have pouches. Female macropods can have joeys of different ages, usually the one from the previous pregnancy is 'kicked out' when the new fetus arrives, but it is not uncommon to have an older joey still nursing whilst a developing joey is in the pouch.

However, most breeders remove the joey once it is weaned or eating mainly solid food, so that there is only one joey being nursed at any time. Breeders tend to keep one male with several females to keep them continually pregnant. In captivity, food and water are abundant, and the weaned joey is removed, so reproduction is different from in the wild, where breeding is dependent on environmental conditions and food sources. Most breeders produce 2–3 joeys from a female wallaby for several years, before it is exhausted. Most pet owners have the males castrated, and some also have the female neutered, primarily to reduce urine marking and obnoxious or aggressive behaviours in intact animals.

Preventive healthcare

Sugar gliders

An annual health examination is recommended, particularly if animals are being used for breeding. This includes: physical examination (palpation, auscultation, dental examination); complete blood count (CBC); serum biochemistry, including calcium; a pouch swab for yeast or bacteria; faecal parasite examination; urinalysis (may pick up subclinical urogenital tract infections, performed by cystocentesis due to potential cloacal faecal contamination if a free-catch sample is used); and radiography to assess bone density.

Virginia opossums

Virginia opossums are carriers of potential **_zoonotic diseases_**, which may be harmful to immuno-compromised humans.

- Virginia opossums have been documented as carriers of *Leptospira*, *Borrelia* (relapsing fever; tick-borne), tularaemia, *Erysipelothrix rhusiopathiae*, *Trypanosoma cruzi* (Chagas' disease), *Sarcoptes scabiei*, *Trichophyton* and *Sarcocystis. Sarcocystis neurona* is a major pathogen of horses (equine protozoal myeloencephalitis) and hoofstock; the Virginia opossum is the definitive host. Horses become infected by ingesting feed or water contaminated with faeces from the opossum. It should be noted that Virginia opossums rescued as infants and reared in captivity may not carry these diseases.

- *Salmonella* spp. has been recovered from clinically normal Virginia opossums.
- Fleas, ticks and mites are found and can be treated as with other small mammals. The wild-caught adult opossum may be heavily parasitized and requires multiple treatments. Most show no clinical signs.
- Nematodes of the gastrointestinal and respiratory tract can be treated with levamisole, thiabendazole, mebendazole or ivermectin. Any treatment needs to be repeated multiple times.
- Canine treatments for heartworm seem to be effective, but diagnostic tests for heartworm have not been validated for the opossum.
- Cestodes and trematodes can be treated with praziquantel using cat regimens.
- Coccidiosis is treated with sulfadimethoxine.

Handling and restraint

Sugar gliders
Restraint of a sugar glider can be done by grasping the scruff of the neck, although they may twist around. They can be held in a towel for examination (Figure 5.19).

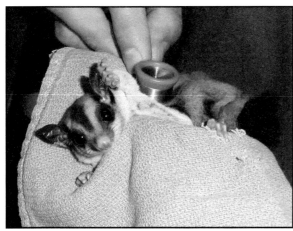

5.19 Sugar glider being restrained in a towel for examination.

South American (Brazilian) short-tailed opossums
Handling and restraint of short-tailed opossums (Figure 5.20) is similar to that used for rats or hamsters (see Chapter 1).

Virginia opossums
Wild Virginia opossums should be handled with gloves and tend to defecate when picked up. They should not be picked up by the tail, but it can be used to help stabilize the animal during restraint by clasping it close to the body and gently lifting the pelvis. The animal should be grasped around the shoulders and thorax with one hand, whilst the other hand holds the pelvis and tail. It should then be placed in dorsal recumbency. These animals can bite, and

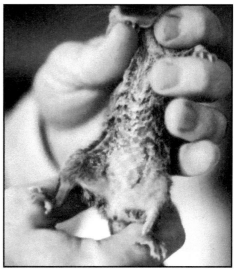

5.20 Female short-tailed opossum being restrained for examination. Note the lack of a pouch.

leather gardening gloves are recommended for the handler. Tame Virginia opossums can be handled in a similar manner to cats (Figure 5.21). These animals tend to squirm and gurgle/hiss when held for nail trimming and do not appear to like to lose contact with a surface; most do not like their feet being handled. To facilitate examination, a Virginia opossum can be wrapped in a towel ('burrito') in a similar manner as restraining a rabbit.

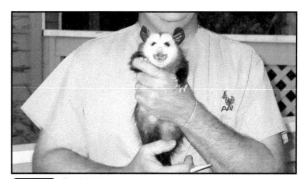

5.21 Pet Virginia opossums can be handled and restrained in a similar manner to cats.

Wallabies
Clinicians need to be familiar with proper handling in the clinic environment. It is usually advantageous to administer diazepam (0.5–1 mg/kg i.m.) or midazolam (0.4–0.5 mg/kg i.m.) immediately to decrease the anxiety of the animal and the potential for future muscle necrosis. Vitamin E administered orally at 500–1000 IU is recommended following capture, transport and handling to prevent myopathy.

Restraint is best done by first securing a firm hold on the base of the tail, then supporting the rest of the body much like one does with a fractious cat (Figure 5.22). Wallabies can do considerable damage with the nails of their hind feet. To prevent injury to itself or the handler, the hind feet can be wrapped in a large towel and secured with tape to prevent kicking. They may also bite. Vocalizations of stress and anger include a loud hissing, accompanied by thumping and whacking the floor with feet and tail.

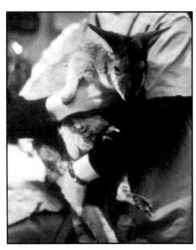

5.22
Restraint of a pet Tammar wallaby is easily achieved, particularly if the animal is used to being handled.

Diagnostic approach

Sugar gliders
In general, physiological parameters such as CBC, serum biochemistry and urinalysis follow those of other small carnivore/insectivore species such as dogs, cats and ferrets.

Imaging
Radiographic positioning is similar to that used for rodents. For lateral positioning, the patagium can be pulled away from the body wall and taped to decrease artefact (Figure 5.23).

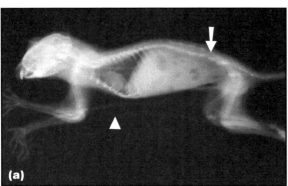

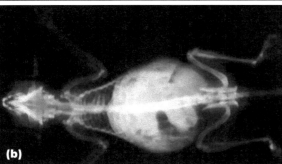

5.23 **(a)** Lateral radiograph of a sugar glider with the gliding membrane pulled away from the body (arrowhead). Note the lumbar vertebrae lucency (arrowed) and spondylosis. This sugar glider was presented due to collapse and inability to eat. Note the poor bone quality and anorexia. The sugar glider had been fed unlimited fruit and *ad libitum* cat food. **(b)** Ventrodorsal radiograph of a sugar glider with fatal enteritis and peritonitis. It had been fed primarily fruit with cat food, mealworms and yoghurt.

Blood sampling
Blood draw sites for volumes up to 1 ml/100 g bodyweight in a healthy sugar glider (less should be drawn if the animal is ill) include the cephalic, lateral saphenous, femoral, ventral coccygeal or lateral tail veins, or medial tibial artery. Tail vessels are more easily utilized if the tail is warmed and the vessels dilated. The jugular vein and cranial vena cava can be used for larger volumes (up to 1 ml in larger, healthy adults) but general anaesthesia is required.

South American (Brazilian) short-tailed opossums

Blood sampling
Blood draw sites, injection sites and volumes are similar to those used in sugar gliders and rats of a similar size.

Virginia opossums

Blood sampling

- Blood can be obtained from the lateral tail vein in younger opossums without scarring the tails. Ventral veins lie on either side of the coccygeal artery and can be accessed in a slender tail (Figure 5.24).
- The cephalic and tibial (saphenous) veins can also be accessed.
- The female has pouch veins that can be accessed both for blood sampling and for injection.

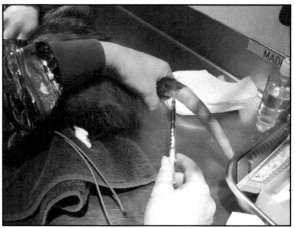

5.24 Blood can be drawn easily from either the ventral or lateral tail vein in Virginia opossums.

Wallabies
When performing a physical examination of a pet wallaby (Figure 5.25), a towel or other supportive material should be placed on the examination table to provide the animal with a secure footing.

- A full dental examination requires sedation (as with rabbits and rodents).
- Cloacal temperature is best taken using a flexible probe, which can be passed up into the rectum, rather than with a short rigid electronic thermometer.

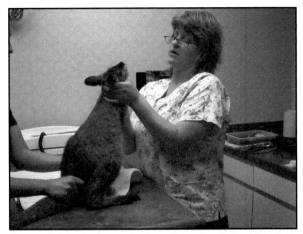

5.25 Physical examination of a pet wallaby. Note that the head of the tail is being held by an assistant to help control the animal.

- The abdomen can be difficult to palpate as it is largely filled with the forestomach.
- The bladder can sometimes be palpated.
- The pouch needs to be thoroughly examined as many pet macropods do not clean the pouch well, resulting in a waxy sour-smelling build-up; this can be due to a yeast and/or bacterial infection. If such material is present, the walls of the pouch should be swabbed for aerobic culture and sensitivity testing. It should then be gently cleansed with dilute chlorhexidine surgical scrub and rinsed with warm water or saline. If infection is present, both topical and systemic medications are usually needed. If the animal is nervous about the examination process, a low dose of an

anxiolytic such as diazepam or midazolam should be administered.

Blood sampling
Blood sampling sites are essentially the same for most macropod species. They include the cephalic vein (Figure 5.26) and the lateral caudal vein (just dorsal to lateral of the vertebral processes on either side of the tail).

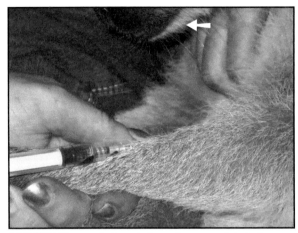

5.26 The cephalic vein is easily accessible in the macropods for blood draws and catheter placement. (For orientation, the muzzle is arrowed.)

Common conditions

Sugar gliders
Figure 5.27 lists common conditions of sugar gliders, their causes, diagnostics and treatment.

Condition	Cause	Diagnostics	Treatment
Behavioural disorders (self-injurious behaviour, overgrooming, aggressiveness, cannibalism of young)	Stress; improper husbandry; lack of social interactions; self-injurious behaviour most often seen in solitary pets; lack of space/areas for exercise; adult males confined together; incompatible pairs	Husbandry history; culture (wounds); CBC/biochemistry; radiography	Treat wounds as in other animals: NSAIDs, analgesics, antimicrobials. Correct deficiencies of husbandry, social patterns. Antidepressant medical therapy and/or benzodiazepines if self-injurious behaviours/overgrooming continues. Neuter overly aggressive males
Cataracts	Vitamin A deficiency; hyperglycaemia (dietary or diabetes); congenital/hereditary?	Ophthalmic examination; history (diet, husbandry, pedigree/breeding); CBC/biochemistry; urinalysis	Cataract removal may be possible. Correct diet to lower blood sugar. If true diabetes, manage as in cats. If possibly inherited, do not breed
Ear margin canker	Mite with secondary bacterial infection	Skin scraping; culture	Ivermectin; appropriate topical antimicrobial. NSAIDs or anti-inflammatory if pruritic
Gastrointestinal disease (rectal prolapse usually with marked tenesmus, diarrhoea, enteritis/enteropathy)	Bacterial (e.g. *Escherichia coli*, *Clostridium*); parasitic (nematode, cestode, protozoal including *Giardia*); diet; foreign body ingestion; prolapse exacerbated by abdominal muscle weakness, overall poor health, pregnancy, age	Faecal flotation; direct smear; Gram stain; culture; CBC/biochemistry; radiography (contrast study); diet/husbandry history, including breeding status	Appropriate antimicrobials/antiparasitics. Surgical correction of prolapse. NSAIDs. Analgesia. Fluid therapy. Nutritional support. Enterotomy if foreign body/obstruction. Adjunctive therapy of intestinal protectants: bismuth subsalicylate
Reproductive disease (weak/not thriving/dying joeys, infertility, pouch/reproductive tract infections, mastitis) (Figure 5.28)	Inadequate nutrition; overbreeding (too many litters/year); poor husbandry; chronic bacterial/yeast infection; retained/mummified fetus	Diet/husbandry history; CBC/biochemistry; radiography; cytology of milk/urogenital mucosa; culture of exudates/reproductive tract/pouch	Correct diet/husbandry. Appropriate antimicrobials, calcium and fluids. Do not breed until healthy. Check male for bacterial/yeast infection

5.27 Common conditions of sugar gliders. (continues) ▶

Condition	Cause	Diagnostics	Treatment
Skin disease (poor hair coat, sebaceous gland/ pouch dermatitis)	General poor health; dietary/husbandry deficiency; lack of grooming; pouch, infections (bacterial, *Candida*)	Diet/husbandry history; skin scraping/biopsy; culture	Correct diet/husbandry. Antimicrobials as indicated. Topical corticosteroids, antihistamines and/or NSAIDs
Trauma (wounds, fractures)	Attacks from mate/rival/other pets; falls/ injuries due to confinement; poor body condition	Radiography; CBC/ biochemistry; culture	Appropriate antimicrobials and wound care as in other animals. NSAIDs. Analgesia. Fracture repair similar to birds/small mammals. Correct diet/husbandry
Urinary tract disease (penile prolapse, necrosis, male urinary tract blockage, bladder rupture, uroliths/ cystitis with haematuria, stranguria, crystalluria, pyelonephritis/nephritis, renal disease/failure)	Lack of territory/ furnishings to mark, leading to urine retention; subclinical dehydration (chronic); improper diet (mineral balance, water/electrolytes, ash content); lack of exercise; poor overall body condition; age; ascending bacterial infection from cloaca	CBC/biochemistry; urinalysis (cystocentesis); culture; radiography; excretory urogram; diet/ husbandry history	Blocked males: relieve blockage via catheterization, flushing, urethrostomy (as in cats), cystotomy for urolith removal. NSAIDs. Analgesia. Fluid therapy. Antimicrobial therapy. Correct diet/husbandry. Treat renal disease/failure as in other animals: fluid administration, phosphorus binding agent, vitamin B complex, potassium, dietary modifications
Weakness/ataxia/paresis/ paralysis/weight loss/muscle wasting/lethargy/reluctance to move/soft jaws/soft teeth/ neurological signs (including tremor)	Improper diet (deficiencies of calcium, protein, vitamins/minerals; excesses of sugar, carbohydrates, fats); ambient temperature too cool (adding to stress of malnourishment); infection (*Listeria*, *Baylisascaris*); bacterial encephalitis from systemic infection; osteomalacia; osteoporosis; encephalomalacia (may be dietary)	CBC/biochemistry; radiography; dietary/ husbandry history; possible serology and culture of CSF (for *Listeria*); necropsy/ histopathology (for nervous system disease)	Immediate therapy: NSAIDs and/or analgesics, parenteral calcium, fluids; gavage feed with high-protein/calcium-rich food. Vitamin/mineral supplementation. Correct diet to include calcium-rich insects, protein; decrease sugars, fats. Increase ambient temperature. Provide exercise. Physical therapy may be needed initially. For *Listeria*: penicillin, antibiotics as indicated from culture/sensitivity testing; **zoonotic potential**. *Baylisascaris*: ivermectin, eliminate exposure to raccoons, skunks

5.27 (continued) Common conditions of sugar gliders.

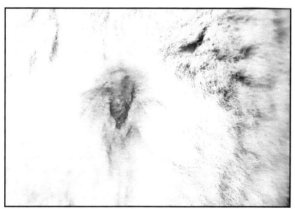

5.28 Exudate from the pouch of a non-breeding intact female sugar glider. There was a sour smell and *Candida* was isolated. The animal responded well to cleaning of the pouch and topical treatment with a dilute chlorhexidine solution.

South American (Brazilian) short-tailed opossums

In general, short-tailed opossums are fairly hardy. In pets, malnutrition, obesity, chilling, injury from falling or handling, and mange mites have been seen. Endocrine alopecia has been frequently noted in aged females, and is usually associated with pituitary adenoma (prolactinoma). Uterine leiomyomas, skin lipomas, adrenal gland phaeochromocytomas and liver carcinomas (most common) have been documented. Most neoplasia is found in short-tailed opossums older than 22 months.

The principal spontaneous disease problems occur in the digestive system, with most involving the liver. The most common cause of death from digestive system disease is rectal prolapse (Figure 5.29). Enteritis of the small intestine may cause gaseous distension. Short-tailed opossums are also prone to atherosclerosis following hyperlipidaemia and hypercholesterolaemia. The second most common system with disease is the urogenital system, with the kidney most frequently affected with nephritis.

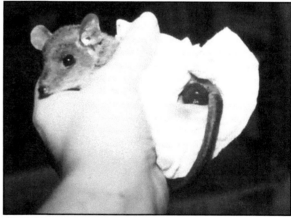

5.29 Short-tailed opossum restrained for in a small towel for examination of the rectal/cloacal prolapse.

Cardiovascular disease is fairly common, with congestive heart failure developing in males more frequently than females. Heart disease is generally found in animals averaging 37 months of age. Figure 5.30 lists common conditions of short-tailed opossums, their causes, diagnostics and treatment.

Condition	Cause	Diagnostics	Treatment
Alopecia: Non-pruritic (particularly on the rump)	Endocrine neoplasia (pituitary adenoma, prolactinoma); ectoparasites; fungal infection	Serum prolactin/oestradiol levels; skin biopsy	Correct husbandry/diet. For sex hormone elevation: deslorelin or leuprolide acetate depot formulation (as per ferrets). No commercial tests for endocrine disease are available. Treat ectoparasites and fungal infections as for sugar gliders
± Pruritus	Ectoparasites (mites, fleas)	Skin scraping; biopsy; clinical observation	Ivermectin for mites. Treat other pets for fleas. Change bedding. Clean cage
Gastrointestinal disease (distension, ileus, diarrhoea, staining of the perineum)	Diarrhoea; diet; inappetence; abdominal bloating; pain; rectal/cloacal prolapse; bacterial/protozoal (rare) infection	Faecal cytology; Gram stain; culture; sensitivity; radiography; diet history	Appropriate antimicrobials. Bismuth subsalicylate. NSAIDs. Analgesia. Fluid therapy. Nutritional support
Heart disease (cardiomyopathy, congestive heart disease, atherosclerosis)	May be due to ageing; dietary deficiencies (information not yet published); exercise intolerance; cold extremities; cyanosis; dyspnoea; ascites; hyperlipidaemia; hypercholesterolaemia	Physical examination; auscultation; radiography; echocardiography; abdominocentesis; cytology; haematology; serum biochemistry	Medical therapy for cardiomyopathy (as for other species). Enalapril. Pimobendan. Furosemide. Potassium supplementation if indicated. Supportive care. Correct diet to reduce fat/cholesterol
Neoplasia (weight loss/gain, abdominal enlargement, dyspnoea, exercise intolerance)	Ageing	Clinical examination; radiography; ultrasonography; laparotomy; biopsy	Surgical removal of mass (if possible). Oncology therapeutics as for other species. Palliative and supportive care
Nephritis/pyelonephritis/nephrosis (polyuria/polydipsia, haematuria, pyuria)	Bacterial infection ascending from the cloaca and reproductive tract	Urinalysis; cytology; culture and sensitivity; CBC; biochemistry; radiography; excretory urogram; ultrasonography; renal biopsy; histopathology	Appropriate antimicrobials. Fluid therapy. Correct potassium/electrolytes. Phosphorus inhibitor. Diet modification (if renal function compromised)
Rectal prolapse	Enteritis/enteropathy; lack of dietary roughage; ageing (particularly females)	Faecal flotation/smear; Gram stain; culture; diet history; cloacal examination; cytology	Surgical reduction of prolapse with cloacal suture (similar to birds); avoid urogenital slits. Antimicrobials. NSAIDs. Analgesia. Treat underlying enteropathy. Diet correction
Wounds/lacerations/fractures	Falls; fighting	Radiography; culture and sensitivity; Gram stain	Treat as for other small mammals. Appropriate antimicrobials, NSAIDs and analgesia. Separate incompatible animals

5.30 Common conditions of short-tailed opossums.

Virginia opossums

Common clinical conditions of Virginia opossums, their diagnostics and treatment are listed in Figure 5.31.

Condition	Cause	Diagnostics	Treatment
Alopecia: ± Acanthosis/exfoliation	Dermatophytosis (*Trichophyton* spp.); ectoparasites	Skin scraping; fungal culture; biopsy	*Trichophyton*: topical griseofulvin. Ectoparasites: topical pyrethrins; ivermectin
Rump (endocrine pattern)	Females: chronic genital tract infection; pituitary adenoma (prolactin elevation?)	Physical examination; skin scraping; biopsy; cytology/culture; CBC/biochemistry; endoscopic examination of genital tract	Broad-spectrum antibiotics. NSAIDs. Consider antihormonal treatment as in ferrets (not proven)
Anorexia	Endoparasites; septicaemia; heart disease; renal disease; gastroenteritis; neoplasia	Faecal examination; CBC/biochemistry; radiography; faecal/blood culture	Treat underlying cause (guidelines as for cats)
Cardiomyopathy (dilated or hypertrophic; common in opossums over 2 years of age)	Likely consequence of ageing	Echocardiography; ECG; blood pressure; radiography; CBC/biochemistry useful to assess other organ function	Treatment regimens based on cats: supplement with omega-3 fatty acids, co-enzyme Q10, L-carnitine, taurine and vitamin E

5.31 Common conditions of Virginia opossums. (continues) ▶

Condition	Cause	Diagnostics	Treatment
CNS disease (circling, torticollis, ataxia, tremors, clonic convulsions, lethargy, coma, death; aged opossums develop neurological deficiencies with clinical appearance similar to Parkinson's disease in humans, although different pathology/aetiology)	Meningitis; microabscesses in CNS (*Streptococcus, Nocardia*); heavy metal toxicosis; histoplasmosis; geriatric neuropathy	CBC/biochemistry; CSF evaluation; radiography; MRI; cytology	Palliative care. Heavy metal toxicosis: edetate calcium disodium, other chelators, diazepam to stop seizures. Microabscesses: may respond to parenteral antimicrobials. Geriatric neuropathy: acetyl carnitine, vitamin B12, omega 3 fatty acids may be helpful but it is progressive and terminal
Crusty ear (also called 'crispy ear')	Acariasis; *Streptococcus* infection; poor vascular perfusion/vasculitis	Skin scraping; culture	Topical ivermectin. Aggressive antibiotic therapy. Stimulate circulation with massage. LED/laser light therapy being tried
Dermatitis	Acariasis; ectoparasites; secondary bacterial infection; septicaemia; *Besnoitia*, dermatophytosis; *Pseudomonas pyocyanea*; *Staphylococcus*; *Actinomyces dermatonomus*	Skin scraping; cytology; bacterial/fungal culture; CBC/biochemistry	Appropriate antibacterials, antifungals, antiparasitics
Dermatophytosis (sparse, scaly lesions, generalized over skin)	*Trichophyton mentagrophytes*	Culture; cytology	Antifungals. **Zoonotic potential**; discuss with owner for precautions
Dyspnoea: With cyanosis and heart murmurs	Cardiomyopathy including vegetative endocarditis; hypervitaminosis D (calcification of aorta, atherosclerosis); heartworm	Auscultation; physical examination; radiography; ECG/echocardiography; blood culture; CBC/biochemistry; diet history	Endocarditis: follow guidelines for cats: amoxicillin for active vegetative endocarditis due to *Streptococcus*; discontinue vitamin D supplementation; correct diet. Heartworm: follow guidelines for dogs
With coughing, cyanosis, nasal discharge, sneezing, fever and left shift leucocytosis	Parasitic/bacterial pneumonia; pulmonary adenoma; neoplasia (metastasis)	Physical examination; radiography; CBC/biochemistry; faecal examination; culture/cytology of exudates/discharge	Appropriate antibiotics. Supportive care including nebulization. No treatment for pulmonary adenoma or neoplasia but palliative therapy with specific medications may be tried. Euthanasia is an option
Emaciation: General	Parasites; septicaemia; malnutrition	Physical examination; CBC/biochemistry; diet history; faecal examination; faecal/blood culture	Treat underlying cause. Supportive care
With ataxia, paraplegia, dyspnoea and diarrhoea	*Mycobacterium avium*; *M. bovis*; atypical mycobacteria	Tubercle lesions may be visible on radiography/ultrasonography, nodules may be palpated, cutaneous granulomas may be identified during physical examination; acid-fast organisms on stained smears of contents of tubercles; palpebral test	Not recommended as *Mycobacterium* is a reportable disease and most public health authorities advise not to treat. There are no validated therapeutic regimens for this species. Euthanasia is recommended/required due to **zoonotic potential**. Reportable disease in most public health districts
Gastrointestinal disease (emesis, diarrhoea, anorexia, depression, abdominal pain)	Endoparasites; foreign body ingestion; neoplasia; ulceration (stress?); renal failure; histoplasmosis	Physical examination; faecal examination; radiography; CBC/biochemistry; urinalysis	Treat underlying cause (guidelines as for cats). Supportive care
Haematuria (males: dysuria, constipation, local pain, fever)	Prostatitis; cystitis	Physical examination; rectal palpation; ultrasonography; urinalysis	Antibiotics. NSAIDs. Analgesia. Antihormonal therapy (can try as in ferrets)
Icterus	Endoparasites; leptospirosis; liver disease/neoplasia	Faecal examination; serology (leptospirosis); CBC/biochemistry; ultrasonography	Treat underlying cause. **NB Leptospirosis** is **potentially zoonotic** and is a reportable disease in many public health districts

5.31 (continued) Common conditions of Virginia opossums. (continues) ▶

Condition	Cause	Diagnostics	Treatment
Neoplasia (oral with non-healing tissue or bleeding common (Figure 5.32), pain, anorexia)	Abscess; bacterial/fungal granuloma; foreign body penetration; epulis is sometimes seen as an oral lesion with gingivitis and may resemble a true tumour	Physical examination; palpation; radiography; ultrasonography; biopsy; CBC/biochemistry	Surgery if possible. Other protocols based on cats/ferrets per type of neoplasia and overall condition
Obesity	Overfeeding; lack of exercise	CBC/biochemistry; radiography; possibly cardiac assessment	Diet control
Organomegaly (may have CNS signs)	Histoplasmosis; splenomegaly; hepatomegaly; anaemia; emaciation; leucopenia; diarrhoea	Cytology of blood smears/ regional lymph nodes; histoplasmin skin test; ultrasound-guided biopsy	Parenteral amphotericin B. Antifungal agents
Scaly tail	Ectoparasites; lack of humidity	Skin scraping; husbandry history	If low humidity, increase relative humidity to >50%. Topical medicated ointment. Ectoparasites: pyrethrins, topical ivermectin
Septicaemia/'poor doer' joey/pouch expulsion	Pouch infection; septicaemia of dam; heavy parasite load; dam inexperience; stress	Physical examination; CBC/ biochemistry; blood culture; faecal examination; husbandry/diet history; culture pouch	Appropriate antimicrobials. Husbandry/diet correction
Soft bones/swollen limbs/jaws/ paraplegia/ataxia/anorexia	Metabolic bone disease; renal failure	Physical examination; diet history; radiography; CBC/ biochemistry	Analgesia. Correct diet. Calcium supplementation. If renal involvement: lower protein diet, fluid therapy, phosphorus-binding agent (cimetidine) as in cats
Urinary tract disease (± polyuria/ polydipsia, haematuria, crystalluria, dysuria, cystic calculi)	Cystitis; cystic calculi; bladder carcinomas; urethritis; nephritis; pyelonephritis; interstitial nephritis; glomerulonephritis; acute renal infarction; renal adenoma (nephroblastoma); amyloidosis	Physical examination; urinalysis; radiography; contrast excretory urogram; renal biopsy; CBC/ biochemistry	Treat underlying cause (guidelines as for cats)
Uterine prolapse	Ascending infection; neoplasia (e.g. mammary carcinoma); endometritis; metritis; traumatic vaginitis; mammary hyperplasia	Physical examination; CBC/ biochemistry; vaginal cytology; biopsy; laparotomy; endoscopic examination of genital tract following reduction of prolapse	Surgical reduction of prolapse. NSAIDs. Analgesia. Broad-spectrum antibiotics. If neoplasia, perform ovariohysterectomy. Hormonal suppression therapy (deslorelin or leuprolide acetate depot) may prevent recurrence and reduce mammary tissue

5.31 (continued) Common conditions of Virginia opossums.

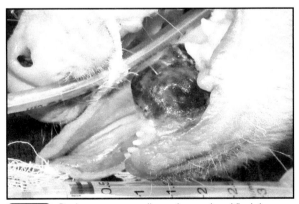

5.32 Oral squamous cell carcinoma in a Virginia opossum.

Wallabies

Common diseases of macropods, their diagnostics and treatment are listed in Figure 5.33.

Dental disease

Captive macropods fed insufficient roughage may have a chronic problem with the tooth eruption process. In the normal 'dental mill', molars erupt posteriorly in the jaw and migrate anteriorly, before being lost adjacent to the diastema. Improper movement and wear may leave openings for bacteria to get into the jaw, and can result in a condition known as 'lumpy jaw' (Figure 5.34). Coarse, sharp foods such as oat awns should be avoided, since they can cause trauma to the mouth and the tissues can be invaded by bacteria such as *Actinomyces bovis* and *Bacteroides* spp. Provision of materials such as long dry grass or fibrous tree bark for the animals to chew on appears to reduce the incidence of the disease. Chewing on these presumably toughens the oral mucosa. It may also be important in providing the molar teeth with sufficient work to enable them to be shed properly.

Condition	Cause	Species/ susceptibility	Clinical signs	Diagnostics	Treatment
Candidiasis	*Candida albicans*	Pouch young or artificially-reared joeys	Act hungry; won't suckle; white curd-like encrustations in mouth/lips/gums/ tongue margins; depression; painful mouth	Cytology; culture	Pouch young: remove joeys, clean out the pouch and teats twice daily with chlorhexidine scrub, rinse and dry using cotton wool. Give oral nystatin/ antifungal agents to joey before replacing Artificially-reared joeys: improve sanitation of bottles, teats and utensils. Give oral nystatin/ antifungal agents
Cystitis/urogenital infection	Ascending bacterial urinary tract infection; pyometra; uroliths (reported in males)	All; intact females	Haematuria/polyuria (small amounts frequently); pawing at lower abdomen; increased grooming of cloaca; protrusion of phallus; pain; anorexia; restlessness or refusal to move; decreased water intake (outdoors/ cold water)	History; urinalysis (note macropods urinate same volume of urine whether dehydrated or not); radiography; ultrasonography; culture urine (cystocentesis sample – as it is not possible to catheterize a male macropod and urine obtained from the cloaca is likely to be contaminated)	Uroliths: surgery may be needed. Infection/ neoplasia: ovariohysterectomy including vaginas. Endoscopic exploration of urogenital tract (female) for biopsy or foreign material removal. Fluid therapy. Broad-spectrum antibiotics. Supportive care
Diarrhoea ± anorexia	Gastrointestinal obstruction due to ingestion of foreign material (e.g. cloth bedding) or improper diet; bacterial imbalance/overgrowth; insufficient roughage; coccidiosis; other illness	All	Bloating; pawing or constant grooming of abdomen; restlessness; flatulence; soiled vent/ ventral tail; dehydration	Faecal cytology; culture; radiography (including contrast study); CBC/ biochemistry	Surgery to remove foreign body. Treat underlying cause (as for rabbits)
Herpesviruses	Herpesvirus	Parma and Tammar wallabies	Transient infertility; eye/nasal discharge; lingual ulcers; depression; anorexia; death	Serology; histopathology; virus isolation	No therapy yet. May try aciclovir?
Lumpy jaw (necrobacillosis, actinomycosis) (Figure 5.34)	*Bacteroides*; *Fusobacterium necrophorum*; *Actinomyces*; *Corynebacterium*	Macropods in captivity; rare in wild	Swelling of mandible or maxilla; poor prehension; gingivitis/ osteomyelitis; exudate production; depression; weight loss; pain	Odour; culture; radiography	Debridement. Parenteral antibiotics, NSAIDs. Local disinfection. Reduce overcrowding. Clean environment. Correct diet
Mycobacteriosis	*Mycobacterium avium*; *M. intracellularis*; *M. scrofulaceum*	Wallabies	Abscesses of skin/ bone; visceral organs may be involved; purulent arthritis	Acid-fast stains; culture	Non-responsive to treatment. Zoos have tried isolation of endangered macropods. For common species, due to potential **zoonoses** and reporting requirements, euthanasia is recommended
Pasteurellosis	*Pasteurella multocida*; *P. haemolytica*	All	Rhinitis; haemorrhagic septicaemia; bronchopneumonia	Clinical signs; culture	Parenteral antibiotics. NSAIDs. Reduce stress/fighting

5.33   Common conditions of macropods. (continues)   ▶

Condition	Cause	Species/susceptibility	Clinical signs	Diagnostics	Treatment
Pneumonia	*P. multocida*; *Klebsiella*; various organisms	All; more common in winter or in wild-caught animals (wet conditions, ambient temperature <15–16°C, body temperature <35°C)	Dyspnoea; coughing; frothy nasal/oral discharge; death	Clinical signs; auscultation; radiography	Parenteral antibiotics. Bronchodilators. NSAIDs. Supportive therapy
Pouch infections	*Pseudomonas aeruginosa*	All females	Dirty pouch; odour; brown, thick discharge	Clinical signs; culture	Disinfection and cleaning. Topical and systemic antibiotics
Salmonellosis	*Salmonella*	Young more commonly affected	Diarrhoea; depression; enteritis; septicaemia	Faecal/oral culture	Parenteral antibiotics. Electrolytes. Fluid therapy. **NB public health significance and potentially zoonotic**
Toxoplasmosis	*Toxoplasma*	All macropods, particularly urban wallabies	CNS signs; ataxia; anorexia; wasting	Serology; CSF cytology/PCR; history of exposure to cats	Atovaquone. Supportive care. Prognosis guarded to poor for full recovery

5.33 (continued) Common conditions of macropods.

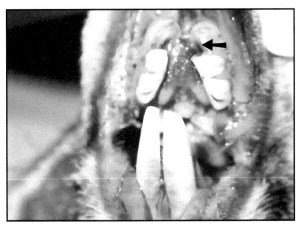

5.34 Bennett's wallaby with extreme wear and necrosis of the pulp of the central maxillary incisors (arrowed). These teeth were also loose, and when extracted there was considerable abscessation and involvement of the underlying bone. There is also uneven wear and a build-up of calculus on the mandibular incisors. Note the minor ulceration of the mouth at the canthi. Oral surgery included a gingivectomy and removal of abscessed teeth and bone. The area was packed with a synthetic bone matrix material mixed with clindamycin and sutured. The area healed completely.

Supportive care

Injection sites

Sugar gliders

- Intramuscular injection sites include the quadriceps and biceps/triceps.
- Subcutaneous injections are given in the scapular area as in other animals, but fluids may end up pooling in the gliding membrane.

- The saphenous vein has been used for intravenous injections.

Virginia opossums

- Intramuscular injections can be given into the anterior thigh, biceps or triceps.
- Subcutaneous injections can be given in the intrascapular and flank area.
- Intravenous injections can be given into the cephalic, lateral tail or pouch veins.
- Intraosseous catheters can be placed in the femur or tibia as in other mammals.

Wallabies

- Intramuscular injections can be made into the anterior thigh, biceps or triceps muscles.
- Subcutaneous injections can be suprascapular or given into the flank or rump.
- Intravenous injection is usually easiest into the cephalic vein, but the saphenous vein can be used in an anaesthetized macropod.

Anaesthesia and analgesia

Sugar gliders

- Preoperative medications include: glycopyrrolate (0.02 mg/kg s.c.); butorphanol (0.2 mg/kg i.m.; repeated postoperatively i.m., s.c. or orally q6–8h as needed); midazolam (0.4 mg/kg i.m.).
- Induction is with isoflurane.
- Postoperatively, meloxicam (0.2 mg/kg s.c. or orally q24h for up to 3 days) seems adequate. Buprenorphine has also been used postoperatively instead of butorphanol as it appears to last 10–12 hours (0.01–0.03 mg/kg s.c. or orally).

Common surgical procedures

Orchidectomy

Orchidectomy is the most common elective surgical procedure (Figure 5.35). In marsupials the testicles in the scrotal sac are attached via a short stalk to the mid-ventral body wall. The procedure is the same for all male marsupials.

1. Under general anaesthesia, perform a local nerve block using 50:50 lidocaine and bupivacaine diluted with sterile water. (For sugar glider: 0.05 ml 2% lidocaine plus 0.05 ml 6% bupivacaine diluted with sterile water to 0.2 ml). Infiltrate the base of the stalk and the incision area.
2. Make an incision longitudinally on the stalk, approximately 1 cm from the body wall.
3. Use blunt dissection to expose the blood supply and vas deferens.
4. Ligate the blood supply and vas deferens.
5. Remove or ablate the testicular sac.
6. Close the skin with subcuticular buried sutures.

It should be noted that sugar gliders are adept at suture removal unless adequate analgesia is provided and the sutures are buried.

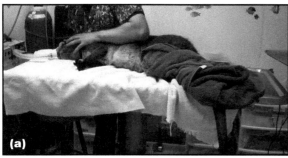

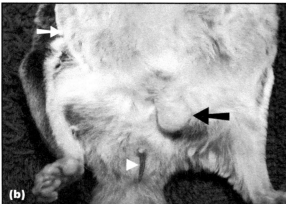

5.35 **(a)** Bennett's wallaby being prepared for castration. Although heavily sedated prior to delivery of isoflurane via facemask, the hindlegs can still inflict injury, and have been secured in a towel to prevent injury to the animal or handler. **(b)** Sugar glider being prepared for castration. It is common for the penis (arrowhead) to extend as the animal is anaesthetized. The sugar glider had only one descended testicle and abdominal surgery was required to locate the other. The undescended testicle was much smaller and lay close to the body wall where the spermatic cord, blood vessels and nerve of the descended one exited. There is no inguinal ring or canal. The testicular sac is denoted by the large arrow, and the gliding membrane by the small arrow.

Ovariohysterectomy

This may incorporate the lateral vaginas, but care must be taken to separate the ureters that loop in between the central and lateral vaginas (Figure 5.36). These are often difficult to differentiate and separate from fat and other tissues. If the female has not had a litter, then only the ovaries and uterus may be removed, leaving the lateral and central vaginas. These atrophy, and the author has not seen any pathology associated with leaving them. There is a potential for urine reflux only if the female has been pregnant and the vaginal orifice into the cloaca is opened.

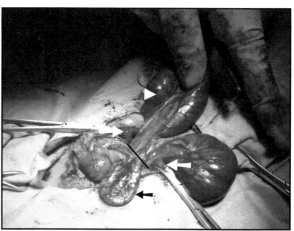

5.36 Exteriorized reproductive tract of a female marsupial, showing the ovaries (large white arrows), uterus and vaginal canals. This female Virginia opossum was in oestrus. The enlarged uterine horn is denoted with an arrowhead. The junction of the two horns of the uterus with the two lateral canals (small black arrow) and the central vaginal canal is shown by a black line.

Preoperative medications include glycopyrrolate, midazolam and butorphanol. An intravenous catheter can be placed in the cephalic vein for continuous-drip warmed isotonic fluids. The abdominal incision is made through the pouch, carefully avoiding the pouch veins. Induction is with isoflurane and the animal can be intubated similarly to a dog. A local incisional anaesthetic block with lidocaine is carried out. There may be a need to scrub the pouch more intensively with chlorhexidine due to the build-up of waxy material within it. Postoperative analgesia includes meloxicam and buprenorphine.

Drug formulary

Figure 5.37 presents a drug formulary for marsupials.

- Pain resulting from an injection can cause the rapid induction of shock in small species.
- Sugar gliders, short-tailed opossums and Virginia opossums have carnivore/omnivore gastrointestinal tracts: carnivore guidelines for antibiotic choice should be followed.
- Brushtail possums and macropods are herbivores with digestion dependent on gastrointestinal flora: guidelines for rabbits and guinea pigs for antibiotic choice should be followed.

Drug	Dose	Comments	Species	Reference
Analgesics/sedatives				
Acepromazine + Butorphanol	0.2 mg A + 0.2 mg B orally once	Sedation; analgesia; postoperative	SG	Johnson (1997)
Buprenorphine	0.01–0.03 mg/kg i.m./i.v./s.c. q10–12h	Analgesic	Various	
Butorphanol	0.1–0.5 mg/kg i.m./s.c./orally q6–8h prn	Analgesic	Various	Johnson (1997); Johnson-Delaney (1997)
Butorphanol + Acepromazine	1.7 mg/kg B + 1.7 mg/kg A orally; dilute with saline to administer once	Postoperative sedative; analgesic	SG	Pye (2005)
Diazepam	0.5–2.0 mg/kg i.m./orally/i.v. as needed up to every 2 hours	Sedation; higher dosages i.v. for seizures	Various	Johnson-Delaney (1997)
Ketamine	15–30 mg/kg i.m.	Immobilization (animal still alert, no muscle relaxation)	W	Finnie (1986a); Johnson-Delaney (1997)
	30–50 mg/kg i.m.	Immobilization (animal still alert, no muscle relaxation)	BP; various phalangers	Shima (1999)
Ketamine + Acepromazine	30 mg/kg K + 2 mg/kg A i.m.	Immobilization with some sedation	BP	Finnie (1986a); Johnson-Delaney (1997)
Ketamine + Medetomidine	2–3 mg/kg K + 0.05–0.1 mg/kg M i.m.	Immobilization with sedation; hypotensive; reverse M with atipamezole 0.05–0.4 mg/kg i.v.	Various	Shima (1999)
Ketamine + Midazolam	10–20 mg/kg K + 0.35–0.5 mg/kg Mi i.m. Dosage depends on excitability of animal and procedure	Immobilization with good sedation; anxiolytic; relaxant; use as pre-anaesthetic (add analgesic) or to facilitate examination/diagnostic procedure; give M first, then K after 5–10 minutes	W; various	
Ketamine + Xylazine	10–25 mg/kg K + 5 mg/kg X i.m.	Immobilization with sedation; hypotensive; reverse X with yohimbine 0.2 mg/kg i.v.	W	Shima (1999)
Meloxicam	0.2 mg/kg s.c./orally q24h for 3–4 days	Postoperative analgesia	VO	
Midazolam	0.25–0.5 mg/kg i.v./i.m.	Anti-anxiety; sedative; preoperative analgesic	Various	
Tiletamine/Zolazepam	3–10 mg/kg i.m.	Immobilization with some sedation; results variable	W	Shima (1999)
	10–20 mg/kg i.m.	Immobilization with some sedation; results variable	BP	Shima (1999)
Antimicrobial agents				
Amikacin	10 mg/kg i.m. q12h for 5 days	Gram-negative pneumonia	W	Blyde (1993)
Amoxicillin	30 mg/kg orally/i.m. q24h for 14 days	Dermatitis; general	SG; do not use in herbivores	Hough *et al.* (1992)
Amoxicillin/Clavulanate	12.5 mg/kg s.c. q24h	Injectable form not available in USA	SG; do not use in herbivores	Pye (2005)
Cefalexin	30 mg/kg s.c. q24h		SG; do not use in herbivores	Pye (2005)
Chloramphenicol	50 mg/kg i.m./orally q12h	Broad-spectrum antibiotic	W; BP; SG; VO	
Enrofloxacin	2.5–5 mg/kg orally/i.m./s.c. q12–24 h (may cause tissue necrosis s.c./i.m.)	Antibiotic	Various	Johnson-Delaney (1997)
Gentamicin	1.5–2.5 mg/kg s.c./i.m./i.v. q12h	Antibiotic; fluid support required	Various	Johnson-Delaney (1997)

5.37 Drug formulary for marsupials. Dosages are anecdotal as reported in the literature except where noted. BP = Brushtail possum; SG = Sugar glider; SO = Short-tailed opossum; VO = Virginia opossum; W = Wallaby/macropod. (continues)

Drug	Dose	Comments	Species	Reference
Antimicrobial agents continued				
Lincomycin	30 mg/kg i.m. q24h for 7 days	Dermatitis	SG	Hough *et al.* (1992)
Metronidazole	80 mg/kg orally q24h	Antibacterial and antiprotozoal	SG	Hough *et al.* (1992)
Nitrofurazone	4.5 mg/kg orally q8h for 4–7 days	For enteric infection	W	
Penicillin	22,000–25,000 IU/kg i.m./s.c. q12–24h for 14–30 days	Susceptible infections; give with oral *Lactobacillus* or probiotics suitable for rabbits, guinea pigs or llams (not proven effective)	W	Wallach and Boever (1983)
Sulfadimethoxine	5–10 mg/kg orally q12–24h	Antibiotic; make sure patient is well hydrated	Various	Johnson-Delaney (1997)
Tetracycline	10 mg/kg i.m. per day in divided doses for 5–10 days	For haemobartonellosis and eperythrozoonosis	W	
Trimethoprim/ Sulphonamide	10–20 mg/kg i.m./orally q12–24h	Antibiotic; make sure well hydrated; subcutaneous administration may cause necrosis	Various	Johnson-Delaney (1997)
Antifungal agents				
Fenbendazole	20–50 mg/kg orally q24h for 3 days	Anthelmintic	BP; SG	Booth (1999)
Griseofulvin	20 mg/kg orally q24h for 30–60 days	Antidermatophyte for *Trichophyton*	Various	
Nystatin	5000 IU/kg orally q8h for 3 days	Candidiasis	W	Finnie (1986b); Blyde (1993)
Antiparasitic agents				
Amprolium 9.6% solution	1 ml/7 kg orally q24h for 5 days	Coccidiosis	W	
Atovaquone	100 mg/kg orally q24h; mix with 2x volume canola oil; treat for 2–12 months	Toxoplasmosis	W	
Carbaryl powder (5%)	Topical agent: apply sparingly, also in nest boxes	Ectoparasites	SG	Pye (2005)
Ivermectin	0.2–0.4 mg/kg orally/s.c. once	Anthelmintic	BP; SG; W	Blyde (1993); Booth (1999)
Levamisole	10 mg/kg orally	Anthelmintic	Various	
	6 mg/kg s.c.; repeat q3–4wk		VO	
	3 mg/kg orally/s.c. q3–4wk	Immune stimulation; adjunctive therapy	VO	
Mebendazole	25 mg/kg orally q24h for 2 days	Gastrointestinal and respiratory nematodes	VO	
Oxfendazole	5 mg/kg orally once	Anthelmintic	BP; SG	Booth (1999)
Piperazine	100 mg/kg orally	Anthelmintic	Various	
	15 mg/kg orally q12h or 50–57 mg/kg orally q24h, depending on patient/owner compliance and type of parasite		SG	Pye (2005)
Pyrethrin powder	Topical product; use at same dosage/ frequency as for kittens (follow manufacturer's instructions)	Ectoparasites	SG	Pye (2005)
Sulfadimethoxine	50 mg/kg orally q24h for 10 days	Coccidiosis	W	Johnson-Delaney (1997)

5.37 (continued) Drug formulary for marsupials. Dosages are anecdotal as reported in the literature except where noted. BP = Brushtail possum; SG = Sugar glider; SO = Short-tailed opossum; VO = Virginia opossum; W = Wallaby/macropod. (continues)

Drug	Dose	Comments	Species	Reference
Antiparasitic agents continued				
Tiabendazole	50–100 mg/kg orally once; repeat as necessary	Gastrointestinal and respiratory nematodes	VO	
Toltrazuril	2–25 mg/kg orally q24h for 3–5 days	For coccidiosis; not available in the USA	W	
Anti-inflammatory agents				
Dexamethasone	0.2 mg/kg i.v./i.m./s.c. q12–24h	Anti-inflammatory; corticosteroid	Various	Johnson-Delaney (1997)
Meloxicam	0.1–0.2 mg/kg orally/s.c. q24h	Anti-inflammatory; analgesic; NSAID	Various	
Prednisolone	0.1–0.2 mg/kg i.m./s.c./orally q24h	Anti-inflammatory; corticosteroid	Various	Johnson-Delaney (1997)
Cardiovascular agents				
Aspirin	18 mg/kg orally q72–96h	Cardiac disease	VO	
Digoxin	0.0011–0.0012 mg/kg orally q24h	Cardiac disease; congestive heart failure; monitor as for cats	VO	
L-Carnitine	100 mg/kg orally q12h	Cardiac disease	VO	
Enalapril	0.22–0.44 mg/kg orally q24h	Cardiac disease, monitor as for cats	All	
Furosemide	1–4 mg/kg s.c./i.m./i.v. q6–8h or 1–5 mg/kg orally q12h	Diuretic; pulmonary oedema/ascites treatment; initial dose i.v. and then use as needed	All	
Pimobendan	0.3–0.5 mg/kg orally q12h	Dilated cardiomyopathy; congestive heart failure	All	
Propranolol	0.55–1.10 mg/kg orally q12–24h	Cardiac disease; monitor as for cats	VO	
Miscellaneous				
Atropine	0.02–0.04 mg/kg i.m./i.v./s.c. once	Control salivation during sedation; part of a pre-anaesthetic regimen	Various	Finnie (1986a); Shima (1999)
Cisapride	0.25 mg/kg orally/i.m. q8–24h	Gastrointestinal motility enhancer	Various	Johnson-Delaney (1997)
Dexamethasone	0.5–2 mg/kg i.v./i.m./s.c. once	Shock	Various	Johnson-Delaney (1997)
Flunixin	0.1–1 mg/kg s.c./i.m. q12–24h; short-term use only	NSAID (may have long-term renal effects even from a single dose); hypotensive	Various	Johnson-Delaney (1997)
Glycopyrrolate	0.01–0.02 mg/kg i.m./i.v./s.c.	Control salivation during sedation; part of a pre-anaesthetic regimen	Various	Shima (1999)
Metoclopramide	0.05–0.1 mg/kg i.v./i.m./s.c./ orally q6–12h prn	Gastrointestinal motility enhancer	Various	Johnson-Delaney (1997)
Vitamin B complex	0.01–0.02 ml/kg i.m. Be very careful of 'sting'; administer under anaesthetic or dilute	Vitamin	Various	Johnson-Delaney (1997)
Vitamin E	25–100 IU per animal q24h; 400 IU post-capture restraint in macropods	Vitamin	W; various	
Vitamin K	2 mg/kg s.c. q24–72h	Adjunctive therapy in cardiac/liver disease	VO	

5.37 (continued) Drug formulary for marsupials. Dosages are anecdotal as reported in the literature except where noted. BP = Brushtail possum; SG = Sugar glider; SO = Short-tailed opossum; VO = Virginia opossum; W = Wallaby/macropod.

Acknowledgements

I would like to thank: Paul of Paul's Place, Kangaroo Island; Ray Ackroyd; Rosemary and Kevin Dohnt; Dr Anita Henness (posthumously) for her tireless work with opossums; staff of the Northern Territory Zoo, Darwin and Exotic Pet & Bird Clinic, Kirkland, WA, USA.

References and further reading

Blyde D (1993) Common diseases and treatments in macropods. *Proceedings, American Association of Zoo Veterinarians,* pp. 168–170. St Louis, Missouri

Booth R (1999) General husbandry and medicine of sugar gliders. In: *Kirk's Current Veterinary Therapy XIII,* ed. JD Bonagura and RW Kirk, pp.1157–1163. WB Saunders, Philadelphia

Fadem BH, Trupin GL, Maliniak E, *et al.* (1982) Care and breeding of the gray, short-tailed opossum (*Monodelphis domestica*). *Laboratory Animal Science* **32**, 405–409

Field KJ and Griffith JW (1990) Corneal lesion in a grey short-tailed opossum. *Laboratory Animals* **19**, 19–20

Finnie EP (1986a) Restraint. In: *Zoo & Wild Animal Medicine, 2nd edn,* ed. ME Fowler, pp. 570–572. WB Saunders, Philadelphia

Finnie EP (1986b) Viral diseases. In: *Zoo & Wild Animal Medicine, 2nd edn,* ed. ME Fowler, pp. 576–577. WB Saunders, Philadelphia

Fowler ME (1986) *Zoo & Wild Animal Medicine, 2nd edn.* WB Saunders, Philadelphia

Hough I, Reuter RE, Rahaley RS, *et al.* (1992) Cutaneous lymphosarcoma in a sugar glider. *Australian Veterinary Journal* **69**, 93–94

Hubbard GB, Mahaney MC, Gleiser CA, *et al.* (1997) Spontaneous pathology of the gray short-tailed opossum (*Monodelphis domestica*). *Laboratory Animal Science* **47**, 19–26

Hume I (1999) *Marsupial Nutrition.* Cambridge University Press, Melbourne, Australia

Johnson SD (1997) Orchiectomy of the mature sugar glider (*Petaurus breviceps*). *Exotic Pet Practice* **2**, 71

Johnson-Delaney CA (1996) Marsupials. In: *Exotic Companion Medicine Handbook for Veterinarians,* ed. CA Johnson-Delaney, Suppl.1, pp. 1–52. Wingers, Lake Worth, FL

Johnson-Delaney CA (1997) *Exotic Companion Pet Handbook for Veterinarians.* Wingers Publishing, Lake Worth, FL

Johnson-Delaney CA (1998) The marsupial pet: sugar gliders, exotic possums and wallabies. *Proceedings, Annual Conference and Expo of Association of Avian Veterinarians,* pp. 329–339. St. Paul, Minnesota

Johnson-Delaney CA (2000) Therapeutics of companion exotic marsupials. *Veterinary Clinics of North America: Exotic Animal Practice* **3**, 173–181

Johnson-Delaney CA (2002) Reproductive medicine of companion marsupials. *Veterinary Clinics of North America: Exotic Animal Practice* **5**, 537–553

Johnson-Delaney CA (2005) What every veterinarian needs to know about Virginia opossums. *Exotic DVM* **6**(6), 38–43

Johnson-Delaney CA and Ness R (in press) Sugar gliders. In: *Rodents, Rabbits and Ferrets,* ed. Quesenberry and Carpenter. Elsevier, Philadelphia

Kuehl-Kovarik MC, Ackermann MR, Hanson DL, *et al.* (1994) Spontaneous pituitary adenomas in the Brazilian gray short-tailed opossum (*Monodelphis domestica*). *Veterinary Pathology* **31**, 377–379

Pye G (2005) Sugar gliders. In: *Exotic Animal Formulary, 3rd edn,* JW Carpenter, pp. 347–358. Elsevier Saunders, Philadelphia

Shima AL (1999) Sedation and anesthesia in marsupials. In: *Zoo & Wild Animal Medicine Current Therapy, 4th edn,* ed. ME Fowler, pp. 333–336. WB Saunders, Philadelphia

Smith A and Hume I (1996) *Possums and Gliders.* Surrey Beatty & Sons Pty Limited/Australian Mammal Society, Chipping Norton, NSW, Australia

VandeBerg JL, Cothran EG and Kelly CA (1986) Dietary effects on hematologic and serum chemical values in gray short-tailed opossums (*Monodelphis domestica*). *Laboratory Animal Science* **36**, 32–36

Wallach JD and Boever WJ (1983) *Diseases of Exotic Animals: Medical and Surgical Management.* WB Saunders, Philadelphia

6

Ferrets, skunks and otters

Nico J. Schoemaker

Introduction

The family Mustelidae contains the weasel-like carnivores (subfamily Mustelinae – including polecats, weasels, stoats, mink) and the otters (subfamily Lutrinae). The skunk used to be classified in the subfamily Mephitinae but has recently been reclassified in a separate family, Mephitidae. Ferrets are domesticated polecats and are popular pets and working animals. Otters and skunks are less commonly presented in veterinary practice but are increasingly kept in small private or zoological collections.

Ferrets

Ferrets have traditionally been kept for hunting purposes but in recent years they have increasingly been kept as pets. Besides hunting rabbits in the field, ferrets can be used to control rat populations in areas where shooting is too risky, such as in buildings. The latter was the original reason why ferrets were taken to the USA, though there are now many states where working with ferrets and keeping them as pets is not allowed. Since the fear of a new influenza pandemic, ferrets have also become more frequently used as laboratory animals as they are highly susceptible to the influenza virus and therefore are considered a good model for research studies.

Some people believe that the ferret (*Mustela putorius furo;* Figure 6.1*)* should not be kept in captivity. This animal, however, can be considered a domesticated creature for which no wild counterpart exists. Its closest relatives in the wild are the European polecat (*Mustela putorius)* and possibly the Steppe polecat (*M. eversmanni).*

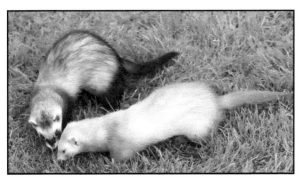

6.1 Domestic ferrets, showing the characteristic long thin body shape and some colour variation. (Courtesy of J. Chitty; reproduced from the *BSAVA Manual of Rodents and Ferrets.*)

Skunks

The striped skunk (*Mephitis mephitis*), native to North America, is becoming increasingly popular as a pet (Figure 6.2), despite the following drawbacks:

- They may be very 'friendly' at an early age, if well socialized, but tend to become less social with age
- They spray from their anal scent glands, and it is illegal to 'de-scent' animals without a medical need in many European countries
- Skunks may be carriers of the roundworm *Baylisascaris columnaris.* The larvae of this worm can also migrate in humans towards nervous tissues and there is no treatment for people infected with migrating larvae. The eggs remain infectious in the environment for years.

Based on these features, keeping skunks as pets should be discouraged.

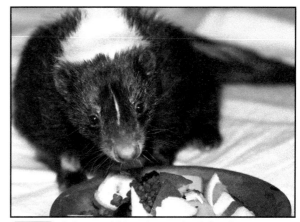

6.2 A 5-year-old female pet skunk feeding on a combination of ferret food and fruits.

Otters

The information in this chapter will focus predominantly on the Asian small-clawed otter (*Aonyx cinereus*). Information on veterinary care and rehabilitation of the European otter (*Lutra lutra*) can be found in the *BSAVA Manual of Wildlife Casualties.*

The Asian small-clawed otter (Figure 6.3) is the smallest of the 13 otter species, and is the one most commonly kept in zoos. In 2004 its conservation status was classified as approaching vulnerable. Asian small-clawed otters are very social and may live in groups of over 20 individuals in the wild. They live in

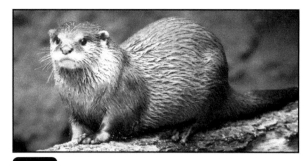

6.3 An Asian small-clawed otter in a zoo.

areas where shallow waters exist, with some vegetation along the shore. They have good climatic adaptability, and occur from tropical regions up into the Himalayan mountains. An extensive overview on captive management, reproduction, health and behaviour can be found in the *Asian Small-clawed Otter Husbandry Manual* (Lombardi and O'Connor, 1998).

Biology

Ferrets

Ferret anatomy is essentially very similar to that of other carnivores, such as the dog and cat. Although most of the ferret's biological features are comparable with other pet carnivores, there are some differences. The ferret's lifespan is a little shorter than that of the dog and cat, but much longer than for most other small mammal pets. For detailed information on ferret anatomy and physiology, see the *BSAVA Manual of Rodents and Ferrets*. Biological data are summarized in Figure 6.4.

Lifespan (years)	8–10 (max. 15); 5–7 in the USA
Average bodyweight (g)	Males: 1200 Females: 600
Rectal temperature (°C)	38.8 (37.8–40)
Heart rate (beats/min)	200–250
Respiration rate (breaths/min)	33–36

6.4 Biological data for the ferret.

Skunks

As noted above, the skunk does not belong to the family Mustelidae but has recently been reclassified. Biological data are summarized in Figure 6.5.

Lifespan (years)	8–10
Length (cm)	Head and body: 20–28 Tail: 28–43.5 (often carried over the back)
Bodyweight (kg)	0.75–4.0 Note: very fat skunks are frequently seen in practice
Body temperature (°C)	37.0–38.9
Heart rate (beats/min)	140–190
Respiratory rate (breaths/min)	35–40 (will pant when excited or hot)

6.5 Biological data for the skunk.

Otters

Biological data are summarized in Figure 6.6.

Length (cm)	Approximately 90
Bodyweight (kg)	Usually <5
Body temperature (°C)	37.2–39.4
Heart rate (beats/min)	80–300
Respiratory rate (breaths/min)	16–60

6.6 Biological data for the Asian small-clawed otter.

Husbandry

Housing

Ferrets

The size of a ferret's cage is not important as long as the owners regularly let their animals play, under supervision, outside the cage. However, based on laboratory animal recommendations, the cage should have an area of at least 4500 cm^2 (males need at least 6000 cm^2 per ferret) and be at least 50 cm high.

More important than size, the housing should be built in such a way that escape is impossible, as these animals are notorious escape artists. The housing should be high enough to allow the ferret to stand on its hindlegs to investigate its surroundings, and big enough to provide a sleeping area (nest box), a litter box, a feeding area and some room to play. Solid materials are preferred for the bottom of the cage. Litter boxes should be placed away from the food and water and sleeping area.

Water can be provided in either a bowl or a bottle. Most owners prefer bottles because ferrets tend to play with bowls and make a mess. Bottles should be thoroughly cleaned and refilled daily. Food can be provided in a bowl attached to the cage or in a bowl heavy enough to prevent the ferret from tipping it up.

The sleeping area should be some kind of box for them to hide in. Cloths, towels or old t-shirts can be used for bedding material. Hides are also commercially available. Hay, straw and wood shavings are not recommended for ferrets as inhalation of dust may lead to chronic irritation of the upper respiratory tract.

Ferrets can be housed either indoors or outside. When housed outdoors ferrets should be provided with protection against the elements. They are highly susceptible to heatstroke as they cannot sweat, so housing should not be placed in direct sunlight. The resting area should be dry and clean and give insulation against freezing conditions. Ferrets are extremely social animals and most are not kept as a solitary animal. Ferrets tend to pile together when sleeping, often in very cramped spaces, rather than sleep alone. Ferrets of either sex or age may accept conspecifics; it often depends on the personality of the individual.

Under supervision, ferrets can be kept with dogs and cats but not with rabbits or rodents.

Skunks

The housing of skunks is comparable to that for ferrets. Both species can be very inquisitive and like to climb into cabinets, and dig in potted plants. When not confined to a cage, the rooms to which the animals have access should be modified accordingly. Suggested minimal dimensions of the cage are 90 x 60 x 60 cm per skunk. A hiding box, such as a dog carrier, can be used as a secure sleeping area. Water should be provided in a bottle as skunks will tip over their water bowl. As young skunks may be trained to use a litter box, this should be available as well. Skunks may be housed together socially if raised together, particularly littermates that have been neutered. Introduction of neutered adults may or may not be successful, depending on the individual temperaments of the skunks. Many skunks raised individually, and that are well integrated into a home (perhaps with other pets), may not accept another skunk.

Otters

In captivity Asian small-clawed otters need plenty of land (at least twice the area of the pool) to rest, groom, explore and eat large prey animals. They need a burrow or nest box to hide and sleep in, with dry grass or hay, reeds and leaves as bedding. In addition to a pool the otters should also have access to fresh drinking water. Since otters are good climbers and diggers, this should be taken into consideration when designing their enclosure. They are highly social and therefore best kept in breeding pairs or in same-sex groups if breeding is not desired.

Diet

Ferrets

The ferret is a carnivore and can therefore be maintained on a good quality high-protein (35–40%) diet. The fat content can vary from 9 to 28%, but both the carbohydrate (<25%) and fibre (<2.5%) fractions should be low. Specific ferret diets as well as good quality cat diets are suitable for ferrets. Some ferrets fed specific diets seem to have firmer stools that smell less strongly. Although ferrets can be fed canned products, dry pellets are preferred. These stay fresh longer and seem to decrease the amount of dental calculus formed. Fresh water should be available, especially when pellets are fed. Because ferrets have a short gut and a fast gut transit time it is commonly recommended to feed them *ad libitum*. In recent years it has become popular to feed ferrets the more natural diet of whole rodents, rabbits or pigeons (Figure 6.7). Dental wear is thought to be less on the latter diets.

Skunks

In contrast to ferrets, skunks are omnivorous animals which consume a combination of whole prey, insects, and fruit and vegetables. Although there is no consensus on what the best diet is for skunks, it is clear that they need a mixture of either formulated dog or cat food, fruits and vegetables. One recommendation is to give a third dog food, a third cat food and another third of fruit and vegetables. Since cat

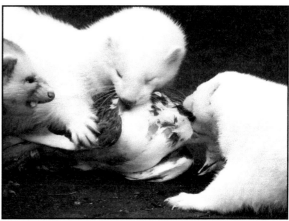

6.7 Ferrets eating a frozen/thawed whole pigeon. (Courtesy of B. van de Laan.)

food tends to contain more fat than dog food, others prefer to feed two-thirds of dog food and one-third fruit and vegetables. In captivity many skunks are fed too much, leading to severe obesity. The amount of food provided should therefore be restricted. It is also recommended that food is provided inside enrichment toys, such as those intended for dogs, to encourage exercise.

Otters

The natural diet consists of crabs, crustaceans, snails, molluscs, frogs and small fish. In captivity it is recommended that they be fed twice a day to accommodate their high metabolic rate and rapid digestion. There is no consensus on what exactly to feed Asian-small clawed otters in captivity. A fish-based diet seems to be the preferred choice, with supplementation of vitamin E and thiamine. To maintain dental health, it is recommended that bones and/or other hard diet items are provided.

Breeding and contraception

Ferrets

Female ferrets (jills) are seasonal breeders and come into oestrus under the influence of light. Day length exceeding 12 hours induces oestrus, which continues until day length decreases to <12 hours. Therefore, under natural light conditions the oestrous season in the northern hemisphere is approximately from March until September. A firm stimulant, in the form of dragging by the scruff of the neck and mating, is necessary for ovulation to occur. Reproductive data are summarized in Figure 6.8.

In the past few years the author has gained a lot of experience with the use of implants containing 4.7 mg deslorelin as an alternative to surgical neutering. At the time of writing, more than 200 ferrets have received such an implant: in the males (hobs), the effect of implants was similar to that of surgical castration for up to 2 years; in jills, a short oestrous period (maximum 2 weeks) may occur after giving the implant, and pseudopregnancy occurred in a small percentage. The use of these implants is recommended over surgical castration, as they may help prevent hyperadrenocorticism.

Sexual maturity	First Spring after birth
Breeding season (Figure 6.8a)	Northern hemisphere: March–September Southern hemisphere: August–January
Gestation period	41–42 days
Average litter size	8
Weight at birth	8–10 g
Eyes open at	4–5 weeks
Eruption of deciduous teeth	3–4 weeks
Eruption of permanent teeth	7–10 weeks
Weaning age	6–8 weeks (preferably 8)

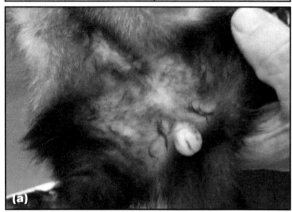

6.8 Reproductive data for the ferret. **(a)** Swollen vulva of the in-season jill. This animal has been in season for a while, hence the ventral alopecia. (Courtesy of J. Chitty; reproduced from the *BSAVA Manual of Rodents and Ferrets*.)

Skunks

Female skunks come into oestrus in February/March, and after a gestation period of 62–66 days produce a litter of approximately six pups. These pups have a birth weight around 14 g. The lactation period will last up to 6 weeks, and 2 weeks later the pups can be weaned. As with ferrets, skunks may have an extended oestrus and any neutering should therefore be carried out prior to first oestrus.

Otters

Both males and females reach sexual maturity at 2–3 years of age. Asian small-clawed otters pair for life and usually produce two litters of young per year. The gestation period is approximately 62 days, and litter size can vary between one and six, although the average is two young per litter. At birth, otters weigh approximately 50 g and are altricial. Both parents care for the kits. Eyes open at 5–6 weeks old and they leave the nest at 9–10 weeks. They start to swim and begin to eat solid foods at 11–12 weeks.

Preventive healthcare

Ferrets

Ferrets are susceptible to canine distemper and rabies. Rabies vaccination is advised as for other mammals in areas where rabies is endemic, and is necessary for ferrets travelling within the European Union under the UK Pet Passport scheme, in addition to treatment for ticks and tapeworms. In many public health districts in the USA vaccination against rabies is required, and there is a 1-year licensed vaccine for use in ferrets available, The US Animal Health Association Rabies Compendium lists ferrets in the same category as dogs and cats concerning post-bite incidence. Young ferrets should be screened for Coccidia, ear mites and fleas.

As canine distemper vaccination requires a series of injections, the veterinary surgeon can use these opportunities to assess growth, tooth development and advise the owner on preventive dental care, diet and the importance of annual examinations. At 3 years of age, because of the incidence of dental disease, heart disease and neoplasia, many practitioners recommend twice yearly check-ups. Regular dental prophylaxis is similar to that for dogs and cats.

Skunks

Skunks are susceptible to canine distemper, rabies and canine adenovirus, and some have recommended vaccination against these agents, and against feline panleucopenia and leptospirosis. None of the available vaccines, however, has been approved for use in skunks. Recombinant vaccines would be preferred but are not available in Europe. Care should be taken when (modified) live vaccines are used, as they may result in vaccine-induced disease.

Skunks should be wormed on a regular basis to decrease the risk of shedding of *Baylisascaris columnaris* eggs. Recommendations for fenbendazole (50 mg/kg orally q24h for 5 days) vary from once a month to twice a year.

Otters

Otters are susceptible to canine distemper. It has therefore been advocated that they should be vaccinated against this virus. Vaccine-induced disease is a risk when using (modified) live vaccines. The risks and benefits should therefore be discussed prior to vaccination.

Handling and restraint

Ferrets

Most pet ferrets are used to being handled, so the risk of being bitten is no greater than with a cat or dog. Ferrets should be picked up by placing one hand around the thorax and supporting the hindlegs with the other hand (Figure 6.9a). Ferrets struggle if their hindlegs are held too firmly. If struggling is excessive, the neck should be gripped more firmly. Scruffing of the loose skin at the back of the neck may be necessary for restraining difficult ferrets (Figure 6.9b).

Ferrets can be distracted by applying a liquid diet to the abdomen; most owners can manage to clip the nails of their pets whilst they are licking the food (Figure 6.10).

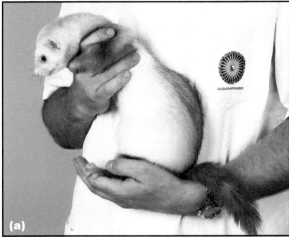

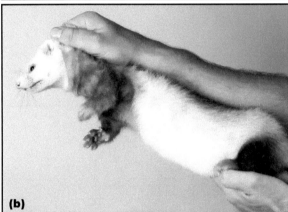

6.9 **(a)** Gently handling a ferret by placing one hand around the thorax and supporting the hindlegs with the other hand. **(b)** Scruffing the loose skin at the back of the neck may be necessary for restraining difficult ferrets.

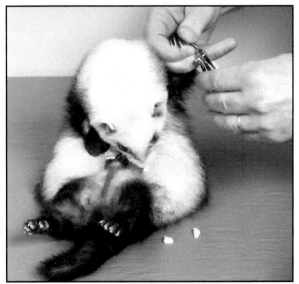

6.10 By applying a liquid diet to the abdomen most owners can clip the nails of their ferrets while they are licking the food.

Skunks

Although skunks may seem friendly at times, one should always be aware of the possibility of being bitten. This is especially true when the skunk is being restrained. Some sources state that it is possible to scruff the animal, but this is not easy in obese skunks. The use of special gloves is advised in animals that are not commonly handled. Some animals will need anaesthesia to allow a thorough examination.

Otters

As otters are not domesticated it is not advisable to handle them without chemical restraint (see below).

Diagnostic approach

Ferrets

History and observation

As with any consultation a thorough case history is mandatory. Alertness and attitude should then be assessed. In the carrier the ferret may appear quite sleepy, but once out of the carrier it should be highly active. Ferrets normally arch their backs when they walk or run.

Clinical examination

Physical examination of the ferret is basically similar to that of the dog and cat. Handling of the ferret may alter its body temperature, heart/pulse rate and respiratory frequency. The author therefore prefers to measure respiratory rate while the ferret is still in the carrier. The ferret is then handled to measure the pulse at the femoral artery. This is best achieved when the ferret is placed on the arm and not on a table. The rectal temperature can then be measured, preferably with a digital thermometer. Reference values can be found in Figure 6.4.

Checking the hydration status of any small mammal is one of the most important features of a physical examination, and can be performed by assessing: the skin turgor of the upper eyelids; skin tenting in the neck; and the moistness of the oral mucosa. While checking the oral mucosa, attention should also be paid to the teeth, which should be free from tartar. The capillary refill time (CRT) can be assessed by pressing on a non-pigmented footpad.

Since ferrets often have ear mites, special attention should be paid to the external ear canals. Pigment in the pinna and canal can often be associated with chronic ear mite infestation. Normal ferret wax is dark brown and should be checked frequently for mites, particularly if the ferret exhibits pruritus when the ear is touched.

The neck, axillary, inguinal and popliteal lymph nodes should be checked. They may appear enlarged in overweight animals. If they are also firm, a fine needle aspirate should be taken to check for lymphoma.

Both auscultation of the thorax and abdominal palpation are finally included in the standard physical examination. An enlarged spleen is a common finding on palpation but is seldom of clinical importance.

Electrocardiography (ECG) can be helpful. Electrocardiographic parameters determined in 29 healthy ferrets are given in Figure 6.11.

Parameter		Range
Heart rate		175–265 beats/min
Heart axis		85–102 degrees
Measurements in lead II	P-wave duration	0.01–0.02 s
	P-wave amplitude	0.09–0.20 mV
	PR-interval	0.04–0.07 s
	QRS-complex duration	0.02–0.04 s
	QRS-complex amplitude	1.4–4.4 mV
	QT-interval	0.11–0.16 mV
	ST-segment	0.02–0.05 mV
	T-wave duration	0.06–0.11 s
	T-wave amplitude	0.15–0.4 mV

6.11 ECG parameters determined in 29 healthy, awake ferrets.

Sample collection

Blood: As a general rule, blood can be collected up to 1% of the bodyweight of a healthy ferret, although usually far less is required. Most laboratories can do haematology and full biochemical analysis with 2 ml of blood.

Techniques for 'bleeding', such as toenail clipping and cardiac or periorbital puncture, should be considered obsolete. Much better locations are the lateral saphenous vein or cephalic vein for small amounts of blood (up to 1 ml) and the jugular vein or the cranial vena cava for larger amounts. The author prefers a 26-gauge needle and a 2 ml or 5 ml syringe for drawing blood. The jugular vein is approached as for cats and can be sampled in docile ferrets without anaesthesia (Figure 6.12). The ventral tail artery can also be used for samples up to 1 ml.

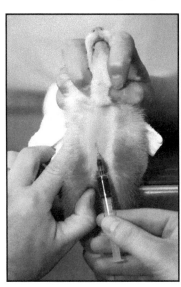

6.12 Blood collection from the jugular vein. The technique is similar to that used in cats and dogs. Some prefer to roll the non-anaesthetized ferret in a towel for optimal restraint.

The cranial vena cava is best sampled under anaesthesia, although this is not necessary in debilitated ferrets. Isoflurane anaesthesia can artificially lower the red blood cell count and PCV by up to 40%; these return to normal after approximately 45 minutes

of anaesthesia. The ferret is placed in dorsal recumbency and the needle inserted into the thoracic inlet just cranial to the connection between the manubrium and the first rib, and then directed towards the contralateral hindleg at a 30-degree angle (Figure 6.13). As the heart is located relatively caudally within the thoracic cavity and the needle is only 1.2 cm long, there is no risk of cardiac puncture from this technique.

Figures 6.14 to 6.16 show reference ranges for haematological and biochemical parameters.

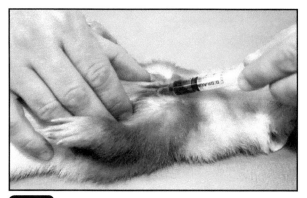

6.13 Blood collection from the cranial vena cava.

Parameter	SI units	Range
WBC	x 10⁹/l	3.8–14
RBC	x 10¹²/l	7.1–11.4
PCV	%	36–57
Hb	mmol/l	7.7–11.4
MCV	fl	44.8–53.9
MCH	fmol	0.95–1.08
MCHC	mmol/l	18.8–21.6
Platelets	x 10⁹/l	206–937
Reticulocytes	%	0.3–3.0
Lymphocytes	x 10⁹/l	1.2–8.4
Monocytes	x 10⁹/l	0.1–0.5
Neutrophils	x 10⁹/l	0.9–9.7
Eosinophils	x 10⁹/l	0.1–0.7
Basophils	x 10⁹/l	0.0–0.2

6.14 Reference ranges for haematological values in 50 ferrets (determined at the University Veterinary Diagnostic Laboratory at Utrecht University).

Parameter	SI units	Range
PT	seconds	9.4–12.4
APTT	seconds	15.1–22.2
Fibrinogen	g/l	1.0–3.5
AT3	%	> 94.4
D-dimer	ng/ml	< 250

6.15 Reference ranges for blood coagulation values in 47 ferrets (determined at the University Veterinary Diagnostic Laboratory at Utrecht University).

Parameter	SI units	Range	Mean
BUN	mmol/l	0.2–16.1	10.4
Creatinine	μmol/l	8.8–106	53
AF	IU/l	14–144	41
ALT	IU/l	48–292	138
AST	IU/l	46–118	68.3
LDH	IU/l	222–377	278
Bile acids	μmol/l	1–28	9.1
CK	IU/l	98–564	245
Glucose	mmol/l	6.66–7.99	6.69
Calcium	mmol/l	1.9–2.4	2.04
Total protein	g/l	43–60	52
Albumin	g/l	34–48	39
Globulins	g/l	2–24	13

6.16 Reference ranges for plasma biochemistry values in ferrets. (Data from Fudge, 2000.)

Common conditions

Ferrets

Viral infections

Canine distemper: On a worldwide basis canine distemper (caused by a paramyxovirus) is the most serious viral infection of ferrets and is almost always fatal, although seldom seen in ferrets nowadays owing to vaccination.

The classic signs are dermatitis on the lips and chin and around the inguinal region, 7–9 days after infection. Other common signs are mucopurulent ocular and nasal discharge, pyrexia (>40°C), sneezing, coughing and anorexia. Just as in dogs, ferrets can develop hyperkeratosis of the footpads (hardpad).

Diagnosis is based on fluorescent antibody tests on conjunctival smears and/or brain tissue. As vaccination is performed with a modified live virus, vaccinated ferrets give a positive result with this test and therefore only non-vaccinated ferrets should be tested.

In the USA a canine distemper vaccine is registered for use in ferrets and contains a recombinant canarypox vector expressing certain glycoproteins of the virus (PureVax Ferret, Merial Inc., Athens, GA). Unfortunately, this vaccine is not available in Europe. Standard modified live vaccines developed for use in dogs can be used in ferrets, provided they are derived from non-ferret cell lines, as ferrets subjected to these can develop distemper from the vaccine. Manufacturers will provide veterinary surgeons with data on the use of their products in ferrets and many of these products have been used safely in hundreds of ferrets.

Influenza: Ferrets are highly susceptible to several strains of human, avian and swine influenza virus and therefore should be considered a zoonosis. Humans can infect ferrets and *vice versa*. Veterinary surgeons or staff with minor symptoms of influenza either should not handle or treat ferrets, or should wear a mask to prevent the spread of the virus.

Many of the clinical signs of influenza are similar to those of canine distemper but less severe. Nasal discharge is mucoserous instead of mucopurulent, there is more sneezing and coughing, and the fever is usually over before the animal is presented to the veterinary surgeon. Just as in humans, the infection is self-limiting and usually not fatal.

Aleutian disease: Aleutian disease is caused by a parvovirus, unrelated to that causing bloody diarrhoea in dogs. Of the Mustelidae the mink is the most susceptible, but a ferret-specific strain has been found (Porter *et al.*, 1982). Aleutian disease is considered more of a problem in the UK than elsewhere. An outbreak of Aleutian disease was seen in the Netherlands after the import of ferrets from New Zealand. A serological survey among 1436 Dutch ferrets, performed by Dr J. Moorman-Roest, found in 4.6% of ferrets antibodies against Aleutian disease. Ten out of 22 ferrets from the latter group died within 1.5 years after detection of antibodies. Aleutian disease has been diagnosed in ferrets in the USA, and screening of 500 clinically normal ferrets housed in shelters in northern America resulted in the detection of antibodies against Aleutian disease in about 10% of the animals.

Aleutian disease is an immune complex-mediated condition, resulting in multiple organ failure. Clinical signs in mink include wasting, hepatomegaly, splenomegaly, melaena, recurrent fevers and eventually hindleg paralysis and other neurological signs. Most mink die within 5 months of infection. Ferrets seldom develop such severe clinical signs. A serum countercurrent immunoelectrophoresis is necessary to confirm the diagnosis. Hypergammaglobulinaemia together with chronic wasting signs, used to be very suggestive for Aleutian disease. Hypergammaglobulinaemia, however, has recently been associated with infectious peritonitis in ferrets as well.

As with almost all viral infections there is no specific treatment, but antibiotics and steroids have been reported to give some relief.

Ectoparasites

Ear mites: The ear mite *Otodectes cynotis* is the most common ectoparasite found on ferrets. Massive infestations can cause pruritus, but many ferrets have low-grade infestations without showing many signs. Mites may be seen during a routine otoscopic examination but can also be easily overlooked. The best diagnostic technique is to place a sample scraped from the ear canal on to a microscope slide with potassium hydroxide (KOH). Under a stereomicroscope the mites can be seen moving around.

For treatment, the author prefers the topical application of selamectin at the base of the skull. Although no side effects have been reported in ferrets after using selamectin, this drug is not authorized for use in ferrets. An advantage of topical selamectin is that it does not need to be administered within the ear canal and there is therefore no risk of an ototoxic effect if the eardrum is not intact.

Fleas (*Ctenocephalides felis*): Ferrets are just as sensitive to flea infestations as are dogs and cats, and the clinical manifestations are similar. Signs of flea-bite hypersensitivity may be seen in some animals, such as papulocrustous dermatitis over the tailbase, ventral abdomen and caudomedial thighs. As for dogs and cats, treatment of the environment is just as, if not more, important than treatment of the ferret alone. Owners who regularly wash their ferrets use a flea shampoo containing permethrin for this purpose. Selamectin can also be used for flea control. Imidacloprid has been used safely and effectively (Kelleher 2001) and lufenuron appears to be effective when given at cat dosages (Orcutt, 2004).

Helminthiasis

Ferrets are usually free of gastrointestinal parasites. Routine worming is therefore not recommended. If worm eggs are found in the faeces, selamectin can be given. Therefore, this drug can be used in young animals for the combined control of ear mite infestations and possible worm infection.

Endocrine disease

Persistent oestrus: If the jill is not mated, she will not ovulate, as ferrets are induced ovulators. This results in increased levels of oestradiol, which remain high until the end of the oestrous season. Continued high levels of oestradiol can lead to alopecia and bone marrow suppression, resulting in a pancytopenia and eventual death. Some ferrets show pancytopenia within the first oestrous season. Oestrous prevention can be accomplished through neutering within the jill's first year, before the oestrous season begins (usually in January or February in the northern hemisphere); however, there is strong evidence that neutering can induce hyperadrenocorticism. Alternatively, proligestone (50 mg/kg i.m.) or a deslorelin implant can be used.

Insulinoma: Insulinomas, small tumours of the pancreatic beta cells resulting in hypoglycaemia, are a common finding in ferrets. They are equally distributed among the sexes, and animals are affected at a median age of 5 years (range 2–8 years). Clinical signs vary from slight incoordination and weakness in the hindlimbs to complete collapse and coma. Episodes of salivation and a glazed look may be noticed by owners, and are most often seen when the ferret has not eaten for some time. The episodes do not usually last long and they clear up when the ferret is given food or a calorie-rich beverage. Insulinomas are commonly found incidentally during surgery for other conditions such as hyperadrenocorticism. Diagnosis is usually based on serum glucose levels <3.4 mmol/l. Plasma insulin levels can be measured and are usually elevated. An insulin concentration within the reference range is still considered increased if the plasma glucose concentration is below its reference range.

Surgery is the most definitive treatment option, as this removes the cells producing the excess insulin. The tumours are, however, small (5–7 mm) and sometimes difficult to remove; they may be undetectable at surgery. Diabetes mellitus can also occur if too much pancreas is removed, and this should be avoided – medical management of insulinomas is far easier than that of diabetes mellitus. Although adenocarcinomas of the pancreas have been reported, most insulinomas are benign.

If an owner prefers medical treatment, diazoxide (5–30 mg/kg q12h orally), an insulin-inhibiting agent, or prednisolone (0.2–1 mg/kg q24h orally) may be prescribed. This author advocates diazoxide because this agent has the most specific effect, and fewest side effects.

Prognosis is considered better in ferrets than in dogs. Metastases are seldom found in ferrets in the Netherlands, whereas insulinomas almost always metastasize in dogs. A literature survey (unpublished data) revealed that insulinomas in dogs have already metastasized in 46% of cases by the time of surgery. Although metastases are rare in ferrets, multiple tumours and recurrent signs are common. Recurrent signs are probably due to the development of new tumours rather than to metastasis of the earlier tumour. Animals remain disease-free for about 10 months after surgery, and the average survival time is 1.5 years.

Hyperadrenocorticism: Although hyperadrenocorticism is now considered one of the most common diseases in ferrets, it was first reported as recently as 1987. Since that time a lot of research has been done. Results have shown that hyperadrenocorticism in ferrets is different from that in dogs and in humans, where increased plasma cortisol levels are characteristic of Cushing's disease. In contrast, in ferrets plasma androstenedione, 17-hydroxyprogesterone and oestradiol concentrations are increased, but not cortisol.

Researchers in the USA have hypothesized that adrenal tumours may develop in ferrets due to early neutering, based on reports in mice. Ferrets are commonly neutered in the USA at 6 weeks of age. However, because hyperadrenocorticism is common in the Netherlands and yet ferrets there are neutered at a much older age (>6 months), the author does not believe that neutering has to occur early for adrenal tumours to develop. It is, however, likely that neutering does play a part in the aetiology of hyperadrenocorticism, and a temporal correlation has been found between the time of neutering and the time of diagnosis of hyperadrenocorticism (Schoemaker *et al.*, 2000). It has been shown that the depot gonadotrophin-releasing hormone (GnRH) agonists leuprolide acetate and deslorelin can control the signs of hyperadrenocorticism. It is hypothesized that the negative feedback of testosterone and oestradiol on hypothalamic GnRH is lost due to castration. This results in an uninhibited secretion of GnRH followed by the secretion of luteinizing hormone (LH) and follicle-stimulating hormone (FSH). These hormones, together or separately, continuously stimulate the adrenal glands, resulting in hyperplasia and tumour formation. Recent studies have shown that LH is the most important gonadotrophin hormone in the aetiology of this disease.

Prominent clinical signs of hyperadrenocorticism in ferrets include: symmetrical alopecia (Figure 6.17); vulvar swelling in neutered jills; stranguria due to

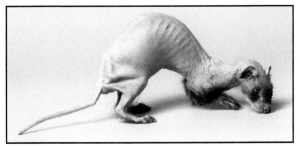

6.17 Extensive alopecia in an elderly ferret with hyperadrenocorticism.

prostate gland hypertrophy in hobs; and pruritus of unknown origin. No sex predilection could be found in a study in the Netherlands. Diagnosis can usually be based on clinical signs. Since ferrets commonly have concomitant diseases (such as lymphoma) it is advisable to perform abdominal ultrasonography in all ferrets with signs of hyperadrenocorticism. Ultrasonography may also demonstrate ovary remnants and allows the prostate gland to be evaluated. Assessment of the size of the adrenal glands also helps to monitor the progression of the disease. In the USA (University of Tennessee) androstenedione, oestradiol and 17-hydroxyprogesterone can be measured; an increase in one or more of these hormones is considered to be diagnostic (in the author's opinion androstenedione is the most sensitive indicator). However, the most likely differential diagnosis, a non-ovariectomized jill or remnant ovaries, cannot be differentiated using the hormone test.

Surgery used to be the treatment of choice: the left adrenal gland can be removed fairly easily but the right adrenal gland is attached to the caudal vena cava and resection is difficult. However, recent experience has shown that depot GnRH agonists (leuprolide acetate and deslorelin) block production of LH so that the adrenal cortex is no longer stimulated and the signs disappear. An advantage of medical treatment is that stimulation of the contralateral adrenal gland is also stopped, which may prevent the development of a tumour in this gland. In young animals (approximately 3 years of age) it may therefore be advantageous to remove the affected left adrenal gland and give a depot GnRH agonist.

Diabetes mellitus: Diabetes mellitus has been documented in ferrets but is considered rare. It is most often seen after debulking of the pancreas for the removal of insulinomas. Clinical signs are identical to those in dogs and cats, with polyuria and polydipsia the most prominent signs. Plasma glucose concentrations >22 mmol/l are considered suggestive of diabetes mellitus. Regulation has been attempted, starting with 0.1 IU of insulin twice daily (Hillyer and Quesenberry, 1997).

Helicobacter mustelae gastritis

Many ferret owners (and veterinary surgeons) commonly suspect that a ferret has an infection with *Helicobacter mustelae*. Confirmation of disease, however, is very difficult; as 80% of all ferrets are carriers of the bacterium, PCR and serology are of no use in diagnosis. It is thought that ferrets are infected at an early age and remain infected until they are treated. Disease is thought to occur when the ferret is in a state of immunosuppression. A ferret with a *Helicobacter* gastritis may be presented with lethargy, anorexia, salivation, vomiting and melaena, the last two being the most important signs. Gastroscopy and gastric biopsy are necessary to confirm the presence of gastric ulcers. Different treatment protocols are available. One protocol that has been found to be effective consists of the oral administration of clarithromycin (50 mg/kg), metronidazole (75 mg/kg) and omeprazole (4 mg/kg). The author prefers to add sucralfate to this protocol.

Cardiovascular disease

Congestive cardiomyopathy is a common cardiac disease of ferrets. Clinical signs are often non-specific and include lethargy, dyspnoea and coughing. Physical examination may reveal bradycardia, tachycardia, a systolic murmur or muffled heart sounds. Both pleural effusion and ascites can be seen with cardiomyopathy. Ultrasonography is the best diagnostic technique, showing results similar to those in other species (increased ventricular dimensions, decreased fractional shortening and enlarged left atrium). ECG is useful for choosing, and monitoring, the medication.

Treatment is similar to that for other species. When ascites or pleural effusion is present furosemide is indicated. A small amount of fluid may be removed to improve respiration. To improve cardiac function digoxin, enalapril and or pimobendan can be given.

Lymphoma

Lymphomas are the third most common tumours found in ferrets after adrenal tumours and insulinomas. Lymphomas occur in both juvenile and adult ferrets but the disease is much more aggressive in juveniles than it is in adults. Preliminary data suggest that the juvenile form may be caused by a virus (Erdman *et al.*, 1995). Clinical signs are often non-specific and may include loss of appetite, weight loss and enlargement of the peripheral lymph nodes. More severe clinical signs, as seen in juvenile ferrets, may include dyspnoea and coughing caused by pleural effusion. Lymphoblastic leukaemias have also been diagnosed in ferrets.

Although radiography can detect pleural effusion and masses in the anterior mediastinum, ultrasonography is more precise for diagnosing individual masses and can also detect masses in the abdomen. Ultrasonography is also useful as a guiding tool for taking samples by fine-needle aspiration (FNA). These samples are essential for confirming the diagnosis, but false-negative results (reactive lymph node) do occur. A full thickness biopsy or surgical removal of enlarged external lymph nodes may therefore be necessary to confirm the diagnosis. Lymphomas of juvenile and young adult ferrets are often immunoblastic, with a high mitotic index, whereas those of adults are mixed cell lymphomas with a much lower mitotic index.

The most effective treatment is difficult to determine, though ferrets initially often respond well to glucocorticosteroids. Different chemotherapy protocols have been developed, with mixed results: a period of remission can be achieved, but a cure is not likely. Administration of glucocorticoids to ferrets may result in resistance of lymphoid cells; ferrets receiving glucocorticoids for treating insulinoma or immune-mediated diseases may therefore be refractory to chemotherapy.

Splenomegaly

This can be found in healthy ferrets and in animals with seemingly unrelated diseases. In severe cases the spleen can extend all the way to the pelvic inlet, but total and differential blood counts do not show any abnormalities. The most common histological diagnosis is extramedullary haemopoiesis. Tumours of the spleen do occur, however. Therefore, when a ferret is presented with non-specific clinical signs and a large spleen is palpable, abdominal ultrasonography is recommended. In cases of lymphoma the spleen usually has an irregular aspect on ultrasonography. An ultrasound-guided biopsy is mandatory to confirm the diagnosis prior to surgery. The only indications for splenectomy are if the spleen contains a tumour (lymphoma) or there is discomfort.

Skunks

Metabolic bone disease

Metabolic bone disease is commonly encountered. Animals are frequently presented with the complaint of a gradual decrease of activity and difficulty walking. When the animals move they may show signs of discomfort or pain. Diagnosis is based on radiographs (Figure 6.18) and blood chemistry. Hypocalcaemia, which is best diagnosed by measuring ionized calcium, can further confirm the diagnosis. Treatment consists of the administration of painkillers and correction of the diet.

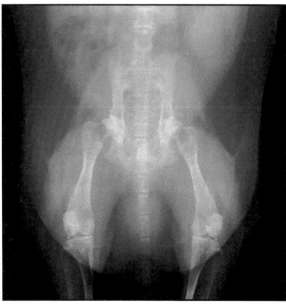

6.18 Ventrodorsal radiograph of an obese skunk, showing severe demineralization of the skeleton due to metabolic bone disease.

Otters

Renal calculi

Renal calculi are very common in otters and may occur in as many as 75% of the population. This is not only true for the Asian small-clawed otter, but has also

been reported in the European otter (*Lutra lutra*). The stones primarily consist of calcium oxalate and are located in the renal pelvis. Some may be seen in the bladder. Initially the stones do not seem to cause any problems, but at 4–5 years of age the urinary flow decreases and azotaemia may be found. No successful treatment has been described. Although uroliths can be surgically removed, they usually recur. Although the formation of stones has been associated with feeding meat-based diets, this is controversial, as the stones are found in animals being fed a range of diets. Some strategies have been developed to prevent renal calculi, but none has proven to be effective.

Supportive care

Ferrets

Drug administration

Oral medication: Tablets and capsules are not easily accepted by ferrets. Capsules are usually too big for them to swallow and will fall apart, and because ferrets have a low bodyweight no commercial capsule contains the right amount of drug. Tablets can be split into quarters for more accurate dosing, but most tablets are still too concentrated for use in ferrets. The author therefore prefers to use liquids and suspensions for oral treatment. These are easily accepted by ferrets and can be dosed accurately. It is recommended that practices dealing with ferrets and other small exotics should keep a stock of methylcellulose for the preparation of suspensions.

Injection sites: Ferrets can receive intramuscular injections, but total muscle mass is a limiting factor. If injections have to be given, the subcutaneous route is preferred (Figure 6.19).

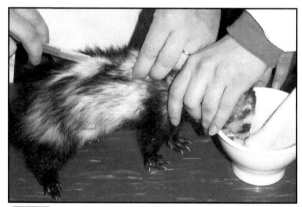

6.19 Subcutaneous injections are fairly easy to administer when the ferret is fed a favourite liquid diet.

Intravenous catheterization: The cephalic vein and lateral saphenous vein are suitable for the placement of indwelling catheters.

Fluid therapy

Although the intravenous and intraosseous routes are the most direct for fluid therapy, the subcutaneous and intraperitoneal routes are also suitable for most ferrets.

Anaesthesia and analgesia

Ferrets

Because ferrets have a relatively fast gastrointestinal transit time, a fasting period of about 4–6 hours prior to sedation or anaesthesia is usually sufficient.

Sedation

For non-painful simple procedures, such as taking blood from the vena cava or abdominal ultrasonography, ferrets can be simply sedated with isoflurane. Sedation or light anaesthesia by mask induction with 100% oxygen and 4% isoflurane, and maintenance with 2% isoflurane, enables procedures to be performed quickly. In a study performed by the author only a slight increase of stress hormones was seen after mask induction, whereas collecting blood without anaesthesia resulted in much higher levels of stress hormones. Ferrets recover quickly from such anaesthesia, so owners can take their pet home soon after the procedure.

Medetomidine can also be given: 100 µg/kg is usually sufficient for sedation of about 30 minutes. Atipamezole can be used to reverse the effects of medetomidine; a practical dosage is 2.5 times that of medetomidine in micrograms (i.e. half the volume dose). After short procedures the author usually doubles the volume of atipamezole to allow an even faster recovery.

Anaesthesia

The standard anaesthesia protocol used at Utrecht University for ferrets is to premedicate with 100 µg/kg medetomidine, followed by the placement of a catheter in the cephalic vein through which 1–3 mg/kg propofol is given for induction. Anaesthesia is maintained with isoflurane. Ferrets are always intubated (inner diameter 2–2.5 mm) for long surgical procedures.

Different combinations of injectable anaesthetics have been investigated. A practical combination is medetomidine at 0.08 mg/kg plus ketamine at 5 mg/kg s.c or i.m. Ferrets should be kept warm both during and after anaesthesia as hypothermia can occur easily.

Analgesia

The use of analgesics is an important part of good veterinary practice. During general anaesthesia both ketamine and medetomidine provide analgesia, but the addition of buprenorphine (0.01–0.03 mg/kg) may reduce the dosages of ketamine and medetomidine necessary.

The analgesics meloxicam (0.2 mg/kg orally) and carprofen (5 mg/kg i.m) have proven to be useful in ferrets.

Skunks

Anaesthesia and analgesia are as for ferrets.

Otters

To sedate the animal an injection of tiletamine/zolazepam or a combination of ketamine plus medetomidine can be given intramuscularly by blowdart or when the animal is restrained in a squeeze cage. The dose of tiletamine/zolazepam adequate for immobilization varies greatly between individuals and ranges from 5.5 to 9 mg/kg i.m. The combination of ketamine

(4–5.5 mg/kg) with medetomidine (40–55 µg/kg) has been described, and has the advantage that the medetomidine can be reversed. For longer procedures otters can be intubated and maintained on isoflurane anaesthesia.

Common surgical procedures

Ferrets

Castration

Castration reduces dominance characteristics of male ferrets, but most importantly reduces secretion from the sebaceous glands during the breeding season, resulting in less odour. Both open and closed techniques have been described for castration. This author used to prefer the open technique, in which the spermatic cord and vessels are ligated with 1.5 metric (4/0 USP) monofilament suture material. The scrotal sac does not need to be closed. Surgical castration, however, results in elevated concentrations of gonadotrophins, which are associated with the aetiology of hyperadrenocorticism in ferrets. Therefore, the use of a depot GnRH agonist is preferred as an alternative to surgical castration.

Ovariohysterectomy

The technique is similar to that used in cats but a complicating factor in ferrets is the large amount of fat in the mesovarium. At Utrecht University incisions of at least 3 or 4 cm are advised so that there is good vision during surgery. As mentioned above, ovariohysterectomy results in elevated concentrations of gonadotrophins, which are associated with the aetiology of hyperadrenocorticism in ferrets. The use of a depot GnRH agonist as an alternative to surgical neutering is therefore advised.

Foreign body removal

Ingestion of foreign bodies should be considered in any lethargic, especially young, ferret that has anorexia and diarrhoea. Although vomiting may occur, this may not be mentioned by the owner. In most cases the foreign bodies contain rubber because ferrets appear to like its taste. Diagnosis by abdominal palpation is possible when a foreign body is stuck in the small intestine but may be difficult if the object is still in the stomach. Radiography and ultrasonography can help to confirm the diagnosis.

The ferret must be stabilized prior to surgery. A midline approach can be used to inspect the gastrointestinal tract, followed by a gastrotomy or enterotomy similar to that in other small species. The stomach can be closed in two layers with 2 metric (3/0 USP) or 1.5 metric (4/0 USP) monofilament suture material, and the intestines can be closed in one layer with 1.5 (4/0 USP) or 1 metric (5/0 USP) monofilament suture material. Water and liquid food can be given again after 12–24 hours.

Removal of anal glands

In the USA most ferrets are bred in large breeding farms where they are neutered and have their anal glands removed at 6 weeks of age. The anal glands are removed because of the false belief that they are responsible for the ferret's strong odour (in fact it is the sebaceous glands). Unless for medical reasons, it is illegal to remove the anal glands from ferrets in the UK and the Netherlands.

Euthanasia

The author prefers to sedate animals prior to euthanasia because most agents used for euthanasia are irritating to the tissues, and ferrets may react to them. Most owners also appreciate seeing their animals sedated. If no post-mortem examination of the peritoneal cavity is necessary, an intraperitoneal injection of any of the barbiturate agents may be given. Cardiac puncture may be too distressing to perform in the presence of the owner (for humane reasons, this technique should only be performed in a sedated or anaesthetized animal). If post-mortem examination is required, an intravenous injection is mandatory.

Drug formulary

A drug formulary for ferrets is given in Figure 6.20. These doses can also be extrapolated to use in skunks and otters.

Drug	Dose
Analgesics	
Buprenorphine	0.01–0.03 mg/kg s.c./i.m. q8–12h
Butorphanol	0.1–0.5 mg/kg s.c./i.m. q4h
Carprofen	2–4 mg/kg orally/s.c. q12h–24h
Meloxicam	0.1–0.2 mg/kg orally q24h
Tramadol	3–5 mg/kg orally q8–12h
Antibacterial agents	
Amoxicillin/Clavulanate	10–20 mg/kg orally/s.c. q12–24h
Cefalexin	15–25 mg/kg orally q8–12h
Chloramphenicol	50 mg/kg orally/s.c./i.m. q12h
Clarithromycin	12.5–25 mg/kg q12h
Enrofloxacin	5–15 mg/kg orally/s.c./i.m. q12h
Metronidazole	10–20 mg/kg orally q12h
Oxytetracycline	20 mg/kg orally q8h
Penicillin G procaine	20,000 IU/kg i.m. q12h
Tetracycline	25 mg/kg orally q8–12h
Trimethoprim/Sulphonamide	15–30 mg/kg orally/s.c. q12h
Tylosin	10 mg/kg orally q12h
Antifungal agents	
Griseofulvin	25 mg/kg orally q24h
Antiparasitic agents	
Ivermectin 1% (1:10 diluted in propylene glycol)	0.2–0.4 mg/kg topical
Pyrethrin products	Topical

6.20 Drug formulary for ferrets. These doses may be extrapolated to use in skunks and otters. (continues) ▶

Drug	Dose
Antiparasitic agents continued	
Selamectin	15 mg topical
Miscellaneous	
Chorionic gonadotrophin (hCG)	100 IU i.m.; repeat in 2 wks
Cimetidine	10 mg/kg orally/s.c./i.m./i.v. q8h
Cisapride	0.5 mg/kg orally q8h
Deslorelin	4.7 mg s.c. once every 2 years
Diazoxide	5–30 mg/kg orally q12h
Digoxin	0.005–0.01 mg/kg orally q12–24h
Enalapril	0.25–0.5 mg/kg orally q24–48h
Famotidine	2.5 mg/kg orally q24h
Furosemide	1–4 mg/kg orally/s.c./i.m./i.v. q8–12h
Leuprolide acetate, 30-day depot preparation	Females: 0.1 mg/kg (females) i.m. monthly Males: 0.2 mg/kg (males) i.m. monthly
Metoclopramide	0.2–1 mg/kg orally/s.c. q6–8h
Omeprazole	4 mg/kg orally q24h
Pimobendan	0.15 mg/kg orally q12h
Prednisolone	0.2–1 mg/kg orally q24h
Proligestone	50 mg/kg s.c./i.m. once
Propranolol	0.5–2 mg/kg orally/s.c. q12–24h
Ranitidine	3.5 mg/kg orally q12h
Sucralfate	25–125 mg/kg orally q8–12h

6.20 (continued) Drug formulary for ferrets. These doses may be extrapolated to use in skunks and otters.

References and further reading

Erdman SE, Reimann KA, Moore FM *et al.* (1995) Transmission of a chronic lymphoproliferative syndrome in ferrets. *Laboratory Investigation* **72,** 539–546

Fox JG (1998) *Biology and Diseases of the Ferret, 2nd edn.* Williams and Wilkins, London

Fox JG, Pequet-Goad ME, Garibaldi BA and Wiest LM (1987) Hyperadrenocorticism in a ferret. *Journal of the American Veterinary Medical Association* **191,** 343–344

Fudge AM (2000) *Laboratory Medicine: Avian and Exotic Pets.* WB Saunders, Philadelphia

Hillyer EV and Quesenberry KE (1997) *Ferrets, Rabbits and Rodents: Clinical Medicine and Surgery.* WB Saunders, Philadelphia

Jenkins JR and Brown SA (1993) *A Practitioner's Guide to Rabbits and Ferrets.* American Animal Hospital Association, Lakewood, USA

Keeble E and Meredith A (2009) *BSAVA Manual of Rodents and Ferrets.* BSAVA Publications, Gloucester

Kelleher SA (2001) Skin diseases of ferrets. *Veterinary Clinics of North America: Exotic Animal Practice* **4**(2), 565–572

Ko JC, Heaton-Jones TG and Nicklin CF (1997) Evaluation of the sedative and cardiorespiratory effects of medetomidine, medetomidine-butorphanol, medetomidine-ketamine, and medetomidine-butorphanol-ketamine in ferrets. *Journal of the American Animal Hospital Association* **33,** 438–448

Lombardi D and O'Connor J (1998) *Asian Small-clawed Otter Husbandry Manual.* Columbus Zoological Gardens & Asian small-clawed otter Species Survival Plan®, Silver Springs, USA

Orcutt C (2004) Dermatologic diseases. In: *Ferrets, Rabbits and Rodents: Clinical Medicine and Surgery, 2nd edn,* ed. KE Quesenberry and JW Carpenter, pp. 107–114. Saunders, St Louis

Porter HG, Porter DD and Larsen AE (1982) Aleutian disease in ferrets. *Infection and Immunity* **36,** 379–386

Schoemaker NJ, Schuurmans M, Moorman H and Lumeij JT (2000) Correlation between age at neutering and age at onset of hyperadrenocorticism in ferrets. *Journal of the American Veterinary Medical Association* **15,** 216(2):195–197

Simpson VR and King MA (2003) Otters. In: *BSAVA Manual of Wildlife Casualties,* ed. E Mullineaux *et al.,* pp. 136–146. BSAVA Publications, Gloucester

7

African pygmy hedgehogs

Dan Johnson

Introduction

The African pygmy hedgehog (*Atelerix albiventris*) is native to West and Central Africa. It occupies a wide range of habitats, including grassland, scrub, savannah, and suburban gardens. Hedgehogs live in brush piles, rock crevices and burrows; they are able to climb, dig and swim. African pygmy hedgehogs will enter a torpid state during periods of extreme temperature, and then re-emerge during ideal conditions. Unlike other species of hedgehog, the African pygmy hedgehog does not hibernate.

Biology

Hedgehogs are generally solitary and nocturnal. When threatened, hedgehogs curl up into a ball, extending their spines, puffing up, and emitting high-pitched hissing sounds. African pygmy hedgehogs exhibit a unique behaviour known as 'self-anointing' (Figure 7.1), which is usually triggered by a novel or irritating substance. The substance is licked until frothy saliva accumulates, and the saliva is then placed on to the spines with the tongue. This elaborate process may continue for up to 20 minutes; its purpose is unknown, but theories include self-defence and pheromonal communication.

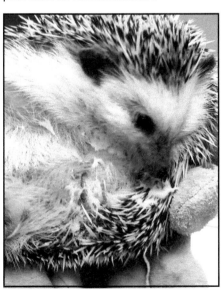

7.1 Hedgehogs 'self-anoint', spreading thick, frothy saliva on to their spines with their tongue, when they encounter a new object or scent.

Hedgehogs have acute senses of smell and hearing, especially in the ultrasonic range. Vision is less well developed.

Anatomy and physiology

The dorsum (or 'mantle') of a hedgehog is covered with spines. There is an orbicularis muscle around the rim of the mantle, which the hedgehog is able to contract in order to roll up. Beneath the mantle is a large subcutaneous space that contains fat, including the brown fat utilized during torpor or hibernation. Hedgehogs have a simple stomach and no caecum. A vomiting reflex is present. The gastrointestinal transit time averages 12–16 hours. Biological data for the African pygmy hedgehog are given in Figure 7.2.

Bodyweight (g)	Males: 400–700 Females: 300–600
Life expectancy (years)	5–7; up to 10 recorded
Rectal temperature (°C)	36.1–37.2
Heart rate (beats/min)	180–280
Respiration rate (breaths/min)	25–50

7.2 Biological data for the African pygmy hedgehog.

Dentition

Hedgehogs have 36 teeth, with the dental formula: I3/2, C1/1, PM3/2, M3/3. The teeth are sharply cuspidate (Figure 7.3).

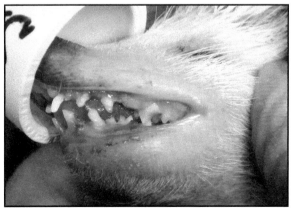

7.3 Hedgehog teeth are sharply cuspidate, an adaptation for prehending and consuming insects and other prey. Hedgehogs are susceptible to tartar and periodontal disease (as shown here), and should receive dental prophylaxis.

Sexing

Males have a prominent penile sheath opening cranially on the abdomen; the testes are intra-abdominal. Internally, males also possess complex accessory reproductive glands, which may account for as much as 10% of bodyweight during the breeding season. In females, the anogenital distance is very short.

Husbandry

Housing

Hedgehogs are best housed individually, although young animals that are raised together may tolerate each other as adults. Fighting is most common between males. Hedgehogs prefer quiet, dim environments, and may react with fright to loud noises or bright light.

Housing should be as large as possible to allow for movement and exercise; a minimum of 60 cm x 90 cm is recommended. Hedgehogs are able to climb and escape through small holes, so the enclosure must be secure or smooth-walled. A shelter such as a hide box or hollow log should be provided to reduce stress. Soft absorbent bedding such as recycled newspaper or aspen shavings should be used and the substrate should be changed often. Some hedgehogs can be trained to use a litter box.

Hedgehogs should be maintained on a 12-hour light/dark cycle. Excessively low or high temperatures may induce torpor or heat stroke, respectively. The preferred temperature for hedgehogs is 24–30°C. Under-tank heating pads and radiant heat emitters are recommended in order to control cage temperature.

To prevent obesity and related disorders such as pododermatitis, and to prevent leg trauma, a solid-walled exercise wheel should be provided (Figure 7.4).

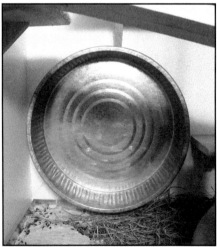

7.4 Solid-sided exercise wheel suitable for a hedgehog.

Diet

Hedgehogs are monogastric insectivores/omnivores. Their natural diet includes insects, arachnids, worms, snails, slugs, small vertebrates, eggs and fruit. The nutritional requirements of hedgehogs are not known. They can be successfully maintained on canned, low-fat cat or dog food, or special hedgehog diets, which should be supplemented with earthworms, mealworms, crickets, and a small amount of chopped fruits and vegetables. A larval insect-only diet can lead to calcium/phosphorus imbalance and metabolic bone disease, and should therefore be avoided. Nuts and grains occasionally become wedged against the roof of the mouth, and milk may lead to diarrhoea; these items should not be given.

Food should be offered in the evening. Depending on the animal's weight and activity, food may need to be rationed to prevent obesity (see below).

Hedgehogs can learn to drink water from a bottle or a bowl. Fresh water should be supplied daily. Heavy crocks and food bowls that cannot be tipped should be used.

Breeding

Hedgehogs are naturally solitary and rarely come together in the wild except to breed. African pygmy hedgehogs breed year-round in captivity, with mating occurring at any time of day. It is suspected that ovulation is induced. Reproductive data for the African pygmy hedgehog are summarized in Figure 7.5.

Age at sexual maturity	61–68 days possible; first breeding generally not until 6–8 months
Oestrous cycle	Seasonally polyoestrous (wild), breed all year round (captive); induced ovulators
Duration of oestrus	3–17 days with 1–5 days dioestrus
Gestation period	34–37 days
Litter size	1–7 (usually 3–5)
Birth weight	8–13 g
Eyes open	13–24 days
Weaning	4–6 weeks (start eating solids at 3 weeks)

7.5 Reproductive data for the African pygmy hedgehog.

Parturition generally occurs in the late night or early morning. The female may cannibalize, kill or abandon her newborn young if she is disturbed or stressed. Therefore, the male must be removed prior to parturition and the mother should not be disturbed for 5–10 days post-partum. Dystocia is rare but should be treated as for other mammals. The young are born with soft spines, which harden over the first 24 hours. Passive transfer of immunity occurs through colostrum in the first 24–72 hours of life. Orphaned young can be raised on puppy or kitten milk replacer.

Handling and restraint

Hedgehog spines may cause discomfort to handlers but can do little harm. Light leather gloves are occasionally required (Figure 7.6a). Young hedgehogs generally do not resist being held, while adults frequently roll up in defence or struggle to escape. Well socialized hedgehogs can sometimes be restrained by the scruff or cupped in the hands without using gloves (Figure 7.6b).

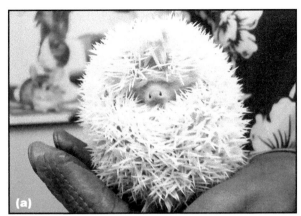

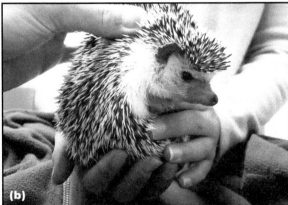

7.6 **(a)** Leather gloves are sometimes required to handle hedgehogs. This coloration is called 'snowflake' and may have either dark or albino eyes. **(b)** Well socialized hedgehogs can be examined while cupped in the hands.

A shy hedgehog can usually be coaxed to open up by placing it in shallow (<2 cm deep) water, pressing a blunt probe over the lumbar region, or gently extending the rear legs in wheelbarrow fashion (Figure 7.7). Placing a finger under the hedgehog's chin may discourage it from rolling up completely.

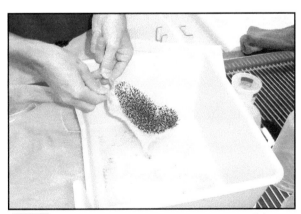

7.7 Hedgehogs can be encouraged to unroll for examination by placing them in 1–2 cm of water and/or by gently extending the hindlegs into a 'wheelbarrow' posture.

For inspecting the face, feet and ventrum, the hedgehog can be placed in a clear aquarium and viewed from below. A wire mesh terrarium lid or tennis racquet can be used for the same purpose and may also permit nail trimming to be performed (Figure 7.8).

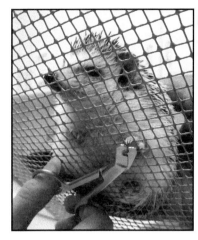

7.8 A wire terrarium lid allows visual examination of a hedgehog and nail trimming.

Diagnostic approach

Hedgehogs normally emit a wide variety of squeals, snuffling, grunts and sneezes. These should not be confused with abnormal respiratory sounds. Anaesthesia or sedation is usually required for complete physical examination or for diagnostic testing.

Imaging

Radiography usually requires anaesthesia or sedation. Dorsoventral radiographs may be hard to interpret due to the overlay of the spines. For lateral radiography, positioning is the same as used in other mammals, but with the mantle pulled dorsally (Figure 7.9).

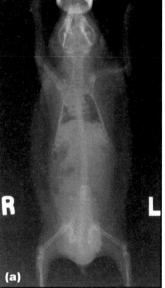

7.9 Normal radiographs:
(a) ventrodorsal view;
(b) lateral view, with the mantle pulled dorsally.

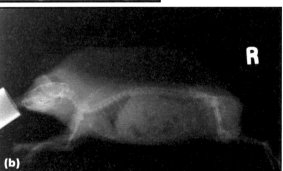

Sample collection

Blood

Sedation or anaesthesia is almost always required for safe and reliable venous access. Venepuncture of the lateral or medial saphenous, cephalic, jugular and femoral veins is possible.

The cranial vena cava approach is preferred for larger volumes of blood. A short (1/2–5/8 inch) small- (25 or 27) gauge needle is used on a 1 or 3 ml syringe. The needle is inserted at the notch formed by the manubrium and the first rib, and directed caudally at 30 degrees from the midline, aiming at the opposite hip.

Haematology and biochemistry reference ranges for hedgehogs have been published (Larson and Carpenter, 1999; Ness, 1999; Ivey and Carpenter, 2004). They are similar to those in domestic dogs and cats, but hedgehogs normally have higher blood urea nitrogen and lower sodium values.

Urine

Urine may be obtained by free catch, catheterization or cystocentesis. Urinalysis is interpreted as for dogs, cats and ferrets. Urinary abnormalities are not well documented in the veterinary literature, but kidney disease is frequently diagnosed post-mortem in hedgehogs.

Common conditions

Eye disease

The hedgehog's shallow orbits and wide palpebral fissures appear to predispose it to proptosis and ocular injuries. Trauma from hedgehog spines (their own or others') or cage furnishings, tooth root infections, neoplasia, retrobulbar abscesses, and ectoparasitism may all contribute. Diagnosis and treatment for ocular disease are as for other small mammals.

Ear disease

Otitis externa has been reported; its signs include purulent discharge, odour and increased sensitivity of the ear. Differential diagnosis includes bacterial or yeast infection; and some cases may be secondary to acariasis or neoplasia. Diagnosis and treatment for ear disease are as for other small mammals.

Dental and oral disease

Dental disease is fairly common. Teeth may become abscessed or fractured. Affected hedgehogs may exhibit weight loss, anorexia, ptyalism, halitosis and pawing at the mouth. Radiography may help in the diagnosis. Extraction and systemic antibiotics are indicated. Periodontal disease is also very common, and traditional dental prophylaxis is indicated. Squamous cell carcinoma and other oral neoplasms (see Figure 7.12) may mimic periodontal or gingival disease, and are relatively common. If traditional dental prophylaxis and antibiotics do not resolve the lesions, histopathology of a biopsy sample is recommended. Oral neoplasms are frequently aggressive locally and cause loss of teeth and appetite.

Gastrointestinal and hepatic disease

Salmonella infection is well documented in hedgehogs. Clinical signs include anorexia, mucoid diarrhoea, dehydration and weight loss. Other bacteria may cause gastroenteritis, hepatitis, pancreatitis and peritonitis, with signs including anorexia, emesis, diarrhoea and abdominal discomfort. Diagnosis is based upon faecal culture. Treatment includes supportive fluid therapy, hand-feeding and broad-spectrum antibiotics. Pet owners should be advised of the **zoonotic potential** for *Salmonella* and that hedgehogs can be non-clinical carriers. *Salmonella* infection may be a reportable disease in some public health districts.

Gastrointestinal parasitism, foreign body obstruction (most often by hair, carpet fibre or rubber), and lymphoma are also reported.

Hepatic lipidosis is relatively common in hedgehogs. Other potential causes of liver failure include hepatic neoplasia and infection by human *Herpes simplex* virus 1 (HSV1). Owners experiencing active cold or canker sores should refrain from handling their hedgehogs until the lesions subside.

Respiratory disease

Hedgehogs are susceptible to respiratory pathogens such as *Pasteurella*, *Bordetella bronchiseptica* and *Corynebacterium*. Dyspnoea, nasal discharge and sneezing may result. Diagnostic procedures include radiography and culture and sensitivity testing. Treatment should include broad-spectrum antibiotics, fluid therapy and other supportive care measures. Oxygen, bronchodilators and nebulization therapy should be provided as indicated. Prevention is through proper husbandry, nutrition and sanitation.

Cardiovascular and haematological disease

Dilated cardiomyopathy leading to congestive heart failure has been reported. Clinical signs and diagnostic approach are the same as for other small mammals. Therapy with digoxin or pimobendan, furosemide and enalapril may be helpful initially; the long-term prognosis is poor.

Severe anaemia may be encountered in female hedgehogs secondary to uterine bleeding (see below).

Urogenital disease

Uterine neoplasia can occur in females as young as 12 months. Affected females present with haemorrhagic vulvar discharge. Treatment involves supportive care and ovariohysterectomy. Histopathology will allow an accurate diagnosis: endometrial hyperplasia has a very similar presentation. The overall prognosis depends upon the stage and aggressiveness of the tumour. Metastasis is not uncommon. Dystocia occurs and is treated as in other small mammals.

Kidney disease appears to be common in hedgehogs. Tubulointerstitial nephritis is the most common histopathological finding. Lethargy, weight loss, polyuria and polydipsia may occur. Urolithiasis may be linked to cat food-based diets. Diagnosis is by radiography and urinalysis.

Blood and crystals in the urine are abnormal. Urolithiasis can occur in addition to crystalluria. Male hedgehogs may have an urethral obstruction. Radiographs are useful for diagnosis of stones. Treatment for urolithiasis, crystalluria and cystitis are as for other species: the obstruction should be relieved and a cystotomy performed to remove larger stones once the animal is stable. Catheterization and retrograde flushing into the bladder may be necessary to resolve urethral obstructions. Changing to a hedgehog/insectivore-specific diet may help to eliminate recurrence.

Neurological disease

Ataxia may be caused by: a state of torpor; neurodegeneration (see below); trauma; toxins; hepatic encephalopathy; infarcts; heart disease; malnutrition; or neoplasia.

Head tilt or circling may be caused by otitis media or primary neurological conditions. Neurological signs from hypocalcaemia, intervertebral disc disease, rabies and *Baylisascaris* are other possibilities.

A neurodegenerative disease has recently been described which occurs in approximately 10% of pet African hedgehogs in North America. 'Wobbly hedgehog syndrome' (WHS) is characterized by progressive ataxia and weight loss, leading to paralysis and death. The age of onset can vary widely but is typically 2 years or less. Affected animals exhibit ataxia and paralysis, beginning in the hindlegs and gradually ascending until only the head can move. Progression of clinical signs of WHS varies from weeks to months, but the majority of hedgehogs are completely paralysed within 15 months of onset of clinical signs. While there is no definitive treatment and no aetiological agent has been found, pedigree analysis suggests a familial tendency. Affected hedgehogs should receive hand-feeding and other supportive care. The prognosis is poor and the disease is generally fatal. Euthanasia should be considered if the hedgehog can no longer eat, drink and maintain hygiene. Diagnosis is confirmed by necropsy and histopathology. Differential diagnoses for WHS include trauma, neoplasia and arthritis.

Musculoskeletal disorders

Long bone fractures most commonly occur when a limb becomes entrapped in a wire cage or running wheel. A smooth-walled exercise wheel helps to prevent leg trauma. Splinting and surgical correction are possible, but repairs must be able to withstand the strong rolling-up mechanism. Lameness may also be caused by ingrown toenails, arthritis, constriction of an appendage by a string or fibre (Figure 7.10), neoplasia, pododermatitis, nutritional deficiency or neurological disease. Vertebral spondylosis is a common finding in older individuals.

Skin disease

Dermatophytosis caused by either *Trichophyton* or *Microsporum* has been reported, and **zoonotic** transmission has been documented. Infections are characterized by crusting around the base of the spines. Dermatophytosis may be secondary to mite

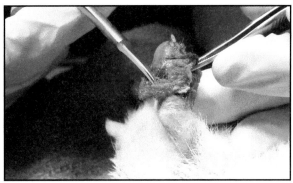

7.10 Fibrous foreign bodies often become entwined on hedgehogs' feet or toes, leading to strangulation injury. Rope, hair, string and frayed linens should be strictly avoided as bedding for hedgehogs.

infestation, trauma, bacterial skin disease or other stressors. Microscopic examination of spines for debris, epithelial cells and spine fragments, cytology from skin scrapings and dermatophyte test medium (DTM) culture are diagnostic. Treatment is with griseofulvin, ketoconazole or lime–sulphur dips; any underlying causes should also be treated. If one individual hedgehog in a group is diagnosed, the entire group should receive treatment.

Mite infestations with *Caparinia* or *Chorioptes* are very common. Most infestations are subclinical, but in severe cases seborrhoea, crusting and flaking of the skin, and loss of spines results (Figure 7.11). The patient may exhibit lethargy, anorexia and weight loss as a result. Diagnosis is by direct examination of the skin under magnification and by skin scraping. The author recommends every hedgehog

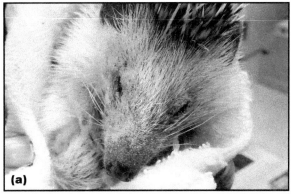

(a)

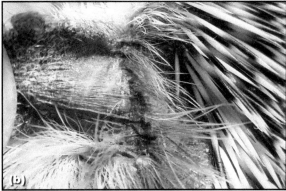

(b)

7.11 **(a,b)** Mites are most easily found on the face, around the eyes and behind the ears.
(continues) ▶

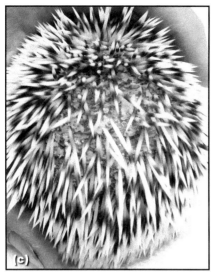

7.11

(continued)
(c) Serious infestations can lead to dandruff and spine loss.

be closely examined for mites at the initial examination. Treatment options include ivermectin, selamectin and fipronil spray.

Hedgehogs are also susceptible to fleas and ticks, which respond to treatment with fipronil, as above. For all ectoparasite infestations, environmental clean-up is advisable at the beginning and end of treatment in order to eliminate 'stragglers'.

Pododermatitis is common where cage substrate is allowed to become wet or soiled. Prevention is by providing clean soft bedding and changing substrate often.

Neoplasia

Neoplasia is common in hedgehogs, and has been reported in all body systems. The incidence is highest in individuals over 3 years old. Lethargy, anorexia and weight loss are the most common clinical signs. Mammary gland and uterine tumours (see above) are common in females and most are malignant. Haemolymphatic neoplasias (e.g. alimentary lymphosarcoma, multicentric lymphosarcoma, myelogenous leukaemia) are common. Oral tumours (Figure 7.12) are common; oral squamous cell carcinoma may mimic dental disease. Skeletal sarcomas affecting the jaw and long bones carry a poor prognosis; early

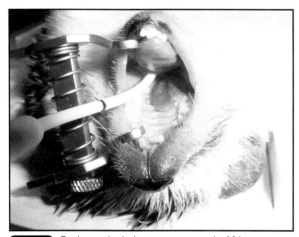

7.12 Oral neoplasia is very common in African hedgehogs and can closely resemble periodontal disease.

amputation is recommended. Some association between these sarcomas and retroviral disease may exist. Lipomas, fibromas and adenomas have also been reported. Diagnosis is via fine-needle aspiration, cytology, biopsy and histopathology, as for other mammals. Complete surgical excision of tumours is preferred. Chemotherapy has not been extensively studied in hedgehogs.

Nutritional disease

Ad libitum feeding, over-consumption and inactivity commonly lead to obesity. The problem can become so severe that the patient can no longer roll up fully (Figure 7.13). Obesity can lead to other metabolic derangements and health problems, including hepatic lipidosis. Treatment is through gradual reduction of food quantity until the amount offered is consumed overnight. Foods high in fat (e.g. mealworms, waxworms) should be limited. Live insects should be offered to promote normal hunting and burrowing activity. Exercise should be encouraged by offering time outside the enclosure; if offered a running wheel (see Figure 7.4), hedgehogs will often use it for much of the night. Owners should be asked to weigh their hedgehog often, using an accurate scale.

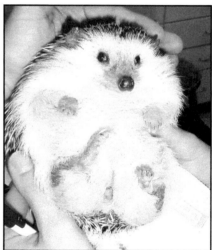

7.13

Obesity can become so severe that the hedgehog cannot roll up completely.

Supportive care

Drug administration

- Subcutaneous injections may be administered into the flank or beneath the mantle, and large quantities of fluid (up to 100 ml/kg, divided into several sites) can be administered beneath the mantle, if necessary.
- Intramuscular injections may be given into the thigh or triceps muscles (may require sedation), or into the orbicularis muscle of the mantle.
- Intraperitoneal and intravenous injections require sedation.
- Intravenous catheters may be placed into the lateral saphenous or jugular veins. If these are too small to access, then an intraosseous catheter can be placed in the tibial crest or the femur using a 20–25-gauge hypodermic needle.

- Oral administration of drugs is preferred when feasible. Animals accustomed to being handled will take pleasant-tasting oral medications (e.g. cherry, banana or chicken flavoured) willingly.

Although oral medication is preferred, injectable medications may be easier to administer; hedgehogs can be given subcutaneous or intramuscular injections even while rolled up. When possible, choose once- or twice-daily dosing regimens (see Figure 7.14).

Torpor

Sick hedgehogs lose their ability to regulate heat and become torpid. Do not assume the hedgehog is in shock or near death. An accurate assessment may not be possible until warmth, fluids and nutritional support have been tried for 24 hours or more. The ambient temperature for sick hedgehogs should be raised to 27–30°C and a quiet, dim environment provided. Warmed crystalloid fluid therapy should be given at 50–100 ml/kg/day.

Assisted feeding

Animals requiring assisted feeding can be syringe-fed with: Carnivore Care® (Oxbow Animal Health, Murdock, NE); soaked and blended commercial insectivore diet; or strained meat baby foods. A gavage needle may be necessary to reach the oral cavity, since hedgehogs tend to roll up. An alternative is to offer live food such as mealworms, which sick hedgehogs may be tempted to eat.

Anaesthesia and analgesia

As with other species, hedgehogs should be sedated with an anxiolytic (such as midazolam) prior to the induction of anaesthesia to reduce stress and prevent the elevation of heart rate and blood pressure and the release of catecholamines. An induction chamber or facemask allows the hedgehog to be rapidly anaesthetized with isoflurane or sevoflurane. Atropine may reduce hypersalivation. Intubation is possible with a 1–1.5 mm uncuffed endotracheal tube, Teflon i.v. catheter or feeding tube. Injectable anaesthetic agents (see Figure 7.14) are less reliable and seldom indicated. Supplemental heat with a circulating warm water heat pad or forced air heating system is essential. Preoperative fluids and analgesia should be administered.

Common surgical procedures

Because hedgehogs are usually maintained singly, elective castration or ovariohysterectomy is usually not indicated. Castration may be performed using an inguinal approach, and ovariohysterectomy is routine. Subcuticular skin sutures are preferred. Small-gauge monofilament absorbable suture (1.5 metric (4/0 USP)) is recommended.

Enucleation may be indicated in cases of severe ocular trauma, and is performed as for other species.

Euthanasia

Hedgehogs may be euthanased by intravenous, intraperitoneal or intracardiac injection of barbiturate. General anesthesia prior to the euthanasia procedure is advised.

Drug formulary

A drug formulary for the African pygmy hedgehog is presented in Figure 7.14.

Drug	Dose	Comments
Antimicrobial agents		
Amikacin	2.5–5.0 mg/kg i.m. q8–12h	Antibacterial. Maintain hydration
Amoxicillin/Clavulanate	12.5 mg/kg orally q12h	Antibacterial
Cefalexin	25 mg/kg orally q8h	Antibacterial
Ceftiofur	20 mg/kg s.c. q12–24h	Antibacterial
Chloramphenicol	30–50 mg/kg orally q12h	Antibacterial
Ciprofloxacin	5–20 mg/kg orally q12h	Antibacterial
Enrofloxacin	2.5–10 mg/kg orally/s.c./i.m q12h	Antibacterial
Erythromycin	10 mg/kg orally/i.m. q12h	Penicillin-resistant Gram-positive cocci, *Mycoplasma, Bordetella, Pasteurella.* May induce nausea
Gentamicin	2 mg/kg s.c./i.m. q8h	Antibacterial. Maintain hydration
Gentamicin ophthalmic drops	1 drop topically to cornea q8h	Corneal injury
Oxytetracycline	50 mg/kg orally q12h	Antibacterial
Penicillin G	40,000 IU/kg s.c./i.m. q24h	Antibacterial
Piperacillin	10 mg/kg s.c. q8–12h	Antibacterial

7.14 Drug formulary for the African pygmy hedgehog. (continues) ▶

Drug	Dose	Comments
Antimicrobial agents (continued)		
Tetracycline ophthalmic ointment	Apply a small amount topically to cornea q12h	Corneal/conjunctival lesion
Trimethoprim/Sulphonamide	30 mg/kg orally/s.c./i.m. q12h	Antibacterial; coccidiosis
Triple antibiotic ophthalmic ointment	Apply a small amount topically to cornea q12h	Corneal/conjunctival lesion
Antifungal agents		
Griseofulvin	25–50 mg/kg orally q24h for 30 days	Dermatophytosis
Itraconazole	5–10 mg/kg orally q12–24h	Systemic mycosis
Ketoconazole	10 mg/kg orally q24h for 6–8 weeks	*Candida*
Nystatin	30,000 IU/kg orally q8–24h	Yeast infections
Antiparasitic agents		
Fenbendazole	25 mg/kg orally, repeat at 14 and 28 days	Nematodes
Fipronil topical spray (0.25%)	Apply lightly q14d for 3 treatments	Ectoparasites
Ivermectin	0.2–0.4 mg/kg s.c. q14d for 3 treatments	Acariasis
	0.2–0.4 mg/kg orally; repeat at 14 and 28 days	Nematodes, including lungworms
Levamisole	10 mg/kg s.c.; repeat after 48 hours; q14d	Nematodes, including lungworms
Metronidazole	25 mg/kg orally q12h for 5 days	Protozoal infections
	20 mg/kg orally q12h	Anaerobic infections
Praziquantel	7 mg/kg orally/s.c.; repeat after 14 days	Cestodes
Selamectin	6–18 mg/kg topically q30d for 2 treatments	Acariasis
Sulfadimethoxine	2–20 mg/kg orally/s.c. q24h for 2–5 days; skip for 5 days and then repeat course	Coccidiosis
Analgesics/anaesthetics/sedatives		
Atipamezole	0.3–0.5 mg/kg i.m.	Reversal of medetomidine
Atropine	0.02 mg/kg s.c./i.m.	Pre-anaesthetic
Buprenorphine	0.01–0.05 mg/kg s.c./i.m. q6–8h	Analgesic
Butorphanol	0.2–0.5 mg/kg s.c./i.m. q 6–8h	Analgesic
Diazepam	0.5–2.0 mg/kg i.m/i.v.	Sedative; seizures
Isoflurane	3–5% for induction; 0.5–3% for maintenance	Anaesthesia. Can use in induction chamber, then mask/intubate
Ketamine	5–20 mg/kg i.m.	Sedation/anaesthesia. Use in combination with other agents. Recovery may be prolonged and/or rough. Do not administer in neck area where brown fat located
Ketamine + Diazepam	5–20 mg/kg K + 0.5–2.0 mg/kg D i.m.	Anaesthesia
Ketamine + Midazolam	5–20 mg/kg K + 0.3–0.5 mg/kg M i.m.	Administer midazolam 5 minutes prior to ketamine for smoother induction
Medetomidine	Light sedation: 0.05–0.1 mg/kg i.m. Heavy sedation: 0.2 mg/kg i.m.	Reverse with atipamezole. Usually used in combinations. Hypotensive
Medetomidine + Ketamine	0.1 mg/kg M + 5 mg/kg K i.m.	Anaesthesia. Reverse medetomidine with atipamezole
Medetomidine + Ketamine + Fentanyl	0.2 mg/kg M + 2 mg/kg K + 0.1 mg/kg F s.c.	Anaesthesia; good muscle relaxation. Reverse medetomidine with atipamezole at 1 mg/kg i.m. Reverse fentanyl with naloxone at 0.16 mg/kg i.m. Note: reversal removes analgesic effects
Meloxicam	0.2 mg/kg orally/s.c. q24h	Non-steroidal anti-inflammatory agent
Midazolam	0.3–0.4 mg/kg i.m./i.v.	Sedative/pre-anaesthetic
Naloxone	0.16 mg/kg i.m.	Reversal of fentanyl

7.14 (continued) Drug formulary for the African pygmy hedgehog. (continues) ▶

Drug	Dose	Comments
Analgesics/anaesthetics/sedatives (continued)		
Sevoflurane	To effect	Anaesthesia
Tiletamine/Zolazepam	1–5 mg/kg i.m.	Sedation/anaesthesia. Recovery may be prolonged and/or rough
Xylazine	0.5–1.0 mg/kg i.m.	Anaesthesia. May be given with ketamine. Hypotensive
Yohimbine	0.5–1.0 mg/kg i.m.	Reversal of xylazine
Miscellaneous		
Calcium gluconate 10%	0.5 mg/kg i.m.	Fracture repair. Higher/repeated doses for hypocalcaemia
Cimetidine	10 mg/kg orally q8h	Gastric ulcers
Dexamethasone	0.1–1.5 mg/kg i.m.	Inflammation, allergies. **Do not use in liver disease**
	1–4 mg/kg s.c./i.m./i.v.	Shock
Digoxin	0.01 mg/kg orally q12h, can decrease to 0.01 mg/kg orally q24h	Positive inotrope for dilated cardiomyopathy and congestive heart failure; serum levels difficult to monitor
Enalapril	0.5 mg/kg orally q24h	Cardiomyopathy
Erythropoietin	100 IU/kg s.c. q48–72h	Anaemia
Furosemide	2.5–5.0 mg/kg orally/s.c./i.m. q8h	Diuretic in oedema, cardiomyopathy
Glycopyrrolate	0.02 mg/kg s.c./i.m. once	Part of a pre-anaesthetic regimen; alternative to atropine
Iron dextran	25 mg/kg i.m. once	Anaemia
Lactulose	0.3 ml/kg orally q8–12h	Liver disease; constipation
Metoclopramide	0.2–0.5 mg/kg orally/s.c. q4–8h	Anti-emetic
Pimobendan	0.3 mg/kg orally q12h	Positive inotrope for dilated cardiomyopathy and congestive heart failure; better tolerated that digoxin
Prednisolone	2.5 mg/kg orally/s.c./i.m. q12h	Allergies
Sucralfate	10 mg/kg orally q8–12h	Gastrointestinal ulcers, inflammation. Best if given 5–10 minutes before a meal
Theophylline	10 mg/kg orally/i.m. q12h	Bronchodilator
Vitamin A	400 IU/kg orally/i.m. q24–48h	Skin disorders; excessive spine loss. Use only one or two parenteral doses then correct diet and add to food
Vitamin B complex (small animal formulation)	1 ml/kg s.c./i.m.	CNS signs, paralysis/paresis; anorexia
Vitamin C	50–200 mg/kg orally/s.c. q24h	Adjunct in gingival disease, infections

7.14 (continued) Drug formulary for the African pygmy hedgehog.

References and further reading

Bennett RA (2000) Husbandry and medicine of hedgehogs. *Proceedings, Association of Avian Veterinarians: Exotic Small Mammal Medicine and Management Program* pp.109–114

Garner M and Graesser D (2006) Wobbly hedgehog syndrome. *Exotic DVM* **8**(3), 57–59

Graesser D, Spraker TR, Dressen P *et al.* (2006) Wobbly hedgehog syndrome in African pygmy hedgehogs (*Atelerix* spp.). *Journal of Exotic Pet Medicine* **15**, 59–65

Ivey EI and Carpenter JW (2004) African hedgehogs. In: *Ferrets, Rabbits and Rodents: Clinical Medicine and Surgery, 2nd edn*, ed. KE Quesenberry and JW Carpenter, pp. 339–353. Elsevier/Saunders, St. Louis

Johnson-Delaney C (2006) Common procedures in hedgehogs, prairie dogs, exotic rodents, and companion marsupials. *Veterinary Clinics of North America: Exotic Animal Practice* **9**(2), 415–435

Larson RS and Carpenter JW (1999) Husbandry and medical management of African hedgehogs. *Veterinary Medicine* **94**, 877–888

Lennox AM (2007) Emergency and critical care procedures in sugar gliders (*Petaurus breviceps*), African hedgehogs (*Atelerix albiventris*), and prairie dogs (*Cynomys spp*). *Veterinary Clinics of North America: Exotic Animal Practice* **10**(2), 533–555

Lightfoot T (1997) Clinical techniques of selected exotic species: chinchilla, prairie dog, hedgehog, and chelonians. *Seminars in Avian and Exotic Pet Medicine* **6**(3), 100–102

Lightfoot T (1999) Clinical examination of chinchillas, hedgehogs, prairie dogs, and sugar gliders. *Veterinary Clinics of North America: Exotic Animal Practice* **2**(2), 454–459

Ness RD (1999) Clinical pathology and sample collection of exotic small mammals. *Veterinary Clinics of North America: Exotic Animal Practice* **2**(3), 591–620

Simone-Freilicher EA and Hoefer HL (2004) Hedgehog care and husbandry. *Veterinary Clinics of North America: Exotic Animal Practice* **7**(2), 257–267

Smith AJ (1999) Husbandry and nutrition of hedgehogs. *Veterinary Clinics of North America: Exotic Animal Practice* **2**(1), 127–141

8

Primates – callitrichids, cebids and lemurs

Nic Masters

Introduction

Primates are not kept as pets very commonly in the UK, although the removal of several species from the list of animals requiring a licence may alter this (Dangerous Wild Animals Act 1976 (Modification) (No. 2) Order 2007; see Chapter 22). In many parts of the USA it is illegal to keep them as pets. Primates most likely to be presented as patients from private or small zoological collections include: Callitrichidae – marmosets, tamarins and Goeldi's monkeys; Cebidae – squirrel monkeys (*Saimiri* spp.), capuchins (*Cebus* spp.) and possibly titi monkeys (*Callicebus* spp.); and Lemuridae – lemurs (Figure 8.1).

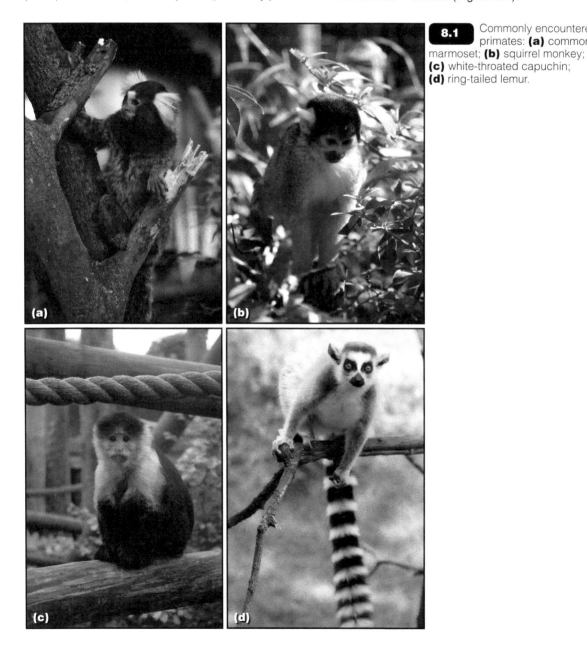

8.1 Commonly encountered primates: **(a)** common marmoset; **(b)** squirrel monkey; **(c)** white-throated capuchin; **(d)** ring-tailed lemur.

Biology

Cebids and callitrichids are commonly referred to as New World (NW) monkeys. They are adapted to arboreal living, with five digits on hands and feet, tails and an excellent ability to climb and manipulate. The skeleton is generally quite upright although they are quadripedal. They have stereoscopic vision and high brain development. Sexual dimorphism is generally limited and all females have two pectoral mammae. These species are omnivorous – they eat fruit predominantly but with significant augmentation by invertebrates, small vertebrates, leaves, flowers and exudates. As such they exhibit limited structural specialization of the gastrointestinal tract between species – for example, marmosets show caecal enlargement as a result of eating plant exudates, whereas squirrel monkeys have especially short tracts suited to a high level of insectivory.

Lemurs are prosimians unique in the wild to Madagascar. They retain biological characteristics considered more primitive than other primates, including prominent scent glands, a bicornate uterus, and a small cranium. Commonly seen species in captivity are *Lemur catta* (ring-tailed lemur), *Eulemur* spp. (black and brown lemurs) and *Varecia* spp. (ruffed lemurs). Unlike most other prosimians, these lemurs are diurnal. Lemurs are predominantly herbivorous with lower metabolic rates than other primates, hence their thick coats and basking and huddling behaviours to conserve energy. Lemurs move on all fours through the trees or on the ground of their forest habitats. Unusually, members of the genus *Varecia* have three pairs of mammae.

All primates have deciduous and permanent dentition (the latter erupting after skeletal maturation) comprising incisors, canines, premolars and molars. NW monkey incisors have spatula-like crowns but cone-shaped canines. The lower incisors of marmosets are elongated with a similar crown length to the canines as an adaptation to eating plant exudates.

Incisors and canines have single roots whilst premolars and molars have two or three roots and cusped crowns. Lemurs have lower incisors and canines that point forward and form a comb for grooming.

All young have slow growth rates and late sexual maturation. This allows for prolonged adolescent learning of behaviours (social, territorial, parenting and food choices) in a family group without sexual competition. Biological data for commonly seen species are given in Figure 8.2.

Husbandry

Groups and housing

Any captive habitat for primates should meet the species' basic requirements for life, but also take into account its natural history. The European Association of Zoos and Aquaria (EAZA) Husbandry Guidelines for the Callitrichidae (Carroll, 2002) state that 'the form and structural configuration of the exhibit should mimic the habitat of these animals in the wild', and this rule holds true across all species. All primates are intelligent and social – they require stimulation (Figure 8.3) and should not be kept alone for long periods, but ideally in groups that reflect their natural social structures (see Figure 8.2). Multi-species housing creates more complex disease and husbandry issues, and different groups of the same species should not be in visual contact with each other. The facility must be structurally sound with tamper-proof locks. The enclosure and food storage areas must exclude rodents, birds and cats – all potential sources of infectious disease.

Space

Primates should have access to outdoor and indoor enclosures. There should be adequate space and refuge for subordinate animals in order to minimize hierarchical stress.

	Common marmoset (*Callithrix jacchus*)	Squirrel monkeys (genus *Saimiri*)	Capuchins (genus *Cebus*)	Ring-tailed lemur (*Lemur catta*)
Average lifespan (years)	15	20	50	27
Average weight (g) Males: Females:	Up to 350 Up to 300	600–1100 500–700	3500–3900 2500–3000	2200–2900 2200–2500
Heart rate (beats/min)	200–350	200–350	165–225	168–210
Respiratory rate (breaths/min)	30–70	20–50	30–50	30–60
Rectal temperature (°C)	39–40	37–38.5	37–38.5	37.9–38.1
Wild groupings	Family group of 3–15. Dominance hierarchy with single breeding female	10–35. Dominance hierarchy with core group of females	3–30. Dominant male	Up to 30. Dominance hierarchy with core group of females
Wild diet	Omnivorous: fruit, exudates, invertebrates, small vertebrates	Omnivorous; high intake of insects	Omnivorous: fruit, nuts, seeds, invertebrates, eggs, small vertebrates	Omnivorous: fruit, leaves, flowers, exudates, insects, small vertebrates

8.2 Biological data for commonly seen primates.

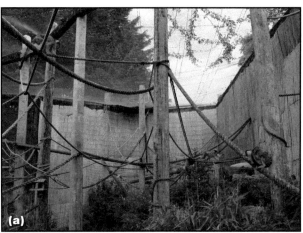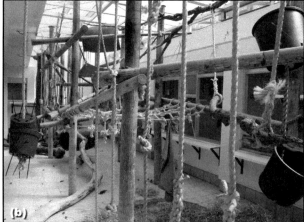

8.3 **(a)** Outdoor enclosure comprising a mix of natural plants, substrates and barriers. The structure and furniture provide a varied and mobile three-dimensional space. **(b)** Indoor enclosure comprising a mix of impervious shelving and surfaces with multiple branches, ropes and other man-made furniture. This more traditional housing is easier to clean and alter in terms of configuration.

Recommendations for callitrichids:

- Minimum height 2.5 m.
- Total three-dimensional space no less than 22.5 m³.
- Indoor enclosures should have a minimum floor area of 3 m² and outdoor enclosures no less than 10 m².
- More space should be provided for groups greater than five.
- Any animal doors and tunnels must be at least 1.5 m above the substrate, since it is unnatural for callitrichids to travel close to the ground, and there must be at least two routes between enclosure areas so that subordinates can not be prevented access by dominant animals.
- Doors and slides need to be controllable from outside the enclosure.

Recommendations for squirrel monkeys:

- Floor space at least 20 m² for a group of 20 animals.
- Height at least 2.5 m, with furniture at 2.2 m so animals can look down on people.
- The outside enclosure for such a group should be at least 40 m² and 3 m high.

Recommendations for lemurs:

- Indoor floor space of no less than 5 m x 5 m.
- Significantly larger outdoor space.
- Both at least 2.5 m high.

Materials

Non-toxic, impervious and robust materials (concrete, wood, plastic, brick) are needed for the construction of indoor enclosures. These allow for correct control of temperature, humidity, ventilation and pests or predators. Adequate cleaning is important but not to the detriment of olfactory cues that are an essential part of communication in all species. Outdoor enclosures are best constructed of similar materials and must include some shelter and shade. Any glass should be made temporarily opaque when first introducing animals to a new enclosure to prevent injury.

Wire mesh fencing is an inexpensive but excellent barrier – it provides an extra climbing area and good viewing for health monitoring or sex determination of juveniles. Important considerations with wire mesh include: correct gauge to prevent escape (usually 2–4 cm²); burial of at least 1 m of mesh beneath the substrate or attachment to a solid foundation to prevent predator access; and adequate tension to avoid entanglement. Electric fencing or water moats are not recommended as primary barriers in private collections.

Substrates indoors are ideally of natural materials (wood shavings, bark or mulch) over an impervious floor with a drain. This allows natural foraging behaviour and cushioning in the instance of a fall. Spot cleaning can take place twice a week and complete stripping and cleaning every 6 months. Outdoor substrate should also be natural (grass or soil) and will generally be kept pathogen-free by weather conditions.

Furniture

Callitrichids must have a minimum of one nest box, measuring 25 cm x 25 cm x 25 cm. Any door to it must be a minimum of 10 cm² (to allow access to an adult carrying a neonate). If the door slides, the box can double as a capture device and ideally be removed without entering the enclosure. For groups of more than five, a second nest box is recommended. Smaller lemur species such as ring-tailed lemurs need nest boxes for seclusion.

Furniture is essential to add complexity to the environment and should be easily cleaned or replaced. Some permanent indoor shelves or beams should be provided as resting spots and for access to nest boxes. Temporary and flexible furniture such as branches (of appropriate diameter for species' hand and foot anatomy), ropes and ladders (with appropriate rung spacing) should be provided to stimulate exploration and locomotion. This furniture should also provide shelter and visual barriers, and with multiple fixing points can be quickly altered in configuration to simulate a changing habitat. Absorbent materials will be used for scent marking and so must be preserved or at least only changed sequentially.

Live plants provide excellent cage furniture, and refuge in outdoor enclosures. Natural, non-toxic vegetation attracts insects that will be especially appreciated by squirrel monkeys. Because lemurs are particularly folivorous, careful thought must be given to the choice of live plants and their potential toxicity. The EAZA Husbandry Guidelines for the Callitrichidae (Carroll, 2002) contain lists of plants thought to be toxic and non-toxic to primates. All the non-toxic species listed should be safe for use in primate enclosures.

Feeding and watering
There should be more than one feeding and watering station to prevent dominant animals from inhibiting the access of subordinates. They should be at least 1.5 m above the substrate, with easy access from the furniture provided. If water bottles are used in preference to bowls they should be checked regularly for blockage or leakage. All bowls should be placed to avoid urine or faecal contamination from above, and ideally situated so they can be removed without needing to enter the enclosure.

Lighting, temperature, humidity and ventilation
Natural photoperiod varies between species but should average 12 hours with minimal to no light at night. Since natural sunlight is very important in NW monkey physiology, all indoor enclosures should have windows or skylights, preferably ones that allow ultraviolet (UV) light through. Indoor enclosures can also be furnished with UV-B lights similar to those suitable for reptiles and parrots (see Vitamins and minerals, below).

Indoor enclosures should be maintained at 18–24°C. A basking spot should be provided under a heat lamp or on a heated shelf. Free access to the outdoor enclosure should probably be limited once the ambient temperature drops below 5°C due to the risk of cold weather injury.

Indoor humidity should be maintained at a minimum of 60% and may require the use of humidifiers, misting or moist substrate. Temperature and humidity should be monitored daily.

Adequate ventilation is essential to prevent build-up of odours, ammonia and condensation and may require an active air circulation system.

Diet
In the wild primates are omnivorous, with diets including fruit, leaves, tree exudates, invertebrates and small vertebrates (see Figure 8.2). It is impossible to replicate these natural diets completely in captivity, and it is not necessary to do so. It is better to meet estimated nutrient requirements and provide enough fibre for normal digestive function and enough diversity for behavioural stimulation. Primate pellets/biscuits and gum substitutes are commercially available and can provide a balanced complete diet with minimal supplementation. In practice most primates are additionally fed a variety of fresh produce and further protein. Multiple feeding stations are important in groups to prevent dominant animals consuming preferred foods before allowing others access. Food items should be offered in small pieces (again to prevent monopolization) and fresh water must be available at all times. Good monitoring of intake is important to gauge whether an animal is getting a balanced diet. Poor captive nutrition remains an important factor in common disease processes.

Callitrichids
Callitrichids are frugivores/insectivores. Common marmosets are especially well adapted to gouge holes in trees to feed on exudates, which they digest via microbial fermentation in the caecum. Offering gum to marmosets in captivity is not a nutritional necessity but is considered by some a behavioural one. Tamarins do not require exudates.

Adult callitrichids should consume 5% of their bodyweight daily on a dry matter (DM) basis, or an average of 20% on an as fed basis. Lactating or pregnant females require 1.5 times these quantities. Captive callitrichids are generally fed a mixture of a complete feed (pellet or jelly), produce (fruit and vegetables) and animal protein (invertebrates, eggs, chicken). Commercially available fruits are higher in water and sugar, and lower in fibre, protein and calcium than wild equivalents. Animals feed preferentially on these high-sugar fruits and on insects before consuming vegetables or complete feeds. Thus, any overprovision of fruit invariably results in inadequate intake of protein, vitamins and minerals. It is recommended that produce represents no more than 30% of energy intake. In practice this can be achieved by feeding approximately 70% produce and 30% dry food by weight.

Callitrichids should be fed at least twice daily, offering the complete feed in the morning when they are most hungry, and the produce later in the day. Invertebrates (preferably live) should be offered to all callitrichids – they offer excellent foraging opportunities and are a good source of protein and fat, although low in calcium. Mice are not to be fed due to the risk of infection with lymphocytic choriomeningitis virus (LCMV) (see below). Gum can be included at up to 9% of DM and arguably reduces the incidence of wasting marmoset syndrome (WMS). Excessive feeding can result in obese callitrichids that are more likely to experience dystocia and stillbirth. Some harder and more abrasive dietary items are needed to prevent periodontal disease. Figure 8.4 shows a suggested diet for a common marmoset.

Cebids
Cebids feed predominantly on fruit, leaves and invertebrates. Squirrel monkeys have very short gastrointestinal tracts and dental adaptations that correlate with a high level of insectivory. Observers have recorded single animals consuming more than 300 insects per day. Squirrel monkeys fed too much carbohydrate during pregnancy appear to get dystocia due to large fetuses.

Time	Feed	Preparation	Quantity per animal
0800	**Breakfast pellet mix**		
	e.g. Mazuri NW Primate	Soak in equal volume of water (possibly with flavouring, e.g. Ribena Toothkind)	~ 25 g
1200	**Fruit, vegetables, gum and protein**		
	Fruit and vegetables (25% apple; 25% pear; 25% seasonal; 15% banana; 10% tomato, carrot, cucumber, boiled potato, sweet potato)	Chopped to appropriate size and mixed	~ 75 g
	Acacia gum	Make up to thick liquid consistency by mixing in water	~ 20 ml
	Protein item (e.g. hard-boiled egg in shell, canned cat food, cooked ox heart, cheddar cheese, Mazuri Marmoset Jelly)		~ 10 g of one item daily
1600	**Insects**		
	Mealworms, crickets, locusts	Pre-fed calcium-rich (8%) diet for 48 hours	~ 25 g
	Supplements		
	Vitamin D3 (e.g. IZVG preparation in oil)	Mix into pellet	0.1 ml twice weekly

8.4 A suggested diet for a common marmoset.

Lemurs

Lemurs can be fed on commercially available complete primate diets, supplemented with produce and browse to provide further minerals, vitamins and enrichment. Lemurs are thought to be much more efficient at using dietary calcium because of the paucity of it in their natural diet. Therefore they should not be fed diets too high in vitamin D or calcium, and metabolic bone disease is much less of a concern than in the other primates. Lemurs are also able to produce endogenous vitamin C, and scurvy is not reported. The most common nutritional problem seen in captive lemurs is obesity, and diets with higher levels of browse (and less protein) are most appropriate.

Protein

It is generally considered that NW monkeys have higher protein requirements than Old World (OW) monkeys. Commercial diets formulated for NW monkeys are often >20% protein by DM. Earliest recommendations for NW monkey diets were as high as 27% crude protein on a DM basis, although this is thought by some to be unfounded and a figure of 16% to be ample for all life stages (Oftedal and Allen, 1996). A common reason for not achieving adequate protein intake is oversupplementation with cultivated fruits, as described above. Low protein diets in squirrel monkeys have been associated with poor reproductive rates.

Vitamins and minerals

Vitamin C is probably an essential nutrient for most primates (1–25 mg/kg/day). Because it deteriorates rapidly in complete feeds, produce (including cabbage and citrus fruits) is an important source.

Sufficient amounts of vitamin D are essential in NW monkeys to prevent metabolic bone disease (MBD). NW monkeys are inefficient at utilizing vitamin D2 from plants in comparison to OW monkeys, and thus require high levels of vitamin D3, either through production in the skin after irradiation with UV-B light or through dietary provision. Because most glass excludes UV-B light many captive NW monkeys are inadequately exposed and require artificial sources. There is a lack of knowledge regarding how efficiently dietary vitamin D3 is utilized across species, but it is generally agreed that NW monkeys exhibit tolerance to very high doses without evidence of toxicity. Thus, it is usually recommended that NW monkeys be provided with both dietary vitamin D3 (110 IU/100 g body mass daily) (NRC 2003 recommends 1000–3000 IU vitamin D3/kg dietary DM for primates in general) and artificial UV-B (285–315 nm) lights (placed 1–2 m above favoured resting places and according to manufacturer's instructions), the latter especially during the winter. Serum values of cholecalciferol in common marmosets should be no lower than 50 ng/ml.

Callitrichids may have higher calcium requirements than other mammals (0.5–0.8% of DM for growth and lactation). The Ca:P ratio in NW monkey diets should be between 1:1 and 2:1. Excessive feeding of fruit, muscle meats or insects may dilute the calcium component of the diet sufficiently to cause a problem. Any invertebrates (e.g. mealworms, crickets, grasshoppers) should ideally be fed themselves on an 8% calcium diet for 48 hours prior to being used as food.

Breeding and contraception

With correct husbandry and reproductively healthy animals, captive primates can prove prolific breeders. Reproductive data for commonly seen primates are shown in Figure 8.5.

	Common marmoset (*Callithrix jacchus*)	Squirrel monkeys (genus *Saimiri*)	Capuchins (genus *Cebus*)	Ring-tailed lemur (*Lemur catta*)
Sexual system	Monogamous	Polygamous	Polygamous	Polygamous
Age at sexual maturity Male: Female:	16 months 12 months (no offspring before 20 months)	3 years 2.5 years	7 years 4 years	18–20 months 18–20 months
Oestrous cycle (days)	16–30	6–12	18–23	39
Interbirth interval	6 months	1 year	2 years	1 year
Length of gestation (days)	148	145–155	160–180	135
Average litter size	2 (1–4)	1	1 (twins rare)	1 (twins rare)
Birth weight (g)	35–40	106–127	200–250	65–80
Weaning age (months)	2–4	6	9	4–6

8.5 Reproductive data for commonly seen primates.

If contraception is necessary, ideal methods should be reliable and possibly reversible, easy to administer and cost-effective, with no physiological or behavioural side effects. Vasectomy of the breeding male(s) (see below) is the least invasive and socially disruptive method. Reversible chemical contraception of females using progestogens is possible, although all preparations have some adverse effects (e.g. endometritis, neoplasia) and hysterectomy is preferred if permanent sterilization is required. Most recently, gonadotrophin-releasing hormone (GnRH) agonist implants have entered the veterinary market and are proving useful in primates.

Callitrichids

In captivity callitrichids are effectively monogamous and should be kept only as a single breeding pair with their offspring. This dominant pair invariably suppresses the reproductive activity of all other animals, both behaviourally and physiologically. The incidence of triplets amongst captive callitrichids has reportedly increased, possibly as a result of higher protein diets than experienced naturally. Successful parent rearing of all three neonates is unusual, however, and energy studies demonstrate that help for the dam in the form of neonate carriage and food provision from other group members is essential. Mating is rarely seen, so conception dates are usually unknown. Pregnancy is normally visually obvious 1 month prior to parturition and births invariably occur overnight. Minimization of stress perinatally is crucial, since disruption may lead to abandonment or infanticide. Neonates are entirely carried for 2–3 weeks, care being shared by the group. By 6 weeks locomotion is mostly independent and weaning is well advanced. By 12 weeks infants are independent. Callitrichids have a rapid reproduction rate, with twins being the norm and conception often occurring at post-partum oestrus, only 10 days after parturition.

Keeping callitrichids in family groups is the simplest way to inhibit reproduction, except between the parents. Single-sex groups of 2–3 individuals are often successful socially, especially if formed from related members, or from unrelated males. This does, however, preclude natural mating behaviour. Progestogen-containing implants such as etonogestrel can be inserted subcutaneously. This requires anaesthesia and fractioning of human implants into appropriate lengths (e.g. one-fifth). Ovulation will be suppressed, and although data regarding its use are limited, in the author's experience it is reasonable to expect 2 years of contraception without major adverse effects. The GnRH agonist deslorelin (Suprelorin®: a slow-release implant containing 4.7 mg of deslorelin acetate) appears to provide reliable shutdown of the female reproductive cycle for approximately 6 months and is the reversible contraceptive recommendation for all NW monkeys from the AZA Wildlife Contraception Center. Current data are very encouraging, although duration of action appears to vary by individual. The main side effects are as for gonadectomy – especially weight gain. If permanent contraception is deemed appropriate then surgical sterilization is preferable. Vasectomy and hysterectomy both require anaesthesia but are relatively simple and will preserve normal reproductive behaviour. Castration and ovariectomy are less appropriate since they can affect behaviour too much.

Cebids

Squirrel monkeys are seasonal breeders, with a birth season in captivity in the Northern Hemisphere of June to August. Changes in humidity or group composition are often a stimulus. Outside the mating season males are often peripheral to the core group run by females. During the season males put on weight (up to 250 g), vocalize, engage in dominance behaviour over each other and become attentive to females in oestrus. Zoo-based research has shown captive squirrel monkeys to have poor reproductive success compared to other primates. As for callitrichids, deslorelin is the latest recommendation for reversible contraception. Progestogen preparations are effective, and permanent sterilization is as for callitrichids.

Lemurs

Lemurs exhibit seasonal reproductive cycles and restricted breeding seasons, during which there is significant testicular enlargement. Males have a baculum (os penis) and a pendulous scrotum. Ring-tailed lemurs tend to have single births, whilst ruffed lemurs generally have twins. Contraception can be achieved with injectable progestogen-medroxy-progesterone acetate (MPA) at a dose rate of 5 mg/kg every 6 weeks for the duration of the breeding season only. Permanent sterilization is achievable through vasectomy or hysterectomy as for calli-trichids. Castration may also reduce aggression but reduces natural behaviours and can result in a change of coat colour in some species. The use of deslorelin is still in its infancy in lemurs and evidence regarding efficacy is lacking.

Hand-rearing

Rearing primates outside their natural social structures is not to be undertaken lightly – it is labour-intensive and unless done correctly can produce maladjusted individuals. It should only be attempted in animals that would otherwise not survive and then only when an owner has the necessary resources and knowledge. Fostering should be considered as a better alternative if a suitable dam is available. Triplets in species that would only produce twins in the wild rarely survive. Possible strategies are: to take the strongest for hand-rearing; to take two for hand-rearing (to provide company); or supplementary rearing by rotation (with each neonate being cared for away from the parents every third day).

New World monkeys: Neonates that are being rejected will often be found on the floor or having received bites from the dam. Those that are being cared for but are not suckling will be restless on the parent, then gradually weaken and be seen hanging off, often with a limp rather than a coiled tail. Record-keeping (including feeding times and intake, behaviour and appetite, urine and faeces production, and weight gain) is critical. Initial assessment should include clinging ability, hydration status, body temperature, weight and respiration. Subcutaneous fluids may be appropriate, as may antibiotics if there is trauma or bite wounds. The umbilicus should be treated with iodine solution daily until it drops off.

An incubator is preferable for warmth, although a hot water bottle wrapped in towels is a good alternative. Initial temperature should be maintained at 18°C, or enough to maintain body temperature at 36–37°C. Initial hypothermia can be resolved by holding the neonate next to the human body. A small soft toy or a pair of rolled up socks provides a surrogate mother to cling to.

A 1 ml syringe with a small teat attached is ideal for feeding, since volumes taken can be recorded accurately. Any good quality milk substitute for human neonates will suffice without supplementation. The first feed should be just a glucose solution (1 teaspoon in 28 ml sterile water), the second a dilute solution of the milk substitute, and from then on the substitute made up as the manufacturer's instructions. All solutions must be fed at body temperature or they will be rejected. The neonate should be held vertically during feeding to prevent aspiration, and the milk only given slowly and to demand. Neonates should be fed approximately 10% of their bodyweight per 24 hours (e.g. a 50 g callitrichid would be fed 0.5 ml per feed, for 10 feeds – a total of 5 ml). Once a neonate is consuming all the formula offered, the amount can be increased incrementally (e.g. by 0.1 ml per day). Urination and defecation should be stimulated after each feed by rubbing the anal area with some warm moist cotton wool.

- Feeds should start at 2-hourly intervals, and for the first week the neonate will require feeds throughout the night.
- In the second week this can stop, with feeds between 6 am and midnight only, every 3 hours.
- In the third week this can be reduced to every 4 hours.
- After 4 weeks small quantities of cereal-based infant food can be added to the milk substitute, gradually increased over the next few weeks. At the same time, soft fruits such as pear and banana can be introduced by hand and then left finely chopped in a bowl.
- Weaning age varies with species (see Figure 8.5).

Regular weighing is important; after the first week neonates should gain weight steadily. A transient loss may be noted around the time of withholding milk when weaning.

Constipation may be resolved by replacing a milk feed with a glucose one. Diarrhoea may require an electrolyte solution in place of milk, but if not resolved after a couple of feeds then veterinary intervention may be necessary.

Contact with the rest of the natal group is ideally maintained by keeping the neonate within sight, sound and smell, possibly within the enclosure. Reintroduction should be started as early as possible after the neonate is mobile, with gradually increasing sessions, always observed very closely. If reintroduction to the family group is not successful, mixing with an individual of another species is better than solitude.

Lemurs: Ring-tailed lemurs carry their neonates, whilst ruffed lemurs leave them in a nest. As a result, neonatal ring-tails require surrogates, as for NW monkeys. The normal position for the clinging neonate is horizontal across the lower abdomen or at a slight angle if suckling. Species that leave neonates in a nest should stay with them almost continuously for the first few days. Criteria for intervention are as for NW monkeys.

Hypothermia, hypoglycaemia and dehydration are common problems, and can sometimes be corrected with removal for warming, feeding and/or fluids, before successfully returning a neonate to parental care. Carrying species have dilute milk, low in energy, fat and protein. By contrast, nesting species produce milk of higher concentrations. Generally, human low-iron formulas are recommended. Lack of bloating and normal faecal consistency (semi-formed) indicates tolerance. Lemurs will consume an average of 25% of their bodyweight in formula daily. Ring-tailed and ruffed lemurs should gain 4–8 g daily for the first month, then rates increase. Weaning occurs from 4 months and can be encouraged as for NW monkeys. Diarrhoea due to intolerance of the formula may be improved by a change to soy-based formula and an initial reduction of intake. Lemurs will kill young they do not recognize as their own, so reintroductions must be undertaken with care. For further detail on the subjects of introduction, reintroduction and socialization see Watts and Meder (1996).

Identification

Standard commercial microchips placed subcutaneously between the scapulae are the best method of unique and permanent identification. In this location they can generally be read during manual restraint, although it should be remembered that migration is possible. The use of tissue glue to close the entry hole prevents immediate loss.

Preventive healthcare

The risk of zoonotic infection from primates is high, through bites or scratches, ingestion of body excretions, or aerosol. Common-sense hygiene precautions will largely mitigate these risks – wearing gloves, washing hands frequently, using work-specific clothes, keeping hands away from the face, cleaning and treating any wounds as soon as possible, and the use of viricidal and bactericidal disinfectants. Owners should be encouraged to follow these principles, and surgeries should be treated as contaminated after any primate visit. Vaccinations against pertinent diseases are recommended for veterinary surgeons and staff and for owners, e.g. tetanus, poliomyelitis, measles, hepatitis B, influenza and *Mycobacterium tuberculosis*.

Humans can also pass infections to primates – faecal parasites or bacteria, streptococcal respiratory infections, common-cold viruses and *Mycobacterium tuberculosis*. Some primates are exquisitely sensitive to minor human diseases, e.g. callitrichid susceptibility to *Herpes simplex* virus (HSV).

A preventive approach is essential. The routine screening of any animals entering the group, and on an infrequent basis those already in it, is an important part of establishing and maintaining a disease-free status. These checks should include: individual identification; weight; clinical examination; faecal analysis for parasites and bacteria (to include *Salmonella, Shigella, Campylobacter* and *Yersinia*); and tuberculosis screening (*Mycobacterium tuberculosis* or *M. bovis*). Post-mortem examination, even when cause of death is already established, is important for surveillance of concurrent disease in the group.

Food and water utensils must be cleaned and disinfected daily, and any other equipment (such as nets) after use. Food must be kept out of the reach of rodents, birds, insects and cats, and a pest control programme is essential. Vaccination against some common pathogens in these species is possible (e.g. tetanus, measles, rabies, *Yersinia pseudotuberculosis*), although efficacy is often poorly established.

Handling and restraint

Handling must only be undertaken with due preparation. Primates can inflict serious bites and may harbour zoonotic disease, and restraint is stressful for the primate, so duration should be minimized. **Disposable latex gloves should always be worn for examination.** Leather gauntlets offer some protection and are recommended for catching animals but they can damage primate teeth and also reduce handler dexterity. Catching animals is easiest when they are still in nest boxes. Useful aids for restraint and/or injection of anaesthetic induction agents include nets (often with the addition of a soft broom) (Figure 8.6) and squeeze cages. Primates may be trained to present arms or hips for injection. Otherwise remote systems such as darts and a blowpipe may be necessary, for which a firearms licence is required. Any primate weighing >10 kg must be restrained chemically after initial catching. Correct manual restraint techniques are described below, whilst anaesthetic agents commonly used in primates are listed in Figure 8.14.

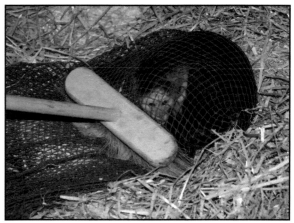

8.6 Use of a net and broom to restrain a white-throated capuchin.

- Callitrichids are restrained by holding the upper body with a thumb and forefinger around the neck, whilst the other hand supports the lower limbs, with a finger between them to prevent pressure damage (Figure 8.7a).
- For cebids, the upper limbs are restrained behind the animal's back with one hand, whilst the other supports the lower limbs, again with a finger between them (Figure 8.7b).
- With lemurs, the handler grasps the back of the neck with one hand and places the other under the neck and mandible to prevent bites (Figure 8.7c). The lemur is allowed to grasp the handler's hand or arm using all four limbs.

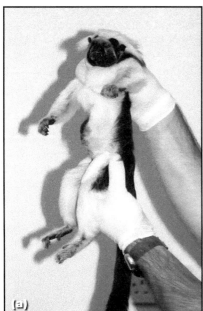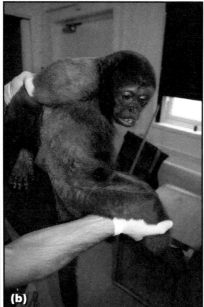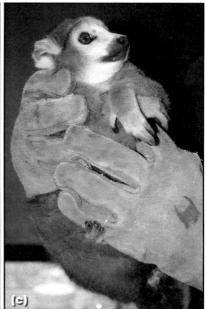

8.7 Manual restraint: **(a)** cotton-top tamarin; **(b)** woolly monkey; **(c)** crowned lemur.

Diagnostic approach

Observation

Owners should observe animals daily for appetite and behaviour. Giving some preferred food items (part of their diet) by hand will allow a closer view of the face and mouth and allow assessment of their general condition including hair, and signs of diarrhoea or pregnancy.

History

Important points for primates:

- Signalment – species; age; sex; wild-caught or captive-bred; parity; hand-reared *versus* parent-reared
- Length of time living with owner
- Husbandry – diet and feeding regime; access to fluids; enclosure (including temperature, humidity, lighting, space, furniture, substrate use and cleaning)
- Social structure – group make-up and changes; reproductive management; level of interaction with owner
- Any previous health issues
- Current clinical presentation – signs; duration; progression; previous treatment if any and outcome.

Clinical examination

A basic understanding of the normal anatomy is important. Although physical restraint is possible (see above), anaesthesia may be a better option if a clinical examination of any detail is to be conducted. This should include the mouth and mucous membranes, palpation of lymph nodes, abdomen and skeleton, auscultation of the heart and lungs, and temperature and weight assessment. Holding the animal vertically may assist abdominal palpation.

Imaging

All imaging requires general anaesthesia.

Radiography

Radiographic settings equate to those for small mammals of comparable weights and dimensions, although it should be noted that the thorax of primates is generally more ventrodorsally flattened and exposures should therefore be adjusted accordingly. Radiographs are used most commonly to assess bone density in suspected cases of MBD (see Figure 8.11), or following trauma. For dorsoventral thoracic radiographs the animal should be placed in sternal recumbency, with the forearms extended cranially and elbows drawn together to remove the scapulae from the thoracic field.

Ultrasonography

Ultrasonography generally requires a 7.5 MHz or higher frequency probe. It can be employed for a similar range of imaging as used in small mammals.

Sample collection

Blood

Samples of up to 1% of bodyweight (i.e. 1 ml/100 g) can be taken from healthy animals. In primates weighing <10 kg the femoral vein is the favoured collection site, and can be readily visualized in most callitrichids. A 2 ml syringe with a 25- or 27-gauge needle is ideal for the smallest species. With the animal in dorsal recumbency and its leg abducted, the femoral artery is palpated and the vein (medial/superficial to the artery) raised with pressure in the inguinal area. The vein is entered just distal to the inguinal canal (Figure 8.8). Haematoma formation is possible and digital pressure following collection is necessary.

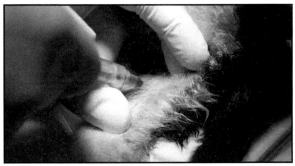

8.8 Collecting a blood sample from a cotton-top tamarin.

The saphenous (popliteal) vein on the caudal aspect of the lower leg is suitable for catheter placement in most primates. Alternative sites for venepuncture include the cephalic and jugular veins (which may be the only feasible site in very small animals). Most commercial laboratories will accept primate blood samples for routine haematology and biochemistry, although interpretation will generally be minimal and specialist tests will require specialist laboratories.

Normal haematological and biochemical data for commonly seen primates are presented in Figure 8.9. It should be noted that serum glucose levels are highly variable in primates, and often significantly raised following stressful restraint and/or induction of anaesthesia.

Urine
Free-catch samples into a clean pan are often the only option. Primates can be trained to urinate on command. Cystocentesis is possible but often difficult due to the small and intrapelvic nature of the bladder, and the tendency of patients to urinate when being caught. Urethral catheterization is possible in both sexes of most species.

Faeces
These need to be handled correctly to diagnose certain infections. For example: multiple samples are needed to culture intermittently shed *Salmonella;* special media are required to grow *Shigella;* and rapid examination is necessary to see *Entamoeba.*

Fluid
CSF can be collected from the cisterna magna with the head in ventroflexion, using an aseptic technique and a 25- or 27-gauge needle. Peritoneal fluid can be collected from the cranial right quarter of the abdomen.

Parameter	Common marmoset (*Callithrix jacchus*)	Common squirrel monkey (*Saimiri sciureus*)	White-throated capuchin (*Cebus capucinus*)	Ring-tailed lemur (*Lemur catta*)
Haematology				
PCV (l/l)	0.45–0.48	0.43–0.56	0.45–0.53	0.44–0.56
RBC (x 10^{12}/l)	6.9	7.1–10.9	5.2–6.5	6.8–8.7
Hb (g/dl)	15.1–15.5	12.9–17.0	14–17	13.9–17.3
WBC (x 10^9/l)	7.0–12.0	5.1–10.9	5.0–24.0	4.9–12.2
Neutrophils (%)	28–55	36–66	55	51
Lymphocytes (%)	43–67	27–55	41	40
Monocytes (%)	0.4–2.1	0–6	1.8	4.4
Eosinophils (%)	0.5–0.6	0–11	1.6	4.0
Basophils (%)	0.3–1.3	<1	<1	0.6
Platelets (x 10^9/l)	390–490	112	108–187	166–390
Biochemistry				
ALT (IU/l)	9.5–10.2	59–99	13–43	40–152
AST (IU/l)	160–182	56–118	21–57	14–76
Bilirubin (µmol/l)	8.5–10.3	1.7–9.0	0–4	3–17
BUN (mmol/l)	9.64	8.21–13.92	8.57–15.71	5.00–10.71
Calcium (mmol/l)	2.4–2.6	2.1–2.4	2.5	2.2–2.66
Cholesterol (mmol/l)	1.4–6.4	3.3–5.4	4.4–6.6	1.6–3.0
Glucose (mmol/l)	7.0–8.3	2.9–6.0	2.4–5.2	3.7–12.0
LDH (IU/l)	799	271–490	121–373	1028
Phosphorus (mmol/l)	0.5–3.3	1.1–2.5	2.3	1.1–2.4
Protein (g/l)	70	69–81	75–87	66–80

8.9 Normal haematological and biochemical data for commonly seen primates. (Data from Carpenter (2005) and ISIS).

Common conditions

Viral infections

Herpesviruses

The majority of primates can harbour host-adapted herpesviruses that cause little or no clinical disease. HSV – the cause of cold sores in humans – is responsible for acute disseminated fatal disease in callitrichids (characterized by oral and cutaneous ulceration and encephalitis). There are documented outbreaks of fatal *Herpes simplex* encephalitis in ruffed and ring-tailed lemurs. Similarly, *Herpes tamarinus*, for which the squirrel monkey is the natural host, can cause fatal disease in callitrichids. Other latent herpesviruses, such as *Herpes saimiri* from squirrel monkeys and Epstein–Barr virus (EBV) from humans, appear able to cause fatal lymphoproliferative neoplasia in callitrichids. Preventing callitrichid herpesvirus infections is best achieved by preventing any direct contact with cebids or humans with clinical signs of HSV (active cold sores) or EBV (sore throat, fever, lymphadenopathy).

Lymphocytic choriomeningitis virus

LCMV is the cause of callitrichid hepatitis, an acute and generally fatal disease characterized by lethargy, anorexia and seizures. Liver enzymes are often elevated and severe hepatic necrosis is often apparent at post-mortem examination. Not feeding mice and excluding wild house mice (the natural reservoir) from enclosures is the only prevention. LCMV is classically reported in callitrichids but can infect, and cause severe disease in, many other species of primate (personal observation).

Measles

Exposure to the human morbillivirus can prove acutely fatal in NW monkeys. Lethargy, erythema and oedema of the eyelids and face, nasal discharge, and lip lesions are common signs. Antibiotics to reduce secondary bacterial infections may help animals seroconvert and survive. Vaccination with human preparations (human live hyperattenuated monovalent vaccine given intramuscularly at 6 months and boosted at 12 months) has been used, but is rarely indicated when good coverage of the human population exists.

Other

Influenza and parainfluenza viruses (from humans) can cause severe and even fatal disease in non-human primates. Consequently, any owner with 'cold' symptoms should avoid close contact with their animals or, at the very least, wear a mask for their duration.

Bacterial infections

Enteritis

Enteric bacteria such as *Salmonella*, *Campylobacter*, *Shigella* and enteropathogenic *Escherichia coli* can cause gastroenteritis and severe diarrhoea in primates. Septicaemia and systemic disease can ensue,

culminating in death, although this normally only occurs in the young, geriatric or immunocompromised. Infection is generally acquired through ingestion of contaminated food or water or through contact with other infected individuals. Diagnosis is generally made on clinical signs and culture of fresh faecal material. Mild infections are usually self-limiting within 2–4 days, in which case supportive therapy (fluids, electrolytes, analgesics) should suffice. Individual nursing of affected animals in warm and quiet conditions may be necessary. Paediatric oral electrolytes (by tube if necessary) are useful for rehydration, or subcutaneous fluids to replace potassium in more chronic cases. Antibiosis should be reserved for severe and/or prolonged cases, and based on culture and sensitivity testing, with treatment extended 5 days beyond resolution. Concurrent use of probiotics (e.g. commercial yoghurts) may assist preservation of normal intestinal flora and prevent yeast overgrowth. Good hygiene is necessary to prevent cross-infection amongst primates and zoonotic transmission.

Yersinia pseudotuberculosis is an enteropathogen carried by, and shed in, the faeces of wild birds and rodents. This bacterium grows especially well (with enhanced virulence characteristics) when ambient temperatures drop. Thus, isolated deaths or outbreaks often occur in the winter and spring. Primates are infected orally from a contaminated environment or by eating infected prey. It is thought that *Y. pseudotuberculosis* can persist in a latent state in soil, water, vegetation and animal waste for prolonged periods. Infections are common in zoological collections. NW monkeys are considered especially susceptible, with juvenile animals apparently at greatest risk due to stress and being out-competed for uncontaminated food. Animals either die acutely with primary enterocolitic lesions (and haemorrhagic diarrhoea if they survive long enough) or lose weight chronically. Infection can persist in a carrier state. It is difficult to isolate the organism from faeces of infected primates because it is not shed into the lumen and cold-enrichment techniques are required. Post-mortem examination often reveals multifocal abscessation of the liver, spleen and mesenteric lymph nodes, from which impression smears of characteristic Gram-negative rods can be obtained. Histology and/or culture are important to differentiate this from tuberculosis or the other enteric bacteria discussed above. It is recommended that all surviving animals be treated immediately with prophylactic doses of potentiated amoxicillin or fluoroquinolones. Some zoological collections have produced vaccines against local strains but the stress of catching and administering vaccine to many individuals, and the unproven efficacy of these vaccines, makes their use questionable. Housing improvements to minimize potential exposure are important, as is stress reduction.

Pneumonia

Bordetella, *Klebsiella*, *Pasteurella*, *Haemophilus*, *Streptococcus* and *Staphylococcus* species are common aetiological agents of respiratory infections in primates. Clinical signs include nasal discharge, sneezing, coughing, dyspnoea, pyrexia and inappetence. High indoor temperatures and low humidity are implicated in occurrence and spread. Outdoor access is beneficial but disease may require supportive therapy and antibiotics. *Haemophilus* can potentially progress to cause meningitis/encephalitis, for which antibiotics that penetrate the blood–brain barrier are essential (e.g. amoxicillin or ampicillin). *Klebsiella pneumoniae* appears to be especially virulent in prosimians, causing peracute pneumonia and death.

Tetanus

Tetanus has been reported in many primates and is generally fatal. If there is a history of infection in a collection, then vaccination is recommended: 40 IU of human tetanus toxoid given by intramuscular injection three times at intervals of 2–3 months, with boosters at 5 and 10 years.

Tuberculosis

Mycobacterium tuberculosis or *M. bovis* can cause tuberculous disease in all primates. Although rare in NW monkeys, and extremely rare in lemurs, they are extremely serious infections and should be considered as differential diagnoses in appropriate cases. Clinical signs include coughing, anorexia, weight loss and lethargy. Transmission occurs through close contact, especially by aerosol from respiratory secretions. Post-mortem examination often reveals granulomatous pulmonary lesions and obvious bronchial lymphadenopathy. Screening ought to be seen as an important part of any preventive medicine programme, and might comprise three tests within 6 months of arrival, then yearly follow-up. Diagnosis has been based historically on an intradermally injected tuberculin test. In the UK it is customary to use 0.1 ml of purified protein derivative (PPD) (0.05 ml in the smallest species) of avian and bovine mycobacteria in the eyelids (avian right, bovine left). There is evidence that non-human primates require higher antigen concentrations to respond and some advocate the use of old mammalian tuberculin (OMT) instead, to increase the test sensitivity, although this can be hard to obtain in the UK. Any delayed hypersensitivity reaction can be read subjectively without catching again, since primates invariably stare back at people. Any swelling seen within 72 hours is considered a positive result. Isolation (including in-contacts) and further testing is then indicated. This should include culture and acid-fast staining (from tracheal and/or gastric lavage samples), thoracic radiography, gamma-interferon or serological tests looking for seroconversion. Successful treatment has been described (Wolf *et al.,* 1988), although public health risk may preclude this.

Septicaemia

This is seen surprisingly frequently as a result of bacterial infection from a variety of sources – gastrointestinal, respiratory and traumatic. Blood cultures are necessary for definitive diagnosis but both *Streptococcus zooepidemicus* and *Pasteurella multocida* have been responsible for fatalities. Aggressive antibiotic therapy and supportive care may be successful.

Fungal infections

Overgrowth of *Candida* in gastrointestinal flora may follow prolonged antibiotic therapy and cause classic 'thrush'. Treatment with nystatin or an azole is recommended. *Cryptococcus neoformans* infection of the respiratory tract and nervous system have been recorded. Cutaneous mycoses are rare. In lemurs that scent mark, alopecia around scent glands (carpi, anogenital and forehead) may be misdiagnosed as dermatomycosis when it is actually caused by excessive rubbing.

Parasitic infections

Protozoa

Many enteric protozoans, including *Entamoeba*, *Trichomonas*, *Giardia* and *Balantidium* species, are detected in primate faeces by direct examination, including in clinically well animals. *E. histolytica* can certainly be pathogenic but its differentiation from non-pathogenic species requires specialist laboratory assistance. Prevention of faeco-oral transmission is important but often difficult to achieve. Metronidazole is routinely used for treatment.

Primates can become infected with *Toxoplasma gondii* through ingestion of cat faeces (sporulated oocysts) or wild rodents (bradyzoites in flesh). NW monkeys are very susceptible, especially squirrel monkeys (Cunningham *et al.,* 1992). Ring-tailed lemurs also appear to be extremely sensitive (Dubey *et al.,* 1985), possibly due to their more terrestrial nature and reduced evolutionary exposure to felids. Disseminated disease often causes peracute death. Less overwhelming infection may result in pneumonia, hepatitis and encephalitis, and infection during pregnancy may cause abortion or stillbirth. Ante-mortem diagnosis is difficult, since clinical signs and pathology are often non-specific. Paired IgG titres measured 2–4 weeks apart showing a 16-fold rise are indicative of active infection, but definitive diagnosis usually comes from histology of post-mortem tissues. Treatment will only arrest multiplication, since no available drugs kill bradyzoites. Potentiated sulphonamides or clindamycin are the drugs of choice but prevention through the exclusion of wild rodents and cats from enclosures and food stores, respectively, is much more effective.

Encephalitozoon cuniculi has been known to cause disseminated microgranulomas in squirrel monkeys. Prevention of faeco-oral transmission and use of anthelmintics such as fenbendazole will prevent it.

Helminths

Tapeworms can cause hydatid disease and mortality in primates. Excluding carnivore hosts and preventing them from contaminating food is essential in control.

Potentially pathogenic gastrointestinal nematodes in NW monkeys and lemurs include species of the oxyurid and ascarid families, and from the genera *Strongylus*, *Strongyloides*, *Enterobius* and *Trichuris*. All are readily identifiable by faecal flotation and can be effectively controlled by reducing faeco-oral transmission and correct use of anthelmintics.

The spirurid nematode *Pterygodermatites nycticebi* can infest the small intestine of callitrichids, resulting in morbidity and mortality. Cockroaches act as intermediate hosts and therefore require control. Treatment is usually based around benzimidazoles or avermectins.

Acanthocephalans have been reported as causing fatal peritonitis following gastric penetration in callitrichids. Cockroach (intermediate host) control is important, and treatment with mebendazole (100 mg/kg) and surgical removal are apparently successful.

Ectoparasites

Mite infestations (*Sarcoptes, Demodex*) have been recorded in callitrichids. Clinical signs include pruritus, alopecia, hyperkeratosis and scaling. Generalized disease can result in loss of appetite and condition. Definitive diagnosis requires skin scrapes and microscopic examination. Treatment options include avermectins and synthetic pyrethroids. The author has found amitraz baths of particular use in the elimination of *Demodex* infestations from groups of red-handed tamarins (Figure 8.10).

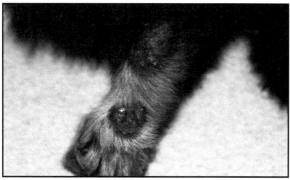

8.10 Demodectic mange on the forearm of a red-handed tamarin.

Nutritional and metabolic diseases

Metabolic bone disease

NW monkeys (particularly young ones) are especially susceptible to MBD (e.g. rickets, osteomalacia, fibrous osteodystrophy). MBD commonly occurs due to incorrect nutrition: dietary Ca:P <1; inadequate dietary vitamin D3; and inadequate dietary protein (see Diet). Insufficient UV-B light and end-stage renal disease are other common causative factors. Clinical signs include lethargy, anorexia, pain, inability to jump ('cage paralysis'), pathological folding fractures of long bones, vertebral damage with spinal cord compression, faecal impaction and facial deformity ('rubber jaw'). Clinical pathology may show raised alkaline phosphatase (ALP) levels and serum cholecalciferol <20 ng/ml. Prognosis depends on radiological assessment (widening of growth plates, thinning of cortices, reduced cortical density, fractures, 'floating teeth', faecal impaction) (Figure 8.11) and treatment should not be attempted if vertebrae have collapsed. Folding fractures of long bones will heal well with correction of the diet and environment and prolonged cage rest (next to cagemates). Splints are not recommended as new fractures often occur at stress points. Radiological reassessment after 6 weeks and then 6 months is necessary.

Wasting marmoset syndrome

Callitrichids are susceptible to a chronic wasting disease of presumed multiple aetiology: poor nutrition; stress; enteric disease (including dysbiosis and *Campylobacter* infection); pancreatic parasites (*Trichospirura leptostoma*) in some recorded cases; and low serum levels of vitamin E. Affected animals lose weight and muscle mass and become ungroomed, lethargic and weak. Accompanying

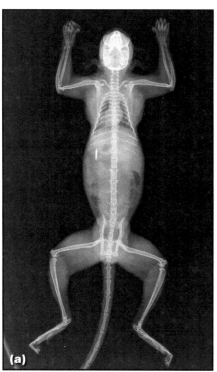
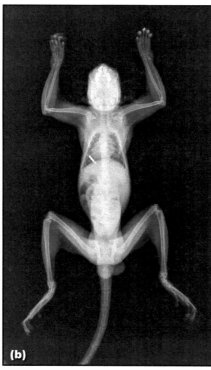

8.11 Radiographs of common marmosets, showing: **(a)** normal skeletal appearance; **(b)** changes indicative of MBD – 'floating' teeth, thinning of cortices and reduced cortical density.

diarrhoea is common, due to enteritis and/or colitis. Investigation must include physical examination and detailed clinical pathology. Blood profiles classically show anaemia, hypocalcaemia and hypoproteinaemia. Many cases will have concurrent MBD. If radiographs demonstrate poor skeletal mineralization, dietary calcium, vitamin D3 and protein should be increased. Other treatments might include broad-spectrum antibiotics, electrolytes and vitamin E and selenium supplementation. The addition of gum to the diet of marmosets may relieve diarrhoea and associated weight loss. Nutritional and environmental improvement is crucial. It can be frustratingly difficult to reverse the course of disease, and prognosis is generally poor.

Iron storage disease

Haemochromatosis has long been considered a problem for captive lemurs. Relative excesses of dietary iron and ascorbic acid, and a lack of iron-binding tannins in the captive diet are thought to be responsible. Naturally available tannins bind iron and reduce its absorption. Ascorbic acid reduces Fe^{3+} to Fe^{2+}, a more readily absorbable form of iron. Thus, reduction of complete diet iron content and the amount of citrus fruit fed with the ration have greatly reduced the incidence of haemochromatosis and the hepatocellular carcinomas that appears to accompany it. Serum iron, transferrin saturation and serum ferritin values appear to be good indicators of systemic iron stores (Crawford et al., 2005). Haemochromatosis is also recognized as a cause of premature death in captive marmosets, in which dietary iron intake should not exceed 180 mg/kg of diet.

Scurvy

Clinical signs of dietary deficiency of vitamin C include loss of bone substance, loose teeth, haemorrhage of the gums and subcutis, and pain on movement. Supplemental vitamin C can be provided but fresh fruit or a complete diet should provide adequate levels.

Colitis

There is some evidence that callitrichids chronically exposed to protein allergens in wheat, soya or milk are at increased risk of developing colitis. Infectious agents are also implicated, including *Helicobacter*, *Giardia* and clostridia.

Diabetes

Type II diabetes mellitus is seen spontaneously in NW monkeys and prosimians, albeit rarely (Greenwood and Taylor, 1977). Clinical presentation varies according to progression of the disease but is broadly similar to that seen in humans. Age, obesity and genetics appear to influence the onset of an initial peripheral insulin resistance, and a resulting hyperinsulinaemia. Gradual insulin depletion leads to borderline diabetes. Overt diabetes follows with severe hyperglycaemia, weight loss, ketosis and acidosis. Useful diagnostic tests include serum glucose (other causes such as stress of capture must be ruled out), urine glucose and ketonuria (primate urine should be negative). Early-stage diabetes can be treated with nutritional management – restricting simple sugar intake and providing a high-protein, high-fat diet but with a reduced caloric intake overall. Oral hypoglycaemic agents may be necessary. For the treatment of overt diabetes exogenous human insulin administration will probably be necessary (Walzer, 1999).

Miscellaneous

Dystocia

Common marmosets and ruffed lemurs appear especially prone to dystocia. All pregnant females should be observed daily for progress (increase in abdominal girth, change in appetite and/or activity levels) so that early intervention occurs in the case of any problem. Primates should give birth at night, so one straining in the morning is an emergency. Immediate Caesarean section (see below) is the only sensible treatment option and, if performed correctly, generally results in a rapid recovery and return to breeding.

Dental disease

Dental disease is regularly seen as a result of incorrect nutrition and/or tooth damage inflicted during catching. The relatively large upper canines are particularly vulnerable to fracture, with resultant pulp exposure and apical abscesses. These cases present as a swelling of the face below the eye (or even facial fistulae) and, although antibiosis will often ameliorate clinical signs, extraction is normally indicated. Leaving the alveolar socket open to drain (Figure 8.12) seems to result in excellent healing. In the larger species endodontics may be appropriate to maintain the integrity of the maxilla or mandible; standard small animal techniques and equipment are suitable. Prolonged delay in treatment may result in chronic bacteraemia, leading to endocarditis and death. Primates with no teeth cope well on a captive diet that is adequately soaked and chopped.

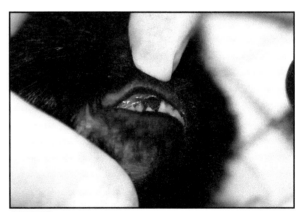

8.12 The alveolar socket of a Goeldi's monkey, left open following extraction of the upper right canine tooth.

Wounds and fractures

Hierarchical or new-group disputes commonly result in wounds, sometimes severe. Even deep wounds are often better debrided, cleaned and left to heal by secondary intention than closed, since most bite wounds become infected. Abscesses may be the first sign, and lancing under anaesthesia and antibiotics (e.g. potentiated amoxicillin) are indicated. Amputation of fingers and tails may be required. Squirrel monkeys appear especially prone to tail trauma, either from others or by self-mutilation due to stress, or as a result of prolonged suboptimal temperature and ischaemic damage. Postoperative management can be extremely difficult due to interference and intolerance of dressings. Subcuticular sutures and NSAID analgesia are useful in these cases. Long-bone fractures can be repaired with internal fixation, or casts may be tolerated.

Intussusception, rectal prolapse and trichobezoars

Animals with severe diarrhoea have been known to develop intussusception and rectal prolapse. The former requires immediate surgical intervention; the latter can be corrected with a purse-string suture but the underlying cause must be identified and corrected (often difficult if stress-related).

Ruffed lemurs are prone to trichobezoars, which will normally respond to laxative therapy (such as oral domestic cat preparations), though surgical intervention may be necessary. Weekly prophylactic laxatives are recommended by some authors (Junge, 1999).

Epilepsy

Neurological disease, head trauma, hypoglycaemia and the ingestion of lead in a high enough quantity to cause toxicity (classically from old paints in enclosures) may all precipitate epileptic seizures. Idiopathic epilepsy is also recognized in primates. When the incidence of seizures becomes unacceptably high, anticonvulsant therapy can be employed.

Supportive care

Although sick primates will respond well to therapy if administration of medication can be well managed, emphasis must be on the prevention of disease.

Drug administration

Therapy can be difficult due to the suspicious nature and manual dexterity of these animals, and their requirement for social contact with cagemates. Individuals can be housed in a 'hospital crush cage' within a social group's enclosure to minimize separation, ease reintroduction and aid injections. Injection sites are illustrated in Figure 8.13. Injectable preparations will ensure drug uptake, although oral ones can generally be administered by gavage to juveniles and callitrichids. Oral suspensions of paediatric human preparations are often useful since they are palatable and can be disguised in food or drink. Due to size, precise calculations are necessary.

Fluid therapy

Fluids may be given intravenously, subcutaneously, intraperitoneally or intraosseously. The subcutaneous or intraperitoneal route is recommended in an emergency.

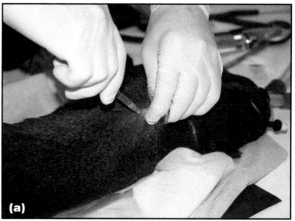

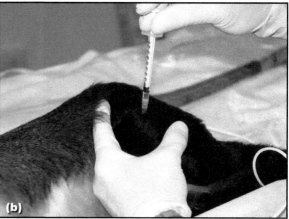

8.13 Injection sites for small primates: **(a)** subcutaneous injection in the scruff of the neck; **(b)** intramuscular injection into the quadriceps muscle. This patient is under anaesthesia.

- Subcutaneous administration is best achieved in the loose skin over the back.
- Intraperitoneal injections are performed with the animal in dorsal recumbency. The abdominal wall is raised by pinching it between the fingers and the needle is inserted just lateral to the midline. Palpation ensures it is not within a loop of bowel.
- Intravenous access is more applicable for fluid administration during elective surgery because of the time it can take to set up and the necessity to remove it once the animal is awake. In most small primates the saphenous vein on the caudal aspect of the lower leg provides the best access.
- Intraosseous catheters can be placed in the proximal femur or tibia if intravenous access is not possible.
- Rates are equivalent to those used in small mammals and a single subcutaneous or intraperitoneal injection would normally represent some 5% of bodyweight (e.g. 15–20 ml in a common marmoset).

Nutritional support

Heating and nutritional support are crucial due to limited reserves, especially in the smaller species. Force-feeding with human liquid food substitutes is possible.

Anaesthesia and analgesia

Anaesthesia, or at least sedation, is essential in most instances for proper clinical examination. Pre-anaesthetic health screening is generally limited to history and close observation, so immediate post-induction physical examination should be undertaken to establish at least airway, breathing, circulation, body temperature, bodyweight and condition, and hydration status. It is best to withhold food from primates weighing <1 kg for no more than 6–8 hours, whilst primates weighing >1 kg should have food withheld for at least 12 hours prior to anaesthesia.

There are many drugs available for the anaesthesia of primates but no single drug, or combination, can be described as safe and reversible in all situations. Oral administration and effect is notoriously inconsistent. Induction chambers can be improvised from plastic containers and used for all relevant species, although manual restraint and mask induction (even through a net) is more controlled. The injectable route is the most reliable but requires prior restraint or remote injection.

A review of agents is beyond the scope of this chapter; readers are referred to Ølberg (2007) and Figure 8.14. **Opioids should be used with caution** since profound respiratory depression can occur, especially with butorphanol. Isoflurane is a commonly used and safe volatile anaesthetic agent for induction and maintenance, although sevoflurane may be advantageous for mask induction due to its non-irritating odour and more rapid effect. Inhalation anaesthesia is safe in most species, although it does cause hypotension. Using oxygen as the carrier gas normally ensures adequate partial pressure of oxygen in arterial blood.

All but the smallest species can be intubated and should be for anything other than short procedures. Positioning in dorsal recumbency with use of a short laryngoscope and extension of the tongue allows good visualization of the glottis. Topical anaesthesia reduces incidence of laryngospasm. All primates have a short trachea and endotracheal tubes must be premeasured (to no lower than the thoracic inlet) to avoid intubation of a mainstream bronchus. Auscultation of respiratory noise in both lung fields will confirm correct placement.

Larger species (>10 kg) require induction with injectable anaesthetic agents, and ideally these agents should be used in the majority of smaller species too. Suppression of thermoregulation, lack of shivering and the large surface-area-to-body-mass ratio of these primates, especially the smallest ones, make preventing hypothermia during and after anaesthesia crucial. This often requires active heating with appropriate pads or hot air/water systems; paediatric forced air systems are ideal. Any intravenous fluids should be given at body temperature. Vascular access is as described for venepuncture, above.

All anaesthetized animals should be monitored closely, including body temperature, heart rate and rhythm, respiratory rate and capillary refill time. Physiological reference ranges are included in Figure 8.2. Pulse oximetry, electrocardiography (ECG), capnography and blood pressure measurements can all be achieved in most patients. Monitoring prior to recovery and then as long as is safe is important. Animals should be prevented from climbing or jumping (e.g. in a pet carrier) until well coordinated. Recovery ideally occurs adjacent to or within the animal's social group, and complete return as soon as it is fully recovered is important.

Drug	Dose rate	Route	Comments
Pre-anaesthetic agents			
Acepromazine	0.5–1 mg/kg	Oral	Tranquillization. No reversal
Diazepam	0.5–1.0 mg/kg	Oral	Sedation. Give in small amount of food or drink 30–60 minutes prior to anaesthesia. Variable effect and recovery prolonged
Midazolam	0.5 mg/kg	Oral	As for diazepam but twice as potent. Half-life of 1–4 hours. More applicable for larger species
Induction and maintenance agents			
Isoflurane	4% induction 1–3% maintenance	Mask or endotracheal tube	Pre-anaesthetic reduces induction stress. Local anaesthetic spray useful to reduce laryngeal spasm. Beware high tracheal bifurcation
Ketamine	5–15 mg/kg	i.m.	Immobilization for examination and blood collection. Minimal cardiopulmonary depression. Poor relaxation for radiography. Seizures in lemurs. No reversal
Ketamine + Diazepam	15 mg/kg K + 1 mg/kg D	i.m.	Surgical anaesthesia of 30–40 minutes. Improved muscle relaxation compared with ketamine alone
Ketamine + Medetomidine	5–7.5 mg/kg K + 0.05–0.1 mg/kg M	i.m.	Use higher doses in smaller primates (e.g. callitrichids). Anaesthesia of 45–60 minutes. Deepen with isoflurane for surgery. Less negative cardiopulmonary effects than in dogs. Excellent muscle relaxation. Reversal with atipamezole (5 times medetomidine dose) produces smooth recovery
Tiletamine/ Zolazepam (Zoletil®)	2–10 mg/kg	i.m.	Commonly used outside UK. Import only with Special Treatment Certificate from VMD. More applicable for larger species

8.14 Anaesthetic agents commonly used in primates.

Lemurs have no active cooling mechanism so capture and handling should take this into account. Folivorous species have a slow rate of gastric emptying but in most commonly seen species withholding food for 8 hours is sufficient. There is a high incidence of seizures in ruffed lemurs when using ketamine alone, and duration of effective anaesthesia is short (10–15 minutes). Darkly pigmented mucous membranes make obtaining pulse oximetry readings difficult and a rectal probe may be necessary.

For primates that can be manually restrained easily, induction and maintenance with isoflurane inhalation anaesthesia alone are possible. The stress of capture and restraint for masking produces tachycardia and hypertension, so some advocate the use of injectable combinations in even the smallest species. For primates weighing more than a few kilograms, and/or which cannot be manually restrained, a combination of ketamine (5 mg/kg i.m.) and medetomidine (0.05 mg/kg i.m.) provides reliable anaesthesia for 45–60 minutes. Supplemental oxygen should be available. Anaesthesia can be extended with isoflurane by inhalation as necessary and already provides a good level of analgesia.

Common surgical procedures

Vasectomy

1. Food is withheld from the animal according to bodyweight (see Anaesthesia and analgesia). Water should only be removed 2–3 hours before the procedure.
2. The animal is anaesthetized and placed in dorsal recumbency.
3. A single dose of carprofen is given subcutaneously.
4. The hair is plucked in the ventral midline cranial to the scrotum (clipper damage impairs healing) and the surgical site prepared.
5. Make a 1 cm midline skin incision over the pubic symphysis, 1 cm cranial to the cranial border of the scrotum.
6. Using blunt dissection lateral to the incision, expose the spermatic sacs and exteriorize.
7. Use further blunt dissection to free the off-white ductus deferens from the spermatic artery.
8. Ligate the ductus deferens twice with non-absorbable suture material and remove a section between the ligations. Histological examination can be used for anatomical confirmation of the section removed.
9. Close the wound with absorbable subcuticular suture material (e.g. 2 metric (3/0 USP) Vicryl). Close the skin with tissue glue or a single mattress suture.

Caesarean section

1. Food is withheld from the animal according to bodyweight (see Anaesthesia and analgesia). Water should only be removed 2–3 hours before the procedure.
2. The animal is anaesthetized, using mask induction with isoflurane if possible.

3. Fluids are given at 5% bodyweight – subcutaneously or intraosseously in smaller species, intravenously in larger species.
4. A single dose of carprofen is given subcutaneously.
5. The animal is intubated and placed in dorsal recumbency.
6. The surgical site is prepared over the ventral midline just cranial to the pubis.
7. The surgical site can be infused with local anaesthetic to reduce postoperative interference.
8. Make a ventral midline incision, being careful not to incise deeper than the abdominal musculature.
9. Exteriorize the uterus and remove the fetus(es) through an incision that avoids the neck of the bladder.
10. Gently remove the placenta. Check the uterine wall for haemorrhage and evidence of placentitis – in the instance of the latter, a swab should be taken for microbiological testing.
11. Close the uterus with a two-layered continuous inverting pattern using absorbable suture material. Oxytocin (2 IU i.v.) given at this stage will hasten involution of the uterus, making closure easier.
12. Close the linea alba with absorbable simple interrupted sutures. A second layer is recommended in older or obese animals.
13. Close the wound with an absorbable subcuticular suture (e.g. 1–2 metric (3/0–5/0 USP) Vicryl, depending on the size of the patient). Along with adequate analgesia this should produce good healing. Alternatively, interrupted mattress sutures in the skin are generally left alone by the animal if not under tension.

Postoperative care
Antibiotic cover should not be necessary, provided surgery was performed without loss of sterility. Further postoperative analgesia can be provided to the dam in the form of oral meloxicam, starting from 24 hours after the procedure at a dose of 0.1 mg/kg q24h, provided hydration status is not compromised and if deemed necessary according to behaviour.

A fetus delivered alive should be left with its dam for maternal rearing (Figure 8.15). It is important to monitor the situation closely; weak or non-feeding neonates require rapid intervention if they are to survive (see Hand rearing, above).

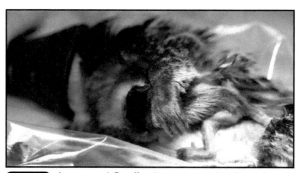

8.15 A neonatal Geoffroy's marmoset is allowed to suckle while the dam recovers on oxygen after Caesarean delivery.

The dam should ideally be kept separate from the group for 5–10 days and be observed closely for any evidence of dehiscence.

Euthanasia

The only recommended method is the induction of anaesthesia by any of the regimens described above, followed by injection of sodium pentobarbital (at dose rates used in other mammals of similar size), preferably intravenously, but alternatively by intracardiac or intraperitoneal routes if necessary.

Drug formulary

A drug formulary for commonly seen primates is given in Figure 8.16.

Drug	Dose	Comments
Antimicrobial agents		
Amikacin	2–3 mg/kg i.m. q24h	
Amoxicillin	11 mg/kg orally q12h or s.c./i.m. q24h	Paediatric suspension available
Amoxicillin/Clavulanate	15 mg/kg orally q12h	Palatable drops useful in small species
Cefalexin	20 mg/kg orally q12h	
Ceftazidime	50 mg/kg i.m./i.v. q8h	
Ciprofloxacin	20 mg/kg orally q12h	Paediatric suspension available. Possible side effects, as for enrofloxacin
Clindamycin	10 mg/kg orally q12h	
Doxycycline	3–4 mg/kg orally q12h	
Enrofloxacin	5 mg/kg orally/s.c./i.m. q24h	Possible side effects: hallucinations in humans; presume similar in primates
Erythromycin	75 mg/kg orally q12h for 10 days	*Campylobacter*-associated diarrhoea and clostridial gastroenteritis. Paediatric suspension available
Metronidazole	25 mg/kg orally q12h	Clostridial gastroenteritis. Oral suspension available
Oxytetracycline	10 mg/kg s.c./i.m. q24h	
Penicillin G, procaine	20,000 IU/kg i.m. q12h	
Trimethoprim/Sulfadiazine	15 mg/kg orally q12h or 30 mg/kg s.c./i.m. q24h	
Antifungal agents		
Fluconazole	18 mg/kg orally q12h	Systemic mycoses
Griseofulvin	20 mg/kg orally q24h or 200 mg/kg orally q10d	
Itraconazole	10 mg/kg orally q24h	Fungal (yeast) gastroenteritis
Nystatin	200,000 IU orally q6h	GI candidiasis. Continue for 48 hours after clinical resolution. Oral suspension available
Antiparasitic agents		
Albendazole	25 mg/kg orally q12h for 5 days	GI nematodes
Amitraz	250 ppm bath for 5 minutes every 14 days or until skin lesion resolution	Demodectic mange in tamarins. Dry but do not rinse. Transient ataxia may be seen
Clindamycin	12.5–25 mg/kg orally q12h for 28 days	*Toxoplasma* infection
Doxycycline	5 mg/kg orally q12h for 1 day then 2.5 mg/kg orally q24h	*Balantidium* infection
Fenbendazole	50 mg/kg orally q24h for 3 days or 20 mg/kg orally q24h for 14 days	GI nematodes and *Filaroides*
Ivermectin	0.2 mg/kg orally/s.c./i.m.	May repeat after 14 days
Levamisole	5 mg/kg orally; repeat in 3 weeks	Spirurids, *Strongyloides, Trichuris*
Mebendazole	40 mg/kg orally q24h for 3 days	*Strongyloides, Trichuris, Pterygodermatites*, acanthocephalans
Metronidazole	25 mg/kg orally q12h for 10 days	Enteric protozoans including *Entamoeba histolytica, Balantidium coli*
Praziquantel	20 mg/kg orally/i.m. once	Cestodes
	40 mg/kg orally/i.m. once	Trematodes
Trimethoprim/Sulfadiazine	15 mg/kg orally q12h	*Toxoplasma* infection

8.16 Drug formulary for commonly seen primates. For anaesthetic agents see Figure 8.14. (continues) ▶

Drug	Dose	Comments
Analgesics		
Aspirin	5–10 mg/kg orally q4–6h	Anti-inflammatory and antipyretic
Buprenorphine	0.01–0.02 mg/kg i.m. q12h	Reversal with naloxone
Butorphanol	0.02 mg/kg i.m. q3–4h	May cause profound respiratory depression. Reversal with naloxone
Carprofen	2–4 mg/kg orally/s.c. q24h/q12h	Anti-inflammatory and antipyretic. Variation in half-life with species. COX-1 selectivity may be an issue
Flunixin meglumine	0.3–1.0 mg/kg s.c./i.v. q24h	Anti-inflammatory and antipyretic
Ibuprofen	20 mg/kg orally q24h	Anti-inflammatory
Morphine	1 mg/kg orally/s.c./i.m./i.v. q4h	May cause profound respiratory depression. Reversal with naloxone
Naloxone	0.01–0.05 mg/kg i.m./i.v.	Opioid reversal
Paracetamol	5–10 mg/kg orally q6h	Antipyretic and minimally anti-inflammatory

8.16 (continued) Drug formulary for commonly seen primates. For anaesthetic agents see Figure 8.14.

References and further reading

Allchurch AF (2003) Yersiniosis in all taxa. In: *Zoo and Wild Animal Medicine, 5th edn*, ed. ME Fowler and RE Miller, pp. 724–727. Saunders, St Louis

Bielitzki JT (1999) Emerging viral diseases of nonhuman primates. In: *Zoo and Wild Animal Medicine: Current Therapy 4th edn*, ed. ME Fowler and RE Miller, pp. 377–382. WB Saunders, Philadelphia

Carpenter JW (2005) *Exotic Animal Formulary, 3rd edn*, pp. 495–532. Elsevier Saunders, St Louis

Carroll JB (2002) *EAZA Husbandry Guidelines for the Callitrichidae*. Bristol Zoo Gardens, Bristol

Crawford GC, Andrews GA, Chavey PS *et al.* (2005) Survey and clinical application of serum iron, total iron binding capacity, transferrin saturation, and serum ferritin in captive black and white ruffed lemurs (*Varecia variegata variegata*). *Journal of Zoo and Wildlife Medicine* **36**(4), 653–660

Cunningham AA, Buxton D and Thomson KM (1992) An epidemic of toxoplasmosis in a captive colony of squirrel monkeys (*Saimiri sciureus*). *Journal of Comparative Pathology* **107**, 207–219

Dubey JP, Kramer LW and Weisbrode SE (1985) Acute death associated with *Toxoplasma gondii* in ring-tailed lemurs. *Journal of the American Veterinary Medical Association* **187**, 1272–1273

Garell DM (1999) Toxoplasmosis in zoo animals. In: *Zoo and Wild Animal Medicine: Current Therapy 4th edn*, ed. ME Fowler and RE Miller, pp. 131–135. WB Saunders, Philadelphia

Greenwood AG and Taylor DC (1977) Control of diabetes in a capuchin monkey with tolbutamide. *Veterinary Record* **101**, 407–408

Hatt JM and Guscetti F (1994) A case of mycobacteriosis in a common marmoset (*Callithrix jacchus*). *Annual Proceedings of the American Association of Zoo Veterinarians*, pp. 241–243

Hrdlicka L and Stringfield C (2002) Tamarins. In: *Hand-rearing Wild and Domestic Mammals*, ed. LJ Gage, pp. 114–117. Iowa State Press, Ames

Hunt RD, Garcia FG, Hegsted DM (1969) Hypervitaminosis D in New World monkeys. *American Journal of Clinical Nutrition* **22**, 358–366

Junge RE (1999) Diseases of prosimians. In: *Zoo and Wild Animal Medicine: Current Therapy 4th edn*, ed. ME Fowler and RE Miller, pp. 365–368. WB Saunders, Philadelphia

Kirkwood JK and Stathatos K (1992) *Biology, Rearing and Care of Young Primates*. Oxford University Press, Oxford

Lewis JCM (2000) Preventative health measures for primates and keeping staff in British and Irish zoological collections. *Report to the British and Irish Primate Taxon Advisory Group (B & I PTAG) May 2000*. British and Irish Primate TAG, London

Montali RJ and Bush M (1999) Diseases of the Callitrichidae. In: *Zoo and Wild Animal Medicine: Current Therapy 4th edn*, ed. ME Fowler and RE Miller, pp. 369–376. WB Saunders, Philadelphia

Morris TH and David CL (1993) Illustrated guide to surgical technique for vasectomy of the common marmoset. *Laboratory Animals* **27**, 381–384

NRC (2003) *Nutrient Requirements of Nonhuman Primates, 2nd edn*. National Academies Press, Washington DC

Nowak RM (1999) *Walker's Primates of the World*. Johns Hopkins University Press, Baltimore

Oftedal OT and Allen ME (1996) The feeding and nutrition of omnivores with emphasis on primates. In: *Wild Mammals in Captivity – Principles and Techniques*, ed. DG Kleiman *et al.*, pp. 148–157. University of Chicago Press, Chicago

Ølberg R-A (2007) Monkeys and gibbons. In: *Zoo Animal and Wildlife Immobilization and Anesthesia*, ed. G West *et al.*, pp. 375–386. Blackwell Publishing, Ames

Sainsbury AW, Eaton BD and Cooper JE (1989) Restraint and anaesthesia of primates. *Veterinary Record* **125**, 640

Schmidt RE (1975) Tuberculosis in a ringtailed lemur (*Lemur catta*). *Journal of Zoo Animal Medicine* **6**, 11–12

Ullrey DE and Bernard JB (1999) Vitamin D: metabolism, sources, unique problems in zoo animals, meeting needs. In: *Zoo and Wild Animal Medicine: Current Therapy 4th edn*, ed. ME Fowler and RE Miller, pp. 63–78. WB Saunders, Philadelphia

Vermeer J (2006) *EEP Husbandry Guidelines for Squirrel Monkeys (genus Saimiri)*. La Vallée de Singes, Romagne

Walzer C (1999) Diabetes in primates. In: *Zoo and Wild Animal Medicine: Current Therapy, 4th edn*, ed. ME Fowler and RE Miller, pp. 397–400. WB Saunders, Philadelphia

Watts E and Meder A (1996) Introduction and socialization techniques for primates. In: *Wild Mammals in Captivity – Principles and Techniques*, ed. DG Kleiman *et al.*, pp. 67–77. University of Chicago Press, Chicago

Williams CV (2002) Lemurs. In: *Hand-rearing Wild and Domestic Mammals*, ed. LJ Gage, pp. 104–113. Iowa State Press, Ames

Williams CV, Glenn KM, Levine JF *et al.* (2003) Comparison of the efficacy and cardiorespiratory effects of medetomidine-based anaesthetic protocols in ring-tailed lemurs (*Lemur catta*). *Journal of Zoo and Wildlife Medicine* **34**, 163–170

Williams CV and Junge RE (2007) Prosimians. In: *Zoo Animal and Wildlife Immobilization and Anesthesia*, ed. G West *et al.*, pp. 367–374. Blackwell Publishing, Ames

Wolf RH, Gibson SV, Watson EA *et al.* (1988) Multidrug chemotherapy of tuberculosis in rhesus monkeys. *Laboratory Animal Science* **38**, 25–33

Yamaguchi A, Kohno Y, Yamazaki T *et al.* (1986) Bone in the marmoset: a resemblance to vitamin D-dependent rickets, type II. *Calcified Tissue International* **39**, 22–27

Useful websites

Contraceptive recommendations: www.stlzoo.org/downloads/NWMonkeys. pdf; www.stlzoo.org/downloads/Prosimians.pdf

Physiological data reference values: International Species Information System: www.isis.org

Acknowledgements

Thanks to Beale Park, Chessington World of Adventures and Zoo, Colchester Zoo, The Living Rainforest and Twycross Zoo – East Midland Zoological Society for access to their primates for photographs in good captive settings and whilst restrained, and to SM Thornton and FM Burns for critical review of the manuscript.

9

Cage and aviary birds

Michael Stanford

Introduction

A diverse range of avian species, including parrots, passerines and exotic softbills, are kept as cage and aviary birds in the UK. A total import ban into the UK of all free-ranging species came into force in July 2007 as part of the avian influenza precautions, but as many species are commonly bred in captivity, aviculture is still popular in the UK, as it is in many other countries.

Biology

Figure 9.1 summarizes the basic information regarding the general characteristics of the most commonly kept species. It is not the purpose of this chapter to cover this aspect in great detail and the reader is referred to the *BSAVA Manual of Psittacine Birds, 2nd edition* and *BSAVA Manual of Raptors, Pigeons and Passerine Birds* for further information.

Family	Weight (g)	Crop capacity (recommended maximum gavage volume, ml)	Comments	Diet	Common problems
Finch (see Figure 9.3a): Zebra Gouldian Green Java sparrow	 10–15 15–20 15–25 20–30	0.1–0.25	Until recently imported in large numbers from Africa and Asia; typically kept in mixed community aviaries rather than cages; easy to breed in captivity; British species and hybrids popular	Primarily granivorous; most species adapt to clean, commercial seed mixtures with a vitamin supplement; grit should be available; useful to offer live insectivore food during breeding season; some purely insectivorous species are kept	Metabolic and nutritional disorders associated with feeding an unbalanced seed diet. Hepatic lipidosis. Cannibalism. Viral disease (paramyxovirus, cytomegalovirus). Bacterial infection (yersiniosis, salmonellosis, *Mycoplasma* spp., *Escherichia coli*). Mycotic infection (candidiasis). Protozoal infection (atoxoplasmosis, coccidiosis, trichomoniasis, *Giardia*). Ectoparasites (*Dermanyssus gallinae, Ornithonyssus sylviarum*). Endoparasites (*Sternostoma tracheacolum*, air sac mites)
Canary (*Serinus canaria*): Roller Norwich Border Red factor	15–40	0.2–0.5	Kept for song or bred specifically for showing; sexually monomorphic, although only males sing well; manipulation of photoperiod commonplace to induce breeding	As for finches	As for finches. Feather cysts
Budgerigar (*Melopsittacus undulates*)	30–60 (pet strains) 50–85 (show strains)	0.5–1.0	Most popular caged bird; easy to tame; good talkers if obtained when young; bred for showing; males have blue cere; females have brown cere; natural colour is green but breeding has selected a variety of colours including lutino and albino	Granivorous; feed good quality boxed seed with a vitamin supplement; offer sprouted seed, grated carrot, apple and chickweed regularly; must have access to grit and an iodine block	Nutritional disease common (obesity; lipomas; thyroid dysplasia, iodine deficiency; bacterial enteritis; hepatitis). Bacterial infection (*Macrorhabdus ornithogaster*, megabacteria; chlamydophilosis). Testicular tumours. Viral disease (polyomavirus; PBFD virus; proventricular dilatation disease). CNS disease. Renal problems

9.1 General characteristics of popular cage and aviary birds. PBFD = Psittacine beak and feather disease. (continues)

▶

Family	Weight (g)	Crop capacity (recommended maximum gavage volume, ml)	Comments	Diet	Common problems
Lovebird (*Agapornis* spp.): Peach-faced Fischer's	40–60	0.5–1.0	Kept in single pairs; bred to produce numerous mutant colour variations	Should consist of 50% formulated diet supplemented by green leafy vegetables or tropical fruits (mango, fig)	As for budgerigars. Reproductive problems common in females
Cockatiel (*Nymphicus hollandicus*)	80–100	0.5–2.0	Popular single pet bird	As for budgerigars; alternatively, feed formulated diet	As for budgerigars. Reproductive disease common
Grass parakeet (*Neophema* spp.): Bourke's Splendid	40–60	0.5–1.5	Aviary birds not pets; sexually dimorphic	As for budgerigars; supplement with insects during breeding season	As for budgerigars. Very prone to endoparasites (*Capillaria* spp.)
Rosella (*Platycersus* spp.) Stanley Golden mantled	100–140	0.5–2.5	Aviary birds	As for grass parakeets	As for budgerigars
Asian parakeet (*Psittacula* spp.): Ringneck Alexandrine	90–150 200–250	0.5–3.0	Aviary and pet birds; small colonies of escapees free-ranging in the UK	As for budgerigars; supplement with fruit; alternatively, feed formulated diet	As for budgerigars
Pionus (see Figure 9.2b): Dusty Maximillian Bronze wing	180–225	2.5–4.0	South American; dwarf parrots; friendly pet bird; beautiful aviary specimens	Should consist of 50% formulated diet supplemented by green leafy vegetables or tropical fruits; soaked pulse diets also highly effective if supplemented with suitable vitamin and mineral mix	As for budgerigars. Hepatic lipidosis common
Poicephalus: Senegal Meyer's	150–180	2.5–3.5	African	Should consist of 50% formulated diet supplemented by green leafy vegetables or tropical fruits	As for budgerigars
Conure: Sun Patagonian	120–180 200–250	2.5–5.0	South American; noisy	Should consist of 50% formulated diet supplemented by green leafy vegetables or tropical fruits	As for budgerigars
Grey parrot (*Psittacus erithacus*) (see Figure 9.2a): Timneh (subspecies)	400–600 300–350	5–10	African; popular pets; historically imported in large numbers; excellent mimics	Should consist of 50% formulated diet supplemented by green leafy vegetables or tropical fruits; provide UV-B light	As for budgerigars. Disorders of calcium metabolism including hypocalcaemic fits and juvenile osteodystrophy common. Feather picking
Amazon (*Amazona* spp.) (see Figure 9.9): Blue fronted Orange winged	400–500 300–350	5–10	27 species; popular pets; ability to talk is limited; can be bad tempered	Should consist of 50% formulated diet supplemented by green leafy vegetables or tropical fruits; pulse diets also highly effective if supplemented with suitable vitamin and mineral mix	As for budgerigars. Hepatic lipidosis common

9.1 (continued) General characteristics of popular cage and aviary birds. PBFD = Psittacine beak and feather disease. (continues) ▶

Family	Weight (g)	Crop capacity (recommended maximum gavage volume, ml)	Comments	Diet	Common problems
Cockatoo (*Cacatua* spp.) (see Figure 9.2c) Sulphur crested Salmon crested Goffin	 500–1250 600–1000 350–450	5–15	Possess erectile crest; most species main body colour white; iris black in males; iris brown in females; destructive; noisy	Should consist of 50% formulated diet supplemented by green leafy vegetables or tropical fruits	As for budgerigars. Behavioural problems associated with sexual maturity commonplace. Feather plucking
Macaw (*Ara* spp.): Hahn's Blue and gold Scarlet Green winged	 150–180 1000–1250 900–1250 1250–1600	5–20	Bare facial area devoid of feathers; despite size gentle birds; dwarf varieties ideal pets; destructive; noisy	Should consist of 50% formulated diet supplemented by green leafy vegetables or tropical fruits; can use large nuts (Brazil, Palm) as training aids or treats	As for budgerigars. Feather plucking
Lory/lorikeet: Red lory (*Eos bornea*)	120–150	2–3	Colourful Asian birds; specialized aviary subjects	Specialized feeders using brush-like papillae on tongue; commercial nectar diets available	As for budgerigars. Bacterial and mycotic infections from contaminated nectar. Iron storage disease
Mynah (*Gracula* spp.) (see Figure 9.3b): Greater Indian Hill	180–230	3–5	Typical exotic softbills; messy; best mimics	Fruit; insects; commercial diets available but keep iron content <30 ppm	Iron storage disease. Hepatic lipidosis. Diabetes mellitus. Amyloidosis. Poxvirus. Yersiniosis. Mycotic infections. Avian tuberculosis
Exotic softbills: Pekin robin Glossy starling	 30–60 50–90	1–2	Mixed community aviary birds	Fruit; insects; commercial diets available but keep iron content <30 ppm	As for mynah birds
Toucan (*Ramphastidae* spp.) (see Figure 9.4) Channel billed Sulphur billed	1000–1300	10–20	Spectacular birds; historically kept in collections but increasing in private hands; dwarf species available	Fruit but avoid those with high vitamin C content; commercial diet with low iron content	Iron storage disease. Metabolic bone disease. Diabetes mellitus. Yersiniosis. Yeast and fungal infections. Avian tuberculosis

9.1 (continued) General characteristics of popular cage and aviary birds. PBFD = Psittacine beak and feather disease.

Anatomy and physiology

Psittacine birds
Parrots are fashionable and expensive pets, mainly kept for their intelligence and potential for training. Many species are excellent mimics. The order Psittaciformes contains parrots, macaws, cockatoos and lories classified into 353 species within 84 genera. Parrots are unmistakably defined by the powerful hooked beaks, short necks and zygodactyl (digits 1 and 4 face caudally, digits 2 and 3 cranially) prehensile feet. Parrots mainly inhabit the tropical and sub-tropical regions of the world, in a variety of habitats, including tropical rainforest, savannah and semi-desert. The group is essentially vegetarian and some species are specialized feeders; for example, lories eat only pollen and nectar. Over the last decade the majority of pet parrots sold in the UK have been captive-bred and hand-reared, rather than wild imports, and this has led to a surge in their popularity as pets (Figure 9.2).

Passerine birds
Passerines (perching or song birds) represent over 50% of the total species of birds in the world, but only three groups are commonly kept in captivity: canaries, finches and exotic softbills such as mynah birds (Figure 9.3). For simplicity, passerines can be divided into two types based on dietary preferences: hardbills and softbills. Passerines have high metabolic rates, with an average body temperature two degrees higher than non-passerine birds, and generally have anisodactyl feet, (digits 2, 3 and 4 face cranially, digit 1 faces caudally). Passerines are kept as individual caged birds, as flocks of the same species in breeding collections intended for showing, or as mixed community collections of different species.

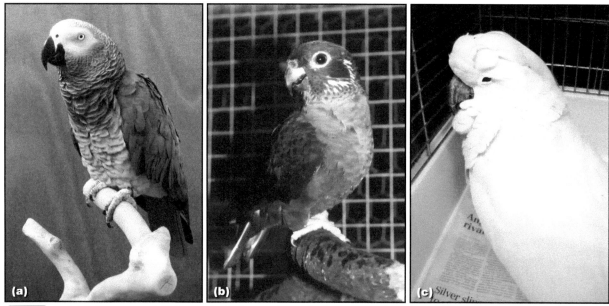

9.2 **(a)** Adult grey parrot. This species is the most popular large parrot kept in captivity in the UK, probably owing to its excellent ability to mimic. **(b)** Dusky pionus typical dwarf parrot, which makes both an excellent pet and attractive aviary specimen. **(c)** Umbrella cockatoo.

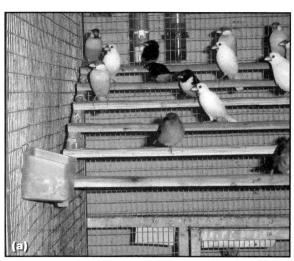

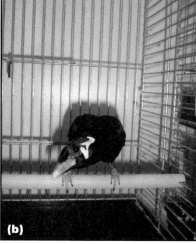

9.3 **(a)** Mixed collection of hardbill finches. These granivorous birds are short-lived and usually kept in community aviaries rather than as single pet birds. **(b)** Mynah bird. This inquisitive softbill, although extremely messy, was historically a popular cage bird owing to its excellent ability to talk; now being bred regularly in captivity, it is regaining its status.

Ramphastids

Ramphastids (toucans and toucanettes) are colourful tropical birds distinguished by a prominent protruding beak, and although historically only found in zoological collections an increasing number are being kept as pets (Figure 9.4).

Sexing

Many cage and aviary birds are sexually monomorphic, but can be sexed by endoscopy or DNA analysis. Common exceptions are:

- Budgerigars – males usually have a blue cere; females have a brown to reddish cere
- Cockatoos – males usually have a black iris; females have a brown iris
- Canaries – can be sexed based on the ability of the male to sing, or the protrusion of the vent during the breeding season.

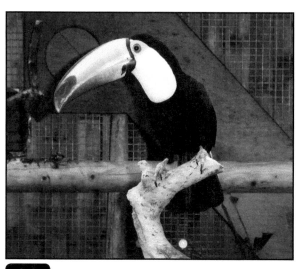

9.4 Sulphur billed toucan.

Either blood or feather pulp (from plucked breast feathers) is suitable for DNA testing, but must be obtained under aseptic conditions to avoid contamination of the sample with DNA from other sources. Endoscopic sexing permits visual assessment of the gonads, which is useful for investigating intransigent breeders; in particular, it can give an indication of sexual maturity. Parrots can be difficult to age, although grey parrots and many macaws possess a dark grey iris at birth. The colour gradually lightens over the first year, finally becoming yellow at maturity. The condition of the beak and feet may also be revealing when assessing age.

Husbandry

Housing
The size of a bird cage is covered in the UK under the Wildlife and Countryside Act 1981, which states that any caged bird should be able to extend its wings in all directions. This should be considered the absolute minimum size for a cage. It is best to permit parrots considerable opportunity to exercise out of the cage (see Figure 9.2a). Cages or aviaries should be constructed from heavy duty (16–18 g) wire for larger parrot species, 19 g wire for passerine birds, and the use of stainless steel or powder-coated wire is advisable to reduce the risk of zinc toxicity from cheap galvanized materials. Aviaries usually consist of an outdoor flight attached to indoor sleeping accommodation. Many passerine birds are kept in cages in single pairs during the breeding season and released into a communal flight at other times. In aviaries, parrots and ramphastids are usually kept in single species pairs, but the smaller passerine birds do well in mixed collections.

Cage bars should run horizontally for ease of climbing and it is preferable to avoid curved cages to ensure maximum space. Commercial cages are normally supplied with unsuitable perches for birds both in terms of size (inappropriate diameter) and material (plastic or smooth wood; see Figure 9.3a). Perches should therefore be replaced as soon as possible with natural tree branches (see Figure 9.2b), which provide an irregular surface of varying diameter. Fruit trees are ideal, providing both environmental enrichment by encouraging chewing behaviour and keeping feet and nails in good condition.

Parrots are highly intelligent creatures so the provision of a variety of toys is recommended. All birds must have constant access to clean water and fresh food. For birds kept indoors, providing a bath or spraying directly with water encourages appropriate preening behaviour and reduces feather dust. Lack of ultraviolet (UV) light can affect the efficiency of vitamin D metabolism and preening behaviour, so UV light should be provided artificially using commercial bulbs for all birds kept indoors. Environmental pollutants, including air fresheners (especially plug-in varieties) and smoke, can lead to dry, brittle feathers, plucking behaviour, and respiratory disease compounded by the dry warm environment associated with central heating. Therefore, the use of air ionizers is recommended. As all birds are extremely sensitive to polytetrafluroethane (Teflon™) they should not be exposed to fumes from Teflon-coated utensils.

Diet
Nutritional disease is common in cage and aviary birds, whatever the species, with most individuals suffering from multiple nutrient deficiencies or excesses rather than problems associated with a single dietary component. The recommended diets for each species group are outlined in Figure 9.1.

Seeds
Until recently, seed-based feeds have been the foundation of most parrot diets, and the resistance of owners to change can be extremely challenging. The pet trade continues to recommend and sell seed mixes as 'complete' diets. Although parrots will survive on seed mixes, they are chronically malnourished and unhealthy with poor reproductive performance. The quality of the seed is frequently substandard and can even be contaminated with pathogens (Figure 9.5). Parrots are likely to become obsessed with individual food items, even if supplied with a varied diet, leading to a nutritional imbalance. Recent studies suggest that the optimal maintenance diet for pet parrots is a complete formulated diet (at least 50% of total food consumed) with some additional fruit and vegetables (Hess *et al.*, 2002).

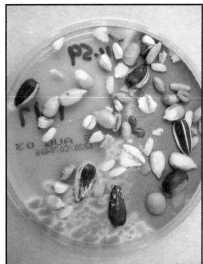

9.5 Culture of a typically poor quality seed mix used to feed parrots and granivorous cage/aviary birds. In addition to the nutrient imbalances expected from these mixes, they are frequently contaminated with fungal spores; in this case *Aspergillus fumigatus*.

However, granivorous passerine and smaller psittacine birds are frequently fed on good quality seed mixtures rather than a formulated diet. For the smaller psittacine birds, this should be supplemented with fresh green vegetables. Commercial insect mixtures and live food are available for supplementation during the breeding season. In the USA, all seed diets are not recommended for budgerigars or other members of the Australian grass parakeet family; pelleted diets supplemented with greens and occasional grains are advised.

Vitamins and minerals
Vitamin and mineral supplementation is widespread in aviculture, although the correction of dietary

deficiencies via supplements is fraught with difficulties. Supplementation often leads both to toxicity and deficiency, since it is not possible to accurately quantify the uptake level of vitamins and minerals by individual birds using water- or food-based supplements.

Grit is a good source of minerals, particularly calcium. In the smaller granivorous birds, such as budgerigars, grit helps digestion by enhancing the grinding action of the gizzard. The lack of grit in budgerigars has been implicated in the fungal disease caused by the avian gastric yeast *Macrorhabdus ornithogaster* (previously known as megabacteria). Provision of grit is also recommended for the large psittacine birds, although no requirement has been demonstrated.

One common nutritional problem in budgerigars is iodine deficiency, which can be prevented by the supply of commercial 'pink' iodine blocks. [Editor's note: commercial pelleted diets are also supplemented with iodine and these are generally advised as the most suitable way of preventing deficiencies in the USA.] A commercial seed diet supplemented with iodine, calcium and other vitamins and minerals is available.

Specialized feeds

Exotic softbills, lories and lorikeets are specialized feeders and considerable attention should be paid to ensure an appropriate diet. Fortunately, commercial diets are available but they should be freshly prepared as bacterial contamination is common, even after just a few hours at room temperature. Haemochromatosis (iron storage disease, ISD) is the most common non-infectious disease in softbills. Mynah birds (and toucans) suffer from haemochromatosis, which is believed to be an inherited metabolic disorder that causes excess iron to be absorbed from the diet and stored in the liver. It is a chronic disease exacerbated by feeding diets with a high iron content. The disease can be prevented by feeding diets with an iron content <30 ppm.

Identification

Birds can be identified by microchips or rings to help pair specific birds or prove the provenance of individuals following escape or theft.

Microchips

Microchips should be of the ISO Standard, and despite being placed intramuscularly do not appear to cause any complications. For some species microchipping may be a legal requirement (see www. defra.gov.uk). The chips should be introduced into the caudal third of the left pectoral muscle mass. Anaesthesia, though not absolutely necessary, is preferable for smaller birds (see below). There is no requirement for suturing, although digital pressure over the injection site will reduce the possibility of the microchip being withdrawn with the needle, and control excessive haemorrhage.

Rings

Rings can be either closed (only applied in young chicks) or split (can be applied at any time, so the legal veracity is negligible). Rings often require

removal, usually due to the placement of an inappropriately sized ring which constricts the leg leading to necrosis. Birds should always be anaesthetized prior to ring removal as it is relatively easy to fracture the long bones during the procedure. The use of specialist jeweller's ring cutters or a rotating dental burr is ideal for removing rings.

Preventive healthcare

Wing clipping

Owners frequently request wing clipping to prevent escape or to provide help, albeit short-term, with training, but the procedure is controversial. The author prefers not to clip as it can lead to psychological problems (particularly in young parrots) or to delayed moulting and eventual feather plucking due to the presence of old, splintered feathers. If the procedure is performed, a bilateral (rather than a unilateral) technique is recommended using a sterile pair of sharp scissors to avoid frayed feather ends. The primary feathers should be cut short so they are protected by the covert feathers, otherwise the birds can be tempted to chew the cut ends. As no wing clip is 100% effective, clear warnings should be given to the client that flight is still possible. An alternative to wing clipping is the use of parrot harnesses and behavioural training.

Claw and beak clipping

Common conditions affecting the beaks and claws of cage and aviary birds include:

- Overgrowth
- Malocclusion
- Disease
- Fractures.

Overgrowth: The overgrowth of beaks and claws is common in small parrot-like birds and is frequently associated with nutritional or liver disease. Overgrown beaks and claws require regularly trimming, preferably using a rotating burr (dremel) rather than clippers. Bleeding should be controlled using a styptic.

General anaesthesia is frequently required; however, many adult birds become familiar with the use of the burr, particularly if regular correction of congenital deformities is required. The bird can be restrained in a towel and the beak/claws shaped using the burr fine sanding cone. The veterinary surgeon should wear a facemask to avoid inhaling the dust. Care must be taken to prevent the burr from heating the beak.

Beaks: Reshaping of the beak should never be required unless there is a underlying problem, as it is normally kept in trim by its own mechanical action or by grinding on objects. In young birds, beak reshaping may be necessary due to congenital malocclusion or traumatic damage. In adult birds, the only reasons for beak reshaping are trauma, disease (e.g. *Cnemidocoptes* in budgerigars) and malnutrition (in particular liver disease as this leads to abnormal keratin metabolism).

Claws: Claw clipping should be unnecessary in most birds if appropriate perches and nutrition are provided. Malnutrition, in particular liver disease, should be suspected in any bird with overgrown claws as this can lead to abnormal keratin metabolism.

Malocclusion: In young parrots malocclusion can be congenital or, more commonly, associated with damage sustained during the hand-rearing process. Most abnormalities can be corrected, but remedial specialist surgery must be performed before the bird is 12 weeks old to be successful.

Disease: The structure of a bird's beak can be damaged by parasitism (*Cnemidocoptes pilae*), infection (psittacine beak and feather disease, PBFD; candidasis) or systemic disease (malnutrition; liver disorders); therefore, appropriate investigations should be carried out if the beak keratin appears abnormal in any way. Metabolic bone disease affecting the bill of toucans is regularly reported.

Fractures: Beak fractures are a common sequel to fighting or trauma; analgesia is imperative. Small wounds should be repaired using dental acrylics or cyanoacrylate adhesives. Supportive feeding may be required. Larger fractures or complete severance of the beak require cross-pinning or application of a prosthesis. Referral to a specialist is recommended.

Handling and restraint

Care must be taken when handling patients as even small psittacine birds are capable of inflicting painful bites, and the larger breeds more serious wounds. Many passerine and rhamphastid birds have sharp pointed beaks, and eye protection should be considered when handling the larger species. Prior to capture, it is important to determine what equipment will be required for the initial stabilization and clinical examination of the bird, in order to minimize handling time.

Larger birds should be caught from their cage/carrier in a calm manner using a towel (Figure 9.6).

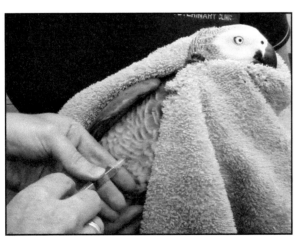

9.6 Method of restraint for parrots. With the parrot restrained, an intramuscular injection into the pectoral muscle can be made.

1. Place your hand in the cage/carrier and once the bird has settled down make a sudden movement to hold it around the neck.
2. Place your thumb under the lower mandible.
3. Attempt to control the rest of the bird, especially the wings, with your other hand. Gloves dramatically reduce manual dexterity and are not recommended.

It is often helpful to place the cage/carrier on the ground and release the bird on to the floor in a darkened room prior to catching it with the towel. Many birds will 'step up' on command on to the weighing scale, from where they are easily picked up and held.

With excitable smaller passerine species it can be useful to dim the lights prior to attempting capture. The birds should be caught in the same way as larger birds; although, a handkerchief or small light cloth can be used instead of a towel. Small psittacine birds, such as budgerigars, can be encouraged to chew on a distracting object like a towel, non-toxic pencil or wooden tongue depressor whilst the examination takes place. Prior to catching the bird, it is advisable to warn the owners that the stress of capture and examination might adversely affect the animal, depending on the nature of the illness. Care must be taken, especially with smaller passerine birds, to avoid restricting sternal movements and hence respiration (Figure 9.7).

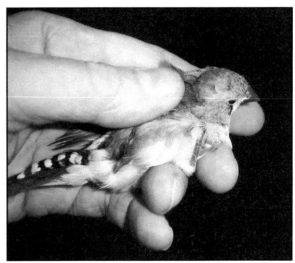

9.7 Small passerine birds, such as zebra finches, should be held with care to avoid restricting sternal movements.

Diagnostic approach

The history taking and clinical examination should follow the same protocol as for other animals. As birds can deteriorate rapidly, an aggressive approach to further investigations and treatment achieves the greatest success. With passerine birds there is a practical limit to what can be achieved diagnostically in the live patient, based on size and economic considerations. Therefore, investigation of disease outbreaks in passerine collections may involve selective culling and post-mortem examination.

History

The key points for taking a history include:

- Species?
- Age?
- Breed?
- Is the bird captive-bred or wild-bred?
- Is the bird kept in an aviary or cage?
- Diet?
- What does the bird actually eat?
- Has there been a recent change in faecal appearance?
- Is there any evidence of increased thirst?
- Is there any evidence of increased respiratory effort?
- Are there any changes in vocalization?
- Have there been any recent introductions into the household?
- Have there been any recent changes in behaviour?

Clinical examination

The clinical examination can be performed in the absence of the owner, especially in tame parrots, to prevent potential damage to the close owner–bird bond, which may happen if the bird associates stressful events with the owner being present. [Editor's note: some owners may not like to be absent for the clinical examination, and many avian veterinary surgeons prefer to carry out procedures with the owner present. Well socialized birds can be examined in the consulting room with minimal stress.]

A standard approach to the clinical examination should be taken, including:

- Observation of posture, attitude, droppings, general condition and respiration prior to removing the bird from the cage. If the bird will stand on the clinician's hand, balance, strength of grip, visual tracking (attention) and hydration status can be assessed
- Examination of the head, including nares, eyes and ears, palpation of the sinuses surrounding the eyes and face
- Examination of the oral cavity, including inspection of the choanal slit with an auriscope or pen torch
- Palpation of the crop
- Auscultation of the dorsum for abnormal lung sounds, the ventral abdomen for air sac noise, and the pectoral region to assess the heart
- Palpation of the abdomen for evidence of pain, swelling or masses
- Examination of the cloaca
- Examination of the long bones of the wings and limbs, palpation along all limbs, and over the back, pelvis and tail head (uropygial gland if present)
- Examination of all surfaces of the feet.

Imaging

Radiography

Radiography is an essential component of the diagnostic repertoire, especially for assessing the respiratory system, gastrointestinal system, size and shape of internal organs, mineral densities, and to diagnose heavy metal toxicity, reproductive problems and fractures. The small size of avian patients and the fine anatomical structures makes radiography a challenge, and the use of mammography film/screen combinations can be highly beneficial. Anaesthesia is necessary for most radiographic studies and although various racks are available commercially to position the bird, adhesive tape is a simple alternative.

The two standard views, taken at 90 degrees to each other, are ventrodorsal (VD) and lateral. For the VD view, the bird is placed in dorsal recumbency with both the legs and wings extended to avoid superposition. For the lateral view, the bird is usually placed in right lateral recumbency with the legs extended caudally and the wings pulled dorsally.

Contrast studies are easy to perform in the avian patient and are frequently helpful diagnostically, particularly for the investigation of gastrointestinal disease. A dose rate of 10 ml/kg bodyweight of a standard barium sulphate suspension (25–45% concentration) can be given directly into the crop. Contrast media can assist in the identification of abdominal organs.

Endoscopy

The regular use of diagnostic rigid endoscopy has transformed modern avian medicine and surgery. Due to the presence of an air sac system, birds have a naturally inflated body cavity, and it is possible to visually examine all the internal organs of a sick bird laparoscopically in one procedure. Endoscopy is normally performed with the bird in right lateral recumbency with the legs pulled backwards and the wings raised dorsally (Figure 9.8).

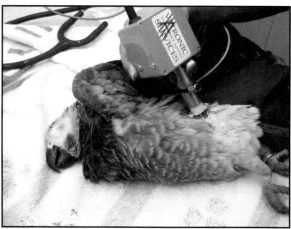

9.8 A 'cut off' endotracheal tube placed intra-abdominally behind the last rib will enter the air sac system. This is a useful emergency technique for birds with signs of acute upper respiratory disease. In this case, the endotracheal tube has been connected to a ventilator. The same surgical approach is used for endoscopy.

The procedure involves a small incision between the last two ribs, allowing a 2–4 mm endoscope to be inserted. The endoscope will usually enter the cranial abdominal air sac and immediately the gonad, kidney and adrenal gland can be visualized through the air sac wall. It is then useful to examine the coelomic cavity, assessing all the abdominal organs prior to directing the endoscope cranially to assess the lung, heart and cranial air sacs. The cloaca can be assessed by passing the endoscope *per cloaca*. Visualization is greatly enhanced by using water or air through the endoscope sheath to dilate the cloaca. Endoscopes can also be used *per os* to examine the trachea (particularly the syrinx) and the gastrointestinal tract.

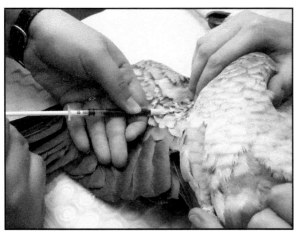

9.9 Venepuncture of the brachial vein. The bird should be anaesthetized prior to the procedure. An assistant should raise the blood vessel and prevent haematoma formation (via digital pressure) following sample collection.

Ultrasonography

Ultrasonography has limited use in birds due to the presence of air sacs, but can be used to assess the liver and heart, and to differentiate between fluid and masses in cases with coelomic distension.

Sample collection

Blood

Blood sampling in birds is simply achieved via the brachial (Figure 9.9), medial tarsometarsal (larger species) or jugular (smaller species) vein, using a 25–27-gauge needle. The author uses the brachial vein whenever possible, due to ease of visualization. The venepuncture site should always be checked before the bird is released back to its enclosure to ensure no post-collection haemorrhage has occurred. A large haematoma will form at the venepuncture site unless is it compressed firmly after the blood sample has been taken.

Although samples can be taken in the conscious bird, anaesthesia is advisable (see below). Approximately 1% of the patient's bodyweight in blood can be safely taken from a healthy bird (e.g. 5 ml of blood from a 500 g patient). The author recommends making a smear immediately after sample collection, and that heparin should be used as the anticoagulant. Pathology laboratories familiar with bird samples should be used whenever possible to ensure correct interpretation, as there are large variations in biological and haematological data between avian species. Basic haematological and biochemical data for common species are summarized in Figure 9.10.

Parameter	Zebra finch	Canary	Budgerigar	Lovebird	Cockatiel	Sun conure	Pionus	Senegal	Grey parrot	Amazon	Cockatoo	Macaw	Red lory	Mynah bird	Toucan
Haematology															
WBC ($\times 10^9$/l)	3.0–8.0	4.0–9.0	3.0–10.0	3–16	5–11.0	7.13–16.4	4.0–11.0	5.6–14	3.3–10.3	5–17	9.0–16.0	5.1–17.5	8.0–13.0	3.57–17.67	2.4–24.0
RBC ($\times 10^{12}$/l)	2.5–4.6	2.5–3.8	3.77–4.60	3.0–5.1	3.47–4.11	3.58–4.25	2.4–4.0	2.07–3.96	3.0–3.6	1.96–2.5	2.3–3.4	2.0–3.4	3.25–3.94	2.77–4.59	2.5–4.5
PCV (%)	45–62	37–49	43–56	44–57	45–56	46–53	35–54	41–51	45–53	41–53	45–56	33–47	41–55	40–48	32–65
Heterophils (%)	20–65	50–80	45–70	40–75	40–60	40–70	50–75	55–75	45–73	3.1–7.1	40–55	45–75	39–60	25–65	35–65
Lymphocytes (%)	20–65	20–45	20–45	20–55	20–70	20–50	25–45	25–45	20–50	2–6.7	29–83	20–50	22–69	20–60	25–50
Monocytes (%)	0–1	0–1	0–2	0–2	0–1	0–3	0–2	0–2	0–3	0–0.2	0–9	0–2	0–2	0–3	0–2
Eosinophils (%)	0–1	0–2	0–2	0–1	0–2	0–3	0–2	0–1	0–2	0–0.1	0–3	0–1	0–3	0–3	0–4
Basophils (%)	0–5	0–1	0–1	0–6	0–2	0–5	0–1	0–1	0–5	0–0.2	0–2	0–1	0–3	0–7	0–5

9.10 Haematological and biochemical data (normal ranges) for a variety of cage and aviary birds (Data supplied by Pinmoore Laboratories, Tarporley, Cheshire). (continues) ▶

Parameter	Zebra finch	Canary	Budgerigar	Lovebird	Cockatiel	Sun conure	Pionus	Senegal	Grey parrot	Amazon	Cockatoo	Macaw	Red lory	Mynah bird	Toucan
Biochemistry															
Total protein (g/l) [a]	30–50	28–45	21–43	24–46	21–48	26–40	32–46	23–31	27–44	33–53	28–43	33–53	49–78	21–44	24–50
Albumin (g/l)	–	–	9–12	–	8–18	12–16	–	10–14	9–18	12–22	9–15	12–22	8–14	12–25	10–23
Globulin (g/l)	–	–	7–15	–	4–16	14–23	–	11–23	12–36	10–25	12–34	13–19	12–27	11–24	14–30
Uric acid (µmol/l)	200–1000	200–1000	285–765	100–650	202–648	119–750	100–700	183–489	100–500	77–333	190–327	109–231	89–1700	196–1260	95–1369
Total calcium (mmol/l)	2–3.0	2–3.0	2–2.8	1.8–2.4	2.0–2.7	1.8–3.2	2.0–2.8	1.7–2.35	1.65–2.68	1.87–2.42	2.2–2.8	2.2–2.8	1.4–2.2	1.55–2.6	1.85–3.20
Ionized calcium (mmol/l) [b]	–	–	–	–	–	–	–	–	0.96–1.22	–	–	–	–	–	–
ALT (IU/l)	–	–	156–375	–	128–396	128–648	–	143–255	0–500	35–200		58–206	106–918	276–729	130–330
ALP (IU/l)	20–135	–	10–80	10–90	0–346	24–250	12–100	–	12–160			290–750	–	–	–
Bile acids (µmol/l)	23–90	–	32–117	25–95	34–112	<90	–	<80	<80	<80	24–95	<80	20–97	30–96	20–40
Creatine kinase (IU/l)	55–350	–	117–365	52–245	160–420	120–358	–	<700	140–411	64–322		61–531	297–2260	132–968	449–1685
Glucose (mg/dl)	–	–	–	–	–	–	–	–	–	–	–	–	–	–	220–350

9.10 (continued) Haematological and biochemical data (normal ranges) for a variety of cage and aviary birds (Data supplied by Pinmoore Laboratories, Tarporley, Cheshire). [a] Total protein should be measured by electrophoresis in birds wherever possible. [b] Ionized calcium should be measured in preference to total calcium wherever possible, as fluctuating protein concentrations significantly affect the total calcium concentration. The majority of birds would be expected to maintain the ionized calcium concentration between a narrow range: 0.9–1.3 mmol/l.

Common conditions

Gastrointestinal disease

Diseases of the gastrointestinal tract (Figure 9.11) are common but often difficult to differentiate from systemic diseases exhibiting secondary gastro-intestinal effects. Hypovitaminosis A also predisposes to diseases of the gastrointestinal system. The provision of grit to aid digestion is a controversial topic, but the author recommends its use as it should enhance the digestibility of poor diets, and would certainly not be expected to do harm.

Clinical sign	Cause	Diagnostics	Treatment
Regurgitation	Crop infection, especially candidiasis and protozoal infections; crop impaction; foreign body; proventricular dilatation disease; systemic disease	Physical examination; immediate examination of a crop wash/aspirate by microscopy; culture; direct visualization by endoscopy; contrast radiography; faecal examination for megabacteria	Fluid therapy. Treatment for specific infections. Ingluviotomy to remove foreign body
Blood in droppings	Endoparasites; severe bacterial enteritis; coccidiosis; cloacal prolapse; egg binding; papillomatosis; zinc/lead toxicity	Cloacal palpation; faecal microscopy/bacteriology; serum zinc and lead levels	Fluid therapy. Treat specific problem
Watery faecal component	Dietary change; stress; endoparasites; bacterial enteritis; coccidiosis; bacterial hepatitis	Important to differential polyuria from diarrhoea; faecal microscopy/bacteriology	Treat specific infections. Probiotics useful. Nutritional support

9.11 Gastrointestinal diseases of cage and aviary birds. (continues) ▶

Clinical sign	Cause	Diagnostics	Treatment
Undigested food in droppings	Proventricular dilatation disease; endoparasites; pancreatic disorders	Blood tests; faecal microscopy; contrast radiography; crop/proventricular biopsy	Nutritional support. Treat specific conditions
Discoloured faeces	Green indicates potential hepatic disorders; brown suggests bacterial enteritis; red/pink suggests heavy metal toxicity	Faecal microscopy/bacteriology; serum zinc and lead levels	Treat specific condition
Discoloured urates	Bright green highly suggestive of *Chlamydophila*; brown/haemorrhagic suggestive of bacterial infections; pink suggestive of heavy metal toxicity	Faecal microscopy/bacteriology; faecal PCR for *Chlamydophila*; serum zinc and lead levels	Treat specific condition
Absence of faecal material	Obstruction; complete anorexia	Intussusception and foreign bodies common in parrot chicks	Surgery

9.11 (continued) Gastrointestinal diseases of cage and aviary birds.

Dropping analysis

It is important to know the normal variation in bird droppings, both between species and due to the effects of diet on consistency. A normal dropping in most species will contain a central dark green faecal component surrounded by solid urate, together with a small amount of liquid urine. Visual observation of the dropping should allow the clinician to immediately differentiate between renal, hepatic, reproductive and intestinal disease. Genuine diarrhoea, malodour or undigested food material in the droppings are normally indicative of a gastrointestinal condition.

Dropping analysis should involve a wet smear, faecal Gram stain, parasite analysis and culture. For a wet smear, a fresh faecal smear is mixed with saline and examined immediately after the cover slip is in place. Common findings include motile protozoa, budding yeast, endoparasites and avian gastric yeast (megabacteria). The faecal Gram stain can provide important information quickly, as bird droppings should contain only Gram-positive bacteria (predominantly rods), with Gram-negative organisms considered potential pathogens. However, it should be noted that occasionally Gram-positive alpha- and beta-haemolytic *Streptococcus* spp. can cause disease. If an abnormal bacterial or fungal population is detected, culture and sensitivity are indicated, but the routine cloacal culture of essentially healthy birds is unrewarding and expensive.

Diagnostic tests

Radiography, endoscopy and blood sampling often yield vital information, especially with respect to systemic diseases. A crop wash is a useful simple diagnostic test in regurgitating birds.

1. Introduce a catheter or metal tube directly into the crop until its presence can be felt percutaneously.
2. Introduce a small volume of warmed saline into the crop.
3. Aspirate a sample on to a pre-warmed slide and immediately examine for evidence of protozoa.

Respiratory disease

The conditions affecting the upper and lower respiratory tracts are summarized in Figure 9.12.

The paired nares have a cornified flap of tissue protecting them, which should not be mistaken for a foreign body. Birds have a complex sinus system draining into the choanal slit in the roof of the mouth. Thorough examination of the choana using an auroscope should always be performed to look for evidence of inflammation or discharge. Inflammation or swelling of the sinuses may be identified below the orbit.

Birds have 8–10 air sacs which act as bellows, but no transfer of oxygen occurs within them. However, they account for approximately 80% of the respiratory

Cause	Clinical signs	Diagnostics	Treatment
Upper respiratory tract			
Hypovitaminosis A; sinusitis caused by bacterial/viral/fungal/mycoplasma infection; *Chlamydophila*; foreign body; tracheal stricture; tracheal obstruction (aspergillosis, seed foreign body)	Nasal exudates; mouth breathing; periorbital swelling; head shaking; dyspnoea; sneezing	Auscultation; choanal and tracheal swabs; culture; sinus flushing; tracheal wash; endoscopy; radiography	Treat for specific condition. Sinus flushing. Nebulization with F10SC or appropriate antimicrobial/mucolytic agent. Nutritional supplementation. Fit air sac tube in acute obstructions
Lower respiratory tract			
Hypovitaminosis A; air sacculitis/pneumonia caused by bacterial/viral/fungal/mycoplasma infection; *Chlamydophila*; Teflon toxicity; aspergillosis; air sac worms in finches; abdominal organ distension; egg binding	Dyspnoea; tail bobbing; abdominal breathing; increased respiratory noise	Auscultation; radiography; haematology; endoscopy; culture	Treat specific condition. Nebulization with appropriate antimicrobial/mucolytic agent/bronchodilator. Air sac tube placement. Pneumonia carries poor prognosis

9.12 Respiratory conditions of cage and aviary birds.

volume. The air sac system traps pathogenic organisms with ease and, combined with the poor blood supply, results in the air sacs being very susceptible to infection. There is a large spare capacity in the avian respiratory system, so inactive cage birds frequently do not present with respiratory signs until pathological changes are advanced.

Respiratory disease is a common presentation, especially in pet psittacines with *Chlamydophila psittaci* (psittacosis) being the most common cause (see below). Due to the zoonotic potential of *Chlamydophila*, it should always be suspected and ruled out in any respiratory case. Investigation of respiratory disease involves the usual basic principles of avian clinical examination. It is useful to initially examine the bird visually in its cage, in order to assess respiratory rate and depth prior to handling and auscultation. Radiography can be used to evaluate gross lesions of the lungs and air sacs, but in the majority of cases endoscopy is the most useful diagnostic tool as it allows direct visual evaluation of the air sacs, lungs, heart and trachea within a matter of minutes.

Blanket treatment with antibiotics is generally contraindicated and can be dangerous due to the fact that mycotic infections (such as aspergillosis) are also common, so it is vital to make a diagnosis first. Alternatively, birds can be given an antifungal drug as well as an antibiotic. Nebulization is a very useful stress-free method of getting treatments and moisture into the air sacs.

Psittacosis

- A common infectious respiratory disease seen in clinical practice, which should always be considered as a differential diagnosis in all species of caged bird (not just parrots) due to its serious zoonotic potential.
- It is caused by the obligatory intracellular bacterium *Chlamydophila psittaci*.
- Classically, birds present with signs of depression, conjunctivitis, dyspnoea, sneezing, watery green droppings and a profuse nasal discharge. In some cases, sudden death occurs without clinical signs. Psittacosis has been implicated as a cause of feather plucking.
- In the majority of cases, the infection remains latent with no clinical signs and the birds are carriers.
- Carrier animals succumb to the disease, or secrete the organism, after periods of stress (e.g. after change in environment).

- Budgerigars and cockatiels are especially prone to carrying the organism and should not be kept near more susceptible species such as the larger parrots.
- Radiography may indicate an enlarged liver and spleen.
- Routine blood tests may demonstrate a significant leucocytosis (monocytosis) and elevated liver enzymes.
- There are a variety of confirmatory diagnostic tests available, but the gold standard is a PCR test on a 3–5 day pooled dropping sample.
- A bird should never be certified as negative for *Chlamydophila*, but just that it was not excreting the organism on the day of testing. The test used should always be stated.
- Owners should always be warned of the zoonotic potential of the disease.
- Euthanasia should be considered for clinical cases.
- Although enrofloxacin is a reasonably effective treatment, doxycycline is the drug of choice. Therapeutic levels must be maintained for 42 days.
- Post-mortem examination of caged birds should be performed in an approved fume cupboard, and staff should always be made aware of the significance of chlamydophilosis.

Skin disease

The most common presentation of skin disease in parrots is 'feather plucking' (also known as 'feather picking' or 'Feather Destructive Syndrome'), but it should be noted that although the clinical signs are the same in most birds, the aetiology varies considerably. In other cage and aviary birds, ecto-parasitism is relatively common.

Behavioural conditions account for many cases of feather plucking, particularly sexual disorders; however, most 'plucking' birds have an underlying illness that causes the feather picking. If underlying illness is ruled out, these behavioural problems are now classified in the same way as human obsessive-compulsive disorders.

Self-mutilation is a more severe syndrome, where the bird damages the skin not just the feathers. The condition is most common in cockatoos and is extremely painful, thus euthanasia on welfare grounds must be considered. Figure 9.13 provides a structured approach to investigating and treating feather plucking; the reader is referred to more specialized texts for further information.

Treatment	Comments
Treat underlying condition	Infection (viral disease: psittacine beak and feather disease (PBFD), polyoma); bacterial (*Chlamydophila psittaci*) or fungal (*Malezzia*) dermatitis; wing-clipped birds; ectoparasites; trauma from in-contact birds; systemic disease (hepatomegaly, air sacculitis); reproductive conditions; behavioural problems
Improve plane of nutrition	Useful in the majority of cases (see Figure 9.1)

9.13 Structured approach to treating feather plucking in parrots. (continues) ▶

Treatment	Comments
Improve husbandry	Spray or bathe daily to reduce feather dust (water or F10SC 1:250 dilution); provide supplementary UV-B lighting equivalent to natural photoperiod; environmental enrichment (toys, food variety); increased contact with owner but permit enough rest; provide privacy with nesting box; provide avian companion
Apply collar	Do not use as an alternative to diagnosis and treatment; useful for assessing feather re-growth; commercial collars available
Behavioural modification	Vital component of managing most 'plucking' birds
Drug therapy	Use with care to break the plucking cycle or as a last resort when all other routes have failed; sedatives (diazepam) or antidepressants (haloperidol) are useful; with plucking birds demonstrating aberrant sexual behavioural, hormonal therapy is useful; euthanasia should be considered

9.13 (continued) Structured approach to treating feather plucking in parrots.

Reproductive disease

Female reproductive disease is a common presentation in all cage and aviary birds, particularly single pet parrots. Testicular tumours are surprisingly common in male budgerigars; contrast radiography of the gastrointestinal tract is very useful to demonstrate the enlarged testicle. Figure 9.14 summarizes the reproductive disorders in cage and aviary birds.

Neurological disease

Neurological disease is a frequent presentation in avian practice. Patients present with a variety of clinical signs, from an inability to perch to convulsions. Figure 9.15 summarizes the neurological diseases in cage and aviary birds.

Condition	Cause	Clinical signs	Diagnostics	Treatment and prevention
Egg binding	Chronic calcium and/or vitamin D deficiency; oviduct torsion; oviduct infection with torsion; neoplasia with oviduct torsion	Depression; straining; dyspnoea; palpable abdominal mass; blood-stained faeces	Clinical signs; radiography	Oral or parental administration of 5% calcium gluconate. Provide additional heat and UV-B light. Milk egg from the cloaca under anaesthesia. Aspirate egg contents using a hypodermic needle transabdominally, collapse egg and expel shell, assist by gently flushing with warmed saline. Exploratory laparotomy. Review diet to avoid recurrence. Oxytocin use is controversial both in terms of efficacy and potential for inducing side-effects
Egg over-production (common in cockatiels)	Poor husbandry, including excessive dietary fat; over developed owner–bird bond	Persistent egg laying; soft shelled or odd shaped eggs	Clinical history	Improve husbandry by reducing photoperiod and owner–bird bond. Improve diet. Hormone control (leuprolide acetate, deslorelin). Salpingohysterectomy
Prolapsed oviduct	Poor abdominal musculature in malnourished birds; behavioural (masturbation in cockatoos); sequel to egg binding	Depression; blood-stained faeces; straining; appearance of prolapse	Palpation; clinical signs; radiography to rule out abdominal mass	Clean and replace prolapse using a cloacal purse-string suture. Correct initiating cause. Severe cases require laparotomy and cloacopexy (place a suture around the last rib)
Egg peritonitis (common in persistent egg layers)	Poor husbandry	Depression; weight loss; straining; ascites	Clinical signs; radiography; endoscopy	Salpingohysterectomy. In mild cases, antibiosis and hormonal suppression of egg production may be effective
Testicular tumour (common in budgerigars)	Genetic (up to 4% of male budgerigars affected)	Limb paralysis or weakness	Clinical signs; abdominal palpation; contrast radiography	Castration
Behavioural problems (common in larger psittacine birds, particularly cockatoos)	Single birds over-bonded to owner; poor diet	Feather plucking; cloacal prolapse; excessive vocalization; aggression towards owner	Clinical signs; history	Behavioural modification. Consider re-homing or euthanasia in severe cases

9.14 Reproductive disorders in cage and aviary birds.

Condition	Cause	Clinical signs	Diagnostics	Treatment and prevention
Heavy metal toxicity	Associated with parrots chewing items in the environment containing zinc or lead; zinc toxicity is common in birds placed in new aviaries or cages constructed from galvanized mesh ('new wire' disease)	Ataxia; wings stretched out; haemorrhagic gastroenteritis; convulsions; visual deficits; sudden death	Identify metal on radiography; blood tests (blood concentration >31.4 mmol/l for zinc or 2 µmol/l for lead is significant)	Chelating therapy via edetate calcium disodium injections. Treat for 7 days after metal is ground down in gizzard (usually 3 weeks following ingestion). Prevent access to source of metal. Only use good quality toys. 'Treat' new aviaries and cages by wiping down with vinegar before introducing birds
Hypocalcaemia (common in grey parrots)	Calcium and vitamin D deficiency associated with deficient diets and lack of exposure to unfiltered UV-B light	Weakness; seizures; head twitching	Clinical signs; history; blood tests; ionized calcium concentration <0.96 mmol/l is significant	Oral and parental supplementation with calcium. Provide UV-B light. Improve long-term husbandry
Proventricular dilatation disease (affects all Psittaciformes)	Unknown; presumed viral disease (a novel *Bornavirus* has been found in affected birds); increasing evidence that it is an autoimmune syndrome; incubation period up to 5 years	Ataxia; twitching; abnormal vocalization; gastrointestinal signs (particularly young macaws and cockatoos)	Clinical signs; contrast radiography to demonstrate dilatation of proventriculus; confirmed by demonstrating pathognomonic histological changes on crop biopsy (75% reliable); PCR serum test for *Bornavirus* is available	Cox-2 inhibitors (e.g. celecoxib, meloxicam). Palliative therapy for single birds. Cull affected aviaries. Difficult to control by quarantine in collections due to long incubation period
Paramyxovirus (common in finch collections)	PMV-1 (Newcastle disease), PMV-2 and PMV-3 reported in toucans, finches and mynah birds	Depression; weight loss; torticollis; seizures	Clinical signs; viral isolation/ serology; severe pancreatitis on post-mortem examination	Notifiable on suspicion in UK. Culling. Inactivated vaccine available

9.15   Common neurological diseases of cage and aviary birds.

Renal disease

Renal disease is felt to be common but under-diagnosed, as the clinical signs can be non-specific or not recognized by the owner. Common presentation is a polydipsic bird with polyuria or increased urates in the faeces. Unfortunately, owners often mistake the dropping changes for diarrhoea, and do not present the bird until pathological changes are advanced. The aetiology of renal disease is usually infectious or toxic (heavy metal or vitamin D toxicity) in nature (Figure 9.16).

Birds excrete uric acid as the main nitrogenous waste product, and blood elevation is not recorded until function of 30% of the proximal convoluted tubules is lost. Therefore, treatment can be difficult as uric acid levels do not increase until the bird is terminally ill. A rise in uric acid concentration above 600 µmmol/l is consistent with deposition of uric acid

Condition	Cause and clinical signs	Diagnostics	Treatment
Renal disease	Polydipsia; visceral/articular gout in small psittacine birds (uric acid deposited in tissues); uric acid concentrations remain unaltered until disease is severe; renal tumours common	Urine dipstick; blood tests (uric acid not urea); radiography; endoscopy	Allopurinol may be useful as a treatment for gout. Uric acid concentration >1000 µmol/l represents a grave prognosis
Hepatic lipidosis (common in single pet parrots, especially Amazons and cockatoos; most common non-infectious disease of small finches)	Sudden death in finches; other birds become depressed/anorexic; green droppings	Hepatomegaly; lipaemic blood samples; raised blood cholesterol; obesity; radiography; endoscopy; liver biopsy; liver samples float in water	Supportive feeding. Essential fatty acid supplementation (e.g. Sunshine oil®, HBD International). Milk thistle. Lactulose. Antibiosis
Diabetes mellitus (reported in cockatiels and toucans)	Polydipsia; polyuria	Urine dipstick (normal bird urine contains no glucose)	Dietary change. Mammalian insulin ineffective
Teflon toxicity	Polytetrafluroethane (PTFE) poisoning is associated with Teflon-coated cooking utensils or cooking linings; sudden death with acute pneumonia	Post-mortem examination reveals haemorrhage over both lungs	None. Death usually within 20 minutes of exposure. Avoid keeping birds in kitchen areas

9.16   Miscellaneous disease conditions of cage and aviary birds.

crystals in the viscera and joints (gout). Lateral radiographs are useful to assess kidney size and endoscopic biopsy can provide a definitive diagnosis. Excretory urograms are also useful.

Hepatic disease

There are many hepatic diseases in birds but *Chlamydophila* should always be suspected as a differential diagnosis. The presence of bright green droppings, especially with discoloured urates, is highly suggestive of liver disease. Differentiating between the various causes of liver disease is aided by both radiography and endoscopy; however, biochemical changes may be minimal. The most common liver disorders are:

- Hepatic lipidosis (see Figure 9.16)
- Chlamydophilosis
- Bacterial hepatitis
- Toxicosis.

The South American species and cockatoos are most frequently presented. The clinical signs of liver disease are non-specific but include biliverdinuria, polydipsia, polyuria, anorexia and generalized depression. In chronic disease, beak and feather abnormalities develop due to abnormal keratin metabolism. Ascites can develop but may be due to cardiovascular or reproductive disease, rather than hepatic disease. Hepatic encephalopathy can also occur, but is rare in the author's experience.

Demonstration of elevated bile acids is the most useful biochemical diagnostic test. A liver biopsy is often required to confirm the aetiology of the disease. Although liver diseases may have specific treatments, normally the only option available to the clinician is supportive therapy. This includes fluid therapy, lactulose, milk thistle and vitamin supplementation. Milk thistle is believed to support liver cell function, and lactulose reduces pH in the intestine together with decreasing enteric ammonia production. Hepatic lipidosis is an increasingly diagnosed condition and is thought to be due to a combination of feeding of high-fat diets (seeds and nuts) and genetic susceptibility (Amazon parrot species and small passerines).

Haemochromatosis is an important condition of exotic softbills and ramphastids.

Haemochromatosis

- Haemochromatosis or ISD is the most common non-infectious disease of captive exotic softbills and ramphastids.
- The aetiology is uncertain but it is believed to be associated with diets containing an iron content >30 ppm combined with some species having a genetic susceptibility to the condition.
- Iron accumulates in the liver parenchyma, resulting in cell damage, organ dysfunction, chronic disease and eventually death.
- Affected birds include toucans, mynah birds and exotic softbills.
- Clinical signs vary from sudden death in toucans without evidence of previous disease to a chronic condition including weight loss, depression, dyspnoea, hepatomegaly and ascites in other species.
- Histological examination of liver biopsy samples which confirm increased iron deposition is the gold standard diagnostic technique. Prussian Blue stains, specifically for detecting iron deposited in liver cells, are available.
- Radiography is a useful screening test as hepatomegaly is highly suggestive of haemochromatosis.
- Ultrasonography may show distortion of the hepatic parenchyma and increased tissue density. If ascites is present, ultrasound-guided drainage may ease clinical signs of dyspnoea and discomfort.
- Treatment involves the use of iron chelating drugs (deferoxamine) or weekly phlebotomies equivalent to 10% of the bird's blood volume; although, once diagnosed the prognosis is guarded.
- Diets should contain <30 ppm iron and excess vitamin C should be avoided as it decreases iron requirements.

Viral disease

Viral disease is common in all cage and aviary birds (Figure 9.17) and is very important economically in the captive parrot trade. Paramyxovirus can be a genuine problem in outdoor passerine collections.

Condition	Cause	Clinical signs	Diagnostics	Treatment and control
Psittacine beak and feather disease (PBFD) (affects most Psittaciformes; acute form common in parrot chicks; economically important disease)	PBFD virus (circovirus); highly resistant in the environment; spread by feather dust; affects rapidly growing cells in young birds; severity of the disease is proportional to the age of the bird at point of infection	Feather/beak abnormalities in chronic cases; severe immunosuppression in acute form of the disease with death from secondary infections (especially aspergillosis); wild spread in captive breeding units	PCR test of blood sample/ feather pulp; clinical signs; with acute form, severe leucopenia/anaemia commonplace	No reliable treatment, although avian interferon has been demonstrated to be effective. Palliative care for single birds. Cull affected birds in collections and test all in-contact animals. Environmental decontamination vital. Controlled by regime of testing and quarantine of new acquisitions

9.17 Common viral diseases of cage and aviary birds. (continues) ▶

Condition	Cause	Clinical signs	Diagnostics	Treatment and control
Proventricular dilatation disease (affects all Psittaciformes)	Unknown; presumed viral disease (a novel *Bornavirus* has been found in affected birds); increasing evidence that it is an autoimmune syndrome; incubation period up to 5 years	Regurgitation; weight loss; passing undigested seed; permanently hungry; neurological signs (including ataxia); cardiac disease; chronic condition but death inevitable	Clinical signs; contrast radiography to demonstrate dilatation of proventriculus; confirmed by demonstrating pathognomonic histological changes on crop biopsy (75% reliable)	Cox-2 inhibitors (e.g. celecoxib, meloxicam). Palliative therapy for single birds. Cull affected aviaries. Difficult to control by quarantine in collections due to long incubation period
Polyomavirus ('budgerigar fledging disease')	Polyomavirus	Sudden death in budgerigar chicks; feather dystrophy in chronic form; diarrhoea; CNS signs in larger parrots	PCR test on cloacal swab/blood sample	Cull affected birds. Test in-contact animals. Probably undiagnosed in UK bird population
Paramyxovirus (uncommon in single pet birds)	PMV-1 (Newcastle disease) can affect all caged birds	Sudden death; chronic CNS signs (torticollis, paralysis and twitching) together with respiratory/gastrointestinal problems	Virus isolation; serology	Notifiable on suspicion. Cull affected birds
Herpesvirus	Caged birds are susceptible to species-specific herpesviruses;	Pacheco's disease associated with fatal acute hepatitis in imported parrots	Intranuclear inclusion bodies on post-mortem examination; viral isolation	None
Avian pox (almost exclusively seen in canaries; cutaneous form less common, although reported in softbills)	Avipoxvirus spread by biting insects	Mortality rate up to 100% with the acute form; severe respiratory signs	Viral isolation; demonstration of intracytoplasmic inclusion bodies	Vaccine available in Europe. Supportive antibiotics. Fly control
Cytomegalovirus (common in Australian finches; associated with considerable losses in finch collections)	Cytomegalovirus	Respiratory disease; conjunctivitis	Intranuclear inclusion bodies in conjunctiva	None

9.17 (continued) Common viral diseases of cage and aviary birds.

Behavioural problems

Behavioural problems are common in psittacine birds, particularly when they are sexually mature and kept individually. The most common indicators of behavioural disease include:

- Biting
- Excessive vocalization
- Neurosis regarding new objects in the environment
- One-person birds ('Feather Destructive Syndrome')
- Feather plucking
- Separation anxiety
- Territorial behaviour
- Inappropriate sexual behaviour (e.g. masturbation).

The reader is referred to the *BSAVA Manual of Psittacine Birds, 2nd edition* for a more extensive review, but the basic rules for behavioural training include:

1. Ensure humans are the flock leaders by dominating birds satisfactorily.
2. Always train birds on neutral territory (e.g. away from the cage).
3. Teach simple 'step up' and 'step down' commands.
4. Teach simple 'yes' and 'no' commands.
5. Punishments, such as shouting, should not be seen as a reward by birds.
6. Provide opportunities for foraging and entertainment, such as natural branches and toys, to keep the bird exercising and active. This also promotes normal species-specific behaviours.

Supportive care

Hospitalization

Birds should be hospitalized in an easily cleaned cage, which can provide both heat and humidity. Commercial intensive care cages are available and have the advantage of including nebulization ports. A cheaper alternative for first opinion practice is the use of garden propagators (Figure 9.18). The cage should be heated to 40°C with 50–80% humidity. The use of UV-B light appears to be helpful for the well being of most birds (Stanford, 2006). Perches within the cage should be kept low.

Stress to the patient can be minimized by covering the cage. Birds should be kept away from the sight

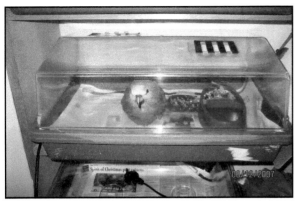

9.18 Garden propagators make effective hospital cages for birds.

and sound of other patients, especially dogs, cats and raptors. The veterinary surgeon should always be aware of infectious disease control, practising barrier nursing where necessary. A 12-hour photoperiod should be maintained if possible. The supply of pure oxygen is useful in cases of severe respiratory disease.

Drug administration

Systemic treatments can be administered by injection, orally or using nebulization.

The preferred intramuscular injection site is the pectoral muscles (see Figure 9.6). The feathers should be parted and the needle introduced into the caudal part of the muscle in the midline, at an angle of 20 degrees. The clinician should ensure that there is no blood vessel present, and large volumes of medication should be split between two sites to prevent skin irritation. Muscle haemorrhage following injection can be a problem in softbills, but can usually be controlled by digital pressure.

Tablets can be crushed and mixed with a small amount of critical care solution or recovery diet and given by crop tube (see below). Nebulization is an excellent stress-free method of medicating birds, particularly in cases of respiratory disease, as it avoids the need for handling. Topical medications can be useful in skin disease, but steroid preparations should be used with great caution as they can cause severe secondary immunosuppressive effects. This includes steroid-based eye drops.

It is not advisable to administer medication via the water supply due to the variation in consumption, especially in unhealthy birds; although, there may be no option in passerine collections. An alternative would be to medicate food.

Fluid therapy

The majority of avian patients are dehydrated.

Crop tube

Oral fluids (e.g. critical care solution) can be administered via a crop tube.

1. Firmly support the bird.
2. Pass a tube over the tongue (avoid the glottis) and enter the oesophagus.

3. Palpate the right-side of the neck to check that the tube is in the correct place prior to introducing the fluid.

Special commercial avian crop tubes are available, but in an emergency situation dog catheters or drip tubing can be used.

Injection

Lactated Ringer's solution is a useful maintenance fluid, which can be administered either intravenously or intraosseously. Intravenous access can be achieved via the basilic, jugular or tarsometatarsal vein using a standard 25-gauge catheter. Although the basilic vein is easy to access for blood sampling, it is very fragile and not recommended for permanent catheter placement. However, it can be used for single bolus injections of fluid. The right jugular vein (Figure 9.19) is easily accessed in most birds and is useful for patients weighing <50 g; for larger species the brachial (see Figure 9.9) or tarsometatarsal vein or an intraosseous method is preferred. The catheter can be sutured in place and most birds appear content to leave it in place. However, all avian veins are prone to severe haematoma formation, and this can be difficult to control in the neck region.

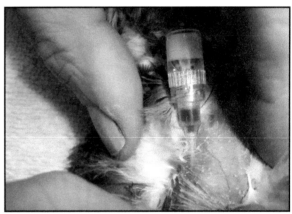

9.19 A jugular catheter is an ideal method of administering fluids, particularly in small passerines.

The placement of an intraosseous needle into the tibiotarsal or ulna bone is a simple technique, and is the author's preferred method of administering fluids in birds. The needle should be placed under anaesthesia as the procedure is considered painful. For ulna placement, the carpus is flexed and the needle advanced through the dorsal condyle of the ulna into the medullary cavity. For tibiotarsal placement, the cnemial crest or 'tibial plateau' of the bone is readily palpated just distal to the stifle joint, and the needle can be simply advanced into the medullary cavity. The needle can be left *in situ* so that repeated bolus volumes (including drugs) can be given throughout the treatment period.

Nutritional support

Anorexia is a common clinical sign in diseased birds. Ill birds need increased energy, fats, proteins, vitamins and minerals in the diet. Commercially prepared juvenile hand-rearing formulae can be used to supply these additional nutrients to diseased adult birds and have the advantage that they can be tube fed. Specific avian recovery diets are now available (e.g. Harrison's recovery formula™).

It is vital to provide adequate nutrition to hospitalized birds, usually by crop tube feeding. The bird should be weighed at point of admittance and then several times daily, so that trends in weight can be followed during the treatment period (Figure 9.20). The bird should be rehydrated and warmed prior to gavage feeding, as crop and gastrointestinal motility are slowed during hypothermia and dehydration.

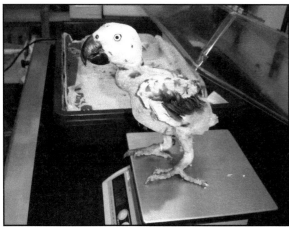

9.20 All birds should be regularly weighed to monitor trends in gain and loss, as it is a useful indicator of condition.

Anaesthesia and analgesia

Anaesthesia should be considered for even simple procedures such as blood sampling, which can be stressful if performed in the conscious animal. Pre-surgical analgesia is advisable to reduce the amount of anaesthesia required. Fluid therapy can be supplied throughout the procedure via an intravenous catheter or intraosseous needle.

Anaesthetic agents
Isoflurane is the agent of choice for induction and maintenance of anaesthesia; although, sevoflurane can be used if it is available. The author has found sevoflurane to be a safe, excellent anaesthetic in birds, with similar properties to isoflurane, but with improved recovery times. The use of halothane is contraindicated due to severe cardiac suppression. Nitrous oxide is also not recommended as it can severely suppress ventilation rates and has been associated with respiratory acidosis. Although propofol has been used to induce parrots, its effects are generally too short lived to be practical.

Injectable (non-volatile) anaesthetic drugs may be useful in certain circumstances, but are normally considered to involve unnecessary risk due to the violent recovery and significant cardiorespiratory depression. There also appears to be considerable species variation in the effectiveness of injectable anaesthesia. If injectable anaesthesia is unavoidable

the use of medetomidine (150–350 µg/kg i.m.) and ketamine (4–10 mg/kg i.m.) appears to be an effective combination in most species.

Equipment
The masks used to deliver inhalation agents to the patient can be created from plastic bottles or syringe cases and made to fit an individual species. Gloves or bandages can be used to make a close-fitting opening in the mask to permit entry of the bird's head in species such as toucans (Figure 9.21). Masks should be used only once to prevent the spread of viruses (e.g. PBFD) via feather debris. Induction chambers can also be used and are particularly useful for smaller passerine species.

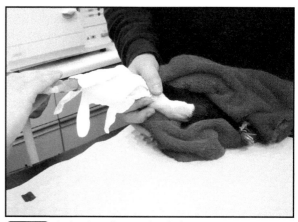

9.21 Induction of anaesthesia in a toucan using an adapted latex glove as a mask.

Induction and intubation
Anaesthesia should be induced using isoflurane at a concentration of 4–5% (6–8% for sevoflurane) and a relatively high oxygen flow rate of 2%, via an Ayres mini T-piece or Bain circuit. Care should be taken not to restrict sternal movements vital for normal inspiration in small passerines.

When the patient reaches a suitable plane of anaesthesia, it can be intubated using an uncuffed latex tube. The smaller tubes specifically made for birds have metal stillettes to aid intubation. The size of tube should reflect the size of the bird – the aim should be to completely fill the trachea, creating an airtight seal, which is fundamental for assisted ventilation. To place the tube, an assistant should pull the bird's tongue forward using a pair of atraumatic forceps. The rima glottidis will be seen at the base of the tongue, which opens and closes as the bird breathes. The tip of the tube should be gently introduced into the glottis and advanced down the trachea.

Monitoring
Unlike those of mammals, birds' eyes remain fixed in position throughout anaesthesia. The corneal reflex is the most useful for monitoring. Lightly touching the eye causes the third eyelid to move across it. This reflex should remain throughout the whole anaesthetic procedure, but it slows with increasing anaesthetic depth. If the anaesthetic plane is too deep, the reflex can stop; as the anaesthetic plane lightens, it speeds up.

An oesophageal stethoscope is a useful monitoring aid; there is also new equipment available which allows an electrocardiogram (ECG) unit to be connected directly to the stethoscope, avoiding the need for wires. ECG units for birds with 2 mm clips, which are atraumatic on the wing and inguinal webs, and accurate up to 700–800 beats per minute, are commercially available. Respiratory rate and tidal volume should be monitored to assess the efficiency of ventilation, and the author recommends the use of a side-stream capnograph to measure end-tidal CO_2.

Ventilation

The use of a commercial mechanical ventilator adapted to fit the Ayres T-piece circuit is ideal, as birds commonly become apnoeic during anaesthesia. If a ventilator is not available, manual intermittent partial pressure ventilation should be considered. During anaesthesia (especially in dorsal recumbency) the bird's sternal excursions are depressed, and this leads to decreased respiratory volume and oxygenation. The use of a mechanical ventilator helps to negate this decreased capacity.

Complications

Hypothermia is a common problem associated with avian anaesthesia. The use of a forced air warmer (e.g. Bair Hugger) is particularly effective at maintaining a bird's body temperature. The use of a single radiant energy source, such as a light bulb, is also an efficient method of providing heat to a patient and reduces the risk of hyperthermia.

Recovery

At the end of the anaesthetic period, the recovering bird should be held until it is able to perch steadily. However, care must be taken not to cause hyperthermia within the towel or cloth. Once the bird can perch, it should be placed in a warm but dark hospital cage and observed constantly until the clinician is satisfied that a full recovery has been made. The veterinary surgeon should ensure that the bird is eating soon after recovery, and certainly within 2 hours.

Euthanasia

Euthanasia should be performed by the administration of intravenous pentobarbital, preferably under general anaesthesia (see above). Intracoelomic injections are very unpredictable, painful and damaging to the tissues. Intracardiac injections are reliable but difficult in all but the smallest bird and should only be carried out under full anaesthesia as they are considered painful.

Drug formulary

A basic drug formulary is presented in Figure 9.22.

Drug	Dose	Comments
Antimicrobial agents		
Amikacin	10–15 mg/kg i.m. q12h	Gram-negative spectrum; least nephrotoxic of the aminoglycosides but maintain hydration during treatment
Amoxicillin	100 mg/kg orally q12h	
Amoxicillin/Clavulanate	125 mg/kg orally q12h	Use contraindicated with allopurinol
Clindamycin	100 mg/kg orally q12h	Useful for bone/joint infections; can tolerate long courses
Doxycycline	*Chlamydophila*: 100 mg/kg i.m. q7d for seven doses Other conditions: 25–50 mg/kg orally q12h Nebulization: 13 mg/ml saline	Drug of choice for *Chlamydophila* and *Mycoplasma* infections; in the UK obtain under authorization from Veterinary Medicines Directorate
Enrofloxacin	5–15 mg/kg i.m. q12h 15 mg/kg orally q12h 200–500 mg/l in drinking water (add fruit juice to disguise taste) Nebulization: 10 mg/ml saline	May be associated with emesis; strongly alkaline so repeated intramuscular injections painful; can cause muscle necrosis
Lincomycin	100 mg/kg i.m. q12h 50–75 mg/kg orally q12h 100–200 mg/l in drinking water	Gram-positive spectrum
Marbofloxacin	10–15 mg/kg i.m. q24h 2.5–5.0 mg/kg orally q24h	Less likely to cause emesis than enrofloxacin
Metronidazole	50 mg/kg orally q24h	Useful antiprotozoal
Oxytetracycline	50–100 mg/kg i.m. q24h 50 mg/kg orally q8h 650–2000 mg/l in drinking water	Can cause muscle necrosis; doxycycline more useful
Tetracycline	40–200 mg/l drinking water	
Trimethoprim/Sulfamethoxazole	10 mg/kg i.m. q12h 10–50 mg/kg orally q24h	Gastrointestinal upset common; contraindicated in liver disease
Tylosin	250–1000 mg/l drinking water	*Mycoplasma*

9.22 Basic drug formulary for cage and aviary birds. (continues) ▶

Drug	Dose	Comments
Antifungal agents		
Acetic acid (vinegar)	16 ml/l drinking water	Useful to prevent/treat gastrointestinal yeast infections
Amphotericin B	1 mg/kg orally q12h	Nephrotoxic, ensure adequate hydration; useful for megabacteriosis
Enilconazole	Topical: 1:50 dilution for 21 days 200 mg/l drinking water Nebulization: 10 mg/ml sterile water	Useful for cutaneous lesions
F10SC disinfectant	Nebulization: 1:100–1:250 dilution	Useful environmental treatment to reduce fungal spore levels; antibacterial and antiviral activity; appears safe by nebulization directly over birds
Itraconazole	5–10 mg/kg orally q24h	Good choice for *Aspergillus* infections; avoid using in grey parrots as toxicity reported
Ketoconazole	20 mg/kg orally q12h	*Candida*; potentially hepatotoxic
Nystatin	300,000–600,000 IU/kg orally q12h for 7–14 days 25,000–100,000 IU/l drinking water or nectar	Drug of choice for *Candida*; treat oral lesions topically; **not** absorbed across gastrointestinal tract
Terbinafine	10 mg/kg orally q12h	
Voriconazole	10 mg/kg orally q12h	Expensive but useful treatment for aspergillosis
Antiparasitic agents		
Fenbendazole	15 mg/kg orally q24h for 5 days	Toxicity reported in some species; can cause feather abnormalities during moult
Fipronil	Spray on skin	Can be used as environmental spray
Ivermectin	0.2 mg/kg orally or topically	
Levamisole	20 mg/kg orally once 80–200 mg/l drinking water for 3 days	Use lower dose rates for finches
Praziquantel	5–25 mg/kg orally, repeated in 2 weeks	Toxic in finches
Toltrazuril	2 mg/l drinking water for 2 consecutive days per week for 4 weeks	Drug of choice for coccidiosis (increase dose to 75 mg/l in canaries with refractory atoxoplasmosis)
Anaesthetics/analgesics		
Alfaxalone	5–10 mg/kg i.m.	Short duration anaesthesia
Buprenorphine	0.05–0.25 mg/kg i.m.	
Butorphanol	0.5–1 mg/kg i.m. q12h	Useful perioperative analgesic
Diazepam	0.5 mg/kg orally 5.5 mg/l drinking water	Useful for calming effect/anticonvulsant
Ketamine	20–50 mg/kg i.m.	Use higher dose rates in smaller species; slow recovery; useful in combination with other drugs (see text)
Medetomidine	50–100 µg/kg i.m.	Usually used in combination with ketamine
Phenobarbital	1–7 mg/kg orally q12h	Anticonvulsant
Hormones		
Delmadinone	1 mg/kg i.m. once	For sexual behaviour problems
Dexamethasone	Shock: 2–4 mg/kg i.m./i.v. Anti-inflammatory: 0.2–1.0 mg/kg i.m.	Use with great care; iatrogenic conditions; side effects common
Gonadotrophin-releasing hormone implant (deslorelin)	4.7 mg/per bird i.m.	
Leuprolide acetate	800 µg/kg i.m. q14d	Use for persistent egg layers; effects variable; expensive medication
Levothyroxine	20–100 µg/kg orally q12h	May induce moult
Nandrolone laurate	0.4 mg/kg i.m. q3wks	
Oxytocin	5–10 IU/kg i.m. once	Should be accompanied by calcium administration
Prednisolone	0.5–1.0 mg/kg i.m. once 1 mg/kg orally q48h	
Prostaglandin F2 alpha gels	Topical: 1 mg/kg	

9.22 (continued) Basic drug formulary for cage and aviary birds. (continues) ▶

Drug	Dose	Comments
NSAIDs		
Carprofen	2–10 mg/kg orally/i.m. q24h	Use higher doses for oral route
Celecoxib	10 mg/kg orally q24h	Useful for proventricular dilatation disease
Meloxicam	0.1–0.5 mg/kg orally/i.m. q24h	Well tolerated
Miscellaneous		
Aciclovir	80 mg/kg orally/i.v./i.m. q8h 240 g/kg in food	Antiviral active against herpesvirus and cytomegalovirus
Calcium gluconate (10%)	5–10 mg/kg i.v./i.m. q12h	
Deferoxamine mesylate	100 mg/kg orally q24h for 12 weeks	Preferred iron chelator for haemochromatosis
Edetate calcium disodium	10–40 mg/kg i.m. q12h for 5 days	Preferred chelating therapy for heavy metal poisoning
Haloperidol	0.1 mg/kg orally q24h	Useful for intransigent self-mutilators
Lugol's iodine	0.2 ml/l drinking water kg	Useful for hypothyroidism in budgerigars

9.22 (continued) Basic drug formulary for cage and aviary birds.

References and further reading

Chitty J and Lierz M (2008) *BSAVA Manual of Raptors, Pigeons and Passerine Birds*. BSAVA Publications, Gloucester

Harcourt-Brown N and Chitty J (2005) *BSAVA Manual of Psittacine Birds 2nd edn.* BSAVA Publications, Gloucester

Hess L, Mauldin G and Rosenthal K (2002) Estimated nutrient content of diets commonly fed to pet birds. *Veterinary Record* **150,** 399–403

Stanford M D (2006) Effects of UVB radiation on calcium metabolism in psittacine birds. *Veterinary Record* **159,** 236–241

10

Racing pigeons

Francis Scullion and Geraldine Scullion

Introduction

Pigeons and doves are in the order Columbiformes, which consists of 8 families, 67 genera, 296 living and 11 extinct species, including 3 of the genus *Dodo*. In general, the term pigeon relates to the larger species of the order, whereas the term dove relates to the smaller species. Pigeons have been kept by humans for over 4000 years and today's domestic pigeons are descended from the rock dove (*Columba livia*).

Selective breeding by enthusiasts, known as fanciers, has resulted in a huge variety of breeds for different purposes, including racing, showing, acrobatic flying displays (tumblers and rollers) and food production. Domestic pigeons are also kept for veterinary and medical research. Racing pigeon fanciers who are interested in, care for and breed racing pigeons (Figure 10.1) far outnumber other fanciers. In Europe there are over 20 million racing pigeons bred each year by almost a quarter of a million fanciers. Individual racing fanciers usually keep between 40 and 200 birds.

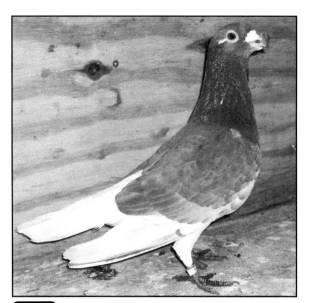

10.1 Racing pigeon.

Racing

Pigeons are instinctively inclined to return to the roost, and their exceptional ability to navigate over long distances forms the basis of the sport of pigeon racing.

Fanciers maintain a loft of birds, which they train to 'home' over gradually increasing distances. On race days competing pigeons are released at a predetermined time and location. The distance between the birds' home loft and the race point is carefully measured by a global positioning system. The birds are fitted with a band containing a chip that can be automatically read using an electronic timing system, immediately the bird returns home. The average flying speed of racing pigeons over moderate distances is around 45 kilometres per hour, but they can achieve bursts of nearly 100 kilometres per hour.

The racing calendar varies depending on location. In many European countries, the adult bird race season begins in early April with weekly races through to July. Flight distances range from 150 kilometres to over 800 kilometres at the end of the season. Some fanciers specialize in the sprints, whilst some breed and train birds for the long distance races. The young bird race season starts in July and extends to September. Race distances range from 80 kilometres at the start to 350 kilometres by the end of the season. The off-season from September to December usually comprises club meetings, shows and sales. This is the time of the year when birds go through an annual moult, and fanciers buy new birds, cull poor racers and decide which adult racers get moved to the stock loft and which young birds go to the adult race loft in preparation for next year's racing season.

Biology

Anatomy and physiology

Pigeons are diurnal birds. They have anisodactyl feet (digits 2, 3 and 4 face caudally, digit 1 faces cranially). Pigeons have a pronounced cere, more so in the males of some varieties. They lack a gallbladder and have rudimentary paired caeca.

Pigeons lack a lateral cervical apterium (featherless tract), making it difficult to visualize the jugular vein for blood sampling without plucking feathers. They lack a well developed uropygial gland and instead produce feather powder (composed of keratin), which protects the feathers from abrasion and gives them the silky grey sheen. Feather powder prevents waterlogging in wet conditions and insulates the body in cold weather. Some fanciers develop an allergic alveolitis in response to inhalation of feather powder, and this is known as pigeon fancier's lung.

Pigeons have a large bilobed crop at the base of the neck. On stripping back the skin of the neck at post-mortem examination, extensive haemorrhage can occur from the well developed subcutaneous vascular plexus which extends from the cranium to the crop. This plexus helps regulate body temperature and is used in sexual and territorial displays. Damage to the plexus can cause fatal haemorrhage, so the authors prefer the sternal apterium for subcutaneous injections. The keel is long and supports well developed pectoral muscles, which makes abdominal palpation difficult. The basic biological data are summarized in Figure 10.2.

Lifespan (years)	20–30
Racing life (years)	7
Bodyweight (g)	400–550
Respiratory rate (breaths/min)	25–30
Breeding span	From 6–8 months and decreasing after 12 years
Clutch size	2 (the second egg is laid within 24–48 hours)
Incubation period (days)	18 – the first egg is only lightly incubated. Both male and female involved in incubation after second egg is laid
Weaning age (days)	Usually 25

10.2 Basic biological data.

Sexing

Males are generally slightly larger than females, and this together with behavioural clues such as fanning and dragging the tail and chasing, usually enables fanciers to determine the sex of the bird.

Husbandry

Housing

Generally, separate lofts are maintained for breeding birds, adult racing birds and young birds. Lofts contain various sections where males and females can be segregated and small groups of race teams can be managed.

Site

In the UK, it is preferable for lofts to face southeast to obtain the full benefit from the sunshine and shelter from the prevailing winds. The possible risk of toxin ingestion or heavy metal poisoning from local vegetation, refuse and building materials, or trauma from collision with power and telephone lines should be considered. Nearby stagnant water can breed flies that allow the spread of disease, such as avian pox.

Structure

The loft construction and design should be suitable in terms of size, insulation, waterproofing and robustness; generally 2–2.5 m³ per bird is acceptable. The loft should contain sufficient sections to allow for the separation of: young birds from adults after weaning;

males and females outside the breeding season; and stock breeding adult birds from adult racers. Ideally, sick or newly purchased individuals should be placed in a completely separate loft.

Regular cleaning and disinfection, including flaming of floors and internal structures, are an essential part of any hygiene programme, and the materials and design of the loft need to reflect this. Deep litter, consisting of different materials such as peat, woodchip and chopped straw, is often used during the off-season, and if well managed is acceptable. Ideally, the substrate should be dry, absorbent and dust free. It can be top-dressed with lime followed by new litter frequently. Badly managed deep litter can lead to a build-up of parasite eggs that will cause recurrent disease outbreaks.

The buildings should be fox and cat proof, and all facilities (including those for food storage) should be vermin proof and dry, with vermin control points positioned so that the pigeons cannot access the poison.

Ventilation

Birds produce water vapour as they respire, and the difference between the temperature inside and outside the loft results in condensation, especially in metal buildings. In addition, dried pigeon faeces, feather powder production and the flapping of wings all contribute to a dusty environment. Any of these conditions can make birds vulnerable to respiratory problems; therefore, adequate ventilation without draughts is important. Vermin proof inlets should be at ground level with baffles to prevent draughts. Outlets should be at the peak of the roof and designed so that rain cannot enter. Opening and closing ventilation inlets allows temperature control in extremes of hot and cold weather, but this must not be at the expense of proper ventilation.

Lighting

Artificial lighting is necessary for inspecting and managing the birds during darkness, but wire-grilled windows and outside flights provide necessary natural lighting for birds housed for long periods.

Ancillary furniture

Utensils: Most fanciers feed their animals once or twice daily, as it is difficult to train birds when food is available *ad libitum*. There should be adequate feed and water points for use by all birds in a section at one time, and it should be ensured that utensils are easily washed and disinfected, and that the facilities for waste disposal are appropriate. Covered food and water utensils help prevent faecal contamination and avoid water spillage, which results in dampness and predisposes to diseases such as coccidiosis.

Perches: Approximately twice as many perching areas as there are birds are required. These are usually staggered on the walls of the loft and positioned so that the birds do not foul one another and are not in direct visual contact, since this encourages aggression. Individual box perches may also be used (Figure 10.3).

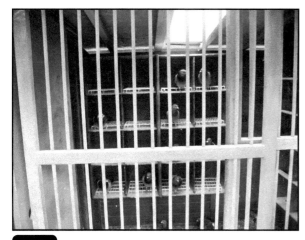

10.3 Individual box perches.

Nest boxes: As well as being a place for laying eggs and rearing young, nest boxes can also provide a retreat for intimidated birds during periods of natural aggression. Nest boxes positioned against one wall of the loft prevent visual contact and reduce aggression. A transparent divider is placed in the nest box when the male is first introduced to the female or during various motivational race management techniques. Nest boxes can have grilled floors for ease of cleaning with nest bowls positioned so that birds cannot disrupt them.

Diet

Pigeons are usually fed 30–50 g of mixed grains and pulses, once or twice daily. The nutrient composition of the feed (3–15% protein; approximately 3% fat) (Vogel *et al.*, 1994) should differ depending on the requirements of the individual bird (breeding, racing, rearing young). A diet that is too high in fat will have a laxative effect. Pigeons usually drink between 20 and 50 ml of water per day, by drawing up water after submerging their beaks. Calcium grit should be made available *ad libitum*, and brewer's yeast and vitamin and mineral supplements may be used by fanciers on a regular basis.

Breeding

Traditionally, racing birds were paired up on 14 February; however, it is now more common in the northern hemisphere to establish breeding pairs in December. Pairing in December results in chicks being hatched in early January, and these pigeons are more mature during the summer young bird racing season (young bird racing involves only birds born in that calendar year).

The first egg is generally laid within 11 days of mating, followed by a second one to complete the clutch within 24–48 hours. The eggs hatch after being incubated, by both adults, for 18 days. Both adults also produce crop milk from desquamated fat-laden epithelial cells, the production of which is under the control of prolactin. Crop milk lacks carbohydrate and calcium, but the adult birds provide these nutrients by regurgitating food to the hatchlings from approximately 4 days old. By day 7, nearly all the food the

chicks (known as squabs) receive is regurgitated. Squabs grow rapidly and reach about 400 g in 3 weeks.

Most fanciers wean young birds at about 25 days old and place them in their own loft. The weaned pigeons are known as squeakers until their voice changes at about 2 months old. Young birds normally go through a moult at 7 weeks old, unless it is curtailed by the fancier using the darkness system.

Management systems

Darkness
Management by rearing young birds in a controlled light environment to delay moulting of flight feathers until after the racing season.

Widowhood
Management by breeding specifically to coincide with particular races to incite a quicker return home to either a receptive partner, eggs or young in the nest. Can be used with both cock and hen birds.

Roundabout
Management similar to widowhood that rotates between cocks and hens being raced.

Fanciers generally take a second round of youngsters from the breeding group to build up the young bird team, and some even take a third round. Domestic pigeons will continue to breed all year if kept together, but from the fourth round health problems can occur in the breeding animals unless extra food supplements (especially calcium) are provided. Chicks may also be bred from racing lofts as part of the strategy for the race team, in the belief that the adult birds will return to the nest faster if they are sitting on eggs or have young to feed (see above). Consequently, the age of birds in the young bird loft can vary by a few months, and this can be one of the stress factors that leads to health problems. Young birds mature from about 6 months of age and their attempts to breed during the young bird racing season add to stress within the loft.

Identification

Pigeons are identified by a closed ring that is placed on the leg before the bird is 5 days old. Rings are purchased for the incoming season from the National Associations and will contain data on the country of origin and year of issue, as well as an individual number.

Handling and restraint

Pigeon fanciers generally remove the bird from its hamper or loft, and hand it to the veterinary surgeon. It is important to keep the wings under control, whilst allowing the bird to rest in the hand with the feet held between the first and second fingers (Figure 10.4). The chest area should not be constricted. Assistance may be required for obtaining samples.

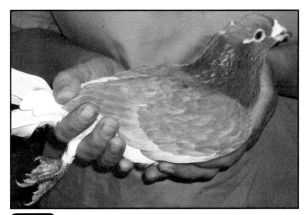

10.4 Restraining a pigeon.

Diagnostic approach

Racing pigeon medicine is best addressed at the population level. The diagnostic approach follows the usual pattern of observation, history, clinical examination and sample collection and testing.

Observation
The starting point is a loft visit. A loft visit affords the opportunity for a discussion with fanciers about the management of their birds. The veterinary surgeon should elucidate what type of racing is being considered (e.g. young birds, sprints, long distance). The lofts should be inspected systematically, starting with the young birds then moving to the race loft and finally the stock loft (Figure 10.5). Footwear should be cleaned and disinfected between lofts. Lofts should also be evaluated with reference to the site, structure and internal design, ventilation, lighting and ancillary furniture (see above).

1. Examine loft and surroundings.
2. Observe birds at a distance without disturbing them.
3. Evaluate hygiene and management standards.
4. Check floors for quantity and quality of droppings; check walls for evidence of expectorations.
5. Look for evidence and quality of pest control.
6. Check food and water quality and storage facilities.
7. Look for evidence of grit supplementation and check fancier's 'pharmacy'.
8. Look for birds that appear fluffed up, sleepy or have noticeable respirations.

10.5 Observation checklist.

Fanciers acknowledge that the fitness of the birds is closely linked to health and may follow a number of anecdotal health protocols within their loft management. In most cases there is little veterinary involvement in the administration of medicines, and much of what is practised is at best empirical treatment with questionably sourced drugs. It should be noted that most fanciers will have administered their own treatment to sick birds before presenting them to a veterinary surgeon.

The nature of pigeon racing carries the inherent risk of continued exposure to transmissible diseases, in particular with regard to the mix of different ages in the young bird loft, mixing of birds from different lofts, and contact with wild pigeons (including fomite exposure) during racing and training. In the adult loft, added stresses associated with racing during or immediately after breeding can predispose birds to contracting diseases. Further, poor weather conditions on race days can lead to 'holdovers', where the release of the birds is delayed, resulting in birds from different lofts being confined in close quarters for a prolonged period. Under these circumstances, food and water are provided but the build-up of faecal contamination and difficulties in maintaining hygiene lead to high levels of disease challenge to all birds.

History
Figure 10.6 lists the questions that should be addressed when obtaining a history.

1. How many birds are housed within the various lofts (young birds, adult, stock)?
2. When were the problems first noticed?
3. How many birds were noticed with problem initially (age, birds from which loft)?
4. How many birds are affected now?
5. Any sick birds? How many?
6. Any deaths? How many?
7. Have the birds been racing/training well?
8. Have any of the birds been regurgitating, sneezing or coughing?
9. Any soft motions?
10. Any lameness (wing or leg) or swelling on limbs?
11. How many birds were paired for breeding this season?
12. How many eggs hatched?
13. How many young were reared to weaning?
14. Have any medications been administered? When? What? How long for? What dose?

10.6 History checklist.

Clinical examination
The approach to the physical examination of an individual bird is summarized in Figure 10.7. The usual range of diagnostic procedures, including endoscopy, radiography and blood sampling for haematology and biochemistry, may be conducted on an individual bird and are similar to those described in other species (see Chapters 9, 11 and 12).

Knowledge of the epidemiology of disease processes can assist the veterinary surgeon in choosing the appropriate laboratory tests (Figure 10.8) and birds from which to collect samples, as random sampling is less effective than testing representative birds. Such birds harbour the more prevalent pathogens within the population and assist in the development of treatment regimens. It is seldom possible to isolate an individual disease-causing agent in a loft, as multifactorial disease is more common. Ancillary tests include:

- Cytology
- Culture and sensitivity
- Histopathology.

A small representative group of the sickest birds should be caught, examined and weighed. The following should be checked:

- The cere for discoloration
- The nostrils and immediate area for evidence of discharge
- The eyes for discharge, conjunctivitis and iris colour
- The feathers over the ears, which may be raised in birds with respiratory disease
- The head for symmetry
- The mouth for excess mucus or focal lesions
- The glottal structures and the skin/mucous membrane junction for abnormal accumulation of exudates
- The choanal slit for spacing and presence of discharge
- The mucous membranes for colour
- The neck and crop region for swellings
- The crop contents, tone and thickness of the crop wall
- The breast musculature to determine body condition
- The wings, which should be examined individually: the joints should be palpated and observed; joint motion, bones and feather coverage from top to bottom should be evaluated

- The feathers for structural integrity and underlying skin problems
- The patagial membrane
- The motion of the wing, by holding the bird upright by both legs at or near the stifle and dropping the hand swiftly to create a reflex wing sweep
- The legs, which should be examined individually: each joint should be moved through its normal range-of-motion; and the soles of the feet and individual pads examined
- The dorsal region to the tip of the tail: the tail feathers should be fanned for inspection
- The abdomen and pelvic bones
- The cloaca and surrounding feathers for signs of faecal staining
- The left and right abdominal air sacs by auscultation
- The lungs by placing the stethoscope on the back between the shoulders
- The heart by auscultating the pectoral region on both sides
- The trachea/syrinx by placing the stethoscope at the thoracic inlet

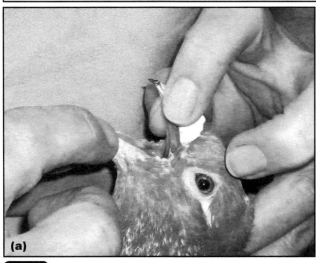 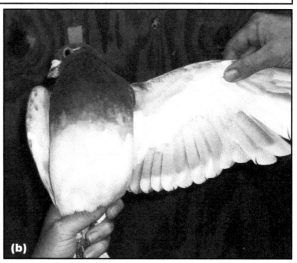

10.7   Physical examination checklist. **(a)** Examining the mouth. **(b)** Examining the wing.

Laboratory test	Conditions that can be confirmed
Ante-mortem	
Crop wash/throat swab	Trichomoniasis; candidiasis; dysbacteriosis
Faecal smear	Coccidiosis; worms; hexamitiasis; candidiasis; dysbacteriosis
Culture and sensitivity	Bacteria (and appropriate therapy)
Virus isolation	Herpesvirus, adenovirus, paramyxovirus, poxvirus
Serology	Salmonellosis, paramyxovirus infection/ vaccination
Droppings (PCR)	Circovirus, chlamydophilosis
Post-mortem	
Culture and sensitivity	Bacteria (and appropriate therapy)
Virus isolation	Herpesvirus, adenovirus, paramyxovirus
Liver (PCR)	Circovirus
Spleen (PCR)	Chlamydophilosis

10.8   Laboratory tests.

Imaging

As with other avian species, radiography is a useful diagnostic tool but requires general anaesthesia. Ventrodorsal and lateral whole body views are standard. More advanced imaging techniques, such as ultrasonography, computed tomography (CT) and magnetic resonance imaging (MRI), are equally applicable but not commonly used in pigeons.

Sample collection

Blood
Venepuncture sites in pigeons are the superficial ulnar/basilic vein (Figure 10.9) or the superficial plantar metatarsal/caudal tibial vein. The jugular vein does not lie under an apterium in the pigeon and is hard to visualize as the overlying skin is thick.

Droppings
Fresh droppings should be examined for evidence of endoparasites, *Candida* and the presence of red blood cells, inflammatory cells and bacteria using smears, salt flotations and Gram/Diff-Quick stains. Collection of loft dropping samples over a 5–10 day period is useful when attempting to isolate or identify organisms such as *Salmonella* or *Chlamydophila* that are intermittently excreted.

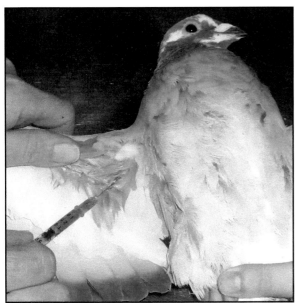

10.9 Venepuncture of the superficial ulnar/basilic vein to obtain a blood sample.

Treatment should be aimed at all of the relevant young bird, adult or race team populations.

Common conditions

Upper gastrointestinal disease

The upper gastrointestinal tract consists of the mouth and its various structures, oesophagus, crop, proventriculus and gizzard. Many conditions present with similar clinical signs, depending on the severity of the disease process. These range from the presence of increased mucus in the oropharynx to visible lesions, which vary from small white spots to yellow caseous focal masses often with underlying ulceration. Crop flaccidity, slow crop emptying, sour crop and regurgitation may also be evident. Common disease conditions include:

- A number of viral conditions, including pigeon poxvirus, adenovirus and circovirus
- Dysbacteriosis
- Candidiasis
- Trichomoniasis
- Nutritional deficiencies.

Pigeon pox

Cause: Pigeon pox is caused by an *Avipoxvirus*. Pigeons are susceptible to pigeon, chicken, turkey and canary strains of the virus. Squabs usually become infected from carrier parents. Blood-sucking parasites and biting insects can spread the disease, and a seasonal occurrence may be related to vector availability. The incubation time from acquisition of infection to development of clinical signs is usually 1 week.

Clinical signs: Clinical disease presents either in a cutaneous or in a diphtheritic form. Epidermal cells are infected in the cutaneous form with swellings developing in unfeathered areas such as the cere, wattles, eyelids and commissures of the mouth. This leads to papule formation followed by vesicular lesions, which enlarge and coalesce. After 2 weeks a scab forms and the clinical course ends when the scab falls off as the epithelium desquamates.

In the diphtheritic form, lesions occur in the oral cavity and may invade the pharynx and trachea, resulting in life-threatening dyspnoea. Affected birds lose weight. Sometimes chronic firm masses (occasionally melanistic) form on the wings or feet. Secondary bacterial infections of pox lesions are common. Morbidity is often >90%. Recovered birds have good resistance for a year or more.

Diagnostics and treatment: Pox disease can be recognized by the history and typical clinical signs. On histological examination, large intracytoplasmic inclusions with ballooning degeneration and bullous formation can be seen. Confirmation is by virus isolation. Treatment is unsatisfactory. Removal of scabs leads to the spread of the infection by release of the virus. Tincture of iodine can be applied to lesions to assist regression. A pigeon pox vaccine is available in some countries in Europe where the problem appears to be more severe. Severely affected birds should be euthanased. Secondary bacterial infection of lesions may benefit from antibiotic treatment.

Adenovirus

There are a number of serotypes of the genus *Aviadenovirus* and conflicting views as to the role in diseases affecting racing pigeons. The most common clinical signs are found in birds with inclusion body hepatitis from which adenovirus has been isolated, and these include anorexia, regurgitation, slimy droppings, polyuria, polydipsia, respiratory disease and death. *Escherichia coli* infection is believed to exacerbate adenovirus infections, and has been isolated from the gut and respiratory tissues of affected pigeons. Treatment of secondary infections with antibiotics (identified by sensitivity testing) can assist recovery, although the final outcome is also determined by the virulence of the adenovirus strain.

Circovirus

Circoviruses were first discovered in the early 1980s and have been associated with disease in a wide variety of animals. In most species, circovirus appears to attack the immune system and multifactorial secondary infections are a feature of circovirus-related diseases. Although the pathogenesis of circovirus infection in pigeons is not yet fully understood, circoviruses are likely to cause immunosuppression in this species. In the authors' practice, circovirus is the primary agent identified and associated with ill thrift and deaths in squabs.

Young bird sickness: This is the term used by racing pigeon fanciers to describe a condition that has occurred regularly in recent years and affects pigeons in the first year of life. It is characterized by slow crop emptying, regurgitation, diarrhoea, weight loss, poor performance and occasionally death. This condition is a complex multifactorial disease, and circovirus is a prime candidate for the initiating factor (Scullion and

Scullion, 2007). The severity of young bird sickness depends on the combination of secondary infectious agents involved. A small number of older pigeons can carry circovirus and spread the disease either directly or through the egg to the next generation.

Diagnostics and treatment: Circovirus infection can be recognized by the characteristic intracytoplasmic botryoid inclusions (i.e. bunch of grapes appearance) in the bursa on histological examination, and confirmed by PCR examination of droppings or tissue samples. The clinical investigation and treatment of young bird sickness should be directed at the many agents that affect the digestive and respiratory systems. Encouragingly, birds affected by young bird sickness early in the race season have responded to such treatment and gone on to win races. The role of circovirus needs further investigation, since at the moment its role in pigeon disease is purely one of association and comparative medicine.

Dysbacteriosis
Dysbacteriosis is defined as an imbalance in the composition of the normal intestinal flora. Bacteria levels frequently rise quickly if a bird's immune system is compromised, and the condition can be an indication of general health impairment or may be associated with some viral infections. In the upper gastrointestinal tract of pigeons, sour crop (caused by a proliferation of a mixed bacterial population) is occasionally encountered. Affected birds are lethargic, have flaccid crops that are slow to empty, and occasionally regurgitate. Numerous morphologically distinct bacterial populations can be seen on cytological evaluation of crop contents; however, culture is often unrewarding. Thus, a quantitative assessment of bacterial levels may be of more value. However, the benefit of culture is that it allows the determination of the antibiotic sensitivity of any organism that is isolated, otherwise treatment is by administration of a broad-spectrum antibacterial drug.

Candidiasis
Candidiasis, caused by the yeast fungus *Candida albicans*, is a disease of the gastrointestinal tract often referred to as thrush by fanciers. Young birds are more susceptible to overgrowth of this normal gastrointestinal inhabitant, but disease also occurs in debilitated adults. Predisposing factors include overcrowding, damp conditions, vitamin deficiencies and prolonged use of antibiotics. Disease can present as unthriftiness and regurgitation with diarrhoea if the organism proliferates in the lower intestine. Severe *Candida* overgrowth causes grey–white loosely attached focal lesions, which can be seen in the oropharynx of the bird. Similar lesions occur in the oesophagus and crop where, in very ill birds, the coalescence of lesions leads to a thick curd-like covering of the crop mucosa. Diagnosis involves examination of fresh smears from the lesions, revealing typical budding yeast bodies. Diff-Quick stain demonstrates dark blue stained bodies and the organism also grows readily on blood agar. Nystatin is an effective treatment.

Trichomoniasis
This protozoal disease, also known as canker, is caused by *Trichomonas gallinae,* a common motile flagellated parasite with an undulating membrane and four anterior flagella. It has a direct lifecycle and can be transmitted via saliva and crop secretions from adults to squabs via crop milk or from bird to bird via common food and water utensils. Young birds are most susceptible as age-related immunity develops, and clinical disease is seldom seen in adult birds. However, in stressful situations such as breeding, racing or overcrowding, the level of canker organisms in adult birds can rise significantly and may lead to decreased racing performance. There are various strains of *T. gallinae* with differing pathogenicity.

Heavy infections cause ulceration of the mouth, oesophagus and crop with some more pathogenic strains spreading to visceral organs such as the lungs and liver. The umbilicus of nestlings can also become infected. Clinically affected birds are unthrifty with signs of regurgitation, diarrhoea and increased mortality. Yellow necrotic material can be found in the oral cavity and sinuses. Diagnosis can be made by examination of fresh smears of crop or lesion material. Treatment with nitroimidazoles such as metronidazole is usually effective. Prevention is best achieved by routine testing of birds at times of increased susceptibility, such as pre-breeding, pre-racing and post-weaning, followed by a course of treatment where appropriate.

Nutritional deficiencies
Pigeons are primarily seed-eaters and are prone to nutritional problems such as hypocalcaemia and hypovitaminosis A.

Calcium: Intake of calcium is important when birds are in lay or in moult. Low calcium levels may play a role in the crop stasis or slow crop emptying that accompanies many upper gastrointestinal problems. Husbandry factors should be evaluated and serum levels of phosphate and total and ionized calcium should be measured. Treatment involves supplementation of the diet. In most cases, this can be achieved by provision of calcium grit.

Vitamin A: Although vitamin A is deficient in some seed diets, the common inclusion of maize to the diet of racing pigeons means that overt disease is uncommon. In hypovitaminosis A there is a lag phase before clinical signs become evident, as liver stores of the vitamin are used. Vitamin A is necessary for proper epithelial integrity, and severe deficiency can lead to kidney and respiratory disease. Sialoliths are believed to be metaplastic epithelial cell blockages of the salivary glands and can be seen in the oropharynx of some racing pigeons, which may indicate a vitamin A deficiency. Diagnosis can be difficult to confirm due to the lack of normal laboratory reference ranges. Epithelial crenation, seen on Diff-Quick stain as shrunken dark pink cells, is also suggestive of hypovitaminosis A. Most fanciers give their birds vitamin supplements but are unsure of what vitamins the mixture actually contains, so treatment should be directed at providing a multivitamin supplement containing vitamin A.

Lower gastrointestinal disease

The lower gastrointestinal tract includes the small and large intestine, liver, pancreas and cloaca. A number of endoparasites, protozoa, bacteria, fungi and viral agents are capable of causing enteritis and associated diarrhoea, which can result in weight loss, poor race performance and in some cases death.

Coccidia

Coccidiosis, caused by *Eimeria labbeana* or *E. columbarum,* is not as common as many fanciers believe. Pathogenic levels of coccidial oocysts can be reached rapidly if the environment is suitable, but fanciers generally keep lofts dry with daily cleaning and frequent torching of floors. Affected birds go off their food and develop diarrhoea as a result of catarrhal enteritis. Polydipsia may accompany the diarrhoea. In some acute cases haemorrhagic enteritis develops, causing weight loss and stunting or death, especially in young birds. Diagnosis is by finding large numbers of coccidial oocysts on microscopic examination of fresh faecal smears or salt flotations. Coccidial infections can be treated with sulfadimethoxine. Prevention is by regular maintenance of a clean dry loft.

Hexamita

Hexamitiasis is caused by the flagellated protozoal parasite *Hexamita columbae*. It is primarily a disease of young birds between 1 and 3 months of age, but it can cause increased losses during training and racing of older young birds. The organism causes small intestinal enteritis and can be a primary pathogen or found in conjunction with other diseases. *Hexamita* infection can result in severe illness characterized by loss of appetite, ill thrift, weight loss, dark green sticky mucoid diarrhoea and death. In a study of young bird sickness, lofts with the highest mortalities usually had hexamitiasis confirmed.

Diagnosis is confirmed by finding characteristic fast-moving 9 µm flagellated protozoa in fresh faecal or cloacal smears. Affected birds may occasionally be negative on smear examination. Post-mortem examination of deep, small intestinal mucosal scrapes obtained from a number of fresh carcasses may be required to confirm the diagnosis, since the organisms do not survive long after the death of the host. Treatment is the same as for trichomoniasis. Prevention involves testing of droppings and cloacal swabs from young birds early in the season with treatment of positive lofts.

Ascarids

Ascaridia columbae are large roundworms between 2 and 6 cm long, which inhabit the small intestine. Ascarid eggs are commonly found in adult bird droppings at routine pre-breeding checks, and may be found in association with *Capillaria* infection. They have a direct lifecycle that takes about 9 weeks to complete. In sufficient numbers they can cause intestinal obstruction, perforation and peritonitis.

Capillaria

Capillaria columbae and *C. longicollis* are fine threadworms which can be up to 2.5 cm long. They are found commonly in adult birds during the winter months and in young birds in the autumn, but can also cause clinical disease in young birds in early summer if the problem is not kept under control in the adult bird loft during the breeding season. These worms inhabit the small intestine and have a direct lifecycle of approximately 4 weeks. *Capillaria* infection can cause severe illness with diarrhoea, weight loss and death if not treated promptly.

Although capable of causing primary disease, an increased burden of round and threadworm eggs is often found in association with many other diseases. Diagnosis is made by examination of fresh faecal smears for the characteristic ova (Figure 10.10). In a racing pigeon loft it is preferable to keep these endoparasites to a minimum level, and treatment is administered when any eggs are found during the qualitative analysis of droppings. Anthelmintics are effective. Prevention involves attention to management, routine droppings analysis, treatment and strict hygiene measures within the loft.

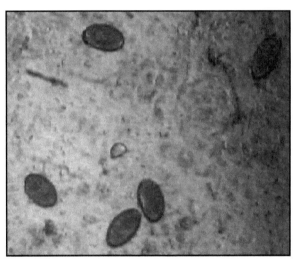

10.10 *Capillaria* worm eggs.

Respiratory disease

Herpesvirus

This disease, caused by pigeon herpesvirus-1 (PHV-1), usually occurs during the breeding season when latently infected adult pigeons excrete the virus. Clinical disease is observed when susceptible birds from virus-negative parents are exposed, or when latently infected birds contract another debilitating condition which allows the latent virus to be excreted. Therefore, the disease is usually seasonal, occurring during the breeding and racing periods.

The main features of PHV-1 infection are upper respiratory tract inflammation with conjunctivitis, nasal discharge and congestion, focal necrosis and ulceration of the mouth, pharynx and larynx. Systemic PHV-1 infection causes hepatitis, which makes affected birds depressed and dull. Intranuclear inclusions may be identified in liver lesions, but can be confused with adenovirus infection. Inclusions in respiratory epithelial cells are occasionally seen on cytological examination of tracheal washes. Swabs or samples can be taken from the pharynx, trachea, lungs or liver of a group of affected birds and submitted for histopathology and virus isolation. Secondary bacterial infections are usually involved and treatment directed at these may assist recovery.

Chlamydophilosis

Cause: The family Chlamydiaceae consists of two genera, *Chlamydia* and *Chlamydophila*, which are obligate intracellular Gram-negative bacteria responsible for a diverse range of diseases in birds and mammals.

Chlamydophila psittaci causes a multisystemic disease affecting principally the respiratory and gastrointestinal organs, with occasional nervous and other system involvement. It is commonly accepted that individual bird species may be infected by *C. psittaci* strains of differing virulence, resulting in variable clinical signs, incubation and recovery times. The severity of the disease also depends on the susceptibility of the host, the route of exposure and the presence of other diseases. In pigeons, the disease appears to be well adapted to its host with up to 90% of lofts testing positive for the organism. Disease may only become evident under times of stress, when the clinical picture may be complicated by the presence of other pathogens such as paramyxovirus, herpesvirus and *Salmonella*. However, the aforementioned high prevalence of chlamydophilosis in lofts means that it is likely to be found during the investigation of any disease outbreak. What is not well defined is its role in the overall health status of sick birds, where it has been associated with other pathogens.

Chlamydophila infection is spread by inhalation of contaminated dust from feathers, or inhalation or ingestion of contaminated faeces or respiratory secretions. In a study on young bird sickness, lofts with severe clinical signs and death of a small number of birds were positive for *Chlamydophila*, diagnosed by PCR testing. Birds from all these lofts showed pneumonitis at post-mortem examination.

Clinical signs: In pigeons, chlamydophilosis can present as a mild chronic disease confined to the respiratory tract, with a resultant decrease in flying performance. Some birds may have a unilateral, clear, ocular discharge and conjunctivitis, giving rise to the so-called 'one-eyed cold' syndrome. Eye infections are non-specific and can also be associated with *Mycoplasma* and *Haemophilus* spp., as well as pox and herpesvirus infections and even trichomoniasis. Diarrhoea is another common sign, associated with weakness and weight loss. High morbidity is more of a feature of chlamydophilosis than high mortality.

Diagnostics: *Chlamydophila* organisms fail to stimulate a sufficient immune response to prevent re-infection, and serological tests for the disease are historically unreliable. *Chlamydophila* DNA can be detected in lofts by PCR testing of faeces collected over a 5-day period or from tissues collected at post-mortem examination, although the virulence of the strains identified remains unknown. Much work needs

to be undertaken to better define the role of less virulent strains of this organism in disease processes.

Treatment: Clinical signs associated with *Chlamydophila* respond well to short-term treatment with tetracyclines, but the drug is only effective during the active growth phase of the organism. Prolonged treatment courses of up to 45 days' continuous therapy are designed to eliminate the organism from all birds, including carriers, by maintenance of constant serum therapeutic levels. Administration of continuous treatment to pigeons during the race season is difficult as they are raced every weekend. There can also be problems with long courses of treatment due to the binding of tetracyclines to essential minerals and the potential for *Candida* to proliferate. One strategy that the authors have found effective is to schedule long-term therapy during the closed season. This does not solve the potential problem of re-infection, but the results reported by fanciers on racing performance of the adult birds have been good, and long-term therapy appears worthwhile in some lofts. In addition, the authors' data (unpublished) show that despite the threat of re-infection, some lofts can remain free from *Chlamydophila* during the race season. More research is required to evaluate the effectiveness of long-term *versus* short-term therapy.

Zoonosis: Chlamydophilosis is a potential zoonotic disease, and its prevalence in over 90% of pigeon lofts would suggest that it should be frequently responsible for illness in fanciers. There are no data to support this, possibly because the disease in fanciers is misdiagnosed or it is less virulent and therefore not diagnosed. It is advisable to err on the side of caution and warn fanciers that there is the potential for severe human disease associated with this organism, and refer them to a doctor if they have any concerns regarding their own health. Avian chlamydophilosis is a notifiable disease.

Other bacterial infections

Streptococcus and *Salmonella* have been associated with respiratory signs in pigeons as part of a multisystemic problem. *Escherichia coli*, in association with adenovirus, has been suggested as a cause of respiratory clinical signs. Diagnosis and treatment is based on culture and sensitivity testing.

Mycoplasma

Three species, *Mycoplasma columborale*, *M. columbinasale* and *M. columbinum*, are shed in the faeces and respiratory secretions of healthy pigeons and pigeons exhibiting respiratory clinical signs. It can be transmitted by inhalation or ingestion. *Mycoplasma* is difficult to culture and there is debate as to whether or not it has a role in pathogenicity, but it is often lauded as a cause of 'one-eyed cold' syndrome. Treatment with tetracyclines can elicit a positive response.

Miscellaneous

Some respiratory signs, such as laboured breathing and increased respiratory effort, may be associated with other factors, for instance anaemia caused by endoparasites. This should be borne in mind when assessing the respiratory system.

Skin and feather disease

Lice and mites

There are a number of species of lice and mites that affect pigeons, including the louse *Columbicola columbae*. Most heavy infestations are associated with underlying problems and a general investigation should be carried out. Treatment is with permethrins.

Neurological disease

Paramyxovirus

Cause: Pigeon paramyxovirus is caused by a type 1 virus (PMV-1) that is recognized as distinctly different from the PMV-1 that causes Newcastle Disease in poultry. As such, it falls outside the international legislation that precludes poultry movement from a PMV-1 infected area to a PMV-1 free area. However, pigeon PMV-1 can cause disease in poultry and because of the similarities in the clinical disease, pigeon paramyxovirus is a notifiable disease in many countries, with movement restrictions on pigeon lofts in the UK imposed for 60 days after the clinical signs abate.

Clinical signs: The incubation period of pigeon PMV-1 infection can be a few weeks and in an outbreak new cases are presented over several months. The main presenting signs are excessive drinking with very watery diarrhoea. This is followed by nervous signs such as head tremors, torticollis, wing or leg paralysis, and poor vision where birds peck at but fail to pick up grain. If birds are affected during moulting, then poor feathering can occur.

Diagnostics and treatment: The disease can be confirmed by serology and isolation of the virus. Birds may be treated symptomatically with careful nursing, but if neurological clinical signs develop then recovery is unlikely. It is recommended that all remaining healthy birds are vaccinated as soon as possible during an outbreak. The highest standards of hygiene must be enforced, along with closure of the loft to visitors and a ban on all bird movements in or out of the loft.

Although pigeon paramyxovirus is endemic in feral pigeon populations, in many countries it is compulsory to vaccinate racing pigeons annually to minimize the impact of potential cross-over of the disease from pigeons to poultry. In racing pigeons, the disease can have a devastating effect on a loft, and vaccination would be highly recommended to fanciers in any case. Veterinary surgeons should also be aware that clinical outbreaks of pigeon paramyxovirus still occasionally occur in vaccinated flocks. Even though the vaccine is a prescription-only medicine (POM), fanciers are permitted to purchase and administer their own vaccine in the UK and Ireland. However, it should be noted that if the correct vaccines are not used, and if they are not stored and administered properly, then apparent vaccine breakdown could occur. It has also been suggested that circovirus infection may affect the immune response to vaccination, although no data are available to support this theory.

Multisystemic disease

Salmonellosis

Cause: Salmonellosis in pigeons is usually caused by *Salmonella typhimurium* variant *copenhagen*, a Gram-negative bacterium. Salmonellosis can affect all ages of pigeons.

Clinical signs: Eggs infected *in utero* or via faecal contamination in the nest may fail to hatch, or result in weakened chicks with poor survival. In young pigeons, infection can lead to enteritis and high mortality. Stressed birds may develop other signs, including weight loss, pneumonia, ocular discharge, peri-ophthalmic swellings, panophthalmitis or loss of colour in one or both irises. Sometimes blindness, head tilting or torticollis due to brain abscesses may be seen. Adult birds are generally more resistant to acute infection but they may be carriers infecting young birds.

Birds become carriers when *Salmonella* naturally persists intracellularly in pigeon macrophages. The prevalence of carriers can be escalated by the injudicious use of antibiotics if an adequate minimum inhibitory concentration is not maintained; unfortunately, the tendency for fanciers to administer medicines without veterinary intervention is problematic in this regard. Chronically infected adult birds can develop arthritic lesions, leading to lameness and wing drooping. If *Salmonella* affects the reproductive organs, infertility may result. Morbidity in young birds is usually higher than in adults. Stressors include breeding, overcrowding and racing. Over time, a variety of the above clinical signs will be seen in an infected loft.

Diagnostics: *Salmonella* infection should be suspected from the loft history and clinical signs. Diagnosis is confirmed by culture of the organism using enrichment techniques. Chronically infected birds and carriers may only excrete the organism intermittently and isolation may take a few attempts, especially if there has been prior treatment with antibiotics. Suspicion of the disease may require post-mortem examination of a sick individual, followed by culture of lesions for confirmation. Affected joints require maceration before culture.

Treatment: Once infection in a loft has been confirmed, it should be made clear to the fancier that elimination of the organism from the loft can be difficult and perhaps impossible. The authors have had success in eliminating recurrence of clinical signs from lofts with salmonellosis using the following method, involving the equally important elements of culling, hygiene and treatment.

- Firstly, cull all clinically ill animals, and attempt to identify any familial lines of ill birds and cull the parent birds.
- Institute a hygiene programme with removal of all droppings, and cleansing and disinfection of all internal structures within the loft.

- The remaining birds are then treated with a 10-day course of an antibiotic to which the isolated organism has been shown to be sensitive.
- Cull any more individuals that have developed clinical evidence of disease and repeat the hygiene programme.
- Administer a further 10-day course of treatment with a different class of antibiotic to which the organism is sensitive.
- A final hygiene programme is carried out at the end of the second treatment.

Although it is impossible to be sure that no carrier birds remain after this regimen, the authors have found that lofts have not reported any clinical signs in the birds for up to 4 years after the *Salmonella* isolation. One loft had continued problems because the fancier found it difficult to cull some of the older birds due to breeding value; this loft instituted an annual *Salmonella* vaccination programme. Although, vaccination against S*almonella* in pigeons is not totally preventive and is not expected to eliminate carrier birds, it is useful to help minimize the number of birds affected with clinical disease over time.

Zoonosis: Salmonellosis is a zoonotic disease and fanciers must be informed that during an outbreak there is an increased need for careful personal hygiene around the birds. Fanciers need to minimize the risk of the disease being passed to others by restricting access to the lofts, appropriate use of disinfectant and correct disposal of carcasses. Depopulating the loft and buying in replacement stock is not an option due to the impossibility of obtaining certified *Salmonella*-free replacement birds.

Streptococcal infection

Streptococcus spp., in particular *S. bovis*, can be isolated from pigeons and the effects can be benign or can cause severe multisystemic disease with a variety of signs resembling salmonellosis. Further, streptococci can localize and cause severe necrosis in muscles, which can result in lameness and wing droop. Some birds with enteritis produce characteristic foamy, slimy faeces accompanied by a swollen abdomen. By far the most common sign is sudden death following septicaemia, with severe inflammation of all the internal organs. Culture and histopathology are required to confirm the diagnosis. This condition can respond well to appropriate antibiotic therapy if caught in the early stages.

Supportive care

Individual sick birds benefit from supportive care. Such birds should be isolated in a warm, darkened area and nutritional support, fluids and electrolytes should be provided via an intraosseous, intravenous, subcutaneous or oral route as indicated. For common treatments, see Figure 10.11. Occasionally, euthanasia may be necessary but the value of the bird in determining possible threats to the loft should not be overlooked. A post-mortem examination should be offered as part of the health management plan.

Anaesthesia and analgesia

Isoflurane is the anaesthetic of choice for racing pigeons. Induction can be achieved by use of an induction chamber. For information on common analgesics used in pigeons, see Figure 10.11.

Common surgical procedures

The requirement for surgery in racing pigeons is uncommon. Foreign body obstruction with resultant perforation and peritonitis can be seen occasionally. Trauma occurs in racing pigeons that fly into electrical or telephone lines, or survive a peregrine attack. Crop tears are common and respond well to appropriate surgery with careful debridement of the necrotic tissue and proper anatomical realignment of structures. Such individuals may be presented for treatment, sometimes after the fanciers have attempted first aid. The individual bird's value may influence whether the fancier funds the necessary surgery, but euthanasia may be required.

Occasionally, keratinized tissue builds up under a bird's leg ring, causing pressure necrosis of the underlying tissues and oedema of the distal limb. The bird shows lameness of the affected leg, usually when the process is advanced. The ring must be removed and the procedure can be safely carried out under general anaesthesia.

1. Carefully saw through the ring on opposing sides. Cutting one side and trying to prise the ring off can cause further irreversible limb damage.
2. Remove the ring in two pieces.
3. Debride and clean the wound.

The healing scar needs to be monitored carefully as it too may cause a constricting pressure necrosis. If the lower limb swelling does not resolve or continues to worsen after ring removal, then it may be necessary to incise the constricting scar tissue by vertical incisions on the medial and lateral aspects of the limb. Regular foot massage in lukewarm water and judicious use of furosemide and non-steroidal anti-inflammatory drugs (NSAIDs) can help alleviate oedema and inflammation and decrease pain, enabling return of use of the foot. Fanciers should be advised to check regularly that leg rings are freely moveable (when handling the birds) and to remove dead and keratinized tissue from underneath rings that are tight.

Euthanasia

Euthanasia can be achieved by the administration of pentobarbital sodium via a suitable intravenous route. If necessary, birds can be initially anaesthetized with isoflurane and euthanased with a percutaneous hepatic injection of a barbiturate.

Drug formulary

A basic drug formulary is presented in Figure 10.11.

Drug	Dose	Comments
Antifungal agents		
Nystatin	10,000–50,000 IU/bird orally q24h	For candidiasis
Antibiotics		
Amoxicillin	20 mg/kg orally/i.m. q24h	For sensitive bacteria
Enrofloxacin	5–10 mg/kg orally/i.m. q24h	For sensitive bacteria
Oxytetracycline	60–100 mg/kg orally/i.m. q24h	For sensitive bacteria; chlamydophilosis; *Mycoplasma*
Tylosin	50 mg/kg orally q24h	For *Mycoplasma*; sensitive bacteria
Antibacterial agents		
Doxycycline	15–40 mg/kg orally q24h or 200–500 mg/l drinking water (soft water only)	For chlamydophilosis
Sulfadimidine	100–120 mg/kg orally q24h	For sensitive bacteria
Trimethoprim/Sulfadiazine	Sulphonamide at 20–40 mg/kg orally/i.m. q24h	For sensitive bacteria
Antiprotozoal agents		
Metronidazole	50 mg/kg orally q24h	For trichomoniasis; hexamitiasis
Sulfadimethoxine	50 mg/kg orally q24h	For Coccidia
Antihelminthic agents		
Fenbendazole	20 mg/kg orally; repeat in 3 weeks	For ascarids; *Capillaria*
Piperazine	100 mg/kg orally; repeat in 3 weeks	For ascarids
Insecticides		
Ivermectin	200 µg/kg orally/i.m.	For lice; mites
Permethrin	1:100 dilution of 4% solution (apply as spray; ensure operator safety)	For lice; mites
Vaccines		
Pigeon paramyxovirus (Colombovac PMV) (Nobivac Paramyxo)	0.2 ml s.c. annually 0.25 ml s.c. annually	For paramyxovirus
Salmonella typhimurium/ S. enteritidis (Salenvac T)	0.2 ml s.c. twice, 4 weeks apart and then once annually	For salmonellosis
Miscellaneous		
Carprofen	2–4 mg/kg orally/i.m. q24h	Anti-inflammatory; pain killer
Furosemide	2–4 mg/kg orally/i.m. q24h	Oedema
2.5% Glucosaline	40–100 ml/kg orally/i.v. q24h	Fluid therapy
Meloxicam	0.1–0.2 mg/kg orally/i.m. q24h	Anti-inflammatory; pain killer
Pentobarbital sodium	200 mg/kg i.v./intrahepatic in anaesthetized bird	Euthanasia

10.11 Drug formulary for racing pigeons.

References and further reading

Scullion FT and Scullion MG (2007) Pathologic findings in racing pigeons (*Columba livia domestica*) with 'Young bird sickness'. *Journal of Avian Medicine and Surgery* **21(1)**, 1–7

Vogel L, Gerlach H and Löffler M (1994) Columbiformes. In: *Avian Medicine: principles and application*, ed. B Ritchie *et al.*, pp. 1200–1217. Wingers Publishing Inc., Lake Worth, Florida

Useful website

Disease fact sheet: Paramyxovirus in pigeons
www.gov.uk/paramyxovirus-infection

11

Birds of prey

John Chitty

Introduction

Falconry has been practised for many centuries, and diseases of birds of prey have been studied and documented for a long time; several Arabic treatises on the subject survive from the ninth century. Many birds of prey are now kept for private falconry, falconry displays, bird control (e.g. at airports and rubbish dumps) and breeding, as well as in zoological collections. Therefore, veterinary clinics will see raptors from time to time, and these birds are often presented in need of emergency stabilization following trauma or acute illness. Wild casualty birds are also frequently presented to clinics. Although this chapter does not specifically cover wildlife rehabilitation, many of the points raised are applicable to both captive and wild raptors.

In the UK, it is illegal to take any raptor from the wild (alive or dead) and keep it, or any part of it, without a licence. If an injured wild raptor is taken, a licence should be obtained immediately from the Department of the Environment, Food and Rural Affairs (Defra), unless the bird is passed to a veterinary surgeon or to a person licensed to treat and release birds. An application to hold a bird unable to be released should be supported by a statement from a veterinary surgeon that the bird would not be able to survive in the wild if released.

Although there is no need to hold a formal licence to own or fly a bird of prey, there are specific legal requirements in the UK to register certain species:

- In the UK there are currently differences in the registration requirements In England, Scotland and Wales for many of the Schedule 4 species, with Scotland and Wales requiring more species to be registered than England. Therefore, when purchasing a Schedule 4 species, or transporting it between countries for falconry, it is important to check with the relevant government department as to the exact registration requirements
- Under Section 7 of the Wildlife and Countryside Act 1981, any bird listed in Schedule 4 of the Act and kept in captivity must be registered with Defra and fitted with an official ring. Of the species listed, those most commonly encountered are the northern goshawk (*Accipiter gentilis*) and the merlin (*Falco columbarius*)
- From 1 April 1998 all species listed in Annex A of EC Regulation 338/97 require Article 10 Certificates if they are to be used commercially (e.g. public display, sale or commercial breeding). The bird must be identified by a closed ring or microchip, and the application should be supported by information to prove that it was legally acquired. Zoological collections can apply for an Article 60 Certificate to cover all their birds for public display, but those used for commercial breeding still require an individual Article 10 Certificate. Species covered by this Annex include most of those commonly used in falconry, with the exception of the Harris' hawk (*Parabuteo unicinctus*)
- If the bird is to be flown at birds not listed in Schedule 2 of the Wildlife and Countryside Act 1981, a quarry licence is required.

Biology

Birds of prey may be classed as raptors and form two groups:

- Diurnal – mainly the Falconiformes (e.g. hawks, falcons, eagles, vultures)
- Nocturnal – principally the Strigiformes (owls).

A wide range of species is kept in zoological collections, from African pygmy falcons (*Polihierax semitorquatus*) to Andean condors (*Vultur gryphus*), but the range of those commonly used in falconry is much more limited (Figures 11.1 and 11.2). Typical bodyweights and other biological data for common species are given in Figures 11.3 and 11.4.

Class	Examples
Hawks ('short-wings')	Harris' hawk (*Parabuteo unicinctus*), the most commonly used falconry bird (see Figure 11.2a); northern goshawk (*Accipiter gentilis*); red-tailed hawk (*Buteo jamaicensis*)
Falcons ('long-wings')	Peregrine falcon (*Falco peregrinus*); lanner (*F. biarmicus*, see Figure 11.2b); Saker (*F. cherrug*, see Figure 11.2c); merlin (*F. columbarius*, see Figure 11.2d)
Eagles	Golden eagle (*Aquila chrysaetos*); Steppe eagle (*A. nipalensis*); martial eagle (*Polemactus bellicosus*)
Owls	Eurasian eagle owl (*Bubo bubo*, Figure 11.2e); Bengalese eagle owl (*B. bengalensis*); barn owl (*Tyto alba*)

11.1 Classification of falconry birds.

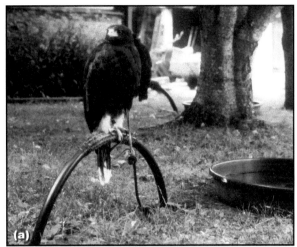

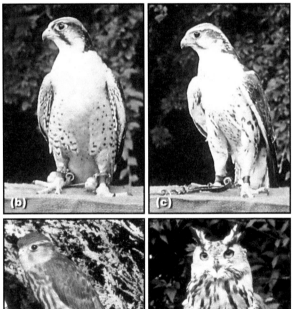

Species	Male (g)	Female (g)
Merlin	160–170	220–250
Lanner	450–600	700–950
Peregrine	550–850	1100–1600
Saker	650–1000	950–1350
Harris' hawk	550–800	850–1300
Goshawk	650–850	950–1200
Golden eagle	2850–4500	3650–6700
Andean condor	11000–15000	8000–11000
Barn owl	200–400	350–500
Eurasian eagle owl	1500–2500	2250–3800

11.4 Typical bodyweight of common birds of prey.

Eagles are used only occasionally for falconry. Owls are rarely flown at quarry, but are frequently kept as breeding birds or as part of a growing 'pet' population.

Sexing

Sexual dimorphism is comparatively unusual in birds of prey, although there is often a size difference. Typically, the female is larger than the male (though this may be reversed in the large vultures). The difference may be very marked; for example, in the peregrine, the falcon (female) is a third larger than the tiercel (male) (Figure 11.5). However, in some species, particularly the buzzards (*Buteo* spp.), there may be some overlap. If there is doubt, sexing may be performed by laparoscopy or by DNA analysis (blood or feather).

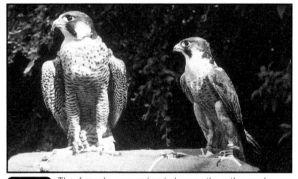

11.2 Some falconry species. **(a)** Harris' hawk tethered on bow perch (note provision of water for bathing and drinking). **(b)** Lanner. **(c)** Saker. **(d)** Merlin. **(e)** Eurasian eagle owl. (© J. Chitty.)

11.5 The female peregrine is larger than the male. (© J. Chitty.)

	Merlins	Peregrine falcons	Harris' hawks	Goshawks	Golden eagles	European eagle owls
Lifespan (years)	10–14	15–20	20–30	15–20	50–60	50–60
Age at sexual maturity (years)	2	3+	3+	3+	5+	2+
Clutch size	2–7	2–6	2–4	2–5	1–3	2–4
Incubation period (days)	28–32	29–32	28	35–38	43–45	32–35
Normal quarry	Skylark	Grouse; partridge; rook	Rabbit; pheasant	Rabbit; hare; gamebird	Rabbit; hare	Rarely used; rabbit (?)

11.3 Biological data for some common birds of prey.

Husbandry

It is useful to have a working knowledge of the many terms peculiar to falconry (Figure 11.6) and of the considerable amount of specialist equipment (or 'furniture') used for falconry birds (Figure 11.7). This equipment should be individually fitted for each bird and carefully maintained. Failure to do so can result in severe injuries.

Housing

There are two basic systems for keeping raptors: tethered and in aviaries.

- Tethered on blocks or perches is for flying birds. They should be taken off daily for exercise, for demonstration flying to the lure or for flying at quarry. Perches must be well maintained. In zoological collections (and recommended for private holders), vultures and owls should not be tethered.
- Aviaries are generally for breeding or exhibition birds, or for flying birds in the closed season, although some birds may be flown from the aviary.

Term	Definition
Bate/ bating-off	Excitable/panicked flight attempt by a tethered bird on fist or block/perch
Cast	1. Two or more birds flown together 2. To grab and hold for examination 3. To regurgitate a pellet
Cast off	To release from the fist
Casting	Indigestible part of the diet
Cope	To trim beak/talons
Crab, to	A term relating to one bird of prey footing another
Creance	Light line used to fly a bird during training
Eyass	Bird taken from the nest in the first year
Foot, to	To strike with the feet
Furniture	Collective term for jesses, bell, telemetry, etc.
Imp	The replacement of a damaged feather by gluing a new tip on to the old broken feather
Keen, to be	When a bird's weight is reduced a little, it responds well and is eager to fly or hunt
Man, to	To tame a bird so it will accept handling and training
Mantle	Spreading wings over food
Mews	Building where trained; tethered birds are kept inside at night or in bad weather, or outside but under shelter
Mutes	Droppings
Rangle	Indigestible material (e.g. stones) sometimes ingested accidentally. Formerly given deliberately to clean out the crop
Rouse	Vigorous shaking of the feathers, usually just before flight
Stoop	The attack method used by falcons, a steep fast dive
Wait on	Falcons circling over the falconer waiting for game to be flushed
Weathering	Area where birds may be placed outside on a perch during the day to sun themselves
Yarrack	As for keen (hungry and ready for work)

11.6   Glossary of falconry terms.

Equipment	Denfition/notes
Aylmeri	Leather anklet secured with a rivet or grommet
Bells	Attached to legs or tail to help track the bird
Bewit	Leather strap for attaching bells to the leg
Block	Solid perch with a padded top (for falcons)
Bow perch	Semicircular bar with a padded region for perching (for hawks, eagles, owls)
Cadge	A portable perch used for carrying several birds together
Creance	Long line attached to jesses and used when training
Hood	Leather 'cap' used to cover the eyes and calm the bird (for falcons and occasionally hawks)
Jesse	Leather strap; passes through the aylmeri (or directly round the legs) to enable restraint
Leash	Attached to swivel; used to secure bird
Mews	Housing for tethered raptors
Swivel	Metal ringed device to link jesses to leash
Telemetry	Radio-tracking device attached to bird's tail when flown

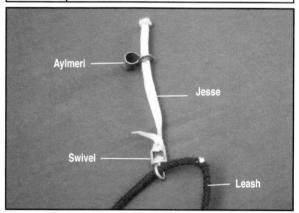

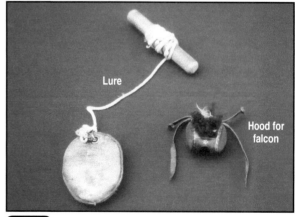

11.7   Falconry equipment. (© J. Chitty.)

In both situations, shelter from inclement conditions should be provided. Further aspects of this subject are provided in the *Code of Welfare and Husbandry of Birds of Prey and Owls* from the British Field Sports Society and in two guidelines from the Federation of Zoological Gardens of Great Britain and Ireland (now the British and Irish Association of Zoos and Aquaria, BIAZA): *Management Guidelines for the Welfare of Zoo Animals: Birds of Prey in Flying Demonstrations* and *Management Guidelines for the Welfare of Zoo Animals: Falconiformes.*

Diet

It is not possible to cover raptor nutrition fully here but there are certain principles:

- Raptors are 'whole carcass' feeders and so should be offered whole carcasses:
  - Evisceration of carcasses will result in loss of essential nutrients
  - Feeding of muscle (e.g. beef) should be avoided, as it cannot provide balanced nutrition (Figure 11.8a)
  - The size of the food item should reflect the size of the bird eating it; for example, the kestrel (*Falco tinnunculus*) cannot cope with rabbit carcasses
  - It is wise to break the long bones of rabbits and hares prior to feeding; if whole legs are swallowed they may cause an obstruction.
- The quantity of food provided should reflect the amount of work the bird is undertaking. Hunting birds have a tightly regulated diet, with performance being closely associated with bodyweight and condition (hunger and 'keenness'). However, aviary birds may have less control over their diet and are exercised less, which may predispose to hepatic lipidosis and/or atherosclerosis (Figure 11.8b)
- Where possible, the food offered should mimic the bird's natural diet; for example, kestrels and barn owls should be offered small rodents, larger owls should receive larger rodents, and the large eagles or vultures may be offered whole rabbit, hare or lamb carcasses
- No single food item will provide all the bird's nutritional requirements at all life stages; therefore, a mixed diet should be fed
- Day-old chicks (DOCs) are the most common staple diet for the majority of raptors, and their value as a food item is considerable:
  - Contrary to previous belief, DOCs have a good Ca:P ratio, good vitamin levels, and not excessive lipid levels
  - It should be noted that this applies only if the yolk sacs are not removed. An exception is when feeding merlins, which are prone to a fatty liver/kidney syndrome (Forbes and Cooper, 1993). This may be due to high lipid levels in the diet or may be due to high avidin levels in the yolk (Rees-Davies, 2000). It is wise, therefore, to feed merlins on deyolked DOCs plus immature rodents
  - Growing or breeding birds should be given a calcium/vitamin D3 supplement.

- Vitamin supplementation should be unnecessary if a correct, well balanced diet is fed:
  - Supplementation may even be counterproductive, as an overdose of one fat-soluble vitamin may lead to deficiency of another because of competitive absorption from the gut
  - However, supplementation may be appropriate at certain times; for example, the use of a high calcium/vitamin D3 supplement prior to the breeding season.
- Good quality food should be used:
  - Carcasses should be fed fresh or properly thawed (and not refrozen)
  - Uneaten food should be removed daily
  - It is wise not to feed roadkill (even if found fresh) or shot game (even if head shot)
  - Feeding fresh pigeon should be avoided, as pigeons may carry many diseases (e.g. trichomoniasis, see Chapter 10). Freezing and subsequent thawing will eliminate some of these diseases, but not all.
- Water is essential. It is often stated that raptors do not drink but this is untrue, although drinking may be infrequent. Birds of prey should always be offered clean, fresh water for bathing and drinking.

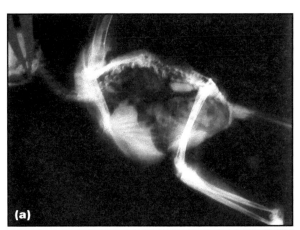

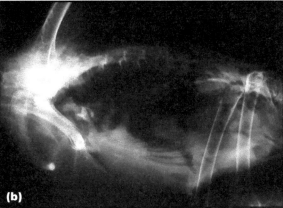

11.8 **(a)** Lateral radiograph showing 'collapsed spine' in a juvenile Bengalese eagle owl reared on a meat-based diet. Failure to provide bone or vitamin/mineral supplementation resulted in nutritional secondary hyperparathyroidism. Spinal deformities appear a common consequence in these large fast-growing owls. **(b)** Atherosclerosis in a falcon. Lateral radiograph showing a thickened aorta. (© J. Chitty.)

- Some birds are messy feeders (especially on DOCs) and fail to clean themselves properly. It is important that food material is removed from under the talons, to avoid the development of skin necrosis and thence deeper infections.

For a comprehensive guide to this subject, see the excellent book *Raptor Nutrition* (Forbes and Flint, 2000) and Chitty (2008).

Identification

Microchip implants should be inserted into the caudal third of the left pectoral muscle mass (Figure 11.9). The feathers should be parted and the site cleaned prior to implantation. Where necessary, bleeding should be stopped using digital pressure and the skin closed using tissue glue or a single suture. Anaesthesia is generally not required for this procedure but should be considered if the implanter is not confident or if the bird is very small.

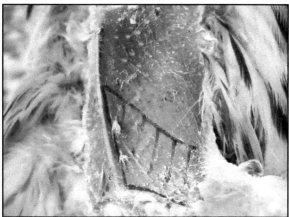

11.9 Microchip implantation site/intramuscular injection site highlighted in the left pectoral muscle of this emaciated kestrel. (Reproduced from the *BSAVA Manual of Raptors, Pigeons and Passerine Birds*.) (© J. Chitty.)

Handling and restraint

It is impossible to examine a bird of prey without handling it.

- With raptors, the feet are more dangerous than the beak (although falcons may give a painful 'nip') and so it is essential to restrain the feet first.
- If handling larger birds (eagles or vultures), the beak may also be capable of causing injury and these birds often require several handlers. In addition, vultures may vomit foul-smelling stomach contents when handled.

To examine a bird, it is 'cast'. If it is used to being hooded, the hood should be fitted first to reduce the bird's anxiety; otherwise, the bird can be taken into a dimly lit room. To cast a typical bird weighing approximately 1 kg (e.g. Harris' hawk):

1. Grasp the bird from behind with both hands, using a towel (*not* gloves). The thumbs should face toward the head.

2. Wrap the towel quickly around the body (taking care not to restrict breathing). Hold the wings in the towel by the thumbs and first two fingers of each hand (Figure 11.10a).
3. With the remaining fingers, grasp each leg as far down as possible to restrict movement (Figure 11.10b).
4. Place fingers between the bird's legs so that it cannot grab itself or damage its legs against each other. With smaller birds, one hand can hold the wings whilst the other holds the feet (Figure 11.10c). With larger birds, it is advisable to have several people helping.
5. If the bird is not hooded, part of the towel can be used to cover the eyes.

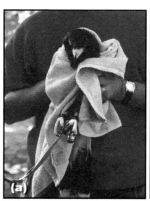 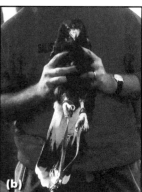
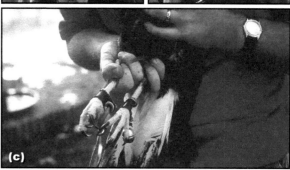

11.10 Casting. **(a)** Harris' hawk cast in a towel. **(b)** Towel removed. Note the position of the fingers holding the legs. **(c)** Holding the feet. Note the fingers between the legs. (© J. Chitty.)

It is important to hold birds firmly so that they do not struggle and damage themselves. Once wrapped in a towel and secured, most birds do not struggle. As many falconers are very adept at handling their birds, it is often sensible to allow them to restrain their own bird.

Diagnostic approach

History

History-taking is a very important aspect of disease investigation and the following points should be covered:

- Species, age, sex (if known)
- When purchased or bred
- Other birds kept
- Disease history of this bird and others in the collection

- Husbandry: aviary or tethered, flying bird or breeding only, when last flown (if at all)
- Diet:
  - What and how fed, and how much
  - Source: wild quarry (shot or caught?) or farmed
  - Supplements used
  - Is casting being fed?
- Weight:
  - What are the normal flying and moulting weights for this bird?
  - Is the weight being dropped deliberately at present (e.g. in training)?
  - Is the bird's weight more or less than would normally be expected at current level of feeding?
- Flying:
  - How keen is the bird to fly?
  - Is it tiring easily?
- Disease history: duration, recent injuries (no matter how minor), medications administered or applied already
- Mutes: do they appear normal?
- Casting: when did the bird last cast and was it normal?

Clinical examination

If at any stage the bird becomes very distressed or still, examination should be discontinued and the bird's condition reassessed. If necessary, the examination should be performed with supplemental oxygen to hand. If the bird cannot be examined without harming it, anaesthesia should be considered.

Head

- Beak and cere: for damage and beak quality (signs of metabolic disturbance or poor diet).
- Nares: for discharge.
- Eyes (Figure 11.11).
- Periorbital sinuses: to distinguish periocular swelling from ocular disease.
- Ears: for discharge or bleeding (post-trauma) (Figure 11.12).

Sinus flushing may be performed for diagnosis or treatment.

Mouth

- Lesions (especially plaques) and *Capillaria* worms at the back of the mouth (Figure 11.13a).
- Choanal slit (Figure 11.13b): discharge and swelling in upper respiratory tract (URT) infection; swabs should be taken from the rostral part of the choanal slit to test for URT infections.
- Glottis: swelling, discharge and *Syngamus* worms.

Eye reflexes
Hard to assess. Threat reflexes are often inapparent and because of the bird's conscious control of pupil size, the pupillary light reflex is unreliable. A consensual light reflex may be apparent, but this is often due to the passage of light directly to the contralateral retina via the very thin bone separating the eyes
Anterior segment
May be examined using routine direct or indirect ophthalmoscopy methods. Consideration should be paid to: • Eyelids and conjunctivae (e.g. swelling) • Nictitating membrane (e.g. trauma) • Cornea (e.g. ulcers, trauma) • Anterior chamber (e.g. presence of blood, pus, 'flare') • Uvea (e.g. inflammation) • Lens (e.g. cataract, displacement).   The nictitating membrane should be lifted to allow examination of the large lacrymal duct opening
Drainage angle
May be directly visualized from the side in large owls
Posterior segment
Examination presents problems as it is so difficult to dilate the pupil. Mammalian mydriatics are ineffective in birds owing to the striated muscle in the avian iris. Topical vecuronium may induce mydriasis but should be used with great care. The most reliable method appears to be to examine under anaesthesia. This is essential in all known or suspected cases of head trauma, as contre-coup injuries result in bleeding from the delicate pecten. This will ultimately result in severe retinal damage and blindness without prompt anti-inflammatory therapy. Without full binocular vision birds will have difficulty hunting

11.11 Ocular examination, an essential part of any clinical examination.

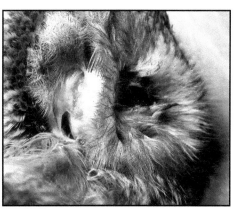

11.12 Bruising on the surface of the globe is visible in the ear of this tawny owl. It can be deduced that there will be haemorrhage within the posterior chamber of the eye. (© J. Chitty.)

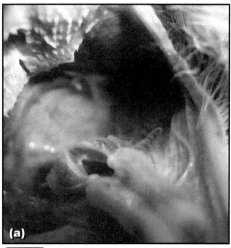

(a)

11.13 **(a)** *Capillaria* nematodes in the pharynx of a tawny owl. (© J. Chitty.) (continues) ▶

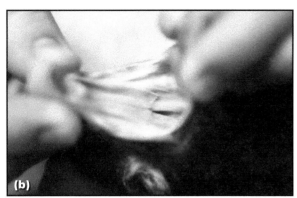

11.13 (continued) **(b)** Choanal slit of a striated caracara. Ideal site for entry of an endoscope or swab in investigation of upper respiratory tract disease. Discharge or haemorrhage from this slit may give information regarding the health of the upper respiratory system. (© J. Chitty.)

Skin and plumage

- Parasites.
- Lesions.
- Quality of feathering (including presence of 'fret' marks).
- Subcutaneous emphysema.
- Uropygial gland.

Abdomen and crop

- Abdomen should be palpated for masses.
- Crop (not present in owls) should be palpated for fluid filling and foreign bodies.

Cloaca

The cloaca should be checked for swelling or prolapse and for soiling of the surrounding feathers. Digital or auriscopic examination can be performed under anaesthesia, or when conscious for large tractable birds.

Limbs

Pectoral and pelvic limbs should be thoroughly examined with all joints flexed, extended and palpated. This part of the examination may need to be performed under anaesthesia in order to assess shoulder and coxofemoral joints fully.

Feet

The feet should be checked for bumblefoot lesions, wounds, talon quality and damage, and the skin underneath any falconry equipment should be checked thoroughly for trauma.

Body condition

Body condition should be assessed by palpation of the pectoral muscle mass. This should be related to species, current weight (often done by the falconer, but should always be checked) and stage of training.

Auscultation

The pectoral area (heart), dorsum between the wings (lung sounds) and abdomen (air sac noise) should be auscultated.

Sample collection

Blood

The preferred site for blood collection is the right jugular vein (Figure 11.14a), which can be found and accessed easily in most species. In larger birds, restraint may be difficult and either the bird should be anaesthetized or the brachial vein should be used. The medial metatarsal vein may also be used, but working close to the feet may be risky in the conscious adult bird. However, it can be a useful site in chicks and vultures (Figure 11.14b).

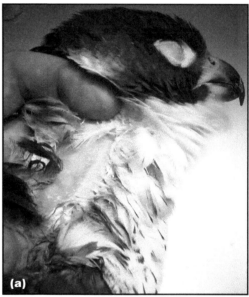

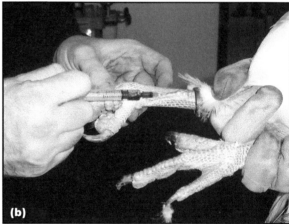

11.14 **(a)** Right jugular vein of a peregrine falcon. Note the large featherless tract under which the vein lies. (© J. Chitty.) **(b)** Venepuncture of the caudal tibial vein of a vulture. (Courtesy of the Hawk Conservancy Trust.) (Reproduced from the *BSAVA Manual of Raptors, Pigeons and Passerine Birds*.)

Samples for both haematological and biochemical analysis should usually be collected into lithium heparin tubes. Ideally, a fresh blood smear should be made at the time of collection. Wherever possible, laboratories with specialized knowledge of raptors should be used. It is wise to consult with the laboratory prior to blood collection to determine the exact requirements. Normal ranges for haematology and biochemistry are given in Figure 11.15.

Parameter	Northern goshawks	Peregrine falcons	Harris' hawks	Tawny eagles	Northern eagle owls
Haematology					
WBC (x10⁹/l)	4–11	3.3–11	4.8–10	5–9.5	3.5–12.1
RBC (x10¹²/l)	2.6–3.48	2.95–3.94	2.63–3.5	1.65–2.35	1.65–2.35
PCV (%)	0.43–0.53	0.37–0.53	0.4–0.55	0.37–0.47	0.36–0.52
Hb (g/l)	121–177	118–188	121–171	108–175	107–180
Heterophils (%)	3.5–6.97	1.4–8.55	2.3–6.71	3.58–6.45	2.2–9.23
Lymphocytes (%)	1.38–1.93	1.1–3.3	0.6–2.36	0.51–2.72	1.5–5.07
Monocytes (%)	0–0.1	0.1–0.86	0.2–1.49	0.2–1.07	0–0.48
Eosinophils (%)	0–0.65	0–0.3	0–0.75	0.3–2.1	0–0.48
Basophils (%)	0–0.35	0–0.6	0–1.55	0–0.4	0–0.35
Biochemistry					
Total protein (g/l)	26.3–42	16.0–38.9 [a] 24–41	31–45.7	29–41.4	30.1–34.5
Albumin (g/l)	8.8–12.4	6.9–14.8 [a] 12.7–22.4	13.9–17	11.1–13.5	11.1–13.5
Globulin (g/l)	18–29.2		21–29.4	25.3–28.4	18.7–22.4
Uric acid (µmol/l)	511–854	170–1250 [a]	533–785	413–576	475–832
Calcium (mmol/l)	2.15–2.69	1.94–2.54 [a]	2.1–2.66	2.21–2.66	2.16–2.61
AST (IU/l)	176–409 0–31 (GOT)	35–327 [a] 34–162	160–348	124–226	
Creatine kinase (IU/l)	218–775	120–442 [b]	224–650		

11.15 Haematology and biochemistry reference ranges. [a] Lierz and Hafez (2006); [b] Lumeij *et al.* (1998).

Common conditions

Common clinical signs and differential diagnoses are summarized in Figure 11.16. The list is by no means exhaustive, nor intended to be, but provides a guide to the more common conditions seen in captive birds of prey. A drug formulary for raptors is given at the end of this chapter.

Clinical sign	Differential diagnoses	Primary diagnostic tests	Secondary diagnostic tests	Comments
Mouth/crop lesions	Trichomoniasis; candidiasis; bacterial infection; capillariasis; hypovitaminosis A; herpesvirus; injury/burn	Wet mount/cytology of lesions; culture/sensitivity of lesions (after debridement); thorough dietary history	Endoscopy of oesophagus and choanal slit; crop flush; haematology; biochemistry; biopsy	Accompanying signs include head shaking, flicking food, dysphagia, regurgitation, acute/peracute death (herpesvirus)
Head shaking	As per mouth/crop lesions; sinusitis; upper respiratory tract infection (bacterial/fungal/protozoal); otitis	As per mouth/crop lesions (if present); sinus flush (cytology with culture/sensitivity) and/or choanal swab (cytology with culture/sensitivity); aural examination and swab (cytology with culture/sensitivity) if discharge present; haematology	Endoscopy of choanal slit/ears; sinus radiography (including positive contrast studies)	
Upper respiratory tract disease (nares, sinuses)	As per head shaking; chlamydophilosis should also be considered if ocular signs present	Choanal swab (cytology with culture/sensitivity); conjunctival smear for cytology if chlamydophilosis suspected	As per head shaking	Clinical signs; ocular/nasal discharge; periorbital swelling; open-mouthed breathing; head shaking; sneezing; exercise intolerance; inspiratory effort

11.16 Common clinical signs and differential diagnoses. (continues) ▶

Clinical sign	Differential diagnoses	Primary diagnostic tests	Secondary diagnostic tests	Comments
Lower respiratory tract disease (trachea, syrinx, lungs, air sacs)	Bacterial/fungal infections; *Syngamus* (gapeworm) infection	Radiography (lateral and dorsoventral views); haematology; biochemistry; endoscopy of trachea/air sacs; faecal parasitology; culture/sensitivity and cytology of discharges and lesion biopsy samples		Clinical signs; change of voice (syringeal); inspiratory or expiratory (lungs/air sacs) effort; dyspnoea; exercise intolerance; weight loss; anorexia; vomition
ADR ('ain't doing right') syndrome (these cases can be among the most frustrating to diagnose)	As per mouth/crop lesions; endoparasitism; aspergillosis; avian tuberculosis; enteritis (including crop/proventriculus infection); hepatic/renal disease	As per mouth/crop lesions (if present); gross examination of mutes; haematology; biochemistry; radiography (lateral and ventrodorsal views); faecal parasitology; culture/sensitivity; acid-fast stain	Based on results of primary diagnostic tests; full range of tests, including laparoscopy and full body radiography will almost always be required	Clinical signs; loss of performance; weight loss; failure to gain weight; sometimes regurgitation/head flick
Regurgitation/vomition	Acute; 'sour crop' (foul-smelling crop/mouth due to bacterial/fungal infection, foreign body (especially long bones), may be secondary to enteritis); trichomoniasis; capillariasis; lead poisoning; air sacculitis (see Lower respiratory tract disease)	Crop wash (cytology, culture/sensitivity); haematology; biochemistry; radiography; faecal parasitology (culture/sensitivity if enteritis present)		As per mouth/crop lesions (if present); if chronic, follow ADR syndrome; if acute, treat as an emergency

11.16 (continued) Common clinical signs and differential diagnoses.

Gastrointestinal disease

Crop stasis

> **WARNING**
> If the crop has not emptied after a suitable period following a feed, it should be seen as an emergency. The time at which the falconer should be concerned will vary from bird to bird, and depends on the diet fed. In short, if the bird has not emptied its crop in the period it would normally (given that diet) then it should be presented for veterinary attention.

Fluids, antibiotics and metoclopramide (if a foreign body has been ruled out) may be effective. Surgical emptying of the crop should be considered if an obstruction is suspected and when medical therapy is not effective.

Loose mutes

Mutes should be collected on paper for examination. Mutes produced whilst travelling or just after should not be used as they are often looser than normal. It should be noted that raptor mutes are normally looser and more voluminous than those of seed-fed cage birds; the faecal portion is not formed.

Polyuria should be distinguished from enteritis and physiological causes (e.g. prior to egg-laying):

- Is the bird drinking?
- Does it have access to water?
- Is the urine discoloured? (Green = biliverdinuria)
- Is there blood in the urine? Clots of blood may indicate haemorrhage in the cloaca or the uterus (females). Blood throughout the urine indicates a renal origin.

Urinalysis (beware of faecal contamination), haematology/biochemistry analysis, radiography and blood lead estimation and, where indicated, organ biopsy should be performed.

Enteritis

Enteritis may be chronic (see ADR ('ain't doing right') syndrome, Figure 11.16) or acute.

> **WARNING**
> **Acute enteritis is an emergency!**

- Fluids and warmth should be given.
- Parasitology, cloacal culture and sensitivity, faecal Gram stain and haematology/biochemistry analysis should be performed.

Seizures and neurological disease

The differential diagnoses for seizures (fitting) and signs of neurological disease include hypoglycaemia, hypocalcaemia, lead poisoning, vitamin B1 deficiency, 'goshawk cramps' (aspergillosis), primary epilepsy (rare), meningitis and terminal state. Certain aspects of the history can give major clues to the diagnosis:

- Hypoglycaemia (during or just after exercise): is the bird's weight low compared with normal flying weight?
- Hypocalcaemia (young growing bird, breeding female): is the diet deficient?
- Lead poisoning: is wild quarry fed (even if not known to be shot, it may have been 'winged' by someone else)?
- Vitamin B1 deficiency: is the diet deficient? Have other causes been ruled out?
- 'Goshawk cramps' (paresis or paralysis of legs only, no fitting): rare in species other than the goshawk.

The veterinary surgeon should check whether the falconer has already given medication, and what the response was. During the clinical examination, the body condition of the bird should be noted and signs of trauma looked for. Lead poisoning is implicated if the feet are gripping each other.

WARNING
Seizures need to be controlled fast!

- Blood samples should be taken (haematology/ biochemistry, especially electrolytes, glucose, ionized calcium (total calcium levels can be misleading in some cases as this parameter will also vary with serum protein levels) and lead).
- Treatment should be given immediately for most likely diagnosis based on history.
- If the treatment is unsuccessful, glucose, calcium, edetate calcium disodium and vitamin B1 should be given by injection.
- If necessary, seizures should be controlled with diazepam or under isoflurane anaesthesia until a diagnosis is made.
- Radiography should be performed (for metal in gizzard).

Feather damage

Fret marks
Fret marks are damage lines on feathers due to dietary or metabolic stress at that stage of feather development.

- Many or all feathers affected.
- Dietary and disease history should be evaluated and a check made for endoparasites.
- If problems are ongoing, haematology/ biochemistry analysis and radiography should be performed.
- The condition often reflects past problems and so there is no treatment other than to wait for the next moult.
- Broken primary, secondary or tail feathers may be replaced by 'imping' a new feather on to the broken stump. Falconers should be encouraged to keep moulted feathers for future imping. If none of the bird's own feathers are available, feathers from other birds may be used but should be frozen for a period to reduce disease transmission.

Ectoparasites
Close examination should show the presence of ectoparasites, which may cause tatty feathers (see below).

Feather damaging disorders
Feather plucking and chewing have only recently been described in captive raptors. Nonetheless, these appear to be growing problems. As with feather destructive parrots, there appear to be many underlying causes (both medical and behavioural) (Jones, 2001; Chitty, 2005).

- Behavioural aspects appear important as the majority of cases occur in 'social' raptors, including Harris' hawks and (in the author's experience) kites and American black vultures.
- Hand-rearing may also be an important underlying factor.
- Many cases appear to occur during training, a particularly stressful period.
- Feather pulpitis also appears to be important, as all cases seen by the author have shown this on cytology and responded fully or partly to antibiosis. However, it is not known whether pulpitis is a primary, secondary or perpetuating factor in these cases. In one Brahminy kite (*Haliastur indus*), cyclical feather plucking appeared to be associated with pulpitis and seemed to recur on a seasonal basis, prompting concerns of an underlying allergic condition. However, it should also be borne in mind that many husbandry systems are also altered on a seasonal basis.
- Chewing of remiges does appear to be linked to bacterial folliculitis and in the author's experience is a primary cause of this sign.

Investigation of these cases should be similar to that undertaken in plucking parrots:

- Full history (including history of the condition): when started, area originally plucked/chewed, spread to other areas, when it occurs, vocalizations during plucking, associated with human/bird presence?
- Signalment
- Management
- Diet
- Clinical examination: dermatological examination and thorough search for ectoparasites, cytological sampling of feather pulp, skin scrapes/ impression smears/acetates of skin lesions, skin biopsy (including feather follicle) as necessary, blood sampling (full haematological and biochemical profile), faecal examination for endoparasites, radiography and other imaging modalities, depending on results of tests.

Elizabethan collars are rarely, if ever, recommended for this problem. Some authors advise use of modified hoods that prevent self-trauma, but these should be reserved for short-term use when the birds are causing active damage to themselves.

Aspergillosis
This is a common fungal disease of raptors. Certain species are especially prone, including the gyr falcon (*Falco rusticolus*), northern goshawk (*Accipiter gentilis*), golden eagle (*Aquila chrysaetos*) and snowy owl (*Nyctea scandinavica*).

Various syndromes are seen, including lower respiratory tract disease, tracheal or syringeal obstruction (change of voice is practically pathognomonic for syringeal aspergilloma; Figure 11.17a) and weight loss or ADR syndrome. The disease process may be chronic (often where latent infection has been triggered by stress, such as training) or acute (often

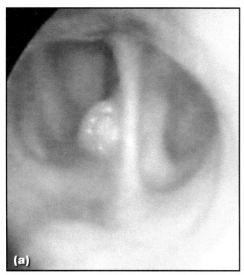

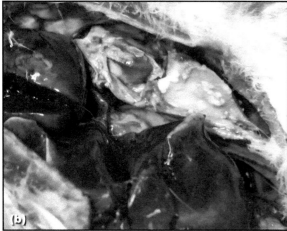

11.17 **(a)** Syringeal aspergilloma in a falcon.
(b) Large aspergilloma in the air sacs of a
falcon. These large encapsulated fungal abscesses will
require months of medical therapy and probably surgical
debridement. It is unlikely the bird will return to full hunting
fitness. Therefore, many falconers will elect for euthanasia
rather than incur the significant expense of treatment.
(© J. Chitty.)

where the immune system has been overwhelmed by
huge quantities of fungal spores). The prognosis is
usually poor.

Diagnosis

Diagnosis is by a combination of clinical examination
and history, radiography, haematology, serum
electrophoresis, endoscopy and tracheal/air sac
culture (current serological tests available in the UK
are of little value). Galactomannan levels show some
promise as a diagnostic test. Galactomannan is a
component of the cell wall of *Aspergillus* and is
released during growth. Detection of galactomannan
in blood is used to diagnose invasive aspergillosis
infections in humans.

Treatment

Individual aspergillomas should be removed
surgically after stabilization of the bird, especially for
the syringeal form; other forms should be managed
medically, at least initially. Therapy consists of
antifungal drugs given orally or systemically and by

nebulization or intratracheally. Therapy should continue for several weeks to months. The author's current preferred combination is oral itraconazole (or
voriconazole) and terbinafine with twice daily F10
nebulization. In severe cases the falconer should
always be warned that, even if therapy is successful,
the bird may not be able to perform optimally after-
wards (Figure 11.17b). Therefore, many falconers
may opt for euthanasia of the bird at an early stage,
especially if it is a young bird or hybrid species. As
ever in complex cases, communication with the falconer is of paramount importance.

Prevention

Prevention consists of avoiding inhalation of spores,
particularly when young birds are in the nest. Rotting
organic matter should be frequently removed from the
environment. Travelling boxes may also be a source of
spores and should be cleaned and disinfected after
each use (but note that cleaning immediately before
use may even induce fungal spore release). Susceptible species may be given itraconazole at times of
stress, e.g. training or travelling. Prophylactic dosing
should be started 5–7 days *before* training, to allow
effective tissue levels to be attained.

Bumblefoot

Bumblefoot is swelling of the plantar metatarsal pad
complicated by secondary bacterial infection. It is
seen in all species of raptor but can be especially
severe in falcons, eagles and owls.

Cause

There are many suggested aetiologies, including:

* Injury
* Self-induced injury
* Incorrect perching
* Poor perch hygiene
* Excess perching weight and inactivity
* Type III or IV hypersensitivity
* Hypovitaminosis A
* Cardiovascular changes.

In general, *Staphylococcus* is involved, although
environmental organisms (such as *Escherichia coli*
and *Proteus*) and *Candida* may be found.

Lesion classification

The most important aspect of bumblefoot is that it is a
two-footed problem. It is frequently seen in both feet,
but when it is unilateral the other ('good') leg should
be thoroughly assessed for injury or lesions that may
lead to increased weight-bearing (and hence bumblefoot) in the contralateral limb.

Various authors have proposed systems of
bumblefoot lesion classification (Bailey and Lloyd,
2008). For reasons of simplicity, the author prefers the
system proposed by Cooper (1978):

* Type 1: a proliferative thickening or degenerative
  thinning of the epithelium (Figure 11.18a)
* Type 2: more extensive combination of acute
  inflammation and chronic reaction. Purulent
  material is usually present (Figure 11.18b)

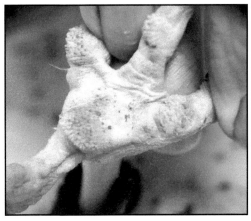
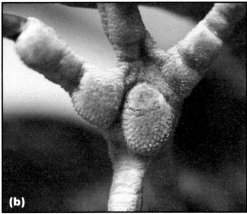

- Type 3: generally a progression of Type 2 into the underlying tissues (bones, tendon sheaths, joints). This type carries a very poor prognosis and euthanasia should be considered.

Diagnosis and treatment

In all cases, the feet should be radiographed to assess underlying damage and, hence, prognosis. All lesions should be swabbed for culture and sensitivity (after curettage in Types 2 and 3). All cases should receive long-term antimicrobials based on culture and sensitivity test results. Prior to obtaining results, therapy may be commenced with clavulanate-potentiated amoxicillin or a combination of marbofloxacin and clindamycin.

Type 1 cases may not require surgery, but the feet should be bandaged (Figure 11.19a). Dressings should be changed every 7–10 days. In unilateral cases, the unaffected foot should be dressed using a ball bandage (Figure 11.19b) to prevent development of lesions. Food should be cut up, as the bird will be unable to tear for itself. Care should be taken not to include rings or falconry equipment in the dressings, nor to push rings up the leg, as constriction lesions may result. Alternatively, perches should be padded; soft leather over Astroturf provides a suitable surface. If necessary, disinfectant solutions (e.g. F10SC or chlorhexidine) may be poured over the padding so the foot is continuously 'bathed'.

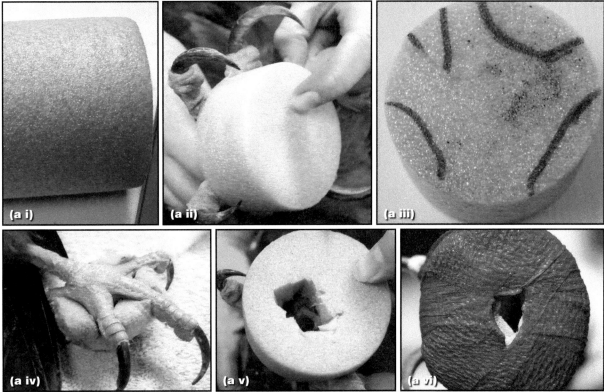

11.19 **(a)** A simple bumblefoot dressing designed to take pressure off the lesion and to allow the falconer to apply daily topical treatment to the lesion. **(i)** Foam swimming 'noodles' are used to create the padding (a thick slice is cut from the noodle). **(ii)** The foam slice is measured against the foot. **(iii)** The outline of the foot is drawn on the foam and space for the toes excavated from the foam. **(iv)** The foam is then placed on the foot. **(v)** A hole is then cut in the foam over the lesion on the ventrum of the foot. **(vi)** The foam is then bandaged on to the foot using cohesive dressing. The hole is left open. (Reproduced from the *BSAVA Manual of Raptors, Pigeons and Passerine Birds*.) (© J. Chitty.) (continues) ▶

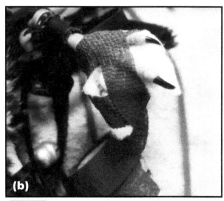

11.19 (continued) **(b)** Ball bandage (suitable for protection of the foot or for therapy of fractured toes). Cohesive bandage is used to wrap the foot around a ball (in this case, a wad of cotton wool). The ends of the toes and the talons are left clear of the bandage, allowing slight movement of the toes. This is important in preventing tendons from becoming incorporated in the toe fracture callus. Ball bandages should never be left on longer than 5 days for this reason. (Reproduced from the *BSAVA Manual of Raptors, Pigeons and Passerine Birds.*) (© J. Chitty.)

More advanced cases require surgery to debride the necrotic tissue. This should not be attempted without a thorough knowledge of the anatomy of the foot, as there is a risk of damaging important tendons and nerves (Harcourt-Brown, 2000). After debridement, swabs should be taken for culture. The wound may be flushed with antimicrobial solutions, or antibiotic-impregnated polymethylmethacrylate beads may be inserted. Where possible primary wound closure should be attempted. Where this is impossible, various forms of granulating dressing are available. For a thorough review of the options available for bumblefoot therapy, see Bailey and Lloyd (2008). Concurrent use of non-steroidal anti-inflammatory drugs (NSAIDs) is strongly recommended in all cases of bumblefoot.

Ectoparasites

The treatment of ectoparasites seen in raptors is summarized in Figure 11.20. Ticks are one of the very few indications for corticosteroids in raptors; general use should be avoided as they cause profound immunosuppression and a 'diabetic-like' syndrome. Other mites (e.g. *Cnemidocoptes* or *Dermanyssus*) may occasionally be found. For a fuller overview of ectoparasites, see Chitty and Lierz (2008).

Endoparasites

Figure 11.21 summarizes the diagnosis of endoparasites seen in raptors. It is strongly recommended that a faecal sample be collected and submitted for parasitological examination twice a year.

Wing tip oedema and necrosis syndrome (WTONS)

In WTONS blood flow to the wing tips appears to be reduced, resulting initially in oedema and then dry necrosis until the wing tip and associated primary feathers are lost (Figure 11.22a). It should be distinguished from 'blaine' (a traumatic carpitis; Figure 11.22b), which is normally unilateral, centred on the carpus and warm to the touch, and from folliculitis where inflammation is around the follicles rather than between them.

Parasite	Clinical signs/significance	Treatment/control
Feather lice/ mites	May result in feather damage; a heavy infestation may be a sign of ill health	Piperonal powder or fipronil spray; apply fipronil via a pad to the base of the neck, tail base and under each wing; **do not** soak the bird (as per dogs)
Louse flies (hippoboscids/ flat flies)	May cause anaemia in very young or weak birds; otherwise of little clinical significance, but may act as vectors for important blood parasites (*Haemoproteus*, *Leucocytozoon*)	As for feather lice/mites
Mosquitos/ gnats	May also act as vectors for blood parasites	Do not keep birds near insect breeding areas; if flown in high-risk areas, apply fipronil spray to bare skin immediately before flying; if mosquitos a problem in aviaries then treat local insect breeding sites and apply fipronil weekly to bare skin on birds during major risk periods (late summer/autumn)
Ticks (Figure 11.20a)	Severe, even fatal, reactions to tick bites are seen; typically a massive haemorrhagic reaction centred on the point of attachment, invariably on the head (many birds will also have ticks on the rest of the body without reaction); unknown whether haemorrhage is related to tick species, an infectious agent, or an inappropriate immune reaction	*Reaction:* prompt use of fluid therapy, broad-spectrum antibiosis and an intramuscular injection of a short-acting dexamethasone compound *Control:* regular applications of fipronil; acaricidal spray may be applied to the environment

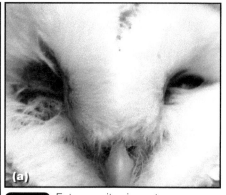

11.20 Ectoparasites in raptors. **(a)** Tick reaction in a barn owl. Note the extensive swelling around the right eye. (© J. Chitty.)

Class	Species	Clinical signs	Diagnostic tests
Nematodes	*Capillaria*	White, necrotic mouth/crop lesions and/or enteric problems; may see head flick or ADR syndrome/weight loss; rarely diarrhoea	Faecal flotation; may see adults in the pharynx or (via endoscopy) in the crop/oesophagus
	Ascarids	Large numbers may cause gut impaction/rupture in young birds; may cause weight loss/ADR syndrome	Faecal flotation
	Spiurid (stomach worm)	Inappetence/weight loss/ADR	Faecal flotation
	Syngamus (gapeworm)	Dyspnoea/cough	Faecal flotation; direct visualization/tracheal endoscopy
Cestodes/ trematodes		Rarely of significance in the UK	
Coccidia	*Caryospora*	Of great importance in falcons, especially merlins; may cause weight loss/ADR; in severe cases results in haemorrhagic enteritis and death	Faecal flotation
Other gut protozoa	*Trichomonas*	White necrotic mouth/crop lesions ('frounce'); inappetence; dysphagia; head flick	Direct microscopy of a (very) fresh wet preparation of lesions for motile protozoa
Blood parasites (becoming more common)	*Haemoproteus*; *Leucocytozoon* (Figure 11.21a); *Plasmodium*	Frequently present collapsed and profoundly anaemic	Examination of a blood smear; *note*: some birds may act as asymptomatic carriers so low numbers of parasites may not be significant (does **not** apply to *Plasmodium* where low numbers can be very significant)

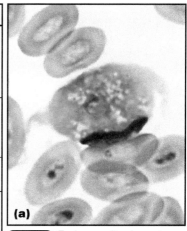

11.21 Endoparasites in raptors. **(a)** *Leucocytozoon* in a peripheral blood smear from a collapsed anaemic Harris' hawk. (© J. Chitty.)

The prognosis is good if the disease is caught early. Therapy involves broad-spectrum antibiosis and vascular stimulants (isoxsuprine orally and Preparation-H® topically). Radiographs should be taken in all cases because in the advanced stages erosive lesions may be seen developing in the second phalangeal bone. This is a poor prognostic sign, as is passage to dry necrosis.

The cause is still unknown, although an underlying inflammatory aetiology is suspected from serum protein electrophoresis results. Low ground temperatures may be involved (at least as a trigger factor). For prevention, no young raptor should be tethered within 45 cm of the ground (without supplying heat) in winter, nor should wet birds be left out at night in winter, whether tethered or in aviaries.

Fracture repair

Fractures are common in hunting birds (Figure 11.23). A full description of raptor orthopaedics is beyond the

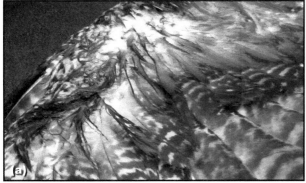
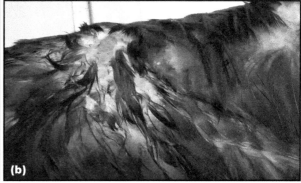

11.22 **(a)** Wing tip oedema in a falcon. Note the oedema between the feather follicles. **(b)** Blaine in a Harris' hawk. Note the swelling is centred on the carpus and is secondary to trauma. This should be distinguished from WTONS. (© J. Chitty.)

scope of this Chapter but is covered by Hatt (2008). The following principles always apply:

1. Attention must be paid to length and rotation of the bone in any fracture repair.

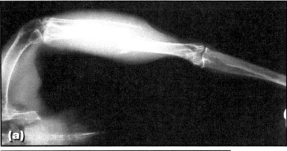

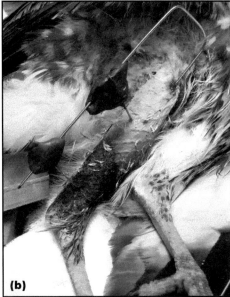

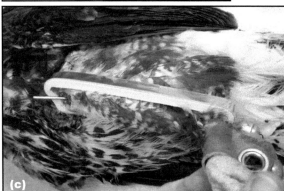

11.23 **(a)** The most common fracture seen is that of the tibiotarsus (there is a thinning and weakness about the point where the fibula ends). Typically, this is a simple fracture approximately one-third to halfway along the bone. It is seen in young, recently jessed Harris' hawks that have been given too long a leash; as they bate off, so they build up considerable momentum when they hit the end of the leash. These are relatively simple to fix, remembering that attention must be paid to bone length and rotation. **(b)** An intramedullary pin tied into a Type 1 external fixator. **(c)** Where cost is an issue, the intramedullary pin can be left 'proud' of the skin and an aluminium finger splint used to make a box around the tibiotarsus (held over the pin above the stifle and wrapped under the flexed tarsus). The splint is removed after 5–7 days and the pin 10–14 days later. (© J. Chitty.)

2. The raptor is a high performance athlete; therefore, any fracture repair must restore full function. This means that the limb restoration must be as near to perfect as possible.
3. Attention must be paid to soft tissue structures in the vicinity of the fractured bone. If limbs (or especially toes) are bandaged for more than 5 days, there is a strong chance that bone callus will start to incorporate neighbouring tendons, thus restricting movement. Bandaging of wings for more than a few days may result in permanent joint contracture. Thus, physiotherapy is an important part of any orthopaedic repair.

Squirrel bites

The typical squirrel bite is on the foot or leg, perhaps 2 mm long, and appears innocuous. Therefore, it is often left untreated, other than staunching blood flow and initial cleaning. Unfortunately, these bites often introduce bacteria, and erosive infections commence. These may often not be apparent for a few weeks, by which time there may be osteomyelitis or tenosynovitis. Tendon rupture post-infection is not unknown. Thus, it is recommended that squirrel bites should be seen as a matter of urgency, the wound thoroughly irrigated and antibiosis instigated, typically with a 14-day course of clavulanate-potentiated amoxicillin in the first instance.

Supportive care

Emergency stabilization of the collapsed bird

1. *Before the bird arrives*: prepare a warmed chamber (approximately 25–30°C) and ensure that oxygen and fluids are available.
2. *Do not keep the bird waiting*: it should be seen at once, in a quiet room away from barking dogs and other stresses.
3. *Perform a brief examination* to find major injuries and lesions.
   • Assess dehydration (brachial vein refill time can be useful; if more than 2 seconds, assume >7% dehydration).
   • Stop blood loss (pressure, clamps).
   The aim at this stage is to assess prognosis; keep the examination brief and stress-free. In case of respiratory distress, supply oxygen by mask.
4. *Give fluids*: preferably by intravenous bolus but if this causes too much distress, use the subcutaneous route.
5. *Place the bird in the warm chamber*, darken the area and observe every 10–15 minutes.

When the bird appears stronger, a full clinical evaluation and sample collection may be carried out. If necessary, this may be performed under anaesthesia (if the bird is unable to cope with being handled when conscious).

Hospital equipment

Most of the equipment required for treating parrots will also suit raptors. Because the beaks of raptors are not as powerful as those of parrots, metal crop or stomach tubes are not essential, and very useful tubes can be made from drip tubing or dog urinary catheters (it should be ensured that the cut ends are smoothed off).

It is essential that hospitalized raptors do not damage wing or tail feathers, as this will reduce their flying ability until the next moult. They should be kept tethered in open areas or in kennels large enough that they do not strike the walls when bating or being caught-up. When handling, the wings should be well restrained. To protect the tail, perching should be provided. A simple wooden block will suffice for short periods but it may be worth purchasing a travelling bow perch (for hawks) or a travelling block (for falcons). These are available from many makers of falconry equipment. If perching is not available, a tail guard can be made from X-ray film, stiff card or autoclave bags and secured at the tail base with tape (Figure 11.24).

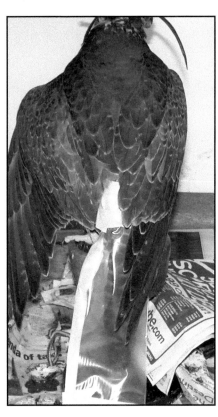

11.24

Hospitalized falcon with a tail guard made from an autoclave bag. (© J. Chitty.)

If the practice does not hospitalize birds often, there is likely to be spoilage of food stocks. The problem can be reduced if the falconer is asked to bring a supply of the bird's normal food, which will also avoid diet change problems. However, it is vital that the diet is assessed thoroughly before feeding (it should be checked for freshness, hygiene and potential toxins). Anorexic birds may be given a liquid diet by crop or stomach tube. In the short term, an amino acid/electrolyte mixture may be used. For longer-term treatment, commercial meat-based diets may be used.

Drug administration

Intravenous

See the section on blood sampling (above) for intravenous access sites.

Intramuscular

Injection into the caudal third of the pectoral muscle masses is recommended. Injection into the leg muscles may be performed but is not advised when using nephrotoxic drugs, due to the presence of the renal portal blood flow (although fears about this may be overstated). Irritant substances may cause muscle damage that may be of great significance in the hunting bird. Irritant compounds (including enrofloxacin (concentrations >2.5% should be avoided altogether) and some of the long-acting oxytetracycline preparations) should be used with care; if long-term administration is required it may be wise to use oral drugs, less irritant compounds, or drugs that need to be given less frequently.

Subcutaneous

This route may be used but is not popular, probably because of concerns regarding the rate of drug absorption.

Oral

This is an easy route in raptors. Liquid compounds may be given directly by stomach or crop tube (although this may cause stress). Tablets are easy to hide in food (e.g. in a chick head) and are usually taken readily.

Nebulization

This is a useful adjunctive therapy in respiratory disease. It may improve drug penetration into the respiratory system and will improve clearance of discharges as well as hydrate mucous membranes.

Fluid therapy

Oral

A crop or stomach tube is suitable for giving maintenance fluids or for medication of mildly debilitated birds. Many falconers are familiar with the technique (Figure 11.25) and often give fluids prior to

Equipment
Tube – either semi-rigid plastic tubing (made from drip tubing or dog urinary catheter) or commercial metal tubes should be used

Technique
Two operators are required: 1. Restrain the bird firmly. 2. Extend the neck fully and open the beak. 3. The glottis lies in the ventral midline, so pass the tube gently dorsolaterally. It may be palpated in the oesophagus or the tip may be seen in the crop. 4. Insert fluid.
To avoid regurgitation, warm the fluid and inject it slowly. The recommended volume (12 ml/kg for diurnal birds; 8 ml/kg for owls) should not be exceeded. If there is resistance to passing the tube, or if fluid appears in the mouth, *stop*, withdraw the tube and reassess

11.25 Stomach and crop tubing.

presenting the bird to a veterinary surgeon. Isotonic solutions should be used, such as Hartmann's solution or various commercial products. Fluids should be given at a rate of 12 ml/kg bodyweight for diurnal birds and 8 ml/kg for owls (which have no crop).

Subcutaneous

This route is commonly used in collapsed birds when it is felt that excessive handling or anaesthesia would be inappropriate until the bird is further stabilized. Isotonic fluid (choice should be based on plasma electrolyte measurements) is given at 20 ml/kg into the pre-crural fold. Typically, this will be absorbed in approximately 15 minutes.

Intravenous

This is the route of choice in the extremely debilitated bird or perioperatively. Either the right jugular or brachial vein may be catheterized. Fluids are then given either as a bolus (10 ml/kg/minute; a useful technique if the bird is collapsed or at the start of surgery) or by continuous infusion using drip apparatus or a syringe pump. It may be tricky to maintain catheters in raptors in the long term.

Intraosseous

Given the difficulties in maintaining intravenous catheters, the intraosseous route is the method of choice for continuing fluid therapy. Specialized intraosseous needles or spinal needles (or even hypodermic needles of an appropriate size) may be inserted into the distal ulna or proximal tibia. Pneumatized bones (e.g. humerus or femur) should *not* be used. A syringe pump or 'Flowline' apparatus must be used. Fluid is given at a rate of 10 ml/kg/hour. The technique is simple but should be performed in a sterile manner to avoid the risk of osteomyelitis. Intraosseous needles appear to be well tolerated.

Anaesthesia and analgesia

As with all species, pre-anaesthetic assessment is essential, although the high safety margin of isoflurane means that many of these assessments are now carried out under anaesthesia. It is difficult to recommend any anaesthetic agent other than isoflurane or sevoflurane. In general, isoflurane is used as the slight advantages given by sevoflurane in quicker induction and recovery times may be outweighed by significantly higher costs. Where isoflurane or sevoflurane are not available or practical (e.g. in the field), anaesthesia using medetomidine (25–100 µg/kg) and ketamine (2–5 mg/kg) may be used (higher doses used i.m., lower ones i.v.). Reversal of the medetomidine with an equal volume of atipamezole may be used. An accurate weight must be obtained first.

Anaesthesia should be induced by facemask, using oxygen as the carrier gas. There appears to be no benefit in adding nitrous oxide.

- For short procedures, the bird can be maintained on a facemask.

- For longer procedures, or where access to the head is required, an endotracheal tube should be placed and an appropriate circuit (e.g. Ayre's T-piece) used.
- For ocular procedures, or those involving surgery of the head and neck, an air sac tube should be placed and anaesthesia maintained via this route.

During anaesthesia, heat should be supplied using a mat or a radiant heat source. Heart and respiratory rates should be monitored continuously. Pulse oximetry, capnography, peripheral Doppler and electrocardiography are also useful. At the end of the procedure, the bird should be lightly wrapped (to reduce flapping in recovery excitement) and placed in a warm quiet environment. Recovery is usually complete within a few minutes. For a fuller description of anaesthesia of raptors and air sac tube placement, see Heatley (2008).

Euthanasia

Euthanasia of the sick bird is an option for the clinician where therapy is not possible, practicable or affordable and the bird is suffering. Whatever the indication, euthanasia must be carried out in a humane manner and the decision taken with sensitivity for the owner. The human–animal bond is rarely as intense as with parrots and their owners, but many falconers are very close to their birds.

- Ideally euthanasia should be by intravenous injection of pentobarbital. It may be useful to induce anaesthesia prior to the injection. Sedation using intramuscular ketamine may also be used.
- Where the body is required for post-mortem examination, euthanasia may be achieved by overdosage of the volatile anaesthetic agent.
- Intracoelomic injection of pentobarbital cannot be recommended. It may result in rapid death, but it often does not and these injections may be associated with considerable pain to the bird. They may also disrupt internal anatomy, thus affecting necropsy findings.
- Intracardiac injection of pentobarbital may be achieved in smaller passerine birds, but inadvertent intrapulmonary injection may cause unnecessary distress to the bird.

In the field situation, such as severe injury to a hunting raptor, other methods may be considered. In these cases, a physical means of euthanasia may be more appropriate to reduce bird suffering than transporting it for injection. Cervical dislocation is rarely easy in larger raptors, but a sharp blow to the head will render the bird unconscious or dead very quickly.

Drug formulary

A basic drug formulary is given in Figure 11.26.

Drug	Dose	Comments
Antibacterial agents		
Amoxicillin	150 mg/kg i.m. q24h (long-acting injection) or 150 mg/kg orally q12h	
Amoxicillin/Clavulanate	150 mg/kg orally/i.v. q12h or i.m. q24h	May cause regurgitation if used orally
Azithromycin	50 mg/kg orally q24h for 5 days	Chlamydophilosis
Cefalexin	40–100 mg/kg i.m./orally q8–12h	
Clindamycin	100 mg/kg orally q24h	Halve dose if used with marbofloxacin
Doxycycline	50 mg/kg orally q12h or 100 mg/kg i.m. every 5–7 days	'Vibravenos' – specific treatment certificate required in the UK
Enrofloxacin	15 mg/kg orally/i.m. q12h	Authorized in companion birds; irritant injection; care with use in working birds due to muscle damage; may cause regurgitation
Lincomycin	50–75 mg/kg orally/i.m. q12h	
Marbofloxacin	10 mg/kg orally/i.m./i.v. q24h	
Oxytetracycline	200 mg/kg i.m. q24h (long-acting preparation) or 25–50 mg/kg orally q8h	
Piperacillin	100 mg/kg i.m./i.v. q12h	Often combined with tazobactam; base dosage on piperacillin dose; preparation should be reconstituted with glucose–saline for improved stability; prepared solution also suitable as a topical flushing agent
Trimethoprim/ Sulphonamide	30 mg/kg i.m. q12h or 12–60 mg/kg orally q12h	
Antifungal agents		
Amphotericin B	1.5 mg/kg i.v. q12h for 3–5 days	Give with 10–15 ml/kg saline
Enilconazole	Dilute 10% solution 10:1 and give 0.5 ml/kg/day i.t. for 7–14 days	
Fluconazole	2–5 mg/kg orally q24h	
Itraconazole	10–20 mg/kg orally q24h (prophylactic) 10–15 mg/kg orally q12h (therapeutic)	
Ketoconazole	25 mg/kg i.m./orally q12h	
Nystatin	300,000 IU/kg orally q12h	Not absorbed from the gastrointestinal tract
Terbinafine	10–15 mg/kg orally q12h	
Voriconazole	12.5 mg/kg orally q12h for 30–60 days	
Antiprotozoal agents		
Carnidazole	25–30 mg/kg orally once; may repeat the next day if required	
Chloroquine/Primaquine	Take one chloroquine tablet 500 mg, add one primaquine tablet 26 mg. Crush them and add 10 ml water. 0.5 ml of this then gives active ingredients of 15 mg chloroquine + 0.75 mg primaquine. Initial dose is 25 mg/kg chloroquine + 1.3 mg/kg primaquine at 0 hours, then 15 mg/kg chloroquine at 12 hours, then 15 mg/kg chloroquine at 24 hours, then a final dose of 15mg/kg chloroquine at 48 hours. Prophylaxis: 26.3 mg/kg orally weekly from 1 month before until 1 month after mosquito season	Avian malaria
Clazuril	30 mg/kg orally once	

11.26 Drug formulary for birds of prey. Note: few of these drugs are authorized for use in these species in the UK. Where authorized, the stated drug dose may be different from that included in the table. It is recommended that clinicians follow the prescribing legislation in their own country and use authorized products at the authorized dose rate in that country before using alternative therapies or alternative dose rates. (continues) ▶

Drug	Dose	Comments
Antiprotozoal agents continued		
Mefloquine	50 mg/kg orally q24h for 7 days	Avian malaria
Melarsamine	0.25 mg/kg i.m. q24h for 4 days	Leucocytozoonosis
Metronidazole	50 mg/kg orally q24h for 5 days	Trichomoniasis
Paromomycin	100 mg/kg orally q12h for 7 days; repeat after 1 week	
Pyrimethamine	0.5 mg/kg orally q12h for 28 days	Leucocytozoonosis
Toltrazuril	25 mg/kg orally weekly for 3 weeks	Coccidiosis
Trimethoprim (40 mg/ml) + Sulfamethoxazole (200 mg/ml)	0.15 ml/kg i.m. q24h for 7 days	Leucocytozoonosis
Antiparasitic agents		
Doramectin	1000 µg/kg orally/i.m. twice 1–2 weeks apart	*Serratospiculum*
Fenbendazole	Nematodes and some cestodes: 25–100 mg/kg orally once Capillariasis: 25 mg/kg orally q24h for 5 days	Blood dyscrasias have been reported at higher doses in vultures and some other raptors
Fipronil	Apply spray preparation via a pad to the base of the neck, tail base and under each wing. **Do not** soak the bird	
Ivermectin	200 µg/kg orally/i.m.; repeat after 2 weeks	
Moxidectin	500–1000 µg/kg orally/spot-on once	Capillariasis
Piperonal powder	Shake over entire bird	
Praziquantel	10 mg/kg i.m.; repeat after 1 week	Cestodes and trematodes
Anti-inflammatory agents Large vultures of the *Gyps* genus appear sensitive to certain NSAIDs, particularly diclofenac. Studies show that meloxicam appears safe at therapeutic doses. However, it would be wise to use NSAIDs with caution in these species, restrict use to meloxicam and ensure use only in normotensive well hydrated individuals		
Carprofen	1–5 mg/kg i.m./orally q12–24h	Care in dehydration, shock and renal dysfunction; higher dose rate appears effective for 24 hours
Ketoprofen	1–5 mg/kg i.m. q8–24h	
Meloxicam	0.1–0.5 mg/kg i.m./orally q24h	Care in dehydration, shock and renal dysfunction; higher dose rate appears effective for 24 hours
Piroxicam	0.5 mg/kg orally q24h	
Anaesthetics/analgesics/emergency agents		
Adrenaline	0.5–1 mg/kg i.v./i.o./i.t.	
Atropine	0.04–0.5 mg/kg i.m.	
Bupivacaine	<2 mg/kg local infiltration	Mix with dimethylsulfoxide (DMSO) for topical analgesia
Buprenorphine	0.01–0.05 mg/kg i.m./i.v. q8–12h	
Butorphanol	0.3–4 mg/kg i.m. q6–12h	
Dexamethasone sodium phosphate	2–6 mg/kg i.m./i.v.	Care with use of corticosteroids in birds; immunosuppression and other side-effects are common
Diazepam	0.2–1 mg/kg i.v./i.m. q12–24h	Control of fitting: lower dose orally q24h may be useful as an appetite stimulant

11.26 (continued) Drug formulary for birds of prey. Note: few of these drugs are authorized for use in these species in the UK. Where authorized, the stated drug dose may be different from that included in the table. It is recommended that clinicians follow the prescribing legislation in their own country and use authorized products at the authorized dose rate in that country before using alternative therapies or alternative dose rates. (continues) ▶

Drug	Dose	Comments
Anaesthetics/analgesics/emergency agents continued		
Doxapram	5–20 mg/kg i.v./i.o./i.t.	
Glycopyrrolate	0.01–0.03 mg/kg i.m.	
Lidocaine	<2.5 mg/kg local perfusion	
Prednisolone sodium succinate	10–30 mg/kg i.v./i.m.	
Miscellaneous		
Aciclovir	333 mg/kg orally q12h for 7–14 days	Herpesvirus
Allopurinol	10 mg/kg orally q12h	Toxicity reported in red-tailed hawks at 50 mg/kg
Colchicine	0.04 mg/kg orally q12h	
Digoxin	0.02–0.05 mg/kg orally q12h for 2–3 days, then reduce to 0.01 mg/kg q12h–24h	
Dimercaprol/BAL (British Anti-Lewisite)	2.5 mg/kg i.m. q4h for 2 days, then q12h until signs resolve	
Edetate calcium disodium	35–50 mg/kg i.m. q12h for 5 days, then stop for 2 days; repeat courses until lead levels normal	
Enalapril	5 mg/kg orally q24h until signs improve, then decrease to 1 mg/kg	
Furosemide	0.1–6.0 mg/kg orally/i.m./i.v. q6–24h	Not in dehydrated or hyperuricaemic birds
Isoxsuprine	Small pinch powder/kg orally q12h	
Kaolin/Pectin	15 ml/kg orally q8–12h	
Lactulose	0.5 mg/kg orally q12h	
Metoclopramide	0.3–2.0 mg/kg orally/i.m. q12–24h	
Oxprenolol	2 mg/kg orally q24h	
ᴅ-Penicillamine	55 mg/kg orally q12h for 10 days	
2-Pralidoxamine HCl (2-PAM)	10 mg/kg i.m. as required	
Propentofylline	5 mg/kg orally q12h	
Vitamin B1 (thiamine)	10–30 mg/kg i.m. q24h	
Vitamin E/Selenium	0.5 mg S + 1.34 IU Vitamin E/kg s.c.; repeat after 72 hours	
Vitamin K1	0.2–2.5 mg/kg orally/i.m. q6–24h	

11.26 (continued) Drug formulary for birds of prey. Note: few of these drugs are authorized for use in these species in the UK. Where authorized, the stated drug dose may be different from that included in the table. It is recommended that clinicians follow the prescribing legislation in their own country and use authorized products at the authorized dose rate in that country before using alternative therapies or alternative dose rates.

References and further reading

Bailey T and Lloyd C (2008) Disorders of the feet. In: *BSAVA Manual of Raptors, Pigeons and Passerine Birds*, ed. J Chitty and M Lierz. BSAVA Publications, Gloucester

Chitty J (2008) Raptor nutrition. In: *BSAVA Manual of Raptors Pigeons and Passerine Birds*, ed. J Chitty and M Lierz. BSAVA Publications, Gloucester

Chitty J and Lierz M (2008) *BSAVA Manual of Raptors, Pigeons and Passerine Birds*. BSAVA Publications, Gloucester

Chitty JR (2005) Feather plucking/chewing in raptors. *Proceedings 26th Conference of the Association of Avian Veterinarians*, pp. 91–93. Monterey, California

Cooper JE (1978) *Veterinary Aspects of Captive Birds of Prey, 2nd edn.* Standfast Press, London

Forbes NA and Cooper JE (1993) Fatty liver–kidney syndrome of merlins. In: *Raptor Biomedicine*, ed. PT Redig *et al.*, pp. 45–48. University of Minnesota Press, Minneapolis

Forbes NA and Flint C (2000) *Raptor Nutrition*. Honeybrook Farm Animal Foods, Evesham

Harcourt-Brown NH (2000) *Birds of Prey: anatomy, radiology and clinical conditions of the pelvic limb* (CD-ROM). Zoological Education Network, Lake Worth, Florida

Hatt JM (2008) Hard tissue surgery. In: *BSAVA Manual of Raptors, Pigeons and Passerine Birds*, ed. J Chitty and M Lierz. BSAVA Publications, Gloucester

Heatley JJ (2008) Anaesthesia. In: *BSAVA Manual of Raptors, Pigeons and Passerine Birds*, ed. J Chitty and M Lierz. BSAVA Publications, Gloucester

Heidenreich M (1997) *Birds of Prey: medicine and management.* Blackwell Science, Oxford

Jones MP (2001) Behavioral aspects of captive birds of prey. *Veterinary Clinics of North America: Exotic Animal Practice* **4**, 613–632

Lierz M and Hafez HM (2006) Plasma chemistry reference values in hybrid falcons in relation to their species of origin. *Veterinary Record* **159**, 79–82

Lumeij JT, Remple JD, Remple CJ and Riddle KE (1998) Plasma chemistry in peregrine falcons (*Falco peregrinus*): reference values and physiological variations of importance for interpretation. *Avian Pathology* **27**, 129–132

Rees-Davies R (2000) Avian liver disease: etiology and pathogenesis. *Seminars in Avian & Exotic Pet Medicine* **9**(3), 115–125

Samour J and Naldo J (2007) *Anatomical and Clinical Radiology of Birds of Prey.* Saunders Elsevier, Philadelphia

Wernery W, Wernery U, Kinne J, *et al.* (2004) *Colour Atlas of Falcon Medicine.* Schlutersche Verlagsgesellschaft, Hannover

Useful addresses

British and Irish Association of Zoos and Aquaria: Regents Park, London NW1 4RY

British Falconers' Club: 5 Tarnaway Avenue, Thornton Cleveleys Lancs FY5 5BB

British Field Sports Society (BFSS): 59 Kennington Road, London SE1 7PZ

Department of the Environment, Food and Rural Affairs (Defra): Global Wildlife Division, Temple Quay House, 2 The Square, Bristol BS1 6EB

Falconers and Raptor Conservation Magazine: PO Box 464, Berkhamsted, Herts HP4 2UR

Independent Bird Register: Tiercel House, Falcon Close, Scotton. N Yorks DL9 3RB. Telephone: 01748 830112/ 0870 6088500; email juliana @ ibr.org.ukwww.ibr.org.uk. Lost/found birds. Information resource. Publishes annual directory of useful addresses

International Falconer Magazine: PO Box 91, Carmarthen, SA33 5YF

The Hawk Board: www.hawkboard-cff.org.uk

Acknowledgements

The author would like to thank Ashley Smith of the Hawk Conservancy Trust and Jim Chick, Hawk Board Chairman, for their help in compiling the data for Figure 11.3.

12

Ostriches, emus and rheas

Thomas N. Tully Jr

Introduction

The Ratites group of flightless birds includes the ostrich (*Struthio camelus*), emu (*Dromaius novaehollandiae*), rhea (*Rhea americana* and *R. pennata*), cassowary (*Casuarius casuarius, C. bennetti, C. unappendiculatus*), and kiwi (*Apteryx australis, A. mantelli, A. ownei, A. haasti, A. rowi*). The name ratite is derived from the large flat sternum that resembles a raft, *ratis* in Latin. All ratites are native to the Southern Hemisphere, but they have adapted to farming and exhibition facilities found the world over. For the veterinary surgeon there are three main ratite species commonly treated; the ostrich, emu and greater rhea (*R. americana*) (Figure 12.1).

Traditionally the ostrich, emu and greater rhea were hunted primarily for food. The feathers were used for ceremonial dress, the hides were tanned for leather products, and the bones used as weapons. The ostrich and emu have the ability to produce a great amount of internal body fat which was considered, even by traditional hunters, a delicacy to be eaten on bread. It was also thought to contain medicinal qualities.

Farming of ratites was noted in South Africa as early as 1775 and continues to this day. Emu farming appears to have its origins in Western Australia, beginning in 1970. From these humble beginnings the possibility of establishing large avian farms that would produce saleable avian meat, leather and fat generated worldwide interest during the late twentieth century. Since the height of ratite production in the 1990s, the number of ratite farms has dramatically decreased in many areas of the world but there are still farms that require veterinary assistance and care for their birds.

Ratites are and have been a popular exhibit animal in zoological parks. In South America, it is not uncommon to see the greater rhea walking free in the park grounds (see Figure 12.1c). The care sought by ratite owners today, other than those found in zoological collections, is based on herd health management. The production practices utilized in ratite farming and the cost of an individual bird makes extensive costly medical work-ups, treatments and surgical procedures unprofitable for most owners.

Biology

Although the ostrich, emu and greater rhea appear to be similar in appearance, they are physiologically quite different. Biological data for common ratites are summarized in Figure 12.2.

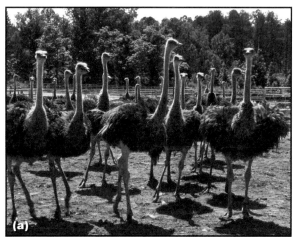
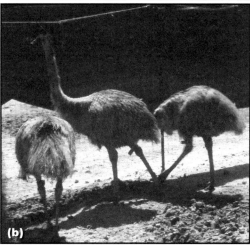
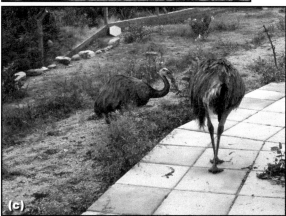

12.1 The three ratites most likely to be seen by the veterinary surgeon: **(a)** ostrich; **(b)** emu; and **(c)** greater rhea.

	Ostriches	Emus	Greater rheas
Bodyweight (kg)	63–104	17–48	20–40
Body temperature (°C)	39.9	38.1	39.7
Heart rate (beats/min)	60–72	41	48
Respiration (breaths/min)	6–12 (resting)	7–10 (resting)	7–10

12.2 Biological data for common ratites.

Anatomy and physiology

Ratites have thick skin relative to other avian species. The feathers attached to the skin have no barbules, and the barbs attached to the central shafts give the feathers a hair-like appearance. Since ratites are flightless they have underdeveloped pectoral muscles, but they have large thigh muscles to allow running.

The digestive system of the three species is significantly different. Both the rhea and ostrich are hindgut fermenters, while the emu digestive system resembles that of a simple stomached animal. Digestive tract transit time averages 50 hours in an adult ostrich, 18 hours in an adult rhea, and 8 hours in an adult emu. The anatomy of the stomach has a significant effect on feed utilization, feed requirements, and disease presentations. Ostriches, and to a lesser extent greater rheas, have a tendency to present with proventricular, ventricular and intestinal impactions, while emus are rarely subject to this disease process.

An unusual anatomical finding occurs in the emu trachea. As with all birds, emus have cartilaginous rings that comprise the trachea. These cartilaginous rings are interrupted in emus by a 6–8 cm cleft on the ventral surface of the trachea, 10–15 cm cranial to the thoracic inlet.

Sexing

All male ratites have an intromittent organ (phallus), which lies on the ventral floor of the cloaca. In adult males the phallus, when flaccid, remains within the cloaca; when erect, it extends outside the cloaca. The erect phallus is introduced into a receptive female's cloaca and guides the semen towards the urodeum and entrance to the oviduct. The phallus does not have a urinary function.

Ostrich, emu and rhea females all have slight tissue prominences that protrude from the genital mound on the ventral floor of the cloaca (Figure 12.3). The female reproductive tracts of ostriches, emus and rheas consist of the left ovary and oviduct (infundibulum, magnum, isthmus, uterus (shell gland), and vagina), after which the egg passes through the urodeum and out of the cloaca.

Husbandry

Housing

All pens should be large enough for birds to run and exercise. Ratites of all ages require exercise to maintain health and physiological wellbeing. Running is especially important for young birds: ratite chicks (Figure 12.4) need exercise through running to reduce

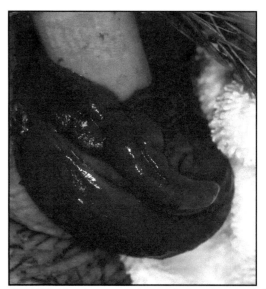

12.3 The tissue prominence in female emus is found in the same location as the male phallus – on the ventral floor of the cloaca.

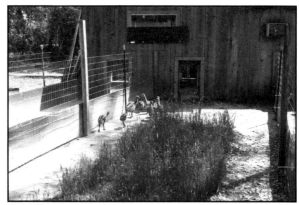

12.4 Young ratites, like these emus, need plenty of room to run and exercise to maintain normal skeletal growth in their legs and prevent excessive weight gain.

rapid excessive weight gain and to maintain normal musculoskeletal development of their legs.

Fencing is very important, both to prevent predation and to keep birds together within a facility (Figure 12.5). Fencing for captive ratites should have high breaking strength, should eliminate the potential for climbing, and have either no or small openings to avoid head, neck or foot entrapment. Most livestock chain-link fencing is suitable, and it should be at least 8 feet tall. It is best to ensure that supporting posts are placed on the outside of the enclosure to avoid high-velocity impacts by frightened birds.

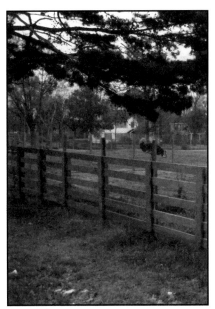

12.5 It is important to build strong fencing around ostrich holding pens to prevent birds from breaking out if startled.

All enclosures should have a shelter that protects birds from the prevailing wind, sun and precipitation. Depending on the environment and weather conditions, shelters can range from roofed three-sided structures to fully enclosed air-conditioned facilities (Figure 12.6).

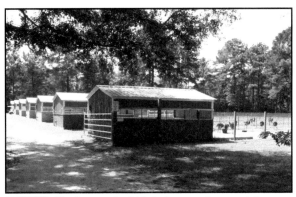

12.6 Shelters protect birds from environmental stresses such as weather.

Food should be placed in containers that are protected from the elements, in an area where birds are not restricted while feeding, and on a surface that does not become muddy after significant rainfall or snowmelt.

All indoor facilities should be well ventilated to prevent respiratory disease. Ratites are susceptible to *Aspergillus* respiratory infections, especially young birds that are housed in dry dusty hay-filled buildings. This type of environment can also lead to ocular disease.

Natural grass substrate is recommended for ostriches, emus and greater rheas. If rocks, sand or gravel are used as substrate in a pen or enclosure there is a potential for gastrointestinal impaction if the birds (e.g. ostrich, rhea) start eating the material in a rapid manner.

Diet

As hindgut fermenters with well developed caeca, ostriches and rheas can utilize grass as a primary food source. Emus and cassowaries have vestigial and non-functional caeca more appropriate for grains, seeds, legumes and non-grass plant material. However, although grazing is recommended to diversify the diet, commercially produced ratite feed is necessary to optimize the bird's growth, reproduction capabilities and health. Grazing is especially important for young ratites to prevent rapid weight gain which could lead to musculoskeletal leg problems. There are many commercially available ratite feeds and these products should be used and recommended through a careful appraisal of the manufacturer and the feed. Although ratites will eat just about any food placed in their feed container, the use of feed not specifically formulated for ratites is arguably the most common cause of disease problems on commercial farms.

Breeding

Reproductive data for the ostrich, emu and greater rhea are summarized in Figure 12.7. Breeding of ratites is best done in group settings to take advantage of economics, fertility and management personnel. In groups managed for maximum reproductive success, the ostrich and rhea should have 20–30% males to hens, while the emu should have 60% males to hens. It has been speculated that failure to copulate due to behavioural problems is the most common cause of infertility in ostriches. Other reproductive diseases that affect fertility include oviduct infections, egg peritonitis, papillomavirus, eggbinding, cystic ovaries, tumours, abnormal egg development, and cloacal prolapse.

Artificial incubation

Artificial incubation is considered 'state of the art' when it comes to increasing the number of successfully hatched eggs. Prior to incubation, the eggs should be cleaned with a soft dry cloth. If water must be used to clean the shell, the temperature of the water should be slightly higher than that of the egg (i.e. 37.5°C). A large, well ventilated incubator that automatically turns the eggs is required to maximize hatching (Figure 12.8).

	Ostriches	Emus	Greater rheas
Age at sexual maturity (months)	24–36	20–24	18–24
No. eggs per year	40–60	20–40	40–60
Egg weight (g)	900–1700	500–700	400–700

12.7 Reproductive data for the common ratites. (Data from Doneley, 2006.)

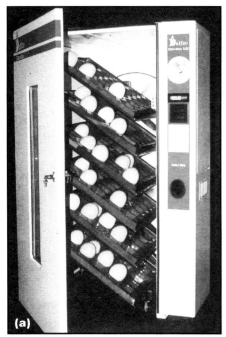

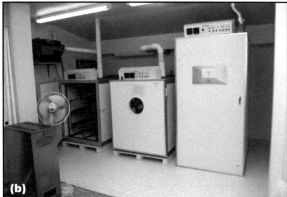

12.8 Artificial incubation. **(a)** This large, well built incubator has been specifically designed to incubate ratite eggs, thereby increasing hatch success. **(b)** Setting up an incubator room allows for better biosecurity and external environmental control.

Problem	Possible causes
Infertility	Incompatible breeders. Sterile or obese male. Distractions around breeder pens. Breeders too young or too old. Deficiencies or imbalances in breeder diet. Inclement weather. Handling or management stress. Early or late in lay cycle. Systemic or reproductive disease
Early embryonic mortality	Delayed egg collection. Storage temperature too high. Storage time prolonged. Infected eggs. Formaldehyde fumigation during 24–96 hours of incubation. Deficiencies or imbalances in breeder diet
Mid-embryonic mortality	Deficiencies or imbalances in breeder diet. Infected eggs. Inadequate egg turning. Rough handling of eggs
Late embryonic mortality	Deficiencies or imbalances in breeder diet. Inadequate ventilation. Infected eggs. Fluctuating incubation temperature
Air cell pip; no hatch	Hatcher temperature too high or too low. Hatcher humidity too high. Inadequate ventilation rate. Lack of social facilitation
Early hatch	Setter temperature too high. Setter humidity too low. Undersized eggs
Late hatch	Setter temperature too low. Oversized eggs
Malposition	Horizontal egg position after first week. Inadequate turning. Rough egg handling around 35 days. Deficiencies or imbalances in breeder diet
Malformed chicks	Setter temperature too high. Deficiencies or imbalances in breeder diet. Rough egg handling. Malpositioned chicks. Genetic factors, especially with related parents. Teratogens
Oedematous chicks	Inadequate circulation in setter. Setter humidity too high. Oversized eggs. Thick shells. Deficiencies or imbalances in breeder diet
Small chicks	Setter humidity too low. Undersized eggs. Thin, porous shells
Sticky chicks	Setter or hatcher humidity too low
External yolk sacs	Premature intervention to assist chick. Infected eggs. Oedematous chicks. Setter temperature too high. Fluctuating setter temperature
Yolk sac infections	Premature intervention to assist chick. Inadequate umbilical disinfection. Contaminated hatcher. Infected eggs
Spraddled legs	Smooth hatcher surface. Oedematous chicks

12.9 Causes of ratite incubation problems.

Incubation problems for ostriches, emus and greater rheas are shown in Figure 12.9. When incubating ostrich eggs, an increased temperature shortens the period by approximately one day for each 0.5°C rise.

- For ostriches the incubation period averages 45 days at 35°C and 42 days at 36.8°C with a relative humidity of 35–40% (chicks should be incubated with a relative humidity of 83–88%).
- For emu eggs, the recommended incubation temperature is 36.5°C, with a relative humidity of 25–30%, resulting in hatching at 51 days.
- For greater rhea eggs, the incubation period at 36.7°C is 42 days with a relative humidity of 20–25%.

Excessive incubation temperatures produce chicks with malformed eyes and limbs and exposed yolk sacs, and result in premature hatching (Figure 12.9). Conversely, low incubation temperatures produce soft weak chicks that hatch late. Humidity settings within the incubator are essential to regulate water loss from the egg. The optimum water loss of an ostrich egg during development is 12–15%; water loss above or below 12–15% will adversely affect the ability of the bird to survive after hatching. Humidity settings should be 25–40% depending on incubation temperature, egg quality and air circulation.

Eggs should be rotated during incubation, and most high-quality incubators will assist with this requirement. Eggs should never be turned in the hatcher or when near to full development (39–40 days for ostriches).

'Candling' eggs is required to distinguish fertile from non-fertile eggs and to identify dead embryos. Any non-developing egg should be removed from the incubator to prevent possible contamination of the remaining viable eggs. Candling is only recommended at Day 14 of incubation and on transfer to the hatcher. Emu eggs are difficult to candle, due to their thick coloured shell, and special devices have been developed that use infrared light.

Eggs should be moved into the hatcher (Figure 12.10) approximately 3 days before the embryo is fully developed. If the chick is fully developed but is having trouble breaking the shell, a 2 cm opening can be created by the veterinary surgeon or owner over the air cell to assist hatching. If the chick is still unable to break out of its shell within 12–24 hours, the shell can be gradually removed, taking care to prevent compromising blood vessels connected to the inner shell membrane.

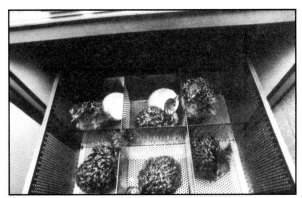

12.10 Young ostriches that have been removed from the incubator and placed in a hatcher.

Handling and restraint

Young birds (<30 days old) can be grabbed by the base of the neck and lifted by supporting the body. Birds that are 20–50 kg can be restrained and moved by straddling the bird's body with both legs (Figure 12.11) and placing both arms around the distal neck area.

Large adult ostriches need at least two people to capture and restrain them. The bird should be caught by quickly grabbing the head, if it will allow a close approach. Once the ostrich's head is grabbed, a hood can be placed to cover the eyes (see Figure 12.12). An ostrich hood can be made out of a long sleeved shirt. If the sleeve, which is to be used as a hood, is worn on the handler's arm then as the head is captured the sleeve can be brought down over the eyes and head. Once captured, the first reaction of the animal is to back up. The head must be held down below the level of the bird's body, allowing the assistant to push from behind as the restrainer with the head leads the bird. If the bird is unable to be approached, a shepherd's crook capture device may be used to pull the patient's head down for capture. This device can damage the bird's neck and/or head and therefore should only be used by an experienced person.

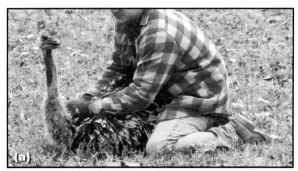

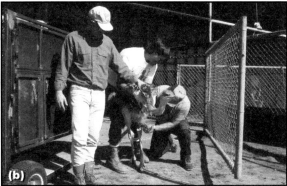

12.11 Handling young ostriches. **(a)** Sitting behind the bird, with its legs folded underneath its body, is an effective way to restrain a bird of this size. Care must be taken not to sit on the body or compress the body cavity. **(b)** Restraint for physical examination.

Larger emus and rheas can be captured in a hinged gate section that works as a squeeze chute (Figure 12.12). A number of homemade devices have been developed to facilitate capture and restraint of larger ratites for physical examinations. For extremely fractious animals, sedation may be needed to allow a physical examination to be performed.

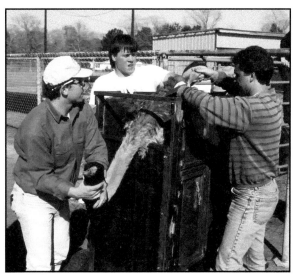

12.12 Hooded adult ostrich being examined in a chute.

WARNING
The large ratite species kick forwards and can kill a human with a vicious strong blow of the leg into the person's body and/or head.

Diagnostic approach

Clinical examination

Included in the external physical examination are an ophthalmological assessment, and oral cavity and dermatological evaluation. The caudal body cavity should be palpated, especially in ostriches (Figure 12.13) and rheas to check for impaction of the gastrointestinal tract. Due to the difficulty in determining body condition score in ratite species, because they lack significant pectoral musculature, ante-mortem assessment of an ill bird is difficult. The best way to assess the body condition of a ratite is to palpate the lumbar musculature. If the dorsal processes of the vertebrae are prominent, then the bird is in poor body condition. In birds suffering from severe gastrointestinal impaction the examiner can often hear 'rocks grinding a significant distance away from the patient'. The legs are examined for musculoskeletal abnormalities and gait problems. To isolate the anatomical area that is causing lameness, nerve blocks of the affected leg are recommended (Figure 12.14). All birds should have faecal parasite examinations – both direct and by flotation.

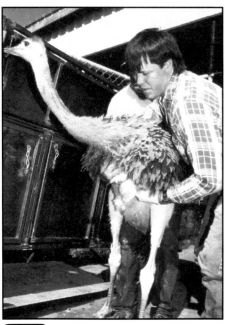

12.13 Palpating a restrained large juvenile ostrich.

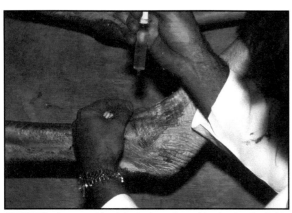

12.14 A nerve block is being placed in the hock of this ostrich to try and localize the site of lameness.

Imaging

Appropriate radiographic views can be taken with the bird in a standing position, or sitting on the cassette for a dorsoventral view (Figure 12.15). As ratites have thick leg muscles, a lateral radiographic view of the coelomic cavity is difficult to interpret. Ingested foreign bodies are common; a single ventrodorsal view of a large bird will often provide adequate information to confirm a diagnosis.

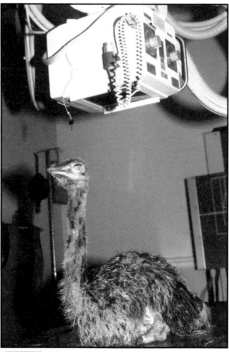

12.15 To examine a bird for gastric impaction or an ingested foreign body, the patient can be placed on the radiographic cassette, under mild sedation, to obtain a dorsoventral view of the coelomic cavity.

Ultrasound imaging on a sedated patient is also useful in ratites. Young ratites with a retained yolk sac and hens that are internally ovulating are two presentations for which ultrasound images are recommended, and for which radiographic films are often non-diagnostic. Although computed tomography (CT) and magnetic resonance imaging (MRI) have been used, they are cost-prohibitive in the majority of cases.

Blood sampling

Blood should be collected prior to physical examination: the right jugular, basilic and median metatarsal veins can be used in most ratites.

- The right jugular vein (Figure 12.16) is the site of choice for collecting blood and placement of intravenous catheters in all ratite species.
- In ostriches and rheas the right and left basilic veins are large enough for both blood collection and intravenous catheter placement (see Figure 12.22). The underdeveloped wing of the emu renders the basilic vein too small for quick easy collection of blood for diagnostic testing.
- The disadvantage of using the median metatarsal vein is the danger of collecting a sample while near the powerful legs of a conscious patient.

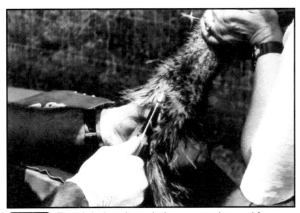

12.16 The right jugular vein is commonly used for blood collection from ratite species.

Once collected, the blood should be placed in heparinized tubes, since ostrich blood is adversely affected by EDTA anticoagulant, which will cause rapid haemolysis. To reduce the occurrence of false results, the whole blood should be centrifuged within 2 hours of collection. Reference ranges for haematology and biochemistry in adult ostriches and emus are given in Figure 12.17.

Parameter	Ostriches		Emus	
	Mean	**Range**	**Mean**	**Range**
Haematology				
WBC (x10⁹/l)	18.65	10–24	14.87	8–21
Heterophils (%)	72.9	58–89	78.8	54–88
Lymphocytes (%)	24.2	12–41	19.8	10–44
Monocytes (%)	2.64	0–4	0.1	0–1
Basophils (%)	0.2	0–2	0.2	0–1
Eosinophils (%)	0.035	0–2	2.58	0–6
Biochemistry				
AST (IU/l)	447.9	226–547	227.2	80–380
LDH (IU/l)	970	408–1236	778.1	318–1243
Creatine kinase (IU/l)	3702	800–6600	428.8	70–818
Uric acid (µmol/l)	513	59.5–862.5	374.7	59.5–814.9
Calcium (mmol/l)	2.67	1.99–3.39	2.77	2.19–3.12
Glucose (mmol/l)	12.04	9.10–18.32	7.44	5.61–13.49
Creatinine (umol/l)	22.98	8.84–61.88	19.45	8.84–35.36
Phosphorus (mmol/l)	1.72	0.94–0.25	0.18	0.12–0.23
Total protein (g/l)	39.3	24–53	39.3	34–44
Albumin (g/l)	17.2	11–23	17	12–24
Globulin (g/l)	22.1	14–31	22.3	14–32
Cholesterol (mmol/l)	2.66	1.01–4.45	3.15	1.76–4.39
Bile acids (µmol/l)	21	2–30	18	2–34

12.17 Haematology and biochemical data for ratites. (Data from Tully and Shane, 1996.)

Common conditions

There appear to be differences regarding susceptibility of the different ratite species to the many diseases a veterinary surgeon may encounter.

Parasites

Parasites should always be considered as possible contributors to, or the primary cause of, a disease condition in a ratite. A thorough evaluation of the appropriate diagnostic samples will lead to a complete appraisal of the case as it relates to parasitic involvement.

Ectoparasites

Ticks, mites, lice and flies have all been found on ratites. As in other hosts, ectoparasites that feed on blood often transmit infectious organisms and haematogenous parasites. The argasid species of tick has been identified as transmitting aegyptianellosis to ostriches from chickens in Africa. The biting gnat *Culicoides crepuscularis* is the primary vector for *Chandlerella quiscali* in North American emus; *C. quiscali* is a nematode that causes neurological disease in an aberrant host.

Endoparasites

Ostriches are susceptible to nematodes, cestodes and trematodes. The ostrich trematode is *Philothalamus gralli* and is commonly referred to as an eye fluke. The 'wireworm' *Libyostrongylus douglassi* is the most pathogenic nematode of young ostriches and is found in the proventriculus. It is imperative in a production facility that *L. douglassi* be prevented from entering the compound through screening new animals and routine worming.

Two species of tracheal nematodes affect ratites: *Cyathostoma variegatum* and *Syngamus trachea*. Clinical signs include head shaking, coughing and bloody froth from the beak. Flotation of faecal material or the bloody froth will often reveal the double-operculated eggs. Ratites ingest nematode eggs that have been shed by infected transport hosts (e.g. waterfowl).

Ostriches and rheas have been diagnosed with cestode infestations. *Houttuynia struthionis* has been found in both the ostrich and rhea, and *Chapmania tauricollis* in the rhea. Praziquantel is highly effective in treating *H. struthionis* and possibly *C. tauricollis* also.

There are many protozoan parasites that cause disease in ratites. The haemoparasites *Leucocytozoon struthionis* (ostrich), *Plasmodium struthionis* (ostrich, rhea) and *Aegyptianella pullorum* (ostrich) have been diagnosed; as noted above, these may be transmitted by arthropods that ingest blood meals. Intestinal protozoans that adversely affect ratites include *Giardia, Histomonas meleagridis, Trichomonas* and *Hexamita*. The tissue protozoan *Toxoplasma gondii* has been diagnosed in rheas.

Viral infections

Encephalitis

Emus appear to be very susceptible to both Eastern and Western equine encephalitis viruses. Eastern equine encephalitis (EEE) causes severe depression and haemorrhagic diarrhoea, whereas clinical signs noted in emus with Western equine encephalitis (WEE) are more consistent with neurological presentations. A definitive diagnosis is obtained through viral isolation from affected tissues (e.g. spleen, liver, blood, intestine). Treatment is mainly supportive and the majority of susceptible birds that are infected die. Emus can be protected using an inactivated commercial equine vaccine. A suggested vaccination protocol for a bivalent vaccine containing antigens against both EEE and WEE is as follows:

1. 6–8 weeks of age.
2. 10–12 weeks.
3. 16–18 weeks.
4. At 6 months.
5. Thereafter in April and September.
6. Birds can also be vaccinated when the virus has been identified in the area, either as a booster or in unvaccinated birds (adult schedule, April and September).

Administration of an equine product represents 'off-label' use and practitioners must obtain consent from the owners before vaccinating their animal(s).

Avian influenza

Both ostriches and rheas are susceptible to avian influenza (AI) virus, but at this time it does not appear that ratites are susceptible to the highly pathogenic strain H5N1. Type A orthomyxoviruses are commonly introduced through wild bird contact but indirect transmission can occur through contaminated equipment, feed bags, and transport of birds. Birds that are susceptible to specific strains of AI die suddenly, after short-term respiratory distress and green diarrhoea. The virus is usually isolated from tracheal and cloacal swabs using specific pathogen-free chicken eggs; PCR testing of swabs may also be used. Birds infected with mild influenza strains can be treated using supportive care and usually show a favourable response. Highly pathogenic strains uniformly cause death, and infection is not easily treated. Often in the event of a declared disease, emergency compulsory depopulation and disposal of carcasses is mandated by the country in which the outbreak occurs.

Newcastle disease

Newcastle disease caused by paramyxovirus type 1 results in high morbidity and up to 50% mortality of infected ratites. The most prominent clinical signs are neurological signs. Diagnosis may be obtained through isolation and identification of the virus, and in most cases treatment is not recommended. In countries where it is acceptable, vaccination is recommended for disease prevention.

Fading ostrich chick syndrome

An avibirnavirus has been identified as the causative agent of 'fading ostrich chick syndrome'. Affected birds exhibit clinical signs that are non-specific (e.g. depression, anorexia, diarrhoea) but, due to their debilitated state, become sternal and die. The virus has been

isolated from dead birds, and only supportive therapy is recommended. Biosecurity practices are the only measure that can be taken to prevent exposure to the virus within a ratite production facility.

Ostrich pox

Ostrich pox (Figure 12.18) presents as raised, circumscribed, often coalescing lesions on the non-feathered areas of the body, most often the head and base of the beak. Avipox viruses are transmitted by mosquitoes or other vectors that feed on a host's blood. The granulomas develop at the site where the blood meal was taken. Haematogenous transfer can also occur if the granulomas are disturbed by a pen mate and there is bleeding and a break in the surface epithelium. Diagnosis is made through identification of the classic intracytoplasmic inclusion bodies (Bollinger bodies) found in histopathological tissue samples of the granulomas. Treatment is supportive and antibiotic therapy is recommended to prevent secondary bacterial infections. The granulomatous lesions may be treated with an antibiotic ointment. Prevention of ostrich pox is best achieved through vaccination using a percutaneous poultry vaccine.

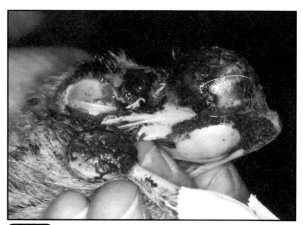

12.18 Avian pox lesions on a young ostrich.

Bacterial infections

Ratite species in their native habitats developed resistance to many infectious diseases, but as they were shipped to other parts of the world the naïve animals became ill from diseases to which they had never been exposed. The stresses of increased population density and intense breeding practices predisposed many birds to infectious disease due to an immunosuppressed state. Maintaining birds in healthy condition and reducing stress within their environment will help diminish illnesses associated with infectious organisms.

Salmonellosis

Birds can be exposed to *Salmonella* organisms through contaminated feed and water. The most common sources of contamination are rodent and, to a lesser extent, wild bird faeces. Clinical signs include diarrhoea, sudden death, severe depression and anorexia. Not only is the primary gastrointestinal infection life-threatening, but the endotoxins produced by the bacteria adversely affect the vital organs, particularly the liver. Supportive therapy is recommended along with fluoroquinolone or sulphonamide-based antibiotics. There is a concern of developing subclinical carriers by treating salmonellosis with antibiotics, and a decision must be made by the owner as to whether treatment is warranted. Preventive measures are the best method to reduce exposure and disease within a production facility.

Erysipelas

Erysipelothrix rhusiopathiae infection has been diagnosed in emus. The birds show acute mortality, possibly preceded by depression; otherwise, no specific clinical signs are noted. Birds are usually exposed through contaminated soil and they become infected through small skin lacerations. If diagnosed early, affected birds may be treated with antibiotics (e.g. fluoroquinolones). Birds that are raised and maintained in areas in which erysipelas is historically present may be immunized with a commercial adjuvant bacterin authorized for turkeys.

Colibacillosis

Emus appear more susceptible than ostriches and rheas to gastroenteritis cause by pathogenic *Escherichia coli*. Embryos can be infected while in the shell if contaminated by older birds. Clinical signs range from non-specific (e.g. depression, anorexia) to gastroenteritis and omphalitis. A definitive diagnosis is made by culture and isolation of the organism. Treatment is supportive plus appropriate antibiotic therapy based on culture and sensitivity testing. Preventing exposure requires the manager of the facility to implement proper hygiene measures for the incubation room and in juveniles and adult pens.

Mycoplasmosis

Mycoplasmosis is caused by *Mycoplasma cloacale,* which has been isolated from swabs from ostriches and emus. *Mycoplasma* organisms are transmitted vertically by the transovarian route and through direct contact with clinically affected and previously infected birds. *Mycoplasma* is an intracellular bacterium that can affect the respiratory, ocular and synovium of leg/foot joints. If a definitive diagnosis is made through the use of a serum plate agglutination test, recommended treatment includes tylosin or a fluoroquinolone antibiotic.

Tuberculosis

Tuberculosis caused by *Mycobacterium avium* has been diagnosed in emus and ostriches (Figure 12.19). Exposure to the causal organism may be through contact with infected birds that are subclinical carriers. A definitive diagnosis is through a positive acid-fast stain of faecal material or observation of acid-fast organisms in tissues obtained at biopsy or necropsy. No treatment is recommended. There is a possible zoonotic risk, particularly for humans or other animals that are immunosuppressed. *Mycobacterium avium* may be a reportable disease in some public health jurisdictions.

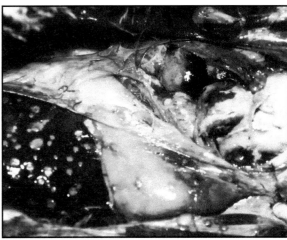

12.19 *Mycobacterium avium* granulomas on the liver of an emu.

Chlamydophilosis

Chlamydophila psittaci is transmitted through direct contact with the respiratory mucosa. Of all ratite species, rheas appear to be the most susceptible. An ante-mortem diagnosis can be made using an avian chlamydophilosis panel that includes PCR testing of a combined choanal and cloacal swab and a blood sample. Serum is also collected to determine antibody titres to see whether exposure and infection have elicited an immune response. Clinical signs are essentially non-specific (e.g. anorexia, depression, nasal discharge, diarrhoea). If diagnosed, treatment recommendations include tetracycline or doxycycline. For individual birds, intramuscular or oral doxycycline is feasible; for flocks, tetracycline in-water administration has been used. In the USA, FDA regulations prohibit the addition of tetracycline to ratite feed. As regulations change, practitioners should consult with governmental agencies concerning acceptable treatment. In some public health jurisdictions, *C. psittaci* infection is a reportable disease.

Clostridiosis

Clostridium perfringens and *C. colinum* have been isolated from the intestines of dead ostriches and emus. Clostridial organisms cause an enterotoxaemia similar to that in poultry cases, which has been confirmed in two zoo ostriches (Lublin *et al.*, 1993). Acute mortality is the primary presentation in most birds. Diagnosis is made through isolation and identification of the organism. Treatment of the penmates of the bird(s) that died should help prevent recurrence. Prevention is through proper management and nutritional offerings to the birds.

Coryza

Ostriches in Israel that presented with upper respiratory disease (e.g. rhinitis, sinusitis) have been diagnosed with infectious coryza, which is caused by the bacterium *Haemophilus* spp. Exposure of susceptible birds is either through direct transmission or via fomites (e.g. contaminated clothing, contaminated equipment, feedbags). A definitive diagnosis is made through isolation of the organism. Infected birds can be treated with trimethoprim/sulphonamide or penicillin/dihydrostreptomycin. Although clinical signs will abate, the birds probably will remain as subclinical carriers of the disease. Appropriate biosecurity measures are required to prevent other birds within the facility from becoming exposed and infected.

Anthrax

Anthrax caused by *Bacillus anthracis* has been diagnosed in South African ostriches (Snoeyenbos, 1965). Birds that become infected usually die without any ante-mortem clinical signs. There are no treatments recommended and ostriches should not be housed on farms with a history of anthrax. In the USA, anthrax is a reportable zoonotic disease.

Fungal infections

Aspergillosis

The most common fungal disease diagnosed in ratite species is aspergillosis (Figure 12.20). The *Aspergillus* organism is ubiquitous within the environment and birds are very susceptible when stressed. Clinical signs include peracute death, dyspnoea and depression. Aspergillosis is identified by the presence of 1–2 mm yellow to green granulomas in the air sacs and lungs. To confirm the diagnosis, the organisms can be identified through histopathological examination of the affected tissues. Treatment is cost-prohibitive when diagnosing an animal that is part of a production facility.

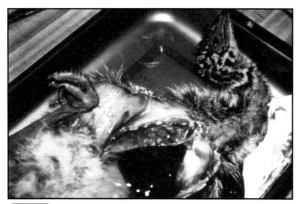

12.20 *Aspergillus* granulomas in the lung of a young emu.

Candidiasis

Candida albicans is usually a secondary opportunistic pathogen associated with a primary disease process but may itself develop into a life-threatening condition. Birds with candidiasis are easily treated but the underlying immunosuppressive condition must be identified to prevent recurrence and facilitate recovery. Diagnosis is through isolation and identification of the *Candida* organism. Treatment includes nystatin and fluconazole: nystatin must touch the lesion, and therefore the organisms, to be effective.

Musculoskeletal disorders

Developmental orthopaedic diseases are common in young growing birds and can be significant in some facilities. Young birds that gain weight too fast and do not exercise through running are predisposed to tibiotarsal rotation and leg deviation problems (Figure 12.21). Because of the rapid growth rate of ratites and their disposition, successful surgical recovery and disease resolution of orthopaedic injuries or abnormalities is often unrewarding. Basic mammalian orthopaedic techniques are applicable to ratites.

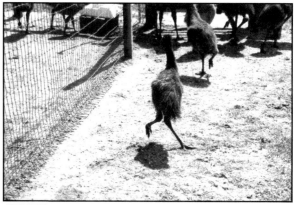

12.21 A young ratite suffering from skeletal leg abnormalities.

Supportive care

Drug administration

- Large ratites will generally swallow pills directly from the hand but oral liquid medication is difficult to administer. Another option is placing medication in food or water; strict adherence to instructions is necessary to ensure that therapeutic levels are attained.
- Although ratites are relatively large, there is no pectoral musculature to serve as an injection site. Intramuscular injection sites should be alternated between the tibiotarsal and thigh muscles of both legs. The lumbar muscles may be used in ostriches if the patient is in good body condition.
- Catheterization is necessary for prolonged intravenous or intraosseous administration but is practical only in a hospital setting. A venous catheter may be placed in the right jugular vein, basilic veins (Figure 12.22) or medial metatarsal veins. An intraosseous catheter may be used in

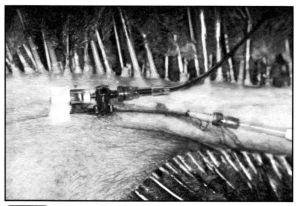

12.22 An indwelling intravenous catheter placed in the basilic vein of an ostrich.

neonates and requires insertion into the proximal aspect of the tibiotarsus or ulna of the ostrich.

- Nebulization therapy is limited to neonates and young juveniles, which are seemingly more susceptible to respiratory disease than adult birds.
- Ophthalmic ointment is preferred over drops, since it often is present for a longer period of time, thereby reducing the number of treatments needed per day.

Fluid therapy

Fluid requirements in ratites may be calculated using the following:

- Fluid maintenance requirement = 50 ml/kg/day
- Deficit = estimated weight x percentage dehydration.

Fluids should be replaced using the intravenous or intraosseous route and the estimated deficit should be replaced over a 48-hour period.

Nutritional support

Anorexic adult ratites can be force-fed using a tube placed directly into the oesophagus, with special attention paid to avoid the glottis. Alternatively, a tube may be inserted using an oesophagostomy procedure through a percutaneous approach: an incision is made approximately midway between the head and thoracic inlet on the left side; after the end of the tube is in position in the proventriculus, it is fixed by insertion of a skin suture. Ratites should be fed at 6-hourly intervals. A slurry of ratite diet can be offered to adults (100 g per 5 kg bodyweight).

Anaesthesia and analgesia

All ratite patients scheduled for anaesthesia should have a complete physical examination prior to the procedure to determine their ability to withstand the associated physiological stresses. Adult ratites should be fasted for 12–24 hours prior to induction of anaesthesia to minimize the risk of regurgitation and aspiration. Pre-anaesthetic and analgesic agents (Figure 12.23) are usually administered intramuscularly, while inhalant gas anaesthetic compounds (e.g. isoflurane, sevoflurane) (isoflurane induction 4.0–5.0% and maintenance 2.0–3.0%) are given via an endotracheal tube (Figure 12.24).

Apnoea during general anaesthesia is not uncommon in ratites. When it occurs, anaesthetic depth should be decreased and ventilation assisted manually or mechanically until spontaneous ventilation is re-established. The cardiovascular system is evaluated by continuously assessing pulse quality and rate, tissue perfusion (mucous membrane colour), electrocardiogram (ECG) and arterial blood pressure. A lead II ECG is recorded, with the right arm and left arm leads placed on the right and left wing webs, respectively. The patient's heart may be auscultated by placing the stethoscope over the lateral aspect of the ribs. Respirations should be slow,

Drug	Dose
Anticholinergics	
Atropine	0.035 mg/kg i.m.
Tranquillizers/Sedatives	
Acepromazine	0.1–0.2 mg/kg i.v. or 0.25–0.5 mg/kg i.m.
Azaperone	0.5–2.0 mg/kg i.m.
Detomidine	1.5 mg/kg i.m.
Diazepam	0.1–0.3 mg/kg i.v. or 0.22–0.44 mg/kg i.m.
Medetomidine	1.1 mg/kg i.m.
Midazolam	0.15 mg/kg i.m.
Xylazine	Sedation: 0.2–1.0 mg/kg i.m. Immobilization: 1.0–2.2 mg/kg i.m.
NSAIDs	
Carprofen	2.2 mg/kg orally q12h
Flunixin meglumine	0.2 mg/kg i.m. once
Metamizole	20–25 mg/kg i.m./i.v./s.c. once
Opioids	
Butorphanol	0.05–0.5 mg/kg i.v./i.m.
Dissociative agents	
Ketamine	Rhea, emu: 20–25 mg/kg i.m. Ostrich: 10–15 mg/kg i.m.
Ketamine + Diazepam	5 mg/kg K + 0.25 mg/kg D i.v. OR 2.2–3.3 mg/kg K i.v. + 0.22–0.5 D i.m. NB Intravenous ketamine given 15–30 minutes after intramuscular diazepam
Ketamine + Xylazine	5 mg/kg K + 1 mg/ml X i.m. OR 2.2 mg/kg K + 0.25 mg/kg X i.v.
Tiletamine/Zolazepam	2–10 mg/kg i.m. or 1–3 mg/kg i.v. High end of dose ranges required for emus and rheas

12.23 Pre-anaesthetic and analgesic agents used in ratites. (Data from Tully and Shane, 1996.)

Patient	Tube size (internal diameter)
Ratite chick (<5 kg)	4–6 mm
Ratite juvenile (5–20 kg)	7–11 mm
Adult rhea/emu (25–50 kg)	12–14 mm
Adult ostrich (>50 kg)	14–18 mm

12.24 Endotracheal tube sizes for ratites.

deep and regular, remaining at or above 8 breaths per minute during a surgical plane of anaesthesia. Oesophageal temperature should be monitored during the anaesthetic period.

For recovery from the anaesthetic procedure, a small dark and quiet environment, free of sharp objects and corners is needed for large adult birds. Hoods may help smooth the recovery of ostriches and the birds should be extubated when a swallowing reflex is observed. During the recovery procedure the bird is placed in sternal recumbency with the head supported until the bird is able to maintain a normal head position unassisted. If recovery is rough, diazepam (0.1–0.2 mg/kg i.v.) may be used. A wrap may also be used around the bird's body to facilitate recovery and reduce the chance of the bird injuring itself.

Common surgical procedures

All basic veterinary surgical procedures need to be followed when treating ratites. Principles of wound management used for mammalian species are applicable.

Proventriculotomy

One of the most common procedures performed on ostriches is the proventriculotomy. This surgery takes place when there is an impaction or ingested foreign body in the proventriculus or ventriculus.

Anaesthesia is induced with xylazine (2 mg/kg) plus ketamine (20 mg/kg) i.m. and then the patient is maintained on isoflurane.

1. Place the bird in right dorsolateral recumbency.
2. Perform a left paramedian approach to access the proventriculus, using as the cranial landmark the cranial aspect of the abducted left leg.
3. Bluntly separate the air sac with the fingers to access the abaxial surface of the proventriculus.
4. Aspirate fluid from the proventriculus through a stab incision, prior to lengthening the incision for removal of foreign material.
5. Remove the contents from the proventriculus.
6. Clean the proventriculus and surrounding tissues with saline-moistened gauze sponges.
7. Lavage the surgery site and clean after each layer of tissue closure.
8. Close the proventriculotomy in layers:
   i. Close the first layer with a simple continuous pattern (3.5 metric (0 USP) polydioxanone)
   ii. Oversew in a continuous Cushing or Lembert pattern
   iii. Close the rectus abdominus with a simple continuous pattern (4 metric (1 USP) polydioxanone)
   iv. Close the skin using a simple continuous pattern (3.5 metric (0 USP) polydioxanone).
9. Place an oesophagostomy tube if required.

Hysterotomy

Hysterotomy is used to relieve egg retention. Anaesthesia is induced with xylazine (2 mg/kg) plus ketamine (20 mg/kg) i.m. and then the patient is maintained on isoflurane.

1. Place the bird in right dorsolateral recumbency.
2. Make a left paramedian incision over the palpable egg.
3. Once the abdomen is entered, exteriorize and isolate the uterine segment containing the egg.
4. Make a small stab incision just proximal to the egg.
5. Aspirate all entrapped fluid in oviduct.
6. Lengthen the incision in the uterus and remove the egg.
7. Flush and lavage the surgical site prior to closure.
8. Close the oviduct in two layers using 3.5 or 4 metric (0 or 1 USP) polydioxanone in a simple continuous pattern, followed by a continuous oversew with a Cushing's pattern.
9. Close the rectus abdominus and skin as described for proventriculotomy.

Yolk sacculectomy

Prior to surgery, antimicrobial therapy should be initiated and continued for 5 days postoperatively. Anaesthesia is induced with xylazine (2 mg/kg) plus ketamine (20 mg/kg) i.m. and then the patient is maintained on isoflurane.

1. Place the bird in dorsal recumbency and prepare the ventral aspect of the body for surgery.
2. Make a 2–3 cm fusiform skin incision around the umbilicus.
3. Tent the rectus abdominus musculature with thumb forceps to prevent incising the yolk sac or abdominal viscera.
4. Exteriorize the yolk sac with gentle bilateral pressure.
5. Clamp around the yolk sac stalk.
6. Use 2 metric (3/0 USP) polydioxanone to place an encircling ligature around the base of the yolk sac.
7. Remove the yolk sac and take a sample from the interior for culture.
8. Close the abdominal wall and skin with 3 metric (2/0 USP) absorbable sutures in patterns of the surgeon's choice.

Euthanasia

It is very dangerous to attempt to euthanase a fully conscious large ratite. Heavy sedation and, preferably, general anaesthesia are recommended prior to administering the euthanasing agent. A commercial pentobarbital solution (0.5 ml/kg i.v.) is the recommended method for euthanasia of a heavily sedated or anaesthetized ratite.

Drug formulary

Knowledge of ratite therapeutics is limited by documented field observation and a lack of subjects for experimental and clinical research. Many ratite owners have limited experience in medicating flocks. A drug formulary is provided in Figure 12.25.

Drug	Dosage	Comments
Antimicrobial agents		
Amikacin	7.6–11 mg/kg i.m. q12h	Animal must be well hydrated
Amoxicillin/Clavulanate	10–15 mg/kg orally q12h	
Ampicillin	4–7 mg/kg i.v./i.m. q8h	
Bacitracin methylene disalicylate	220 mg in 4 litres of drinking water	
Cefotaxime	25 mg/kg i.m. q8h	Young birds
Ceftiofur	10–20 mg/kg i.m. q12h	
Ciprofloxacin	3–6 mg/kg orally q12h	
Doxycycline	2–3.5 mg/kg orally q12h	
Enrofloxacin	1.5–2.5 mg/kg orally q12h	
Metronidazole	20–25 mg/kg orally q12h	
Norfloxacin	3–5 mg/kg orally q12h	
Oxytetracycline	2–5 ml per 50 kg bodyweight i.m. every 3 days	Long-acting; severe muscle necrosis at injection site – use as last resort
Trimethoprim/Sulphonamide	10–15 mg/kg orally/i.m./s.c. q12h	
Antifungal agents		
Fluconazole	Chicks: 5–10 mg/kg orally q24h, up to 15 mg/kg orally q12h for 14–60 days for systemic candidiasis Flocks: 50 mg/l drinking water for 14–60 days	Dose for chicks should be given in an acidic formulation (e.g. apple orange juice). Drinking water for flocks should be acidified to a pH <5
Itraconazole	6–10 mg/kg orally q24h	If neurological signs develop, reduce dosage or discontinue
Ketoconazole	5–10 mg/kg orally q24h	
Nystatin	250,000–500,000 IU/kg orally q12h	Drug must come into contact with lesion or affected area to be effective
Antiparasitic agents		
Albendazole	1 ml per 22 kg bodyweight orally q12h for 3 days; repeat after 14 days	For flagellate and tapeworm parasites
Fenbendazole	5–15 mg/kg orally q24h for 3 days	
Levamisole	30 mg/kg i.m./orally	For *Libiostrongylus douglassi;* give at 1 month of age then once a month for 7 treatments, then 4 times a year
Anti-inflammatory agents		
Dexamethasone	4 mg/kg i.m. q12h for 2 days	Shock
	2 mg/kg i.m. q12h for 2 days	Trauma
Miscellaneous		
Aminophylline	8–10 mg/kg orally/i.m./i.v. q8h	
Cimetidine	3–5 mg/kg orally/i.v. q8h or 5–10 mg/kg i.m. q12h	
Doxapram	4–8 mg/kg i.v. every hour	
Furosemide	0.1 ml q6–12h every 2 days	For oedematous chicks
Mineral oil	15 ml/kg orally	Adult birds – impaction

12.25 Drug formulary for ratites. If the bird being treated is being raised for human consumption, it is the responsibility of the veterinary surgeon to be aware of the withdrawal times required for each drug prior to that animal being processed for food. See Figure 12.23 for anaesthetic and analgesic agents.

References and further reading

Carpenter JW (2005) *Exotic Animal Formulary, 3rd edn.* Elsevier/Saunders, St. Louis

Davies SJJF (2002) *Ratites and Tinamous.* Oxford University Press, New York

Deeming DC (1999) *The Ostrich: Biology, Production, and Health.* CABI, Wallingford

Doneley B (2006) Management of captive ratites. In: *Clinical Avian Medicine II,* ed. GJ Harrison and T Lightfoot, pp. 957–991. Spix Publishing, Palm Beach, FL

Drenowatz C (1996) *The Ratite Encyclopedia: Ostrich – Emu – Rhea.* Ratite Records Inc., San Antonio, TX

Fowler ME (1991) Comparative clinical anatomy of ratites. *Journal of Zoo and Wildlife Medicine* **22**, 204–227

Greve JH and Harrison GJ (1980) Conjunctivitis caused by eye flukes in captive reared ostriches. *Journal of the American Veterinary Medical Association* **177**, 909–910

Griffiths G and Buller N (1991) *Erysipelothrix rhusiopathiae* infection in semi-intensively farmed emu. *Australian Veterinary Journal* **68**, 121–122

Lublin A, Mecham S, Horowitz HI and Weisman Y (1993) A paralytic-like disease of the ostrich (*Struthio camelus*) associated with *Clostridium chauvoei* infection. *Veterinary Record* **132**, 273–275

Malan FS, Gruss B, Roper NA, Ashburner AJ and DuPlesis CA (1988) Resistance of *Libyostrongylus douglassi* in ostriches to levamisole. *Journal of the South African Veterinary Association* **59**, 202–203

Minnaar M (2000) *The Emu Farmer's Handbook.* Schatz Publishing, Blackwell, OK

Snoeyenbos GH (1965) Anthrax. In: *Diseases of Poultry, 5th edn,* ed. HE Biester and LH Schwarte, pp. 432–435. Iowa State University Press, Ames

Stewart JS (1996) Ratites. In: *Avian Medicine: Principles and Application,* ed. BW Ritchie *et al.,* pp. 1284–1326. Wingers, Lake Worth, FL

Tully TN (1994) Examination and joint isolation for lameness in ratites. *Proceedings, Association of Avian Veterinarians Annual Conference* pp. 141–142

Tully TN and Shane SM (1996) *Ratite Management, Medicine, and Surgery.* Krieger Publishing Company, Malabar, FL

Watters CE, Joyce KL, Heath SE and Kazacas KR (1994) *Cyathostoma* spp. infection as the cause of respiration distress in emus (*Dromaius novaehollandiae*). *Proceedings, Association of Avian Veterinarians Annual Conference* pp. 151–156

13

Crocodilians

Darryl Heard

Introduction

Crocodilians should not be kept as pets. All are dangerous and have the potential to maim or kill. Many species are critically endangered. All require large terrestrial and aquatic habitats, as well as warm temperatures for optimum health. Veterinary surgeons are most likely to be consulted for animals housed in zoological or research facilities, or crocodilian farms.

All living crocodilians belong to the family Crocodylidae, subdivided into crocodiles (*Crocodylus*, *Osteolaemus*), false gavial (*Tomistoma*), alligators (*Alligator*), caiman (*Caiman*, *Melanosuchus*, *Paleosuchus*) and gharial (*Gavialis*). Figure 13.1 illustrates some commonly kept species.

Biology

A table of biological data is given in Figure 13.2.

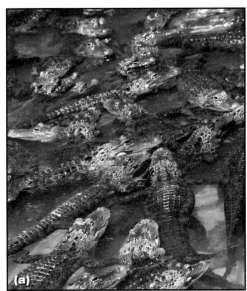
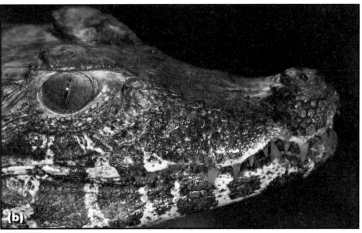

13.1 Crocodilians are not recommended as pets. Some species that may be encountered by veterinary surgeons include: **(a)** American alligator and **(b)** spectacled caiman.

	American alligator (*Alligator mississippiensis*)	Spectacled caiman (*Caiman crocodilus*)	Dwarf caiman (*Paleosuchus palpebrosus*)	Saltwater crocodile (*Crocodylus porosus*)	American crocodile (*Crocodylus acutus*)
Natural distribution	Southeastern North America, extending to northeastern Mexico	Central and South America	South America	Asia, Australia	Florida, South America, West Indies
Habitat	Estuaries, freshwater, venturing into salt water for short periods	Lakes, ponds, marshes, tributaries			
Adult length	Males: >4 m Females: average 2.8 m	2–3 m	1.5 m	6–7 m	Adult body length: 4.5 m
Lifespan (years)	30–50	12–20	15–30	18–45	30–50
Average no. eggs laid	40	30	18–25	53	

13.2 Biological data for some crocodilians. (Data from Webb and Manolis, 1989, and Lane, 2006)

Anatomy and physiology

All living crocodilians are similar in structure; the main differences between species are in adult size, skull structure and skin. The skin is covered with scales or 'scutes', arranged in different patterns for each species. The skin of the skull is closely adhered to the underlying bone. Bony plates (osteoderms) are present in the dorsal as well as ventral scales of some species. These calcified structures may obscure radiographic visualization of internal structures (Figure 13.3) and can interfere with needle placement for blood collection. Although tough and heavily protected, the skin is well innervated with pain, thermal and mechanoreceptors. Paired holocrine glands are present lateral to the cloacal opening (cloacal or paracloacal) and in the posterior intermandibular skin (mandibular or gular). Each large paracloacal gland empties through a single duct. These glands may be mistaken for abscesses during necropsy.

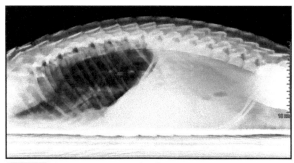

13.3 Lateral radiograph of a dwarf caiman. Note the presence of the osteoderms (bony plates) within the scales.

The external nares are located at the dorsorostral end of the skull, and are closed tightly except during inhalation and exhalation (Figure 13.4ab). The opening to the ear is located caudal to the eye and is covered by a flap (Figure 13.4c). During diving, sphincters close the nares and a depressor muscle closes the auricular flap. The eyes can be retracted and closed tightly, making ophthalmic examination difficult. An opaque third eyelid covers the cornea during submersion (Figure 13.4d).

The homomorphic (same shape) teeth are replaced constantly throughout life, although this process slows as the animal ages. The teeth should be pointed and sharp and are usually white (Figure 13.5). In crocodiles the first mandibular canine is the longest and often extends above the snout. In some animals mandibular incisors penetrate the maxilla to produce 'false nares'. The teeth are surrounded by mechano- and pain receptors, as well as taste buds. The large tongue covers the floor of the mouth, but is attached laterally and is relatively immobile. Crocodiles have salt glands on the dorsal surface of the tongue; in hypovitaminosis A the lingual glands may be altered by squamous metaplasia leading to caseous abscesses. The powerful jaw muscles attach to the medial mandibular surfaces. The jaw articulation is behind the atlanto-occipital joint, allowing a very wide mouth opening. The closing force of the jaws of an adult American alligator is sufficient to crush the shell of a large freshwater turtle.

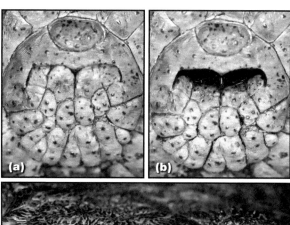
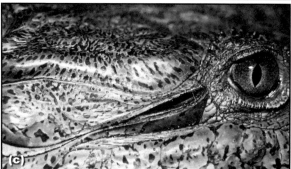
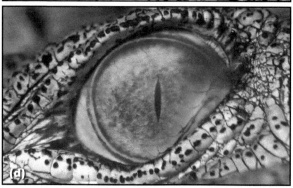

13.4 Adaptations to an aquatic life. Crocodilian nares are kept tightly closed **(a)** except during inhalation and exhalation **(b)**. **(c)** The openings to the ears are covered by the auricular flap. **(d)** The opaque third eyelid covers the eye during diving.

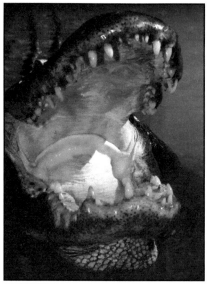

13.5 The oral cavity of an adult American alligator. Note: the large sharp white teeth; the gular flap at the back of the throat; the large relatively immobile tongue; and the wide powerful gape.

The oral cavity is separated from the pharynx by the gular flap (Figure 13.5), which allows crocodilians to open their mouths underwater. The simple glottis lies immediately behind this flap, is linked to the internal nares, and closes during swallowing. Both eustachian tubes enter the pharynx through a common opening slightly posterior to the internal nares. Close to this opening are two lateral mucosal folds containing tonsillar tissue; this tissue is important for sampling during necropsy for evidence of infectious disease. As would be expected, the thoracic inlet is big to allow large portions of unmasticated food to be swallowed. In crocodiles, but not alligators, the trachea bends to the left inside the thorax before its bifurcation.

All vertebrae have dorsal spinous processes, and both the cervical and thoracic vertebrae have ribs. The ribs connected to the sternum are partially cartilaginous, allowing them to collapse during diving. The caudal vertebrae have ventral spinous processes (haemal arches) protecting the coccygeal vessels. The pubic bones are connected to the sternum by a fibrous membrane containing abdominal ribs (gastralia). This membrane supports the abdominal viscera. The humerus, radius and ulna are short; the hindlimbs are twice as long as the forelimbs. The fore- and hindlimbs have five and four toes, respectively. Claws are present on the first three toes of each limb.

The lungs are highly vascularized, thick-walled and multisaccular. They lie in pleural chambers separated by a complete mediastinum. Two transverse membranes divide the thorax from the abdomen. These fibrous and muscular membranes attach the caudal lung to the liver and the liver to the os pubis. During inspiration the liver is pulled caudally, increasing the volume of the lungs and generating a negative pressure. Expiration is both passive and active. Crocodilians make a range of sounds by forcing air through the compressed glottal opening.

The oesophagus has many longitudinal folds to accommodate large chunks of food. The stomach lies to the left, immediately behind the left lobe of the liver. There is a well defined sphincter between the cardia and the oesophagus. The small bulbous pyloric antrum lies slightly to the right of the cardia and opens into the duodenum. The pyloric opening is very small, preventing the escape of foreign bodies. The gastric wall is strongly muscularized, giving the stomach a gizzard-like appearance. Stones are commonly found in the stomach but their function is unknown. The intestine, as in other vertebrates, is composed of duodenum, jejunum, ileum and colorectum emptying into the cloaca. The duodenum is looped, sometimes doubly in crocodiles. The intestinal mucosa is formed into a system of complex zigzagging, ridge-like folds.

The proximal pancreas lies within the duodenal loop, while the distal part surrounds the cranial spleen. The liver is bilobed, the right being slightly larger than the left and separated by the heart. The gallbladder lies between the two lobes and receives bile from both. The pear-shaped spleen lies in the mesentery close to the base of the duodenal loop. The four chambers of the heart are completely separated and crocodilians have two aortic arches.

The two kidneys are firmly attached to the dorsal abdominal wall in the caudal coelom. They lack a capsule and are not embedded in fat. The renal tissue is folded over, in a single fold in the dwarf crocodile and in multiple folds in other species. Crocodilians do not have a urinary bladder; the two ureters open into the cloaca.

Crocodilians are considered to be ectotherms (poikilotherms), requiring external sources of heat to maintain body temperature. Thermoregulation is accomplished, both in water and on land, through heat-seeking or heat-avoidance behaviour. Water serves as a heat reservoir as well as a cooling medium. All crocodilians seek heat (thermophilia) after feeding, to increase the rate of digestion and absorption. As with other reptiles, thermal selection affects the immune status, disease control and overall metabolism.

Sexing

Most crocodilians are not sexually dimorphic, although adult males are usually larger than females. The male gharial develops a protuberance on the end of its nose when sexually mature. The sex of all crocodilian species can be determined by palpation of the anterior cloaca (Figure 13.6): the male has a phallus; females possess a similar, but much smaller, structure. The phallus can occasionally be extruded in juveniles by gently palpating the cloacal area. Males have paired internal testes close to the kidneys. Females have paired ovaries and all species are oviparous.

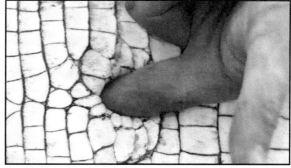

13.6 Crocodilians can be sexed by palpating the cloaca.

Husbandry

Housing

Adult crocodilians should not be housed in mixed-species exhibits. Cannibalism is common when small individuals are housed with larger ones. Compatibility will also change depending on sexual status, housing density, body size and for unknown reasons. Even animals housed together for many years may suddenly turn on each other. This aggression can be reduced by providing adequate hiding areas. Some species, especially alligators and dwarf crocodiles, can make extensive tunnels into the mud banks of aquatic enclosures.

Some crocodilians can tolerate high densities as juveniles (e.g. alligators), but not as adults. For a pair of crocodiles, the land area must have a width that is a minimum of 3 times the largest animal's snout-to-vent length (SVL) and a length that is 4 SVL. The minimum water area must be 4 times the largest animal's SVL wide, and 5 SVL long; minimum water depth must be 0.3 SVL.

Crocodilians are adapted to environments with moderate to high humidity and warm temperatures. Most have a preferred body temperature (PBT) of approximately 30°C (29–34°C). Air temperatures in enclosures can range from 36°C during the day to 20°C at night, but water temperatures are maintained around 27–31°C. It is important that animals do not overheat; temperatures >40°C should be avoided. Conversely, long periods of hypothermia will depress appetite, slow digestion and growth, and impair immune function.

In small to medium-sized enclosures the water can be heated with submersible aquarium heaters capable of using 1 watt of power to heat 1 litre of water. All heaters must: have a thermostat to prevent overheating; be pre-tested before adding an animal to the enclosure; and be connected to a ground-fault circuit interrupter (GFCI). All heaters should be installed so that the animal cannot directly contact it: a strong rust-proof wire mesh or cage material can be used.

At least one basking area over land is required in the enclosure for each crocodilian. A thermostat is used to control the temperature. When environmental temperatures are measured they are taken at the level where the animal's head or back is likely to be. The temperatures to aim for are at the higher end of the PBT. The surface temperature of the substrate must also be measured because a cold surface, even in a warm environment, will make an animal hypothermic. Incandescent bulbs are commonly used as heating elements. Other heat sources suitable for larger enclosures include ceramic heat emitters. Higher wattages require a ceramic lamp holder because the lamps become very hot. To prevent thermal injury it must be ensured that the animals cannot reach the heater. An advantage of a ceramic heat emitter is it can be used at night without emitting light to disrupt the circadian cycle. Many crocodilians are active at night, but do not require a night light.

The land area should be large enough for every animal to emerge from the water into an area either within or outside the basking spot. Most crocodilians require a daylength of 12–13 hours and a night period. Light can be provided by incandescent bulbs or fluorescent tubes, or natural light if the daylength is long enough. Dim light at night can be provided by coloured incandescent bulbs, or natural moonlight when available. Although controversial, it is recommended that a fluorescent light which emits both UV-A and UV-B wavelengths be used for animals not exposed to sunlight. Some species of crocodilians, such as the dwarf caimans (*Paleosuchus*) and the dwarf crocodile (*Osteolaemus*) often spend considerable amounts of their daytime hidden in burrows or under dense vegetation in the wild.

Contaminated water and unclean enclosures reflect poor husbandry practices and predispose the animals to disease. Any uneaten food should be removed from the enclosure as soon as possible, and faeces should be cleaned up immediately. A filtration system is used to keep the water clean. Unless the water is replaced frequently, it is recommended that a bacterial system is used to break down ammonia and other toxic contaminants. Protein films that form on the water surface are removed with skimmers. No matter the type of filtration system, frequent water changes are recommended as for aquarium maintenance, depending on water quality. The enclosure must also be cleaned periodically (every week or two).

Diet

All crocodilians are carnivores. Although the ideal diet should mimic that eaten in the wild, the diet and nutritional requirements of many crocodilian species has not been defined. Dietary supplementation should be unnecessary if the animals are fed a complete balanced diet. Crocodilians can be fed a whole prey item (e.g. rodent, rabbit), a commercial pelleted diet or, in the case of fish-eaters, whole fish or a fish gel. This author recommends the use of commercial pellets because they are balanced, inexpensive and it is easy to monitor the food intake of an animal. Similarly, the fish gels are balanced and less expensive than feeding fresh fish. Contrary to popular opinion, crocodilians do not like eating rotten food.

All crocodilians should have access to water for drinking and bathing. Some species, e.g. the estuarine or saltwater crocodile (*Crocodylus porosus*) can drink salt water.

Breeding

Age at sexual maturity varies between species; for example, 4 years in the spectacled caiman, but around 12 (females) or 16 (males) years in saltwater crocodiles. Captive animals may reach sexual maturity earlier than wild animals, due to optimal feeding and temperature maintenance.

Crocodilians have strong and dramatic courtship behaviours that often occur over several months, increasing during the breeding season in both wild and captive populations. Displays consist of roaring or bellowing and head slapping by both males and females. Copulation mainly occurs in the early morning hours.

Nest building (usually a mound) and egg deposition occur at night. Average egg numbers laid are detailed in Figure 13.2. Most females are fairly docile during the egg-laying process but may become extremely broody and guard the nest aggressively once the eggs have been laid. Incubation time depends on temperature, ranging from 40 to 100 days. Gender determination is also dependent on incubation temperature (Figure 13.7).

	All females	Males and females	All males
Caimans, alligators	28–30°C	31–32°C	32–34°C
Crocodiles	28–30.9°C	31–33°C (males predominate)	>33°C

13.7 Incubation temperature and gender determination.

For artificial incubation, eggs should be collected immediately after laying. When removing an egg from the nest, the top should be marked and the same orientation maintained in the incubator, with the upper surface of the egg remaining exposed to the air. Incubation requires careful temperature regulation, and no disturbance of the eggs. The eggs are *not* rotated during development. Moisture levels need to be close to 100% relative humidity, with good air flow around the eggs. Air should be bubbled through water and humidified before it enters the incubator. Most species can be incubated at 31–32°C for 75–85 days. American alligators have more rapid development and are incubated for only 69–72 days. Temperatures above 34°C or below 29°C cause a number of developmental abnormalities and lead to poor hatchability and survival.

Crocodiles are usually fully developed when they pip from the egg and can be taken out manually, washed with clean warm water, and placed in a hatchling pen. If the yolk has not been fully internalized by hatching, survival rate is lower. American alligators need to hatch themselves fully before being removed from the egg tray. Optimal conditions for hatchlings vary with species, but a suitable ambient temperature for most hatchlings is 30–32°C, with a basking area allowing for body temperature elevation to 35°C. Hatchlings will seek the darkest corner if fully exposed, and will crowd or pile up; smaller and weaker animals may be suffocated or drowned. Loud noises, inability to escape other animals, humans or elevated temperatures will cause stress. Water quality and sanitation must be impeccable for hatchlings to survive, as nitrogenous waste accumulation affects bacterial and parasitic numbers.

Hatchlings should be fed fresh high-quality food. If frozen foods are used, they should be defrosted just before feeding. There are a number of different diets used, but all should contain large amounts of calcium and low amounts of fat. Food must be of appropriate size for the hatchling, but also of a size that does not wash away in the water as the animal eats. Many species take food into the water to consume, making keeping water clean difficult.

Microchipping

The microchip is best placed at the base of the neck. A reader on the end of a pole can then be used to read it.

Handling and restraint

Physical restraint or chemical immobilization (see later) is required for examination and collection of diagnostic samples. Techniques for restraint of juvenile and adult crocodilians are well described by Vliet (2007). If a veterinary surgeon has no experience restraining a crocodilian, especially medium to large animals, they **must** seek help from people who have.

All crocodilians are dangerous. Although the teeth are the most obvious potential cause of injury, the tail can also inflict severe damage. Some crocodilians show behavioural indications of impending aggression (e.g. hissing), but most do not. Aggressive responses are explosive and crocodilians may not immediately respond to touch or a close approach. When restrained they will roll to escape.

Small crocodilians can be caught using protective gloves or a heavy towel. All crocodilians should be approached from behind; the immediate aim of capture is to grasp the animal behind the head and press it down to the ground. The opening force of the jaws is weak and they can be taped shut with electrical tape (Figure 13.8a). The tape must avoid the nares. If the jaws are taped for long periods of time the animal will become dehydrated, even if immersed in water. The legs must not be tied above the back because of the potential for muscle injury. Struggling crocodilians will develop lactic acidosis. Large crocodilians can be restrained using flat boards and strapping (Figure 13.8b). Captive crocodilians may also be trained to enter restraint crates for blood collection and other minor diagnostic procedures.

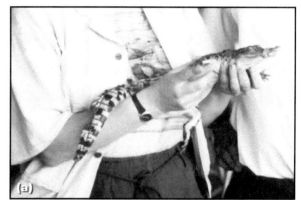
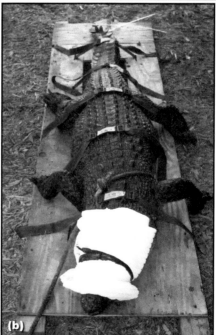

13.8 Restraint. **(a)** Holding a juvenile saltwater crocodile, with jaws taped. (Courtesy of C. Johnson-Delaney.) **(b)** Medium to large crocodilians may be restrained on boards with straps to allow transport and minor diagnostic procedures.

Diagnostic approach

History

The history, especially concerning husbandry, is very important in evaluating crocodilian patients.

Clinical examination

Physical examination first begins at a distance, observing the enclosure and the animal. The animal is assessed for body position, abnormal swellings or discharges, respiration rate, body condition, relationship to its physical surroundings, interaction with other animals in the enclosure, and response to feeding and other stimuli (i.e. noise, approach of a human, touch). Figure 13.9 gives details for systematic examination.

Observation from a distance
Location in relation to water, land, heat sources, other animals Water position – buoyancy, asymmetry, rolling Interaction with other animals, keepers, feeding Abnormal limb position, swellings, discharges, skin discoloration, odour
Skin
Colour Presence of lacerations, swellings, ulcerations, vesicles, crusts Reddened skin (hyperaemia) or haemorrhage in scales suggest vasculitis due septicaemia/bacteraemia Leeches?
Body condition
Cachexia indicated by prominent supertemporal fossae, pelvic bones, tail lying to side, obvious neck Obesity indicated by prominent jowls, generalized body distension
Limbs
Presence or absence of toes or limbs Position Swellings, discharge
Head
Shape Orientation
Eyes
Swelling Colour
Teeth and jaws
Teeth colour, position Relationship of mandible to maxilla
Oral cavity
Colour, ulcers, crusts, other lesions Halitosis
Nares
Open/closed Discharges Colour, ulcerations
Ears
Discharge, swellings, ulceration
Cloaca
Colour, discharge, swelling, ulcerations

13.9 Physical examination.

Supertemporal fossae, located dorsal and posterior to the eyes, are indicative in some species of muscle wasting (Figure 13.10).

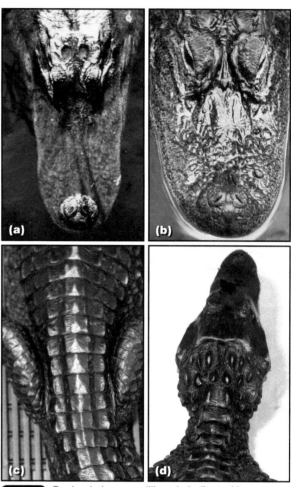

13.10 Cachexia in crocodilians is indicated by prominent supertemporal fossae **(a, b)**, obvious pelvic bones **(c)** and a narrow neck **(d)**.

Imaging

Radiography is an important diagnostic tool but the large size of many crocodilians may exceed the capability of many veterinary radiology units. The osteoderms can also make interpretation difficult (see Figure 13.3). Computed tomography (CT) and magnetic resonance imaging (MRI) can be used in crocodilians and are particularly useful in evaluating lung disease. On plain radiographs the gastrointestinal tract should contain little to no air (see Figure 13.3). Lead fragments ingested in prey items are readily identified on radiographs.

Endoscopy is an important diagnostic tool in evaluating the presence of lung disease in crocodilians. It can be performed in small crocodilians with them awake. It can also be used for evaluating the upper gastrointestinal tract for disease.

Sample collection

Blood

Approximately 10% of the blood volume can be collected safely, assuming the animal is not severely anaemic. In reptiles this is approximately 0.6–1.0% of bodyweight (1 ml = 1 g). For example, 30–50 ml could be collected from a 5 kg animal. Blood for a complete blood count (CBC) and plasma biochemical panel can be collected into a heparinized syringe, and then placed into serum tubes. Alternatively, blood for the CBC can be collected into a non-heparinized syringe and placed in an edetate calcium disodium tube; crocodilian blood appears not to be as susceptible to haemolysis as that of other reptiles. Several air-dried smears should be prepared. One heparinized blood sample should be centrifuged immediately, and the plasma separated, decanted and frozen until analysis.

There are several blood collection sites in crocodilians. These include the supravertebral sinus, and ventral and dorsal coccygeal vessels. All blood collection sites should be cleaned and disinfected before inserting the needle through the skin.

The supravertebral sinus lies immediately above the spinal cord. The indentation immediately behind the back of the skull is palpated and the needle inserted in the midline at the point of greatest depression (Figure 13.11a). Once the needle is inserted through the skin, the plunger of the syringe is pulled back to generate a small amount of negative pressure. The needle is oriented at 90 degrees to the surface of the skull and slowly advanced until blood enters the syringe (Figure 13.11b). The hub of the needle is steadied with one hand resting on the animal. If the animal twitches or clear liquid enters the needle it has gone too far. If the needle contacts bone, the needle is withdrawn and redirected. Needle size depends on the animal. The largest needle required for an adult would be 6–8 cm long, while 3 cm should be adequate for most medium to smaller size crocodilians. The dorsal coccygeal vessels (see below) are an extension of the supravertebral sinus.

The ventral coccygeal vessels are located in the midline immediately below the vertebral bodies. They include both an artery and vein(s) and are protected by ventral spinous processes formed into haemal arches, which angle caudoventrally. The coccygeal vessels can be accessed using a ventral or a lateral approach. For the **ventral approach** the animal is placed either in dorsal recumbency, or left in sternal recumbency and the tail lifted and gently flexed to expose the ventral surface. The needle is inserted in the midline and advanced cranially at a 40–45 degree angle until either the vertebral body or vessels are contacted. If bone is touched, the needle is withdrawn gently with a slight negative pressure and redirected. The **lateral approach** allows the animal to remain in ventral recumbency (Figure 13.12). The transverse process is palpated, and the needle inserted between the process and the ventral midline. The needle is perpendicular to the long axis, but angled upward at 45 degrees. The needle is then advanced until it contacts the bone of the vertebral body, then 'walked' ventrally until it enters the coccygeal vessels.

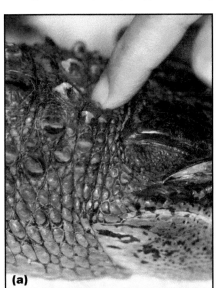

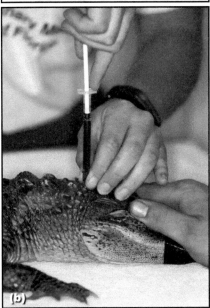

13.11 Blood collection from the supravertebral sinus. After disinfecting the skin, the depression behind the skull is palpated **(a)** and the needle inserted in the midline **(b)** and advanced until blood is aspirated.

(a)

(b)

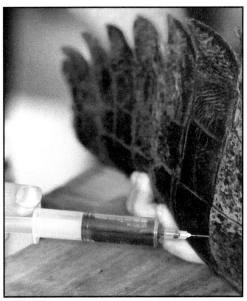

13.12 The ventral coccygeal vessels can be accessed from the ventrolateral surface of the tail.

The dorsal coccygeal vessel(s) can be accessed in the midline, in a similar way to the supravertebral sinus discussed above. The space between the spinous processes on the tail is palpated and the needle inserted in the midline until blood is aspirated.

Although this technique works well for juveniles, in adults the insertion site is protected by osteoderms.

There are several publications of reference ranges for blood values in crocodilians (for example, see Figure 13.13). CBC and plasma biochemical values are similar to those of other reptiles. Electrolyte values are similar to mammals and birds. Mature females are seasonally hyperalbuminaemic and hypercalcaemic, and calcium is elevated in females undergoing folliculogenesis, but a P:Ca ratio >1 suggests renal dysfunction. Normal and abnormal values given by laboratories must be treated with caution as there are no reference data for many species. Massive seasonal changes in normal haematology and biochemical values are also possible.

Parameter	American alligators	Dwarf caimans
Haematology		
PVC (%)	25 (12–40)	22 (16–29)
RBC (x10^{12}/l)	600 (230–1290)	640 (430–890)
Hb (g/dl)	7.8 (3.7–11.6)	7.3 (5.3–8.8)
MCV (fl)	445 (230–1174)	382 (180–540)
MCH (pg/cell)	139 (58–370)	119 (98–140)
MCHC (g/l)	3.2 (1.8–6.5)	3.1 (2.3–3.8)
WBC (x10^9/l)	0 (180–2900)	570 (250–1060)
Biochemistry		
ALP (IU/l)	39 (0–109)	13 (6–29)
ALT (IU/l)	39 (0–154)	52 (24–93)
AST (IU/l)	289 (0–700)	111 (42–221)
Calcium (mmol/l)	2.75 (0–3.89)	2.82 (0.18–3.59)
Chloride (mmol/l)	110 (0–130)	119 (9–137)
Cholesterol (mmol/l)	2.43 (0–6.34)	3.28 (1.71–8.90)
Creatine kinase (IU/l)	2022 (0–8620)	2350 (37–9890)
Creatinine (mmol/l)	35.36 (0–114.92)	17.68 (0–44.2)
Glucose (mmol/l)	5.05 (0–10.99)	4.24 (1.61–10.38)
Phosphorus (mmol/l)	1.42 (0–3.04)	1.71 (0.84–4.39)
Potassium (mmol/l)	3.8 (0–6)	4.6 (3.3–7.9)
Total protein (g/l)	53 (25–94)	55 (36–74)
Albumin (g/l)	16 (8–23)	16 (9–27)
Globulin (g/l)	36 (16–60)	41 (3–54)
Sodium (mmol/l)	146 (0–165)	150 (140–162)
Uric acid (mg/l)	16 (0–57)	22 (7–45)

13.13 Haematological and serum biochemical values of selected crocodilians. (Data from Diethelm and Stein, 2006).

Blood culture: Blood culture (2–5 ml in appropriate media bottles) is useful for identifying circulating bacteria and sensitivity testing can be performed to direct antimicrobial therapy. It is very important that blood for culture is collected as sterilely as possible, to avoid environmental contamination. The skin must be disinfected, sterile surgical gloves worn by the collector, and the needle used for collection changed to a new sterile needle before insertion into the blood culture bottle.

Faeces
Faeces are usually eliminated into the water. Fresh samples collected from water with a dip net may be examined as for any other mammal. Since the sample is from water, care must be taken in interpreting the significance of motile protozoa. Since crocodilians are carnivores, parasites and their ova from prey items will also pass through in the digesta.

Urine
The primary nitrogenous excretory product is ammonia. As crocodilians do not have a bladder, their urine is excreted into water and usually not recoverable. Some crocodilians will void faeces and urine when handled. Crocodiles, unlike alligatorids, are able to tolerate salt water without increases in plasma sodium and chloride.

Cerebrospinal fluid
The subarachnoid space lies immediately below the supravertebral sinus. To obtain a sample uncontaminated by blood it is necessary to use a spinal needle directed through the sinus into the space. The author has used ultrasonography to identify this space and direct a needle into the subarachnoid space. Normal reference ranges have not been defined for cerebrospinal fluid in either crocodilians or other reptiles, but the presence of bacteria or large numbers of white blood cells is likely to signify infection within the nervous system.

Nasal samples
Nasal swabs are indicated when upper respiratory disease is suspected. Unfortunately, it is very difficult to obtain a sample from an awake animal, though it may be possible to wait for inhalation and rapidly insert a swab. Alternatively, in anaesthetized crocodilians a nasal flush is preferable for sample collection.

Common conditions

Figure 13.14 summarizes common disease processes based on body system involved, and can be used as a guide to begin formulating a differential diagnosis list. The most common health problems in captive crocodilians are related to husbandry and trauma. Several nutritional deficiency syndromes have been identified, including metabolic bone disease, hypovitaminosis A and E, and thiamine deficiency. Obesity can also be a major problem. Lead toxicosis is a possible complication of feeding either prey that has been shot or urban wildlife contaminated with lead.

Condition	Cause	Clinical signs	Diagnostics	Treatment
Skin				
Bacterial dermatitis	Usually Gram-negative, occasionally Gram-positive organisms; *Dermatophilus*	Skin discoloration; swollen scales; ulceration; haemorrhage into scales; skin sloughing	Biopsy; culture; PCR	Antimicrobial therapy. Remove from water. Increase environmental temperature. Remove obvious sources of stress
Fungal dermatitis	Many species; mixed mycotic/ bacterial infection common; predisposed by low environmental temperatures	Similar to bacterial dermatitis	Histopathology; culture; PCR	Systemic and/or topical therapy
Leeches	Variety of species	Leeches present in oral cavity, eyelids, under ear flaps or axillae	Visual	Physically remove. Bathe in saltwater
Nutritional disease	Hypovitaminosis A	Hyperkeratosis with build-up of oedematous or unshed skin; secondary bacterial/fungal infection due to dysecdysis	Histopathology; blood retinoic acid levels; dietary review	Vitamin A injection. Dietary correction. Appropriate antimicrobials if infection is preventing proper shedding of skin
Pox	Poxvirus	White to dark brown multifocal crusty lesions	Biopsy (histopathology shows typical intracytoplasmic inclusions); PCR; electron microscopy	No treatment. Antimicrobial therapy for secondary bacterial infection
Trauma	Intraspecific aggression (main cause); cage furnishings/ environmental injury	Lacerations	History; visual	Supportive care. Antimicrobial therapy. Topical cleansing
Eyes				
Blindness	Trauma; panophthalmitis		Cytology; culture; PCR	Treat underlying infections. Enucleation
Conjunctivitis	Trauma; bacteria; fungi	Swollen lids; discharge; discoloration	Cytology; culture; PCR	Systemic antimicrobial therapy. Subconjunctival antibiotic injection
Glaucoma	? Congenital; infectious	Globe distension	Ophthalmic examination; intraocular pressure measurement	Treat underlying infection. Symptomatic therapy. Enucleation?
Third eyelid prolapse	Periocular inflammation	Swollen prolapsed eyelid	Cytology; culture; PCR	Symptomatic treatment
Trauma	Intraspecific aggression	Corneal laceration; ruptured globe	History; visual	Symptomatic wound management
Teeth				
Abnormal mineralization	Dietary calcium deficiency; Ca:P imbalance; inadequate UV exposure?	Translucent teeth, easily damaged or lost	Histopathology; dietary assessment; radiography	Correct nutritional deficiencies
Abnormal position	Dietary calcium deficiency; Ca:P imbalance; inadequate UV exposure?	Malleable jaws ('rubber jaw')	Histopathology; dietary assessment; radiography	Correct nutritional deficiencies
Protruding incisors	Dietary calcium deficiency; Ca:P imbalance; inadequate UV exposure?	Horizontal incisors; swollen jaws	Histopathology; dietary assessment; radiography	Correct nutritional deficiencies
Tooth loss	Normal; trauma; vitamin A deficiency; metabolic bone disease; osteomyelitis	Small broken teeth; no tooth replacement	Histopathology; dietary assessment; culture; radiography	Correct nutritional deficiencies
Gingivitis				
Bacterial	Gram-negative bacteria	Ulceration; swelling	Cytology; biopsy; culture	Dental cleaning and irrigation of gingiva. Appropriate antimicrobial therapy. If dental abscess, remove affected tooth

13.14 Common disease problems by system. (continues) ▶

Condition	Cause	Clinical signs	Diagnostics	Treatment
Gingivitis continued				
Hyperkeratosis	Hypovitaminosis A	Tooth loss; gingival swelling; tongue abscesses	Biopsy; dietary history; blood retinoic acid levels	Vitamin A injection. Correct diet
Pox	Poxvirus	White to dark brown multifocal crusty lesions	Biopsy (histopathology shows typical intracytoplasmic inclusions); PCR; electron microscopy	No treatment. Antimicrobial therapy for secondary bacterial infection
Traumatic	Intraspecific aggression	Lacerations; fractures	Visual	Symptomatic wound management
Stomach				
Gastritis	Bacteria; endoparasites; heavy metal; virus; fungus	Anorexia; weight loss; regurgitation; bloating	History; endoscopy; biopsy; culture; PCR	Antimicrobial therapy. Chelating agents. Antiparasitics
Ulcers	Stress; bacteria; foreign bodies; malnutrition	Anorexia; weight loss; regurgitation; bloating	History; endoscopy; biopsy; culture; PCR	Antimicrobial therapy. Correct husbandry and diet. Remove foreign bodies
Intestines				
Enteritis, hypomotility	Bacteria (mainly Gram-negative); endoparasites (common but rarely cause disease); heavy metal (gunshot (lead) or coins (zinc) tossed into water by public); virus; fungus; depressed immune function due to poor husbandry or malnutrition predispose to secondary infection	Anorexia; regurgitation; weight loss; septicaemia/bacteraemia; diarrhoea; abnormal flotation	Blood electrolytes; acid–base; endoscopy; biopsy; culture; PCR; radiography (including contrast studies); ultrasonography	Depends on cause: antimicrobials; antiparasitics; chelation; laxatives; surgery. General supportive care
Occlusion	Foreign body; severe enteritis; ileus	Anorexia; regurgitation; weight loss; bloating; abnormal flotation	Blood electrolytes; acid–base; endoscopy; biopsy; culture; PCR; radiography; ultrasonography	Antimicrobial therapy if abnormal gut flora. Parenteral fluids. Surgery
Liver				
Adenoviral hepatitis	Adenovirus	Non-specific debilitation	Liver biopsy and histopathology; PCR; elevated AST	Supportive care. Antimicrobial therapy for secondary bacterial infection
Bacterial hepatitis	Gram-negative bacteria	Non-specific debilitation	Liver aspiration/biopsy for histopathology	Antimicrobial therapy
Chlamydial hepatitis	*Chlamydophila* spp.	Non-specific debilitation	Liver aspiration/biopsy for histopathology; PCR; culture	Oxytetracycline, doxycycline, enrofloxacin
Renal system				
Gout	Renal injury – drugs, bacteria	Non-specific debilitation (visceral gout); swollen joints; decreased activity; reluctance to leave water; difficulty in walking; periarticular and articular swelling	Uricaemia (may not be present depending on stage of disease); arthrocentesis and cytology (characteristic uric acid crystals)	Treat renal disease. Symptomatic therapy
Pyelonephritis	Ascending bacterial infection	Non-specific debilitation	Clinicopathological indicators of diminished renal function (difficult); urinalysis; ultrasonography	Antimicrobial therapy
Reproductive system				
Ectopic eggs	Repetitive breeding; metritis; older animal	Non-specific; cessation of egg-laying; debilitation	Radiography; CT; MRI; coelomic aspiration to detect free egg yolk and inflammation	Surgical removal. Antimicrobial therapy for secondary bacterial infection
Uterine prolapse	Egg laying	Tissue protruding from cloaca	Cloacoscopy; ultrasonography	Surgical replacement or removal. Antimicrobial therapy for secondary infection

13.14 (continued) Common disease problems by system. (continues) ▶

Condition	Cause	Clinical signs	Diagnostics	Treatment
Nervous system				
Encephalitis/ meningitis	Bacteria; fungi; *Mycoplasma*; West Nile Virus	Depression; debilitation; ataxia; paresis; paralysis	CSF tap; culture; cytology; MRI; serology	Antimicrobial therapy
Encephalo- malacia	Thiamine deficiency – feeding fish deficient in thiamine and/or endogenous thiaminases	Opisthotonus; depression; debilitation; ataxia; paresis; paralysis	History; clinical signs; CSF tap; culture; cytology; MRI; response to therapy; thiamine blood levels	Thiamine injections. Correct diet
Respiratory system				
Pentastomiasis	Pentastomid worms, several species	Debilitation; secondary respiratory disease	Faecal and tracheal wash, examination for ova; endoscopy of lungs	No drug therapy. Physical removal impractical if large numbers present. Intermediate stages go through fish – do not feed wild-caught fish
Pneumonia	Parasites; bacteria; fungi; *Mycoplasma*; *Chlamydophila* spp.	No clinical signs usually; possible abnormal flotation	Tracheal wash; cytology; culture; radiography; CT; MRI; endoscopy	Antimicrobial therapy. Increase environmental temperature. Remove other stressors. Assess and correct diet
Rhinitis	Trauma; bacteria; fungi; *Mycoplasma*; *Chlamydophila* spp.	Nasal discharge; perinasal ulceration	Cytology; culture; radiography; CT; MRI	Antimicrobial therapy. Increase environmental temperature. Remove other stressors. Assess and correct diet
Musculoskeletal system				
Arthritis	Trauma; bacteria; *Mycoplasma*; fungi	Swollen joints; difficulty or reluctance to move	Radiography; arthrocentesis; cytology and culture	Antimicrobial therapy. Joint lavage/drainage. NSAIDs
Metabolic bone disease	Dietary calcium deficiency; Ca:P imbalance; inadequate UV exposure?	Pathological fractures; hindlimb paresis; muscle fasciculations	Radiography; blood calcium usually normal	Correct diet. Correct UV exposure?
Swollen leg(s)	Bacterial cellulitis secondary to bite wounds; ulcerative pododermatitis	Swollen leg	Radiography; aspiration and cytology	Antimicrobial therapy. Debride necrotic tissue. Clean environment and provide softer substrate
Trauma	Intraspecific aggression (main cause); environmental (cage furnishings)	Fractures; limb swelling; haemorrhage; purulent discharge	Radiography	Fracture repair and wound management: even severe wounds may heal if kept clean. Antimicrobial therapy for secondary infection

13.14 (continued) Common disease problems by system.

Parasites are not usually a major concern, except when animals are exposed to parasites from a different geographical area. This may occur by housing animals from different regions together or from feeding local wildlife (e.g. fish) containing parasite immediate stages. The most important pathogenic parasites are pentastomids. There are several species; all have intermediate stages in fish, and most reside in the lungs as adults. The main infectious causes of disease are Gram-negative bacteria producing bacteraemia and septicaemia. Although other infections have been described (e.g. mycoplasmosis, West Nile Virus, chlamydophilosis), they are usually a problem of large collections or farms.

Zoonoses

Salmonellosis is the most important reptilian zoonosis. West Nile Virus has recently been described in several disease outbreaks in alligator farms in North America and represents a potential for human transmission. *Trichinella* has also been identified in the skeletal muscle of several crocodile species but would only be of significance if the animal were eaten, and even then its zoonotic potential is unknown.

Supportive care

Hospitalization
Crocodilians should be hospitalized in a heated enclosure, especially for long-term management. Medium to large crocodilians require specialized housing, and most will be treated at the facility in which they are housed. The enclosure should be waterproof and easily cleaned. Cat and dog cages are unsuitable for even small crocodilians. For most, a plastic tank with a haul-out area is suitable. Where animals are kept out of water, regular misting is advisable. In humid

environments, plastic mats limit ground contact where excreta may predispose to ventral scale infections. Some crocodilians can be trained to enter chutes or restraint cages, facilitating drug administration and diagnostic sampling.

Drug administration

- The ventral coccygeal vessels can be catheterized for intravenous drug administration; see blood collection sites, above, for details of access.
- Intramuscular injections are preferably given in the forelegs because of the renal portal system. This author, however, will inject medium to large crocodilians in the hindlimbs or tail for handler safety, and because pharmacokinetic studies suggest the clinical effect of the renal portal system is minor.
- Edetate calcium disodium can be administered intracoelomically for chelation of lead. The injection is made off midline into the caudal coelomic cavity.

> **WARNING**
> **Intravenous drugs should not be administered into the supravertebral sinus because of the possibility of accidental injection into the subarachnoid space.**

Fluid therapy and nutritional support

Oral methods

Nutritional support or oral fluid therapy can be given by stomach tubing. This assumes that gastrointestinal motility and gastric emptying are normal. The animal must also be at an appropriate body temperature for normal digestion to occur. Animals that have been anorectic for prolonged periods of time should be fed conservatively, beginning with electrolyte solutions first, then gradually adding in liquefied solids. For longer-term administration of enteral fluids and food it is recommended that an oesophageal tube be placed (Figure 13.15); if this tube is sufficiently long it will allow food administration from behind the animal.

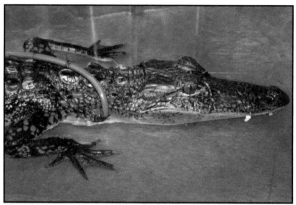

13.15 An oesophageal tube is used for repetitive enteral feeding and drug administration in anorectic crocodilians.

Safe placement of tubes must be done under sedation, with the jaws taped into an open position using a speculum or, in large species, a bite block. When the mouth is opened, the gular fold will be in apposition to the soft palate. It can be depressed using a long wooden spoon or equine laryngoscope, or by the stomach tube itself. The stomach lies approximately midway between the front and hindlegs for approximation of the length of tubing needed.

Non-enteral fluid therapy

Intravenous fluids can be administered through a catheter placed in the ventral coccygeal vessels. Although 'reptile-specific' fluids have been described, this author routinely uses commercially available fluids such as lactated Ringer's solution without adverse effects. Intraosseous fluid administration is difficult, if not impossible, because of the dense bone structure of the appendicular skeleton, even in juvenile animals.

Anaesthesia and analgesia

Anaesthesia always involves some form of physical restraint. Anaesthesia should not be performed in water because of the possibility of drowning. Anaesthetic agents and doses are given in Figure 13.16.

Drug	Dose	Comments
Parenteral anaesthetics		
Medetomidine + Ketamine	100 μg/kg M + 10 mg/kg K i.m./i.v.	
Muscle relaxants	**Not recommended**	No analgesia, animal aware. Succinylcholine causes pain during muscle fasciculations. Low therapeutic index
Propofol	2–6 mg/kg i.v.	Alligators >5–10 kg with good venous access: start with 2 mg/kg
Tiletamine/Zolazepam	4–8 mg/kg i.m./i.v.	Prolonged induction and recovery
Inhalant anaesthetics		
Halothane	Induction: 3–5% Maintenance: 1–2%	
Isoflurane	Induction: 3–5% Maintenance: 1.5–2.5%	
Nitrous oxide	2:1 to 1:1 NO:oxygen	Do not use in hypoxaemia or in animals with closed air spaces

13.16 Analgesics and anaesthetics for crocodilians. Lower dosages should be used in larger animals and for intravenous administration. (Data from Fleming, 2007.) (continues) ▶

Drug	Dose	Comments
Analgesics		
Buprenorphine	0.01–0.03 mg/kg i.m./i.v.	
Butorphanol	0.2–0.5 mg/kg i.m./i.v.	
Meloxicam	0.1–0.3 mg/kg i.m./i.v.	NSAID
Morphine	0.5–3 mg/kg i.m./i.v.	

13.16 (continued) Analgesics and anaesthetics for crocodilians. Lower dosages should be used in larger animals and for intravenous administration. (Data from Fleming, 2007.)

Mask induction of small crocodilians with an inhalant anaesthetic is possible, but may be prolonged because of breath-holding and involuntary excitement. Alternatively, small crocodilians can be physically restrained, a mouth block placed, the gular flap displaced, local anaesthetic applied to the glottis, and the animal intubated and ventilated with an inhalant anaesthetic. Isoflurane and sevoflurane both provide rapid induction and recovery. This author also uses nitrous oxide with these inhalants when there is no evidence of either hypoxaemia or closed gas-filled spaces in the body.

When safety is of primary concern, this author recommends intramuscular administration of a zolazepam/tiletamine combination: induction to safe immobilization is approximately 45 minutes. This drug combination is also recommended for darting animals that cannot be approached closely.

The combination of medetomidine and ketamine has been described for use in alligators, but they seem very resistant and large dosages are required. Alternatively, if intravenous access is obtained, propofol is recommended for induction.

Although muscle relaxants have been used in the past to immobilize crocodilians, this author does not recommend their use in captive animals because of alternatives. Muscle relaxants are not analgesic and the animals are conscious unless other drugs are used. Succinylcholine causes pain during muscle depolarization and may produce hyperkalaemia.

Endotracheal intubation

Once an animal is sufficiently relaxed, a mouth block is placed, the gular flap displaced and the glottis visualized. The endotracheal tube can then be readily placed through the glottis. Since the glottis will usually be closed, the end of the tube is gently placed between the lips of the glottis and then opened.

Monitoring and supportive care

The metabolic rate of crocodilians is very low and the recommended ventilation rate under anaesthesia is approximately 1–2 breaths per minute. Pulse oximetry has not been calibrated for reptiles, including crocodilians. A capnograph is useful for monitoring adequacy of ventilation. A Doppler flow probe can be placed directly over the heart, the eye or into the cloaca to detect blood flow. Occasionally blood flow can be detected on the ventral tail and in the femoral and axillary triangles.

Analgesia

It appears that crocodilians are similar to mammals in having predominantly mu opioid receptors (Fleming, 2007). Since the pharmacokinetics of opiates in crocodilians have not been described, it is recommended that canine doses are given, but less often (see Figure 13.16). Similarly, for non-steroidal anti-inflammatory drugs (NSAIDs) a mammalian dose can be used but given less frequently. Local anaesthetic nerve blocks are recommended for limb amputations, dentistry and biopsy (Wellehan *et al.*, 2006).

Common surgical procedures

Surgery is not commonly performed on crocodilians. The most common indication is for trauma and amputation of injured limbs. Retained infected egg yolks are a cause of poor growth in juvenile crocodilians and can be surgically removed through a midline laparotomy. Exploratory coeliotomy in adult crocodilians is not common. Adult crocodilians have a lot of fibrous adhesions/tissue within the coelomic cavity and abdominal wall dehiscence is common postoperatively. Metal and nylon haemoclips and monofilament suture materials are appropriate for reptilian surgery. Skin sutures may be removed after 4–6 weeks.

Euthanasia

Euthanasia usually involves first anaesthetizing the animal followed by intravenous injection of a commercial euthanasia solution containing a barbiturate. Pithing can be performed only when an animal is unconscious. The use of muscle relaxants to immobilize an animal prior to pithing is inappropriate, since the animal is conscious.

Drug formulary

A drug formulary for crocodilians is given in Figure 13.17. Care must be taken in selecting drug dosages because of the wide range of body size between juvenile and adult animals. In general, the larger the crocodilian, the lower the dosage and frequency of administration. There may also be differences between species. Alligatorids appear to require lower drug dosages than crocodiles of a similar size.

WARNING
Ivermectin must not be used; there are several anecdotal, but unpublished, reports of paralysis and death at recommended therapeutic dosages.

Drug	Dose	Comments
Antimicrobial agents		
Amikacin	2.25 mg/kg i.m. q3–5d	Active against Gram-negative bacteria; no efficacy against anaerobes. Combine with penicillin or metronidazole for broad-spectrum coverage
Ceftazidime	20 mg/kg i.m. q3d	Active against Gram-negative bacteria
Enrofloxacin	5 mg/kg orally/i.m. q5d	Active against Gram-negative bacteria, mycoplasmosis; no efficacy against anaerobes. Avoid intramuscular injection if possible because of tissue injury
Metronidazole	20 mg/kg orally q2d for 5 treatments	Active against anaerobic bacteria, protozoa
Oxytetracycline	10–20 mg/kg i.m. q5–7d	Active against Gram-negative bacteria, *Mycoplasma*, *Chlamydophila*
Procaine penicillin	20,000–30,000 IU/kg q5–7d	Active against Gram-positive and anaerobic bacteria
Trimethoprim/Sulphonamide	20 mg/kg orally q24h for 2 days, then every other day	Active against Gram-negative bacteria; no efficacy against anaerobes
Antifungal agents		
Fluconazole	5–10 mg/kg orally q3–5d	Systemic mycotic infections
Itraconazole	5–10 mg/kg orally q3–5d	Systemic mycotic infections
Antiparasitic agents		
Fenbendazole	20–30 mg/kg orally q24h for 5 days	Nematode parasites
Praziquantel	5–10 mg/kg i.m./orally once; repeat after 2 wk	Cestodes
Sulfadimethoxine	50 mg/kg q2d for 5 treatments	Coccidiosis
Miscellaneous		
Calcium gluconate	10–50 mg/kg i.m./i.v.	Emergency treatment of hypocalcaemic tetany
Edetate calcium disodium	73 mg/kg intracoelomically q24h for 5 days	Chelation therapy for lead, zinc, cadmium
Oxytocin	10 IU/kg i.m./i.v.	Non-obstructive egg binding – use with calcium gluconate, warmth
Thiamine	10 mg/kg i.m. q24h for 5 days	Thiamine deficiency
Vitamin A (retinyl palmitate)	3–6 ml (200,000 IU/ml) i.m. once	Vitamin A deficiency. The palmitate must be metabolized to the active form and, therefore, is safer
Vitamin E	3–6 ml (300 IU/ml) i.m. once	Vitamin E deficiency

13.17 Drug formulary for crocodilians. (See Figure 13.16 for analgesics and anaesthetics.)

References and further reading

Diethelm G and Stein G (2006) Hematologic and blood chemistry values in reptiles. In: *Reptile Medicine and Surgery, 2nd edn*, ed. DR Mader, pp. 1103–1118. Saunders Elsevier, Philadelphia

Fleming G (2007) Crocodilians (crocodiles, alligators, caimans, gharial). In: *Zoo Animal and Wildlife Immobilization and Anesthesia*, ed. G West *et al.*, pp. 655–664. Blackwell, Ames, IA

Huchzermeyer FW (2003) *Crocodiles: Biology, Husbandry and Diseases*. CABI, Wallingford

Jacobson E (2007) *Infectious Diseases and Pathology of Reptiles: Color Atlas and Text*. CRC Press, Boca Raton, FL

King FW and Russell LB (1997) *Crocodilian, Tuatara, and Turtle Species of the World: An Online Taxonomic and Geographic Reference*. Association of Systematics Collections, Washington DC

LaFortune M, Gobel T, Jacobson ER *et al.* (2005) Respiratory bronchoscopy of subadult American alligators (*Alligator mississippiensis*) and tracheal wash evaluation. *Journal of Zoo and Wildlife Medicine* **36**,12–20

Lane T (2006) Crocodilians. In: *Reptile Medicine and Surgery, 2nd edn*, ed. DR Mader, pp.100–117. Saunders Elsevier, St. Louis

Pidcock S, Taplin LE and Grigg GC (1997) Differences in renal-cloacal function between *Crocodylus porosus* and *Alligator mississippiensis* have implications for crocodilian evolution. *Journal of Comparative Physiology B* **167**, 153–158

Richardson KC, Webb GJW and Manolis SC (2000) *Crocodiles: Inside Out. A Guide to Crocodiles and their Functional Morphology*. Surrey Beatty and Sons, Sydney

Vliet KA (2007) Crocodilian capture and restraint. In: *Zoo Animal & Wildlife Immobilization and Anesthesia*, ed. G West *et al.*, pp. 211–221. Blackwell Publishing, Carlton, Victoria, Australia

Webb G and Manolis C (1989) *Graham Webb's Crocodiles of Australia*. Reed Books, Frenchs Forest, NSW, Australia

Wellehan JFX, Gunkel CI, Kledzik D *et al.* (2006) Use of a nerve locator to facilitate administration of mandibular nerve blocks in crocodilians. *Journal of Zoo and Wildlife Medicine* **37**, 405–408

Wellehan JFX, LaFortune M, Gunkel C *et al.* (2004) Coccygeal vascular catheterization in lizards and crocodilians. *Journal of Herpetological Medicine and Surgery* **14**, 26–28

Useful website

Crocodilians: Natural History and Conservation. www.flmnh.ufl.edu/cnhc

14

Tortoises and turtles

Mike Jessop and Tracy D. Bennett

Introduction

The order Testudines represents all modern chelonians; it comprises 14 families and over 300 species. The order is defined by the presence of a bony shell covering the body, into which most chelonians can retract the head and limbs. Chelonians kept in captivity can be described as of two types:

- Tortoises – most are exclusively herbivores and all are strictly terrestrial. Anatomically they are characterized by large hard scales on the forelimbs and thick domed shells
- Turtles/terrapins – all are at least semi-aquatic and omnivorous. Most aquatic species have flattened shells, smooth skin and webbed feet. Less aquatic species, like the North American box turtle, have a more domed shell and can pull the head fully inside.

In the USA most aquatic or semi-aquatic chelonians are called 'turtles'. Most of the terrapin species available for sale in the UK are imported from the USA and hence sold with the common name of turtle.

When treating chelonians it is important to identify the species at hand because:

- Dietary and husbandry requirements vary between species
- Different species should not be housed together – there are increasing examples of infectious disease agents that are more virulent to certain species
- The males of some species will engage in combat.

Figure 14.1 lists the common pet species and their characteristics.

Common name	Latin name	Geographical origin	Physical characteristics	Gender differentiation
Hermann's tortoise (Figure 14.2a)	*Testudo hermanni*	Southern Europe from Spain through Balkans to Turkey (eastern and western subspecies)	Distinct tail tip spur; no thigh spurs; plastron a fixed unit, no hinge; maximum adult size 18–28 cm (depending on species)	Female: short tail Male: longer tail; smaller as an adult
Spur-thighed tortoise: (Figure 14.2b)	*Testudo graeca* (subspecies taxonomy controversial)		Single prominent spur on each thigh; caudal plastron hinged between abdominal and femoral scutes	Female: typically larger than male; shorter tail Male: longer tail; some species have concave plastron
Iberan tortoise	*Testudo ibera*	Greece, Turkey, southern Balkans		
Marginated tortoise	*Testudo marginata*	Greece	Distinct triangular markings on each plastral scute and flared caudal edge of the marginal carapace	Male smaller than female when adult
White's spur-thighed tortoise	*Testudo whitei*	Similar range to Moroccan	Larger than Moroccan	
Horsfield's tortoise (Russian tortoise) (Figure 14.2c)	*Testudo horsfieldii*	From Afghanistan to northwestern China	Fairly circular body shape; convex plastron; thigh spurs present but indistinct; maximum adult size 25 cm	Female: larger than male; shorter tail Male: Smaller than female; longer tail
African spurred tortoise ('sulcata') (Figure 14.2d)	*Geochelone sulcata*	Sub-Saharan Africa	Large heavy chelonian with well developed scutes; pair of prominent spurs present of each thigh; lifespan in excess of 80 years; maximum adult size 90 cm	Female: elongated gular scutes and a deep concavity to the plastron Male: longer thicker tail that folds to the side and a wider scute angle

14.1 Physical characteristics of common pet tortoises and turtles. (continues) ▶

Common name	Latin name	Geographical origin	Physical characteristics	Gender differentiation
Red-eared terrapin (red-eared turtle, red-eared slider) (Figure 14.2e)	*Trachemys scripta elegans*	Southeastern and southern North America	Lifespan in captivity of >30 years; may mature in 5–7 years with maximum nutrition and husbandry; tend to bite and threaten when handled, but can be trained; sales in the USA only legal if the diagonal measurement of the carapace is >10 cm; maximum adult size 30 cm	Female: flat plastron; short forelimb claws Male: smaller; longer forelimb claws; longer tail; more distal vent
Eastern box turtles (Carolina box turtle, three-toed box turtle) (Figure 14.2f)	*Terrapene carolina* (4 subspecies); *T. ornata*	Southeastern, eastern and southwestern USA	Hinged shell; can close up completely; stays fairly small; docile; maximum adult size 15–20 cm (depending on species)	Female: yellow/brown iris; shorter tail Male: red iris; longer, thicker tail; concave plastron

14.1 (continued) Physical characteristics of common pet tortoises and turtles.

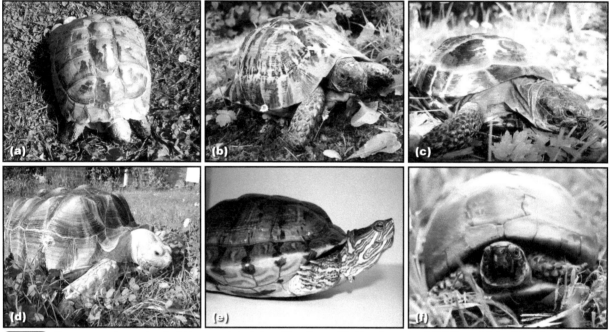

14.2 Common pet species. **(a)** Hermann's tortoise. (Courtesy of L. Handscombe.) **(b)** Spur-thighed tortoise. **(c)** Horsfield's tortoise. **(d)** African spurred tortoise. **(e)** Red-eared terrapin. **(f)** Three-toed box turtle.

Biology

While some turtles are native to temperate climates, most tortoises inhabit desert or tropical zones. Temperate climate-adapted tortoises and turtles in the wild will slow their metabolic rates dramatically in response to cold weather and decreased daylight hours, a dormancy process technically known as 'brumation' (although often referred to as 'hibernation'). Desert-adapted tortoises will aestivate during the hottest months when food is scarce. Life expectancy for tortoises is unknown; age-related disorders occur over 50 years of age.

Anatomy and physiology

The most notable feature is the shell: the upper portion is termed the carapace and the lower portion the plastron. Some species have hinged sections of shell that allow tighter closure of the fossae or in some cases, such as the box tortoises (turtles), complete closure. The shell is composed of bony plates, evolved from modified ribs; these interlock along suture line joints, similar to the mammalian cranium. The outer periosteum forms a modified layer that produces keratin, which covers the bone in an overlapping pattern of scutes that are shed as the animal grows.

Chelonians have a three-chambered heart, with two atria and one ventricle. The lungs occupy a large area just ventral to the carapace and have limited expansion capabilities. They appear sac-like and an obvious reticular pattern is present grossly. Chelonians lack a functional diaphragm. Ventilation is achieved through positive pressure created by the movement of skeletal muscles and by flexion and extension of the limbs.

Reptilian kidneys have no loop of Henle and consequently produce dilute urine. Uric acid is the primary metabolic waste product in terrestrial species but in aquatic terrapins, nitrogenous wastes are released primarily as urea. A urinary bladder is present. Chelonians have a renal portal system which can either shunt blood to the kidney or bypass the kidneys, depending on the position of the portal valve.

Male chelonians have a single phallus and females have a variably sized clitoris.

Digestion in all reptiles is highly temperature-dependent, with the gastrointestinal tract emptying very slowly, or not at all, when the temperature falls below the preferred optimal temperature zone (POTZ) of the species. A gallbladder is present in chelonians.

Sexing

Most chelonians are dimorphic as adults but the characteristics vary widely between species. The sexual characteristics of the animal develop with age and size. The most reliable non-invasive method of gender determination in adults is by examination of the tail (Figure 14.3):

- Male chelonians have a longer tail with the cloaca positioned more distally
- Females generally have short tails with the cloaca positioned close to the body and within the margin of the carapace.

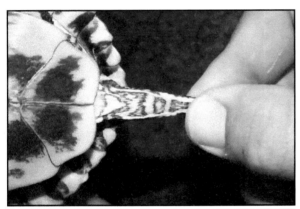

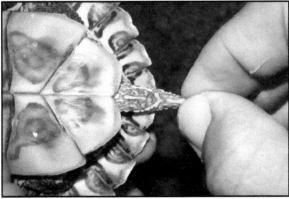

14.3 Gender determination by tail length. In the male (top), the tail is longer and the cloaca is located outside the margin of the shell.

Many other characteristics exist, such as very long front toenails on males of the genus *Trachemys*. Some size differences between males and females exist but these vary widely depending on the species. Some species show a distinct plastron concavity in the male, though some spur-thighed females have a mild concavity. Differentiation is not generally possible in juvenile animals, although an endoscopic technique for determining gender in neonates and juveniles has recently been described (Hernandez-Divers and Mackey, 2008).

Husbandry

Husbandry remains the most important criterion to consider in connection with tortoise and turtle health.

Housing

Terrestrial species

Tortoises are best managed in an indoor facility. This should be an open-topped arrangement that can be deeply littered with substrate to allow burrowing (Figure 14.4). Hay is an ideal substrate but peat or bark mulch are alternatives. The bedding should be digestible if eaten; wood chip bedding should be avoided. Water access is important for drinking and to provide humidity. If used as permanent housing, sufficient space for exercise must be provided.

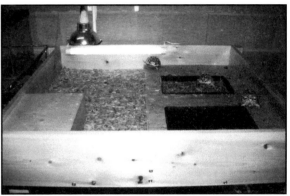

14.4 Tortoise table suitable for terrestrial species. The water tray is shallow enough to allow the tortoise to wade in, but deep enough to allow partial head submersion for drinking through the nostrils.

Where climate allows, many species of tortoise can be successfully managed in largely free-range outdoor facilities; supplemental provision of heat, light, shelter and food may be needed, especially in cooler climates. For animals with access to outdoor space, the indoor facility can be relatively small to provide cold weather protection. Outdoor housing should provide security from potential predators, including dogs, cats, raccoons and coyotes. The tortoise should preferably be supervised when outside.

Tortoise species should be housed separately, and species should not be mixed. Tortoises are not social animals, although similar-sized tortoises can be kept together in non-breeding situations. Smaller animals may be intimidated by larger animals and be kept away from food and water.

Ambient environmental temperatures should be 20–25°C, with basking zones ranging up to 40°C. The minimum night-time/winter temperature should be 15°C, although exact temperatures should be adjusted according to species, age and season. If tortoises are housed indoors for any protracted length of time, there must be some consideration of seasonal variability. It is too easy to maintain the animal on a standard heat/light regimen all year. Planning a seasonal variation to try and mimic the natural variation may be important. Owners should try to mimic known natural lifestyles and may need veterinary help to do this successfully. However, variation may not be important for non-breeding animals, and in addition some pet species come from equatorial areas where day length and temperature are fairly uniform. There is currently a paucity of published research on the natural history of many pet tortoise species, and this adds to the challenge of caring for these animals in a domestic environment.

Semi-aquatic species

Box turtles and other semi-aquatic species require an enclosure that provides them with adequate space for ambulatory exercise, burrowing and soaking. A minimum size would be 60 x 90 cm for two box turtles. Coconut fibre and compressed peat are types of bedding that hold moisture and allow box turtles to burrow. Box turtles need constant access to water. A dish deep enough to allow submersion and large enough for the turtle or terrapin to move around in is sufficient. A glass baking dish works well for this purpose and is shallow enough to allow easy access (Figure 14.5a). Water needs to be changed daily.

Aquatic species

The minimum aquarium size for one animal is a tank four times longer than the turtle's carapace length, or about 90 litres for one turtle under 15 cm. Aquatic turtles can be housed together if they are similar in size. However, aggression does occur in some cases, and aggressive individuals will need to be housed singly. Housing males and females together is not recommended.

The water should be deep enough to allow free swimming. A dry haul-out area is essential to allow the turtle to dry off and bask (Figure 14.5b). Aquarium rocks need to be large enough to prevent ingestion. Aquatic plants should be weighted with rocks or plastic, as metal toxicity can occur from commercial lead weights sold for this purpose.

Water quality is a major issue for turtles and a heavy duty canister filter is recommended. Even with canister filtration, the water needs to be changed completely once or twice a week, depending on the size of the animal and the amount of faeces produced.

For outdoor enclosures, the pool or pond needs to be fenced, covered with mesh, or made deep and large enough to allow escape from would-be predators. A platform can be placed in the middle of the pond to provide a haul-out area in relative safety.

Heat

All reptiles require an external heat source to maintain the optimum body temperature for their species. A radiant heat source is recommended in the form of a ceramic heat emitter. A temperature gradient is necessary for all ectotherms and is specific to each species. For a terrarium a ceramic heat bulb should

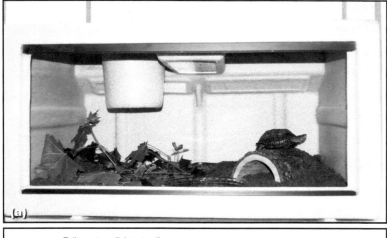

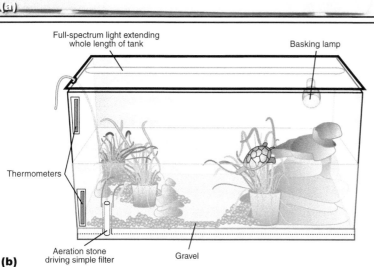

14.5 **(a)** Housing suitable for terrestrial and semi-aquatic species. **(b)** Housing suitable for aquatic species.

be placed above the screen top at one end of the enclosure. The wattage of the bulb will depend on the desired temperature.

Aquatic species must have a water heater in the tank and this must be protected to prevent burns to the turtle. Additionally, a heat lamp should be provided to allow basking in the haul-out area.

At least two thermometers are required to measure the temperature gradient between different sections of the enclosure. Digital thermometers with a probe that extends from the base unit so that two areas can be monitored are widely available from electronics stores and reptile supply companies. Infrared 'temperature guns' that accurately measure surface temperatures instantaneously are useful equipment for any reptile owner.

Lighting

Most chelonians do well with a 12-hour day/night photoperiod, although temperate species used for breeding may need to follow the natural daylight photoperiod. Lighting provided should mimic sunlight as closely as possible. This includes ultraviolet (UV) radiation: UV-A (wavelength 400–315 nm) and UV-B (wavelength 315–280 nm). Normal behaviours and activities modulated by the pineal gland are affected by the intensity and wavelength of light. UV-B light is important for the synthesis of vitamin D, particularly in herbivorous species. Many commercial lights do not provide an adequate amount of UV-B light in the required range. Some types of UV-B light bulbs emit little heat and should be placed within 45 cm of the primary resting place of the chelonian. For bulbs that also emit heat (mercury vapour), the appropriate distance may require close monitoring and adjustment. UV-B lights need to be replaced every 6 months as the UV-B light emitted declines over time.

Recently, metal halide lights have become a popular way to provide UV-B radiation to reptiles. Metal halide lights emit more UV-B radiation and heat than compact fluorescent tubes. These bulbs are not routinely used in chelonian habitats as they produce far more UV radiation than required by more species, and run the risk of overheating and burning the animal. It is important to assess the species requirements when choosing lighting (e.g. a woodland species may need lower UV-B light than a desert species). Metal halide bulbs are available in the UK (Mega-Ray) and in the USA (ReptileUV) in 60–160 W strengths.

Diet

Tortoises

Tortoises are herbivores and require a high-fibre diet. A wide variety of plants should be offerred.

- Grasses, hays and weed varieties should form the bulk of the diet.
- Dandelion, plantain and clovers are eaten readily.
- Lettuce varieties other than iceberg (head) can be used. Iceberg lettuce has minimal nutritional value and an inverse Ca:P ratio, but can be used as part of a balanced diet in obese animals.

- Cabbage, kale, spinach and other greens, along with small amounts of other vegetables can all be fed as part of a broad mixed feed.
- Starchy vegetables, beans, peas, corn should rarely be offered as they are relatively high in carbohydrates and calories.
- Edible flowers can be fed in small quantities, e.g. nasturtium, dandelion, clover.
- Fruit portions should be minimal. Wild varieties (e.g. strawberry) or ancient fruits such as prickly pear and star fruit with a high-fibre, low-sugar ratio are highly preferable to cultivated varieties.
- Some tropical rainforest species, e.g. red-footed and elongate (*Intestudo elongata*) tortoises, may tolerate a greater fruit inclusion.

WARNING
Tortoises allowed to graze outdoors should not be able to access toxic plants such as ragwort, yew, laburnum, rhubarb, rhododendron, and others known to cause problems in livestock.

Calcium supplementation may be needed, depending on the types of foods being consumed. Whilst tortoises are attracted to meat and other animal protein sources (e.g. dog food, cat food) the addition of animal protein will decrease the consumption of needed plant carbohydrate and fibre. Excess protein may contribute to metabolic gout, as it must be eliminated as uric acid. Overfeeding is far more commonplace than underfeeding.

Commercial pelleted diets promoted as tortoise feed are largely composed of grains and may not contain the nutrients needed in the proper formulation. At present, their usage is not recommended.

Tortoises need a constant supply of water, preferably of a depth to allow the head to be fully immersed as most drink through the nostrils as well as the mouth. Most prefer to wallow in their water before drinking. The water tray will also act as a useful source of humidity.

Semi-aquatic species

Box turtles are omnivores and exploit a wide range of food sources in their natural habitat. The diet can be 50% animal protein and 50% vegetation. Foods should be diced together so the turtle cannot choose only favourite items.

- The animal portion can include invertebrates such as earthworms, slugs, silkworms and snails. Whole pre-killed fish should be offered periodically to provide vitamin A.
- The vegetation portion should be composed of foods rich in vitamin A and beta-carotene, such as collard greens, mustard greens, dandelion greens, chard, kale, parsley, squash and carrots. Vegetables can comprise 75% of this portion of the diet. Fruit is readily accepted and constitutes part of the diet of most wild box turtles when it is available. Good choices include berries, apples and tomatoes.

Aquatic species

Freshwater aquatic turtles are primarily carnivores but also feed on aquatic plants in the wild. Adult turtles accept vegetation more readily than juveniles.

* The bulk of the diet may be feeder fish, live or previously frozen, as they contain high levels of vitamin A and constitute a major portion of the wild diet. Invertebrates such as earthworms, tubifex worms, slugs and silkworms should be offered. Crustaceans such as shrimp (with shells) and crayfish are nutritious.
* A small amount of the diet may contain trout or catfish chow and commercial turtle food, though many of these lack appropriate vitamins and may be high in fat.
* Aquatic plants constitute a significant portion of the wild diet, particularly in adults, and vegetation like dark leafy greens or carrots will usually be accepted.

Hibernation

'Hibernation' (or more correctly 'brumation') planned as part of a seasonal variation aimed at mimicking the natural variation is believed by some to be important, and novice tortoise owners may need veterinary help to do this successfully. Owners who do hibernate their tortoises should do so for only 3 months a year. An indoor housing facility is therefore necessary, as temperatures in the northern hemisphere are often below the POTZ for most tortoises for up to 6 months of the year. Tortoises subjected to long hibernation periods (4–6 months) over several years may suffer from poor health.

An advised annual tortoise cycle in the northern hemisphere for captive tortoises is:

December to February	Hibernation
March to June	Regular feeding
July to August	Restricted feeding or natural grazing allowed
September to October	Regular feeding
November	Preparation for hibernation

For a Horsfield's tortoise the schedule may be slightly different:

January to February	Hibernation
March to June	Regular feeding
July	Fasting
August to October	Regular feeding
November to December	Restricted feeding and preparation for hibernation

In the wild, Mediterranean species of tortoises are subjected to near-drought conditions with dry vegetation during the summer months. Spring and autumn bring rain with an abundance of plant growth and food. In northern temperate climates, summer may actually be the 'wet' season and is usually the growing season for grasses and edible plants. Captive tortoises may overeat during the summer months compared with their wild counterparts and subsequently become obese, which is a major health problem. As food is so abundant for tortoises in captivity, restriction of intake may be indicated, following the 'wild' pattern.

During the hibernation period it is recommended that the tortoise be placed on a clean paper towel, with a thermometer probe secured on the tortoise for daily temperature monitoring. Remote temperature sensing devices can also be used as long as they are attached to the soft tissue of the tortoise (e.g. a leg fossa) so that the temperature of the tortoise is monitored rather than the ambient environmental temperature or the reflective surface temperature of the towel or carapace.

The tortoise should then be placed in a container and surrounded by sufficient clean insulating material to ensure good temperature stability at approximately 5°C. The selected insulation should ensure low dust levels and good ventilation (e.g. polystyrene chips or coarse shredded paper). The owner should check the tortoise once or twice weekly and record its temperature on a chart or calendar kept with the container. This will help the owner track start/stop dates as well as any problems with temperature maintenance.

Refrigerator or chiller systems can be used for hibernation. These are especially useful where ambient temperatures may not stay steady below 5°C. In this situation the hibernation compartment needs to be opened a couple of times a week to check and weigh the animal, and to provide ventilation. Additional air circulation can be provided using an air pump, such as those used in fish aquaria, and cutting a small hole into the rubber seal to allow inlet air in and exhaust out. This type of managed hibernation requires close and regular monitoring to ensure good thermostatic control.

Breeding

The number of eggs laid and the preferred nesting/laying site vary between species. Incubation time is usually 2–3 months, with the sex of the offspring dependent on incubation temperature.

* Horsfield's tortoise – incubation: 60–75 days; temperature range: 28–30°C.
* Eastern box turtle – incubation: 70–85 days; temperature range: 28–30°C.
* Red-eared terrapin – incubation: 54–80 days; temperature range: 28–29°C.

Neonates and juveniles show a natural instinct to hide. It is important to maintain humidity for juveniles. Slow steady growth is the aim, and overfeeding is one of the main husbandry problems. Young chelonians are fed the same diet as adults, except the pieces and portions are smaller.

For further information on breeding of tortoises and turtles, see the *BSAVA Manual of Reptiles, 2nd edition*.

Identification

Owners are advised and encouraged to identify their animals with a microchip. In both the UK and the USA the placing of a microchip is considered an act of veterinary surgery. It is not considered safe to microchip animals with a straight carapace length <10 cm, and the site is standardized to the left hindleg. The chip should sit in or above the quadriceps muscle.

1. Surgically scrub the skin.
2. Infiltrate the site with a small dose of local anaesthetic (e.g. 2% lidocaine).
3. Insert the chip introducer needle proximal to the stifle and run up the anterior thigh. In small animals, the chip should be inserted into the quadriceps. In larger animals it will sit subcutaneously.
4. Implant.
5. Withdraw the introducer needle and apply pressure to the site with a sterile cotton bud. The site may bleed and flush the chip out.
6. Once any haemorrhage has abated, close the skin wound with a suture, staple or tissue glue.

Legislation and welfare

In the UK the sale of tortoises is regulated by the Department for Environment, Food and Rural Affairs (Defra), who administer the legislation under the Convention on International Trade in Endangered Species of Wild Fauna and Flora (CITES) regulations (see Chapter 22). The different species of tortoise fall into various categories (Figure 14.6). In addition to CITES, many countries impose strict export controls. This applies, for example, to the export of red-eared terrapins from the USA; once common in UK pet shops, this inappropriate trading has stopped but the pet trade has switched to trading in other turtle species.

CITES Appendix I	Egyptian tortoise (*Testudo kleinmanni*)	Illegal to trade and subject to intense conservation efforts
CITES Appendix II	Moroccan spur-thighed tortoise (*Testudo graeca graeca*) Iberan tortoise (*T. ibera*) White's spur-thighed tortoise (*T. whitei*) Marginated tortoise (*T. marginata*) Hermann's tortoise (*T. hermanni*)	Traded with a Defra licence via an Article 10 certificate
CITES Appendix II	Horsfield's tortoise (*T. horsfieldii*) Leopard tortoise (*Geochelone pardalis*) African spurred tortoise (*G. sulcata*) Red-footed tortoise (*G. carbonaria*) Yellow-footed tortoise (*G. denticulata*)	Not currently subject to trade restrictions. No certification required

14.6 CITES regulations.

Handling and restraint

Tortoises are very amenable to handling (Figure 14.7) and the majority of pet tortoises are benign animals used to close and frequent contact. They should be held firmly above a table. They may struggle and push with their limbs, so should not be held where a loss of grip would cause a fall.

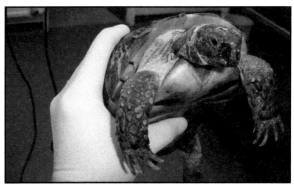

14.7 Handling a tortoise. The tortoise is firmly held over a table. They may struggle and push with their limbs, so should not be held where a loss of grip will cause a fall. Both hands may be needed to lift larger animals.

Occasionally with wild-caught animals or some of the larger species, an animal may be encountered that necessitates extra precautions when handling. The musculature involved in contracting into the shell is very powerful, and care should be taken not to trap the handler's fingers between the patient's limbs and its shell. Some hinged species can trap fingers in the shell closure. Some large specimens have very powerful jaws and care needs to be exercised when examining mouths. Nervous animals will express their bladder.

Aquatic turtles are very active and rarely retreat into the shell. These turtles can be very aggressive, and the handler must be aware that these species can inflict a painful bite. A net can be used to remove aquatic turtles from the water.

When dealing with many chelonians, it is important to ensure good biosecurity from one patient to the next. Use of effective hand sterilization, gloves and equipment sanitization between chelonians will prevent cross-infection. Direct chelonian-to-chelonian contact should be prevented. These considerations are especially important if attending club events such as pre-hibernation health checks.

Diagnostic approach

Most tortoises will allow examination, and significant restraint is not necessary in small to medium individuals. In very large tortoises sedation may be required. An assistant should be present to help with restraint.

In general, most tortoises cannot fully close their shell but instead rely on the large scales on their front limbs to protect their head and neck. In some tortoises and box turtles the patient can retreat almost entirely into the shell. In these animals patience is required to allow them to extend the head or one of the limbs outside the shell. Gentle handling is required to coax the extension of the head, which is firmly grasped and extended gently against the pulsed contraction of the neck muscles (Figure 14.8a). **Excessive force should not be used**, especially in young animals. Sedation may be required. Once the head or any of the limbs is acquired, the patient can no longer retreat into the shell, and examination or treatment can be initiated (Figure 14.8b). If

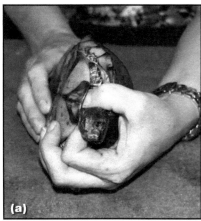 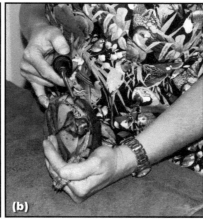 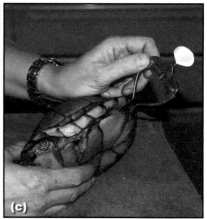

14.8 Physical examination of a tortoise. **(a)** Restraint of the head. **(b)** With the head restrained, the examination can begin. **(c)** Opening the shell using a speculum.

necessary the rear portion of the shell can be gently opened using a mouth speculum (Figure 14.8c). Care should be taken not to use excessive force as damage to the shell or other structures may occur.

History

A thorough history must be taken prior to examination of the patient. The diet, environment, location of purchase or adoption, presence of conspecifics, breeding history and medical history are all crucial to enable diagnosis. As with all exotic pets, many problems encountered by the clinician can be traced to improper husbandry.

Clinical examination

Physical examination is summarized in Figure 14.9.

- A heat pad should be available for sick or chilled patients.
- A soft rubber spatula can be used to hold the mouth open for examination and taking diagnostic swabs.
- An 8 MHz Doppler probe with water-soluble gel should be on hand for evaluating the heart (Figure 14.9a).
- A dremel tool for beak shaping and trimming is often required.

General considerations
Is the animal alert and active? If the shell is closed it should be difficult to open A strong reflex of head withdrawal should be present Limbs should be withdrawn when manually extended

Skin and shell
Examine for ulceration at the beak commissures, top of head, under the lower mandible and on the limbs The scutes of the shell are normally well adhered and dry The shell should be uniform with no active ulceration, erythema or algae The shell should not contact the skin, causing abrasion The nail beds should be smooth and free of hyperplasia or dry necrosis Toenails are normally straight and smooth with normal appearing skin at the interface Beak overgrowth is common – may be indicative of metabolic bone disease and should be corrected as soon as possible

Musculoskeletal system
Good muscle tone should be exhibited and the patient should be able to strongly retract its head and limbs Long bones and jaw are ideally firm and symmetrical The body is normally entirely contained within the shell

Eyes and ears
Use of an ophthalmoscope or transilluminator will reveal any corneal or lenticular opacities The globes and periorbital area should be examined for buphthalmos and asymmetry The conjunctiva should be clear and without erythema The tympanic scales should be flat and symmetrical Use fluorescein dye to assess for corneal ulceration

Cardiovascular system
The mucous membranes of the mouth should be moist and pink in species with non-pigmented oral tissues A Doppler probe can be placed under/over the jugular vein to evaluate heart sounds and rate (Figure 14.9a)

14.9 Technique for clinical examination. (continues) ▶

Respiratory system
Nares are normally open and clear with no discharge: with the mouth held open, the nostrils can be flushed with 5 ml of air to check for any discharges The mouth is closed during respiration Respiration can be observed, as chelonians move the head and limbs to assist in ventilation Audible respiration is abnormal, except sharp exhalations when stressed or surprised

Urogenital system
Many terrapins will urinate when handled, allowing sample collection and visual inspection of the urine The cloaca should be examined for erythema or prolapse A digital internal examination of the cloaca may detect any abnormalities, and in medium-sized tortoises it may be possible to palpate enlarged kidneys Palpation of the coelom through the prefemoral fossa can detect eggs or bladder stones in some patients

Gastrointestinal tract
The oral cavity and tongue should be evaluated (Figure 14.9b) for colour, presence of swellings, ulceration and foreign bodies Check the larynx for discharge Note the eustachian tube openings Faeces vary with lifestyle: aquatic turtles defecate loose stool in the water; tortoises should have firm stools Check the vent for soiling

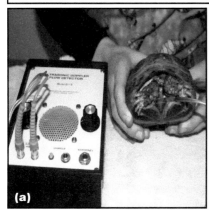 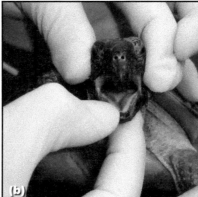

14.9 Technique for clinical examination. **(a)** An ultrasonic Doppler probe can be used to evaluate cardiac sounds and rate. **(b)** Oral examination.

Weight

This is a very useful monitoring tool. A gram scale with 1 g or less weight gradations is essential for small patients (Figure 14.10); a dog or large animal scale can be used for very large patients. All owners should be encouraged to weigh their animal regularly throughout the year; early illness can often be spotted by unexpected weight loss. [Note: ratio assessments should be viewed with suspicion; many, including Jackson's ratio of length to weight, are now considered too inaccurate to be used as health assessments.]

Imaging

Radiography

Chelonians, with their shell, pose challenges for radiography and the internal structures often appear indistinct, necessitating high-detail radiography. Standard rare earth screens allow good detail and fast exposure times, and the use of mammography film will enhance definition. A general 'rule of thumb' is to use the practice exposure settings for a cat radiograph. For digital radiographs a higher mas setting will enhance detail.

The patient can be placed in a clear container, such as a plastic bag or box, if necessary to minimize restraint. Positioning under anaesthesia gives a superior image: the limbs and head can be extended and there is no movement blur.

Where the animal will fit on to a standard radiographic cassette up to 18 x 24 cm, the use of a whole body view is recommended (see Figure 14.11). For larger animals it is sensible to cone the imaging down to selected anatomical areas.

There are three standard views used for tortoises and turtles:

14.10 Use of a plinth to immobilize a tortoise for weighing.

- **Dorsoventral (DV) view.** If very active, the animal can be raised on a plinth, although this may result in loss of limb detail due to movement. Alternatively, chemical restraint can be administered (Figure 14.11). This is preferable if the finer detail of the limbs or head needs imaging and must be extended from the body. The bone of the shell does cause loss of internal contrast. Use of contrast media can be considered for gastrointestinal tract assessment.
- **Lateral view.** This view is primarily for screening the lung or cross-referencing a skeletal lesion. It is not helpful for routine gastrointestinal tract assessment. The animal is best placed on a plinth for this view, to extend the limbs; this can be done with it conscious or under chemical restraint. *The lateral view is best achieved using horizontal beam positioning.* If the X-ray head is fixed, the animal can be taped to a box (Figure 14.12a) or will need chemical restraint and positioning with sandbags and foam wedges (Figure 14.12b) into lateral recumbency. Positional artefacts will appear, since lateral displacement of the coelomic contents causes compression of the dependent lung (Figure 14.12c).
- **Craniocaudal view.** This view is primarily for respiratory assessment but is also useful for shell or vertebral lesions (Figure 14.13). The view is best achieved using horizontal beam positioning. Where this is not possible, the image can be obtained using tape or sandbags as per the lateral view.

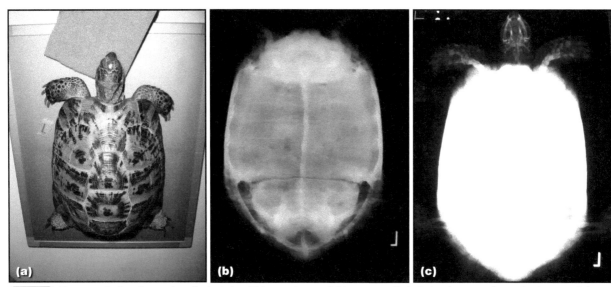

14.11 Dorsoventral radiography of a tortoise. This can be useful for general/whole body screening prior to coned down views of specific areas. **(a)** Positioning under anaesthesia gives a superior image, as the limbs and head can be extended and there is no movement blur. **(b)** View showing body detail. **(c)** View showing limb detail.

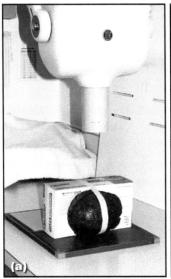
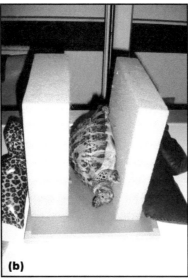
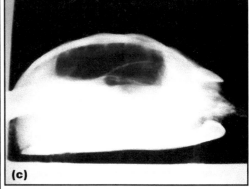

14.12 Lateral radiography of a tortoise. **(a,b)** Positioning for a lateral view. **(c)** Tortoises do not have a diaphragm, which means that the abdominal viscera can expand into the lung field. This view shows the gas-filled stomach floating up into the lung space.

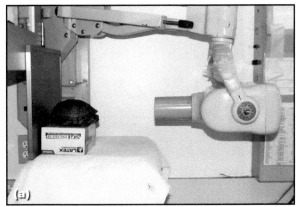

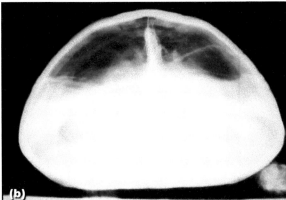

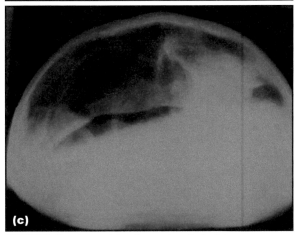

14.13 Craniocaudal radiography of a tortoise.
(a) Positioning for a craniocaudal view using horizontal beam radiography. **(b)** View showing compression of the lung field on the left-hand side by the gas-filled stomach. **(c)** View of a tortoise with severe pneumonia.

Ultrasonography

Given the difficulty of visualizing the coelom with radiography, ultrasonography is very useful for imaging chelonians. A high-frequency probe in the range of 5–8 MHz is ideal for small to medium-sized patients. Very large patients may need lower frequency transducers to increase the depth of penetration. Either microconvex or linear transducers are effective. Patients are usually placed in ventral recumbency, which simplifies imaging and is less stressful to the animal. However, the ultrasonographer may find it is helpful to hold the patient off the table to maximize positioning. A large patient can be placed on a box or plinth that suspends the animal but allows access for probe placement. The

heart and liver are best visualized by placing the transducer medially to the front leg in the mediastinal window (foreleg fossa) (Figure 14.14). The bladder, kidneys and gastrointestinal tract can be visualized through the inguinal window (hindleg fossa).

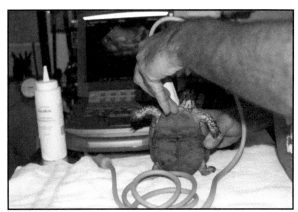

14.14 Ultrasonography using the mediastinal window to visualize the heart.

Sample collection

Blood

Phlebotomy can be performed in most tortoises and turtles using the jugular, subcarapacial, dorsal coccygeal or brachial veins (Figure 14.15). Tortoises do not groom themselves and the scaled skin is heavily contoured, collecting a large amount of debris and dirt, so thorough pre-injection cleansing is extremely important. The use of surgical scrubs applied with toothbrushes or nail brushes, flushing with isopropyl alcohol, and swabbing with cotton wool, gauze or cotton buds until the water rinsed off the area appears clean is advised.

Needle size varies depending on the location of the venepuncture site and the size of the patient; the smallest appropriate size should be used. The blood volume of a reptile constitutes 5–8% of their bodyweight and 10% of this can be taken safely for haematology. Therefore, a 100 g chelonian has 5–8 ml of blood, and 10% of that (0.5–0.8 ml) can be removed. For most animals a 23-gauge needle is sufficient for jugular sampling. For the subcarapacial vein, particularly in larger animals, the use of a one inch needle may be necessary.

The fresh blood sample should be collected into a tube containing heparin. A separate sampling tube may be needed for glucose estimation, but many in-clinic and external laboratories will run all biochemistries from the lithium heparin blood sample. If an immediate glucose level is needed, in-clinic biochemistry units are available. EDTA in blood collection tubes is frequently associated with lysis of chelonian erythrocytes, especially if stored for >24 hours, thus lithium heparin is the preferred anticoagulant. A fresh blood smear should be made before the sample is mixed with heparin. Use of an external laboratory for analysis of the sample is strongly recommended. Analysis of chelonian samples is a very specialized field and it is preferable to have a clinical pathologist familiar with chelonian haematology evaluate the sample.

Site	Location	Technique	Advantages	Disadvantages
Jugular vein (Figure 14.16)	Normally visible with the neck extended. Visualization improved by holding the neck slightly curved toward the opposite side. The right vein is larger in some species	The vessel can be occluded by placing a finger at the base of the neck. Apply pressure after sampling	Provides the best option for avoiding lymph contamination. Straightforward site for tortoises	In turtles usually requires sedation unless patient is moribund. Will cause haematoma formation; post-sampling pressure wraps advised
Subcarapacial space (Figure 14.17)	At the cranial ventral aspect of the carapace	Push the head of the patient into the shell for access. The needle is angled at 45 degrees and directed upwards into the subcarapacial space. The caudal margin can be palpated as a downward projection of the ventral carapace, and the needle directed just cranial. Although applying pressure to the sample site following blood draw is not usually necessary, where warranted a long cotton wool swab can be used	Easily performed on healthy and fully conscious patients. Large volumes can be obtained	Lymph contamination occurs in some instances
Coccygeal vein	At the dorsal ventral midline of the tail, just ventral to the coccygeal vertebrae. The vein is larger cranially	Hold the patient in dorsal recumbency. Direct the needle cranially at an angle dorsally toward the vertebral bodies		Proximal lymphatic vessel can cause sample contamination. Site requires greater pre-sampling cleansing due to faecal contamination
Brachial vein	Laterally located on the antebrachium, along the triceps tendon	With the patient in sternal recumbency, pull the pectoral limb medially to expose the vein. A butterfly catheter may improve placement		

14.15 Location and description of phlebotomy sites in chelonians.

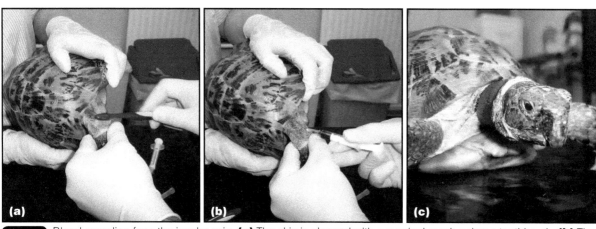

14.16 Blood sampling from the jugular vein. **(a)** The skin is cleaned with a surgical scrub using a toothbrush. **(b)** The blood sample is withdrawn. **(c)** An anti-haematoma scarf is placed.

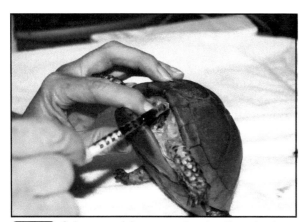

14.17 Subcarapacial venepuncture in a three-toed box turtle (*Terrapene Carolina triungis*).

Haematology and biochemistry: The haemogram should be evaluated for red blood cell (RBC) count and morphology, and for blood-borne parasites. The leucogram may be indicative of an acute or chronic infection of bacterial or viral aetiology. The white blood cell (WBC) count may rise early in an infection, then become depleted. The reptile heterophil is considered equivalent to the mammalian neutrophil. Monocytosis is common in viral infections and may indicate chronicity.

Elevations in serum total protein may indicate dehydration. In reproductively active females, and those with ovarian disorders, there may be disruption in the calcium:phosphorus balance, and elevation in hepatic enzymes. Hepatic lipidosis and/or cirrhosis are difficult to detect through serum biochemistry values. The renal status of tortoises can be evaluated using uric acid levels, along with calcium and phosphorus levels and ratio. Elevations in urea, creatinine and phosphate may occur as renal disease progresses. The clinician should also be aware that the body temperature of the chelonian at the time of blood sampling may affect the biochemistry values; repeated samples may be necessary to detect trends in metabolism.

Reference ranges for haematology and biochemistry are given in Figure 14.18.

Culture and cytology

- For oral sampling the beak can be opened with a rubber spatula in smaller species after the head

is restrained. A culturette swab is used to sample the pharynx and the glottis.
- Cloacal cultures can be obtained after restraint of the tail.

Mini-tip culturettes are useful in small patients or those that allow only limited access to the oral or cloacal space. Large chelonians sometimes require sedation to allow sampling. Aerobic, anaerobic and fungal cultures of samples are recommended.

Common conditions

Figure 14.19 lists common conditions of chelonians, their causes and treatment.

Parameter	Winter	Spring	Summer
Haematology			
PCV	0.33 (0.25–0.45)	0.38 (0.32–0.45)	0.29 (0.2–0.38)
RBC (x10^{12}/l)	0.83 (0.64–1.28)	0.96 (0.73–1.36)	0.67 (0.47–0.87)
Hb (g/dl)	10.1 (8.6–13)	11.3 (9.5–12.8)	9.3 (6.5–12.2)
MCV (fl)	402 (350–432)	408 (331–442)	426 (417–444)
MCH (pg)	124 (101–138)	122 (85–143)	137 (127–146)
MCHC (g/dl)	31.1 (28.6–34.4)	29.8 (25.5–32.6)	32.2 (30.4–33.1)
WBC (x10^9/l)	10.8 (7.5–14)	7.7 (2–13)	9.8 (6–12.5)
Heterophils (%)	66 (42–83)	63 (12–83)	58 (34–80)
Lymphocytes (%)	33 (15–58)	24 (12–50)	41 (20–64)
Monocytes (%)	0.4 (0–2)	2 (0–10)	0.7 (0–2)
Eosinophils (%)	0.6 (0–2)	11 (0–30)	0.3 (0–5)
Biochemistry			
ALP (IU/l)	Range: 196–425		
AST (IU/l)	Range: 19–103		
BUN (mmol/l)	9 (4–14)	103 (58–140)	1 (0–2)
Uric acid (µmol/l)	Range: 125–577		
Cholesterol (mmol/l)	2 (1.2–2.5)	1.9 (1.4–2.3)	3.1 (1.3–4.7)
Glucose (mmol/l)	0.6 (0.5–0.7)	13.8 (6.7–22)	1.5 (0.9–2.1)
Calcium (mmol/l)	Range: 2.7–3.5 (up to 10 in egg-producing females)		
Phosphorus (mmol/l)	Range: 1.7–3.3		
Potassium (mmol/l)	Range: 4.5–5.0 (lower in winter)		
Sodium (mmol/l)	Range: 130–144 (higher in winter)		
Chloride (mmol/l)	Range: 96–115 (higher in winter)		
Total protein (g/l)	73 (51–92)	89 (71–112)	87 (74–103)
Albumin (g/l)	Range: 7–28		
Globulin (g/l)	Range: 10–26		

14.18 Seasonal reference ranges (mean, with range in parenthesis, where available) for haematology and biochemistry in the Hermann's tortoise. (Data from *BSAVA Manual of Reptiles, 2nd edition*.)

Condition	Cause	Clinical signs	Treatment
Anorexia	Multiple causes; renal disease; overlong hibernation	Anorexia (note: seasonal variations); dehydration; poor weight; sunken eyes; dry mouth; high ratio of urate (white thick material) to fluid content in urine Assess carefully for acute *versus* chronic	If recent onset and no obvious cause, consider husbandry changes, especially temperature and water baths. Possible antibiotics and oral vitamin supplements. If critically ill, fluid therapy is paramount
Aural abscesses (Figure 14.20)	Hypovitaminosis A; environmental contamination	Large swellings over the ear, usually unilateral	Surgical removal of purulent debris and flushing. Antibiotic therapy. Vitamin A supplementation
Beak overgrowth	Often related to metabolic bone disease, causing a mismatch of upper and lower jaw development; can be due to over-reliance on soft feeds		Corrective surgery to restore natural anatomy; may need serial treatments. Best done under anaesthesia using high-speed burs or cutters
Cataract	Age-related; high blood glucose levels due to over-feeding of fruit; exposure to freezing temperatures	Opaque lens (commonly mistaken for corneal disease; use magnification glass to ensure lesion is in the lens)	Small size limits surgical removal. Usually cope well
Cloacal/ hemipenile prolapse (Figure 14.21)	Males in breeding condition; gravid females; foreign body ingestion/ obstruction; bacterial/parasitic enteritis		Separate male from potential mates. Treat dystocia if present. Relieve obstruction. Antibiotic/antiparasitic treatment. Decrease inflammation of the prolapsed tissue and replace (if possible) using vertical suture on sides of vent. Surgery
Conjunctivitis (Figure 14.22)	Infection (particularly herpesvirus); foreign body	Inflammation ± chemosis	Antibiotics
Corneal keratitis	Infection (particularly herpesvirus); irritation; tear disruption	Corneal changes	Topical therapy: may include steroids (use with caution if herpesvirus), lubricants and antibiotics
Dermatitis	Environmental contamination; inadequate heat	Ulceration at beak commissures, top of the head, submandibular area and limbs common; dry necrosis of feet, toenails and tail	Topical antiseptics. Systemic antibiotics. Husbandry correction
Dystocia	Improper nutrition; environmental conditions; lack of/inappropriate substrate	Anorexia; straining	Fluid therapy plus calcium. Warm to optimal temperature prior to administration of oxytocin/arginine vasotocin: repeated doses may be required. Antibiotics, NSAIDs, fluid therapy and nutritional support for infection associated with egg retention. Surgery
Foreign body ingestion	Inappropriate substrate/cage furniture	Straining; cloacal prolapse; anorexia; firm object(s) can be palpated in coelom through the inguinal space	Medical therapy including warm water enemas and oral mineral oil. Surgery
Hypovitaminosis A	Dietary deficiency of vitamin A	Ocular swelling; squamous metaplasia; build up of tissue in mouth/beak; aural abscess/swelling; skin sloughing	Dietary correction. Removal of secretions, exudates and sloughed skin. Treat aural abscess. Correct diet and husbandry. Lubrication
Pneumonia	Inadequate heat; poor nutrition; insanitary housing; presence of respiratory irritants	Open-mouth breathing; audible wheeze; blood/mucus in oral cavity	Systemic ± nebulized antibiotics. Increase environmental temperature. Clean environment so it is free of irritants
Ulcerative shell disease	Environmental contamination; inadequate temperature	Ulceration on the shell; erythema on the plastron is common	Debridement of necrotic shell; easily removed manually. Daily scrubbing of shell with a disinfectant. 'Dry docking' of the patient
Upper respiratory tract disease	Normal feature (serous discharge/ bubbles normal in species that drink through the nostrils); hypersalivation; nasal/oral infection (bacterial/fungal/ viral – culture/sensitivity, cytology and PCR required to identify organism)	Nasal discharge	Correct husbandry. Vitamin A supplementation. Nasal flushing. Topical antibiotics if bacterial infection

14.19 Common diseases of chelonians.

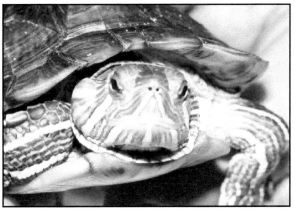

14.20 Aural abscess in a red-eared slider (*Trachemys scripta*).

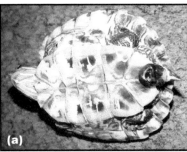
(a)

14.21

(a) Cloacal prolapse in a red-eared slider (*Trachemys scripta*).
(b) Phallus prolapse and organ paralysis in a redfoot tortoise.
(c) Rectal prolapse in a Horsfield's tortoise.

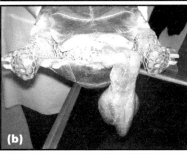
(b)

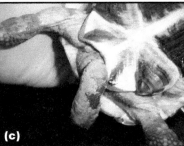
(c)

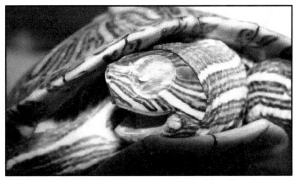

14.22 Conjunctivitis in a red-eared slider (*Trachemys scripta*). The underlying cause in a bilateral condition may be hypovitaminosis A.

Infectious diseases

Viral infections

Herpesvirus is the primary viral infection documented in captive chelonians. Clinically, it is seen in tortoises with upper gastrointestinal disease, usually manifesting as stomatitis (Figure 14.23). Oral lesions can occlude the pharynx and cause respiratory disease. Many non-specific clinical signs can be seen, including anorexia, lethargy, rhinitis, conjunctivitis and regurgitation. Affected individuals may succumb from hepatic disease, pneumonia or severe gastrointestinal ulceration. Most individuals are infected latently, and active disease is mild or subclinical. However, due to the persistent nature of herpesvirus infection, novel individuals should not be exposed to carrier animals. A serological and PCR test (oral swab) are available.

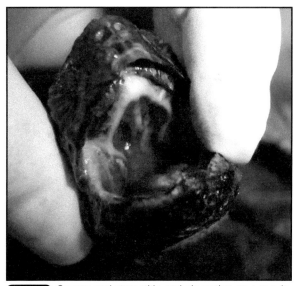

14.23 Severe oral stomatitis and ulceration as a result of herpesvirus infection. The crusting of nasal and oral discharge is evident on the lower jaw.

Bacterial infections

Bacterial infections are common in chelonians, especially secondary to trauma or improper husbandry. Poor water quality, inadequate heat and nutrition are predisposing factors. Husbandry must be corrected or healing will not occur. Most pathogens are Gram-negative, but all reptiles have Gram-negative organisms as part of their normal flora. On culture, therefore, consideration must be given to the species grown and the location from which the sample was obtained. If the clinical signs correlate with the known behaviour of the organism, a presumptive diagnosis can be made. Sensitivity testing is very important, as many common reptile pathogens (e.g. *Pseudomonas*) can have multi-drug resistance. Anaerobic organisms such as *Clostridium perfringens* are frequent pathogens, so anaerobic culture should therefore be requested as well as aerobic. *Mycoplasma* is a common pathogen of tortoises and culture specific for these organisms is recommended. Mycobacteria are occasionally found on cytology or histology in chelonians, but occurrence is rare in captive animals.

263

Bacterial dermatosis can present as ulcerations or abscesses. *Aeromonas hydrophila* is thought to play a role in white patch shell lesions in red-eared terrapins. Abscesses are firm and must be incised and debrided. Systemic antibiotic therapy, in conjunction with topical antiseptics, is recommended in most cases. Respiratory infections, particularly in turtles, are usually bacterial in nature. Pneumonia responds well to systemic antibiotics and, in severe cases, to nebulization therapy. *Salmonella* shedding increases in periods of stress and concurrent illness.

Fungal infections

Fungal infections are less common than bacterial but still observed with regularity in chelonians. Fungal organisms are ubiquitous in the environment and, in general, fungal infection is thought to become established in two ways: either the animal is exposed to an overwhelming dose of fungal spores, or the patient is immunosuppressed. In both of these scenarios husbandry adjustments may form part of the treatment. Dermatoses are the most common presentation and affect both the skin and the shell. When culturing samples from these areas it is advisable to request fungal culture in addition to anaerobic and aerobic bacteria. However, most fungal infections are detected with biopsy rather than culture, which prevents identification of the specific organism involved. Systemic fungal infections are normally seen in severely debilitated patients. A guarded prognosis is associated with widespread systemic fungal infections. Superficial infections often respond well to husbandry correction in conjunction with topical and/or systemic antifungal treatment.

Parasites

Parasitism is very common in chelonians and can be either incidental or pathological, depending on the organism and the host response. Many chelonians in the pet trade are wild-caught or from multi-animal farms and have a wide variety of parasites. Large numbers of ciliate and flagellate protozoans are often see in faecal smears, but these may be normal commensals. Significant parasites are summarized in Figure 14.24.

> **WARNING**
> **Avoid the use of avermectins. Ivermectin is especially toxic to chelonians and there have been many deaths following its use.**

Nutritional disorders

Hypovitaminosis A

Hypovitaminosis A is common in aquatic and semi-aquatic turtles adapted to (but not fed) wild diets high in vitamin A. Clinical signs are attributable to squamous metaplasia and immunosuppression. Mild cases usually present with bilateral periorbital swelling. Aural abscesses (usually unilateral, see Figure 14.20), caseous debris covering the cornea, and respiratory infections are common in more severely affected individuals. Hypovitaminosis A is very rare in tortoises. Affected turtles can be given two injections of vitamin A at a rate of 500–5000 IU/kg s.c. 14 days apart (Mader, 2005). Dietary correction is essential for long-term treatment. Liquid cod liver oil is very high in vitamin A and readily accepted by most turtles.

Metabolic bone disease

Nutritional secondary hyperparathyroidism occurs in rapidly growing juveniles, egg-laying females and aquatic turtles fed mineral-deficient diets. The diet may contain an inverse Ca:P ratio, or be deficient in vitamin D. There may also be a lack of UV-B lighting.

Parasite	Clinical signs	Diagnostics	Treatment
Nematodes			
Capillaria	Weight loss; lethargy	Faecal flotation	Fenbendazole
Strongyloides	Gastrointestinal irritation; diarrhoea; malnutrition	Fresh faecal smear; faecal flotation	Fenbendazole
Ascarids	Heavy loads can cause gastrointestinal irritation and weight loss; larval migration can cause extensive tissue damage	Faecal flotation	Fenbendazole
Oxyurids	Potentially non-pathogenic in tortoises but can cause cloacal irritation and prolapse in box turtles	Faecal flotation	Correct husbandry. Fenbendazole
Ectoparasites			
Fly larvae	Subcutaneous swellings with central opening containing the fly larvae; very common in *Terrapene*	Examination of larvae	Removal of larvae. Flushing affected areas with diluted chlorhexidine or povidine–iodine to prevent secondary bacterial infection
Ticks	May be no clinical illness; weakness; anaemia; clinical signs of vector-borne infections; ticks can transmit zoonotic and reportable diseases	Careful physical examination; ticks can be sent to veterinary parasitologist for identification	Physical removal by grasping the mouth parts with forceps and pulling straight out. Direct application of permethrin at 0.01–0.5% has proven safe and effective. The environment must also be treated. Treatment of any acquired infection

14.24 Significant parasites found in chelonians.

The most obvious clinical sign is softening of the shell. Nutritional secondary hyperparathyroidism can lead to dystocia and pathological fractures. Continued metabolic imbalances may precipitate or exacerbate renal disease. Generalized bone loss is more difficult to appreciate in chelonians than in snakes and lizards, and radiography is required; soft or deformed shell can be marked in severe cases.

Patients can be supplemented with calcium gluconate/glubionate and vitamin D3 while the diet is being corrected. A suggested protocol should include vitamin D3 at a rate of 400 IU i.m. once and calcium glubionate at a rate of 23 mg/kg orally q12h during the first week, along with adjustments in the diet to include calcium-rich foods. In the second week, if there has been significant bone loss and/or little response to treatment (including resistance to diet changes), a second parenteral dose of vitamin D3 may be administered and oral calcium continued. In severe or un-responsive cases calcitonin may be used at a rate of 50 IU/kg i.m. Calcitonin lowers blood calcium levels but inhibits bone resorption, and therefore should not be given without also providing calcium (orally or parenterally) and/or monitoring serum calcium levels. In some cases an additional dose of calcitonin may be given in the third week if there has been little improvement in bone/shell hardness.

Anorexic chelonians may require gavage feeding as well as fluid therapy initially as the animal may be too weak or in too much pain to eat or drink on its own. Additional supportive care including analgesia, restructuring of the environment and continued dietary adjustments are necessary. Monitoring of serum calcium and phosphorus levels, along with radiography, is required to evaluate the progress of bone deposition and renal function, and to determine the endpoint for calcium supplementation.

Urolithiasis

Uroliths are common in chelonians. Improper diet and dehydration are thought to be the main causes. Calculi can consist of different urate salts, such as calcium and potassium. A urolith can occasionally be palpated through the prefemoral fossa with the patient held vertically. Ultimately, the diagnosis of urolithiasis is achieved by radiography (Figure 14.25):

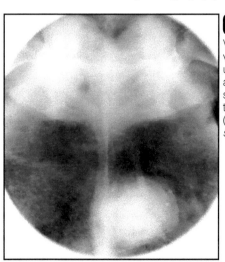

14.25 Ventrodorsal view showing urolithiasis in an African-spurred tortoise (*Geochelone sulcata*).

stones are often large and have a lamellar appearance. Presenting signs vary but may include straining, rear limb paresis and cloacal bleeding or prolapse. Stones are more common in tortoises but do occur in turtles. Treatment is surgical, either using a prefemoral approach (often with the aid of an endoscope and suction in larger chelonians) or by preferred to avoid plastrotomy to directly expose the stone. Cloacoliths also occur and can normally be removed manually through the cloaca.

Supportive care

Drug administration

- Direct oral medication can be difficult in chelonians.
  - A rubber spatula can be used in cooperative patients to open the mouth and deliver the medication.
  - In non-anorectic patients the medication can often be delivered in a favourite food: most box turtles will readily accept medication in a strawberry or other favoured fruits; many tortoises will take medication sprinkled on to the broken vein of a lettuce leaf.
- Subcutaneous injections can be given into the forelimb (Figure 14.26a).
- Intramuscular injections are easy to administer and usually given into the upper forelimb over the humerus (Figure 14.26b).

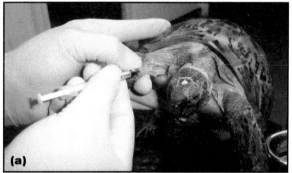

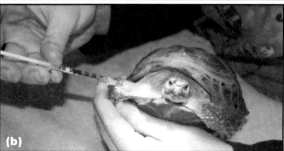

14.26 **(a)** Subcutaneous injection into the forelimb. **(b)** Intramuscular injection into the biceps muscle.

Fluid therapy

The daily maintenance fluid requirement for reptiles has been estimated to be between 15 and 25 ml/kg. Desert-adapted species most likely fall at the lower end of the range.

Dehydration is common in sick chelonians and can be evident on physical examination from the sunken appearance of the eyes and the turgor of the jugular vein. In addition, while difficult to separate from starvation, the apparent weight and density of the patient can be appreciated by a clinician familiar with the normal weight of a healthy chelonian. Many debilitated and dehydrated chelonians experience lactic acidosis. The clearance of lactate is slow in reptiles and so administration of lactated fluids is controversial. Crystalloid fluids such as isotonic saline or dextrose/saline can be used for rehydration. Fluids should be warmed to match the POTZ of the patient. Administration methods are as follows:

- **Oral/cloacal:** many dehydrated chelonians will drink readily if soaked in shallow warm water; fluids are also absorbed readily through the cloaca. The water level needs to be low enough to allow the patient to hold its head above the water without effort. The tray should be filled with warm water to chin level and the animal left for at least 20 minutes. It is important to note that tortoises drink through their nostrils and may hold their head underwater for prolonged periods. This method of administration is appropriate for mild dehydration. Tube feeding water to a debilitated patient is not advised unless the initial deficit has been corrected. Water can then be combined with a tube feeding formula for administration. A thick formula will decrease the chance of aspiration
- **Subcutaneous:** the most accessible area for subcutaneous fluid administration is the skin just cranial to the rear limbs (Figure 14.27). The needle should be directed superficially and be visible under the skin.
- **Intracoelomic:** fluids can be introduced directly into the coelomic cavity for more rapid assimilation. A butterfly catheter is helpful to allow for movement of the patient. The body wall is thin and the needle can be placed shallowly in this location to avoid puncture of the bladder. The patient should be placed in lateral recumbency and the needle angled to sit just under the body wall. Large volumes should not be administered in this fashion to avoid respiratory compromise.
- **Intravenous:** a jugular catheter can be placed in an anaesthetized patient. A cut-down procedure is often required in larger animals or those with

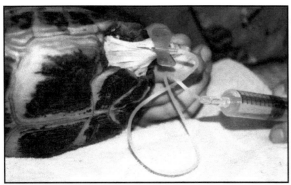

14.27 Subcutaneous fluid administration just cranial to the rear leg.

thick skin in this area. Catheters are easy to place in this location but difficult to maintain. If the catheter is to remain in place after the patient is conscious, it should be sutured in place directly to the skin or to tape placed around the catheter. It may also be necessary to restrict head and neck movement, which could occlude the catheter.
- **Intraosseous:** an intraosseous catheter can be placed into the cancellous bone at the bridge between the carapace and plastron. The preferred location is just cranial to the prefemoral fossa. A small hole can be drilled into the shell and a large-gauge syringe needle or spinal needle placed and secured to the shell. Anaesthesia or sedation with analgesia is required.

Nutritional support

Assisted feeding is not necessary in the early stages of treatment and is only considered after prolonged anorexia. Chelonians, like other reptiles, can tolerate long periods without eating. Calories and vitamins can be supplied through fluid administration. In most cases, once the cause of disease is determined and proper treatment is initiated, the patient will begin eating spontaneously. If anorexia is chronic, the patient can be tube-fed. The patient should be hydrated and at an optimal body temperature prior to tube feeding.

Stomach tube placement

After opening the mouth with a spatula or a mouth speculum, a tube of appropriate size can be passed into the stomach. For tortoises, a 3 mm endotracheal tube can be used; it is important that the tube is well lubricated. The stomach lies in about the cranial third of the body, and it is recommended to measure the tube prior to feeding. In a fully conscious chelonian this can be difficult and sedation may be required. Aspiration and oesophageal trauma are the most common complications of this procedure. Dehydrated tortoises have a very dry mucoid oesophagus, which tears easily; it is therefore best to avoid this technique or limit it to a once-only procedure.

Oesophagostomy tube placement

This is preferable to stomach tube placement for chelonians that require long-term feeding and oral hydration. Wide-gauge tubing can be used. The wide bore allows easy passage of fluids and fibre-based feeds. Some animals will need a tube in place for several months.

1. Use local anaesthesia for very debilitated animals; general anaesthesia otherwise.
2. Position artery forceps on the inside lateral wall of the oesophagus to mark the position to make a small cut in the skin. Take care to avoid the carotid artery and jugular vein.
3. Pierce the oesophageal wall and subcuticular tissues.
4. Open the jaws of the forceps gently to widen the aperture enough to grasp the end of the tube.
5. Draw the tube back out through the mouth and lubricate it.

6. Reinsert the tube down the oesophagus.
7. Tape the free end of the tube to the carapace with zinc oxide tape. It is important to transverse the tube over the neck to the *contralateral* side of the carapace; this prevents forming a loop into which the tortoise can insert its forelimb and pull the tube out (Figure 14.28).
8. Tube placement can be checked using radiography. Always start gavage with plain warm water. Once hydrated nutritional support can be started and, initially, this may be with soluble products (e.g. Reptoboost™ or Pedialyte™).

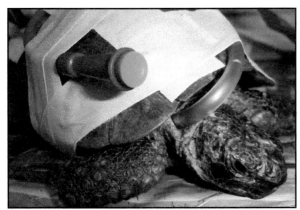

14.28 Use of a wide-gauge lamb feeder tube as an oesophagostomy tube. The non-latex PVC will be 'bound' into the wound and seal. The tube is fastened to the carapace with zinc oxide tape.

The formula offered should address the normal diet of the species. Tortoises can be fed with commercial formulas intended for herbivores. Aquatic turtles can be given a liquid diet formulated for carnivores. For semi-aquatic species, a combination of the two formulas can be used.

Anaesthesia and analgesia

Pre-anaesthetic considerations

A thorough physical examination is essential prior to anaesthesia. Fluid or electrolyte imbalances should be corrected and the patient warmed to its POTZ. For general anaesthesia and prolonged procedures, pre-anaesthetic blood testing and placement of an intravenous or intraosseous catheter for fluids is very beneficial. Atropine and other mucolytic agents are not used. Preoperative analgesia is recommended in the form of butorphanol or non-steroidal anti-inflammatory drugs (NSAIDs) such as meloxicam.

Agents

Injectable induction agents are required, either alone or prior to gas anaesthesia, due to the ability of chelonians to undergo long periods of apnoea. Numerous protocols have been described (Figure 14.29). The injectable anaesthetic is usually delivered intravenously or intramuscularly. In some instances, particularly in large patients, intramuscular delivery can be unrewarding; in these cases, or if rapid induction is desired, intravenous propofol can be given into the jugular or subcarapacial vein. After induction and intubation, inhalant anaesthetic agents (e.g. isoflurane, sevoflurane) can be used, with or without nitrous oxide.

Intubation

Once immobilization is achieved an endotracheal tube can be placed. The glottis in chelonians is at the base of the tongue and positioned caudally in the oropharynx (Figure 14.30). The trachea is short and the tube must be placed carefully to avoid entering the bronchus. Non-cuffed tubes are preferred as the tracheal rings are complete. When the airway is secured the patient is ideally placed on an

Drug	Dose	Comments
Alfaxalone	2–4mg/kg i.v. or 10 mg/kg i.m.	Useful i.v. induction agent. Ultra short-acting but can be used as single agent with top up doses to maintain anaesthesia. Can also be given i.m. but less reliable
Buprenorphine	0.01 mg/kg i.m.	Suitable pre-anaesthetic analgesic
Butorphanol	0.5–1 mg/kg (depending on predicated analgesic needs) i.m.	Suitable pre-anaesthetic analgesic
Ketamine + Diazepam	60–80 mg/kg K + 0.2–1.0 mg/kg D i.m.	
Ketamine + Medetomidine	5–10 mg/kg K + 0.1-0.15 mg/kg Me i.m.	Reverse medetomidine with atipamezole
Ketamine + Midazolam	25–30 mg/kg K + 1–2 mg/kg Mi i.m.	Midazolam is better absorbed from muscles in mammals than diazepam – may also be true for reptiles
Propofol	5–15 mg/kg i.v. Sedation: 10 mg/kg i.v. infusion Anaesthesia: 14 mg/kg i.v. slow infusion (if anaesthesia is induced too quickly, infusion may be stopped at 10 mg/kg)	Gold standard giving approximately 15 minutes anaesthesia per single injection. Can be used as an induction agent or top-up agent (to prolong anaesthesia). Dose to effect
Tiletamine/Zolazepam	4–8 mg/kg i.m.	

14.29 Common anaesthetic protocols used in chelonians.

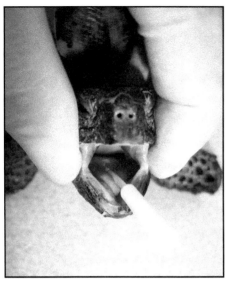

14.30

Intubation of a tortoise.

intermittent positive pressure mechanical ventilator (see Figure 14.31). If the patient is manually ventilated, care must be taken not to overinflate the lungs.

Monitoring

A Doppler flow probe is generally the most useful monitoring device in reptiles. The probe is normally placed over the carotid artery in the neck (Figure 14.31). The probe can be secured using tape or by direct manipulation by the anaesthetist. Pulse oximetry has been used to detect trends in oxygen saturation of the arterial blood, but the accuracy of the values given has been debated. As with other animals, external heat support must be provided; the temperature of the patient can be monitored with a thermal probe advanced into the colon or oesophagus.

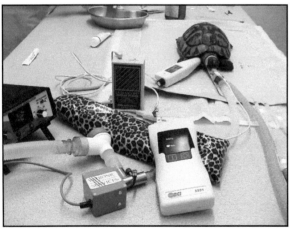

14.31 A Hermann's tortoise maintained under gaseous anaesthesia. Use of a heated water jacket mat. This can be contoured to the carapace if the animal is placed in dorsal recumbency. A Doppler probe is placed deep against the neck to detect blood flow in the heart or large vessels. A pulse oximeter probe (rectal) is placed in the oesophagus. Intermittent positive pressure ventilation is provided by a ventilator. The endotracheal tube and gas circuit are strapped to a wooden tongue depressor and the neck of the tortoise to ensure a stable airway. The endotracheal tube extends just distal to the larynx and is easily dislodged.

Recovery

Body temperature can be maintained during recovery using heat pads and/or lights or by placing the patient in a preheated room or incubator. A thermometer placed with the patient is essential. Aquatic turtles should be provided with appropriate humidity levels. Recovery can be slow in chelonians; patients undergoing general anaesthesia sometimes require overnight hospitalization during the recovery period. Postoperative analgesia can be given with a parenterally administered NSAID.

Analgesia

Pain management in reptiles is controversial and studies to determine appropriate medications and dosages have just begun. Subjectively, it appears that chelonians experience pain under the same apparent conditions as mammals. They possess the appropriate anatomy and physiology for nociception – it is the animal's interpretation of that noxious stimuli that is debated as truly 'feeling pain'. Pre-emptive use of an analgesic before surgery may allow the animal to return to normal function more rapidly, although some analgesics may contribute to the sedative affect of anaesthesia. Local use of lidocaine or bupivacaine appears to decrease pain sensation (as in mammals) and is encouraged for minor procedures or prior to an elective incision. Body temperature, hydration and metabolism contribute to the efficacy of analgesia. As pain may manifest as inactivity, failure to eat, or attempts to struggle away from a noxious stimulus (e.g. injection), the veterinary surgeon should use analgesics in chelonians as they would be used in other animals. It is not appropriate to restrain a patient without analgesia to carry out stressful or painful procedures, which in mammals would be done with analgesia and/or anaesthesia.

Common surgical procedures

Principles

- Preoperative scrubbing needs to be thorough, particularly in tortoises where dirt and debris can accumulate between the scales.
- In general, the skin of a tortoise should be surgically closed in an everting pattern. Use of mattress sutures or staples is effective. Tissue glue is useful for small wounds. Sutures and staples should be left in place for at least 3 weeks. Aquatic species may need additional protective layers such as antiseptic liquid bandages.

Aural abscess removal

The abscessation process in chelonians is different from that in mammals: chelonian tissues attempt to wall off the infection in a fibrin-based clot, and successive layers are added if the infection remains active. Culture of the causative agent is often difficult. Surgical debridement and removal of the abscess 'clot' is the treatment of choice.

The procedure should be performed under general anaesthesia. The area should be prepared aseptically and an elliptical incision made over the central swelling. The debris is normally caseous and can be removed gently with haemostats or small cotton swabs. The ear cavity should be flushed with sterile saline after removal of the debris. A slim section of skin can be removed at the margin of the incision to prevent early closure of the site and allow drainage of the area.

Cloacal/hemipenile prolapse repair

Prolapse of the phallus is common in male chelonians (see Figure 14.21); cloacal prolapse occurs in both genders but is most common in gravid females. Rectal prolapse may be associated with endoparasitism or poor diet. In all cases, if the tissue is not devitalized it can be cleaned and replaced.

Mannitol, 50% dextrose or hypertonic saline can be used to shrink the tissues prior to replacement. After the prolapse has been reduced, simple interrupted non-absorbable sutures can be placed at the lateral aspects of the vent. Purse-string sutures are not used. The patient should be monitored for several hours for re-prolapse. Suture removal is performed 5–7 days after placement if the patient is stable.

If the tissue is devitalized, it must be resected. The tortoise phallus does not contain a urethra and amputation is straightforward; however, it will render the animal incapable of inseminating a female.

Shell repair and wound care

Shell trauma is common in pet chelonians. The damage often creates a full-thickness crack in the shell, exposing the coelomic cavity. Defects that have distracted edges and those which expose the body cavity must be repaired. Superficial lesions may also need repair in aquatic species if the depth is sufficient to expose the deeper layers of the shell to infection in the aquatic environment. All lesions must be thoroughly cleaned prior to repair. Haemostasis must also be achieved.

Bacterial and fungal infections of the shell need thorough debridement, particularly if necrotic tissue is present. The lesions should be left open to granulate, and daily topical antimicrobials applied. Deep or extensive lesions may need to be cleaned and dressed daily, and some may require bandaging during the initial stages of healing.

Many wounds can be treated as for soft tissue/dermal wounds in other species. Once the body cavity is protected, the area can be covered initially with a wet-to-dry antimicrobial dressing, secured on the carapace or plastron with tape. The dressing should be changed at least every 24 hours. Some wounds initially may require more frequent dressing, particularly if the coelomic cavity was exposed.

Many techniques have been described for creating apposition of the shell edges. One method involves using stainless steel or non-absorbable monofilament sutures to appose the edges at the damaged area. Small holes are carefully made at the wound edges with an intramedullary pin to avoid penetration into the body cavity. The suture is then passed between the holes on either side of the defect.

After the defect is closed, the area needs to have a patch placed over the wound to ensure long-term protection while the shell heals. Fibreglass cloth attached with multiple layers of epoxy is an inexpensive method of repair (Figure 14.32a). It should not be placed until contamination and infection are cleared, and there is healthy granulation tissue. The patch must be monitored every 6–12 months in adult animals and monthly in fast-growing juveniles. A dremel tool should be used to remove the patch gradually as the shell heals. Use of a methacrylate polymer (e.g. Technovit™, available as a cattle hoof repair kit) has dramatically improved shell surgery (Figure 14.32b). This product is extremely adherent to keratin. The disadvantage is its exothermic reaction at curing. Good analgesia is advised and it is preferable to use only in anaesthetized animals. The preferred technique is to fill a standard hypodermic syringe with a mix and apply the epoxy. Other dental polymers have been used but they lack the durability of Technovit™.

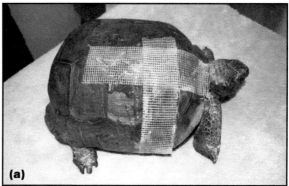

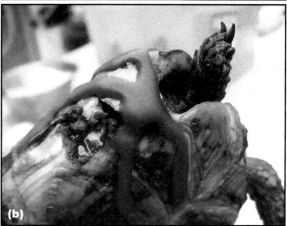

14.32 **(a)** Shell repair of a penetrating carapacial fracture in a gopher tortoise (*Gopherus polyphemus*). **(b)** Use of Technovit™ resin to stabilize a shell fracture but allowing access to the wound for cleansing and dressing. The resin has been applied using a standard hypodermic syringe.

Coeliotomy

The body cavity occasionally requires entry. This may be for foreign body retrieval, reproductive disorders, bladder calculi retrieval or systemic diseases such as neoplasia. Route of entry may be via the prefemoral fossa or via an osteotomy incision through the plastron. The technique requires experience with anaesthesia and a knowledge of chelonian anatomy. It is advised to study more advanced texts, such as the *BSAVA Manual of Reptiles 2nd edition*, before attempting this procedure.

Limb conditions

Fractures are relatively uncommon but hindleg weakness and paresis is not uncommon in tortoises. Trauma and infections are also seen. In extreme cases, amputation may be necessary. It is not easy to apply fixation support to chelonian limbs. A simple solution is to immobilize the limb by lifting it off the ground. To make a tough support, a table tennis ball can be cut and filled with Technovit™ resin, allowed to harden, and then bonded to the plastron (Figure 14.33).

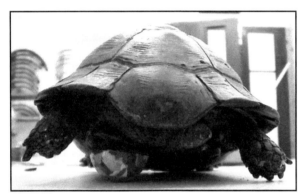

14.33 Use of a half table tennis ball filled with Technovit™ resin provides a durable plinth to immobilize a limb during recovery.

Euthanasia

Injection of a barbiturate is the preferred method of euthanasia for chelonians. Sedation may be required in order to achieve venous access or if the procedure is to be performed with the owners present. Sedation can be achieved with an intramuscular injection of ketamine (100 mg/kg) plus diazepam or tiletamine/zolazepam (25–50 mg/kg). The time period required for sedation to take effect is variable but it is usually accomplished within 30 minutes. Drug absorption is enhanced when the patient is warm. Sick animals can have reduced circulation, resulting in a prolonged period until sedation is evident. Once the chelonian is sedated, the euthanasia solution can be introduced intravenously (usually through the jugular vein), intracoelomically or by intracardiac injection.

The most challenging aspect of chelonian euthanasia is confirmation of death. Doppler ultrasonography can be used, but it may be prudent to ask the owner to leave the patient until death is confirmed by rigor mortis. Once the Doppler probe no longer detects heart activity, death may be assured by pithing the animal with a hypodermic needle in the foramen magnum.

Pithing through the foramen magnum to finalize death should not be done with the owner present. If the owner wishes to take the body home for burial immediately and has been present for the intravenous, intracoelomic and/or intracardiac injections, the clinician can pith the chelonian through the oral cavity using a long, slightly bent hypodermic needle inserted into the base of the cranium. A small amount of euthanasia solution can be injected as well. This should only be done after no heart beat has been detected via the Doppler probe for 10 minutes. Alternatively, the animal can briefly be removed from the room and pithed.

Freezing reptiles is a common method of euthanasia by lay people, but it should be stressed that this method should never be used. It is not a humane form of euthanasia as the brain ceases to function slowly, causing the animals to experience the entire process of freezing. Humane euthanasia is considered to be a method which causes loss of consciousness prior to death and veterinary surgeons need to make lay people aware of the difference.

Necropsy

Necropsy is complicated by the need to incise the shell. In most small to medium-sized chelonians a cutting wheel on a dremel or dental drill works well, combined with strong scissors or shears. A larger cutting device or hacksaw is required for large species. The shell is cut along the lateral margins between the carapace and the plastron. Care must be taken not to damage the internal structures. The soft tissue can be bluntly dissected away from the shell. Once the plastron is removed, the procedure is routine.

Drug formulary

In the UK very few medications are authorized for use in chelonians, and signed consent is advised for all therapeutics. Figure 14.34 gives a drug formulary for chelonians.

Drug	Dosage	Comments
Antiviral agents		
Aciclovir	80 mg/kg orally q24h Topical ointment (5%) also available	Herpesvirus
Antibacterial agents		
Amoxicillin	5 mg/kg orally q24h	Useful for *Staphylococcus*, *Streptococcus* and some anaerobic bacteria
Carbenicillin	400 mg/kg s.c./i.m. q48h	Increased efficacy against Gram-negative bacteria (e.g. *Pseudomonas*)

14.34 Drug formulary for chelonians. [a] Clinicians should be aware of responsible use of third generation cephalosporins and fluoroquinolones. These drugs should only be used where infection is known to exist and it should be remembered that a response to treatment cannot be achieved without other antibiotics. (continues) ▶

Drug	Dosage	Comments
Antibacterial agents continued		
Cefotaxime	20–40 mg/kg i.m. q24h	Can be used with an aminoglycoside to enhance activity against Gram-negative bacteria
Ceftazidime [a]	20 mg/kg s.c. q72h	Currently the recommended antibiotic for chelonian use
Ceftiofur [a]	4 mg/kg i.m. q24h	Useful for bacterial respiratory tract infections (e.g. *Pasteurella*, Gram-negative bacteria)
Cefuroxime [a]	100 mg/kg i.m. q24h	Can be used with an aminoglycoside to enhance activity against Gram-negative bacteria
Clarithromycin	15 mg/kg orally q48–72h	Useful for pasteurellosis and *Mycoplasma*-associated upper respiratory tract infections
Clindamycin	2.5–5 mg/kg orally q24h	Useful for anaerobes and osteomyelitis
Doxycycline	50 mg/kg loading dose, then 25 mg/kg i.m. q72h	Use against *Staphylococcus* and *Klebsiella*. Also likely effective against *Chlamydophila*, *Mycoplasma* and rickettsias
Enrofloxacin [a]	5–10 mg/kg orally/i.m. q24h	Useful for *Pseudomonas*, *Mycoplasma*, *Chlamydophila* and Gram-negative bacteria. Drug causes discomfort and tissue necrosis at site of injection. Oral solution achieves good systemic bioavailability. Associated with occasional regurgitation and excessive salivation. Use with care in juveniles due to damaging effects of fluoroquinolones on growing cartilage
Gentamicin	2.5–5 mg/kg i.m. q72h For Gram-negative respiratory infections: 10–20 mg/15 ml saline and then nebulized for 15–30 minutes q8–12h	May be combined with a third-generation cephalosporin. Ensure adequate hydration and healthy renal function
Marbofloxacin [a]	5 mg/kg s.c./i.m./orally q24h	Good activity against Gram-negative bacteria. Use with care in juveniles due to damaging effects of fluoroquinolones on growing cartilage
Metronidazole	20 mg/kg orally q24h	Useful for anaerobes. May combine with amikacin to broaden spectrum of activity. Duration of treatment usually >10 days, but beware of hepatotoxicity if using q24h
Piperacillin	50–100 mg/kg i.m. q24h for 1–2 wks For respiratory infections: 100 mg/10 ml saline and then nebulized for 15–30 minutes q8–12h	Broad spectrum of activity. May be used with an aminoglycoside to increase activity against Gram-negative bacteria
Silver sulfadiazine cream	Apply topically q24h	Broad-spectrum antibacterial. Some fungicidal activity
Antifungal agents		
Amphotericin B	0.5–1 mg/kg i.v./intracoelomically q24–72h for 2–4 wks For respiratory infections: 5 mg/150 ml saline and then nebulized for 30–60 minutes q12h	Useful for aspergillosis and candidiasis. Potentially nephrotoxic; ensure adequate hydration and renal function
Clotrimazole	Apply topically q12h	Fungal dermatitis/stomatitis
Enilconazole	1:50 dilution with water applied topically q2–3d	Fungal dermatitis
Fluconazole	21 mg/kg s.c. loading dose; then 10 mg/kg s.c. q5d, based on loggerhead turtles	Fungal infection
Ketoconazole	15–30 mg/kg orally q24h for 2–4 wks	Studies in gopher tortoises. Beware hepatotoxicity
Malachite green	0.15 mg/l water as a 1h bath q24h for 2 wks for soft-shelled turtles	Fungal and algal dermatitis
Nystatin	100,000 IU/kg orally q24h for 10 days	Fungal gut infections

14.34 (continued) Drug formulary for chelonians. [a] Clinicians should be aware of responsible use of third generation cephalosporins and fluoroquinolones. These drugs should only be used where infection is known to exist and it should be remembered that a response to treatment cannot be achieved without other antibiotics. (continues) ▶

Drug	Dosage	Comments
Antiparasitic agents		
Chloroquine	125 mg/kg orally q48h on 3 occasions	Blood parasites
Fenbendazole	50–100 mg/kg orally; repeat after 2 wks and 4 wks	Nematodes, some cestodes. Efficacy can be increased by dividing dose over 3 days
Fipronil	Spray on cloth and wipe over reptile surface q7–14d until negative tests for parasites	Ectoparasites, particularly mites and ticks
Levamisole	10 mg/kg i.m. once; repeat q2wks until negative test for parasites	Nematodes. Use with care
Metronidazole	125–250 mg/kg orally once	Protozoans. Beware toxicity at higher doses
Oxfendazole	66 mg/kg orally once; repeat q2wks until negative tests for parasites	Nematodes
Paromomycin	Entamoebiasis: 35–60 mg/kg orally q7d for 2 wks Cryptosporidiosis: 300–350 mg/kg orally q48h for 3 wks; then q5d for 3 months	Long-term cure not proven for cryptosporidosis
Permethrin (10%)	Dilute to 1% solution and apply topically; repeat after 10 days	Mites. Less toxic than pyrethrins, but beware toxicity and ensure adequate ventilation after treatment
Praziquantel	5–8 mg/kg orally once; repeat after 2 wks and 4wks	Cestodes and trematodes
Quinacrine	1 mg/kg orally q7d for 4–8 wks	Protozoans
Sulfadiazine	25 mg/kg orally q24h	Coccidiosis. Ensure adequate hydration/renal function as potentially nephrotoxic
Sulfadimethoxine	90 mg/kg orally once; then 45 mg/kg orally q24h	Coccidiosis. Ensure adequate hydration/renal function as potentially nephrotoxic
Sulfadimidine (33% solution)	0.3–0.6 mg/kg orally q24h for 10 days	Coccidiosis. Ensure adequate hydration/renal function as potentially nephrotoxic
Sulfamethazine	50 mg/kg q24h for 3 days; then no treatment for 3 days; then repeat for 3 days	Coccidiosis. Ensure adequate hydration/renal function as potentially nephrotoxic
Trimethoprim/ Sulfadiazine	25 mg/kg orally q24h for 7 days	Coccidiosis. Dose based on sulfadiazine component

14.34 (continued) Drug formulary for chelonians. [a] Clinicians should be aware of responsible use of third generation cephalosporins and fluoroquinolones. These drugs should only be used where infection is known to exist and it should be remembered that a response to treatment cannot be achieved without other antibiotics.

References and further reading

Ernst CH and Barbour RW (1989) *Turtles of the World.* Rowman & Littlefield Publishing Inc., Lanham, Maryland

Girling S and Raiti P (2004) *BSAVA Manual of Reptiles, 2nd edn.* BSAVA Publications, Gloucester

Hernandez-Divers SJ and Mackey E (2008) Endoscopic determination of gender in neonate and juvenile chelonians. *Proceedings, Association of Reptile and Amphibian Veterinarians*, pp. 3–4

Highfield A (1996) *Encyclopedia of Keeping and Breeding Tortoises and Freshwater Turtles.* Krieger Publishing Company, Malabar, Florida

Hollamby S, Murphy D, Schiler CA, *et al.* (2000) An epizootic of amoebiasis in a mixed species collection of juvenile tortoises. *Journal of Herpetological Medicine and Surgery* 10, 9–15

Klingenberg RJ (2004) Diagnosing parasites in box turtles. *Exotic DVM* **5(6)**, 27–31

Mader DR (2005) *Reptile Medicine and Surgery, 2nd edn.* Saunders/ Elsevier, St. Louis, Missouri

McArthur S, Wilkinson R and Meyer J (2004) *Medicine and Surgery of Tortoises and Turtles.* Wiley-Blackwell, Ames, Iowa

Useful websites

www.britishcheloniagroup.org.uk
www.tortoisetrust.org

15

Lizards

Kevin Eatwell

Introduction

There are over 7200 species within the Order Squamata and there are a large number of hypotheses regarding classification within this Order. Lizards comprise nearly 5000 of these species and form the Suborder Lactertilia. Forty-one families exist, and a dozen or so of these are regularly represented in exotic pet practice (Figure 15.1). However, there are only a few species which are commonly seen, and these are covered in this chapter. More detailed references, such as the *BSAVA Manual of Reptiles, 2nd edition*, should be sought for more unusual species that may present from time to time.

Biology

Anatomy and physiology

Lizards are an anatomically diverse group. Most of the common species seen in practice have a similar anatomy, with a few clinically significant differences.

Many species are highly protected with scale modifications, leading to crests (Figure 15.2), beards and casques. These can be used for defence and for communication between individuals.

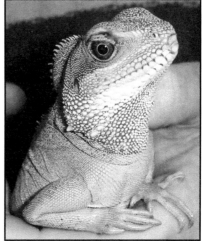

15.2 Male water dragon demonstrating bright coloration and crest.

Family	Common species	Biology	Comments
Agamidae (agamids): 300 species	Bearded dragons (*Pogona vitticeps*)	Diurnal; terrestrial; Australian desert species; omnivorous	Good as a first lizard pet, rarely aggressive; require heat, good UV-B light, low humidity; adults more herbivorous then insectivorous
	Chinese water dragon (*Physiognathus cocincinus*)	Diurnal; arboreal; Asian forest species; carnivorous; often found near water	Quite flighty and can become aggressive; not ideal as a first lizard pet
Chamaelonidae (chameleons): 130 species	Veiled or Yemen chameleon (*Chamaeleo calyptratus*)	Diurnal; arboreal; from mountain regions of Yemen and Saudia Arabia; omnivorous	Can become aggressive; not good as a first lizard pet due to complex husbandry requirements
Iguanidae (iguanas): 34 species	Green iguana (*Iguana iguana*)	Diurnal; arboreal; from South American rainforest; herbivorous; often found near water	Very large when full grown (up to 1.5 metres in length); can be very aggressive; not recommended as a first lizard pet; require good source UV-B light, heat, high humidity
	Uromastyx or dab lizards (*Uromastyx* spp.)	Diurnal; terrestrial; North African and Middle East desert species; omnivorous	Good as a first lizard pet as can become very accustomed to handling
Eublepharidae (geckos): 25 species	Leopard geckos (*Eublepharius macularius*)	Nocturnal; terrestrial; from desert areas in Pakistan and India; insectivorous	Can become aggressive if poorly handled; small lizard; good first lizard pet
Varanidae (monitors): 40 species	Bosc or savannah monitor (*Varanus exanthematicus*)	Diurnal; terrestrial; from savannah in South Africa; insectivorous; carnivorous	Captive breeding is rare for this species; common pet presented; can become aggressive
Other species can be seen, including: day geckos (*Phelsuma* spp.), basilisks (*Basiliscus* spp.), plated lizards (*Gerrhosaurus* spp.), sand lizards (*Lacerta* spp.), anoles (*Anolis* spp.) and a variety of skinks and geckos			

15.1 Common species of lizards presented in practice.

Head

Tongue: All species have a fleshy tongue, but in chameleons this has become extensively modified and is a projectile which can be launched to acquire prey. Bearded dragons have a tongue with a flattened tip which is distinct from the rest of the tongue. Other lizards such as green iguanas have a red-coloured tip to the tongue. These anatomical variations should not be mistaken for pathology.

Eyes: Lizards have good colour vision. The eyes of chameleons are further modified; the eyelids have fused to form a turret with a small hole and the eyes are able to move independently of each other, allowing the animal to scan its environment widely. When an object (such as a prey item) draws attention, binocular vision is used to pinpoint its exact location. Geckos can be either eublepharine (such as the leopard gecko) which have eyelids, or ablepharine (such as day geckos, *Phelsuma* spp.) where the eyelids are fused and transparent and form the spectacle. Iguanas have a parietal eye in the centre on the top of the head, which is linked directly to the pineal gland. This is believed to be important in regulating circadian rhythm.

Ears: The external ear canal is much reduced in all lizards and the tympanum is clearly visible in many species, apart from chameleons.

Cardiorespiratory system

Inspiration and expiration are active processes requiring muscular effort. There is a single coelomic cavity and no diaphragm, so respiratory movements are primarily performed by the intercostal muscles. The trachea is positioned at the base of the fleshy tongue and is made of incomplete tracheal rings, as in mammals. The trachea bifurcates into two bronchi, which enter the lungs in the cranial coelomic cavity. The paired lungs can be quite simple in some species or have multiple chambers. The respiratory surface consists of ediculi (flatter and wider than alveoli), and smooth muscle can assist in elevating the respiratory surface to facilitate gas exchange. The lungs become simplified as they progress caudally. Chameleons have tubular extensions of the respiratory tract (denticular processes) that extend far back in the coelomic cavity.

The heart consists of two atria and one ventricle. The ventricle is functionally split into three chambers. There is communication between the atria and ventricle during systole. In diastole, the arterioventricular (AV) valve occludes the communication between the atria and ventricle. Blood exits the ventricle and enters the left and right aortae. This allows for a differential flow of blood, depending on the physiological state of the animal. When breathing there is a small left-to-right shunt, and when breath-holding there is a right-to-left shunt and the lungs are bypassed. Resistance to anoxia is high. Monitor lizards have a higher aerobic scope and their heart functions like a mammalian heart at all times.

Stance

Lizards have a semi-erect stance and the body is held above the substrate. Chameleons have highly modified limbs and the digits oppose each other. This combined with sharp nails facilitate gripping branches.

Ecdysis

Lizards undergo ecdysis, which is the periodic shedding of the skin. This is an important aspect of growth. A new layer forms from the basal epidermis, and lymph enters the cleavage zone between the layers to separate the old skin from the new. At this stage the lizard may go a dull colour. After 3 days, the lizard abrades the top layer, causing it to split and then be shed. During this time high humidity levels are required. Lizards shed piecemeal and may eat the exuvium.

Iguanas and geckos can shed their tails due to fracture planes in the caudal vertebrae. Iguanas have multiple fracture planes, whereas geckos have only one at the base of the tail (Figure 15.3). Autotomy serves to distract a potential predator, allowing the lizard to escape. As iguanas get older, the shedding planes ossify as the tail is better used in defence. Shedding of the tail is a last resort as the lizard will lose an energy reserve, social status and, thus, potentially mates and territory. The tail does subsequently regenerate over a number of weeks. Regenerated tails usually have a different scalation to the original and a cartilaginous internal support instead of bony vertebrae. Agamids, monitor lizards and chameleons do not shed their tails as they are important in locomotion and defence.

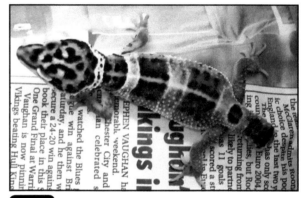

15.3 Leopard gecko after tail autotomy.

Body temperature

Lizards are ectothermic reptiles and require an external heat source to elevate body temperature. This is provided either by solar radiation (diurnal species) or by environmental conduction (nocturnal species). Correct body temperature is critical for survival, and wild reptiles have a specific range within which they can thermoregulate to maintain optimal body temperature. This allows them to elevate and control their metabolic rate for all body functions, and is particularly important for stimulating digestion and immune function. Diurnal species regulate temperature by basking intermittently and seeking shade or burrowing into a cool substrate to avoid overheating. Species close to water may use this both as a refuge and a way to cool and control body temperature. Nocturnal species regulate temperature by varying the amount of body surface contact with the ground or rocks.

Cholecalciferol

Ultraviolet (UV-B) light from solar radiation is important to enable many lizards to synthesize cholecalciferol (vitamin D) in the skin, which is converted by the liver and kidneys into the metabolically active hormone. Species that eat whole prey or are nocturnal can obtain cholecalciferol from prey items. Some species such as the bearded dragon and dab lizard have highly pigmented coelomic cavities to shield them from excessive UV-B radiation.

Water

Water is critical to the majority of lizards and many desert species have evolved methods to conserve water by storing it in the bladder (iguanids) or colon, and using this as a source. Raising blood osmolarity also helps to maintain blood volume. Certain rainforest species (such as chameleons) prefer to take water dripping off foliage.

Metabolic rate

The metabolic rate of lizards is low, and there are a number of ways in which they conserve energy. Lizards elevate body temperature only when there is a need to do so (e.g. after feeding to assist in digestion), and the cost of obtaining food has to be weighed against the energy provided. Many small species are insectivorous and can forage widely due to their small size. However, larger lizards cannot afford to forage as widely, so either take much larger prey items (e.g. monitor lizards) or are herbivorous. In many species there is an ontogenetic shift towards herbivory as the lizard ages. Many omnivorous species take far more vegetable matter than insectivorous prey items.

Behaviour

Communication in reptiles is usually cryptic and so overt behavioural displays are unusual as they lead to increased risks of predation. However, many diurnal lizards that have grown confident in their environment exhibit assertion displays, which can include puffing up their bodies, turning to demonstrate frontal or lateral displays, doing push ups or head bobbing. Captive animals can spend a lot of time defending territories that are too small, and this can be directed against any potential competitor, including the owners. Aggressive behaviour is commonly seen, depending on species. Mouth gaping and vocalization are signs of a particularly offensive individual and many lizards try to whip with their tails, bite and scratch. Cloacal contents may also be voided.

Sexing

Many lizards are sexually dimorphic, and secondary sexual characteristics can be used to distinguish between males and females.

- Male lizards can be more brightly coloured and have more robust bodies and heads than females.
- Femoral and pre-anal pores are far more prominent in male geckos, iguanas and agamids.
- Male lizards also have two hemipenes situated in the tail base, which can be seen as a post-anal bulge resulting in a wider tail base (Figure 15.4).

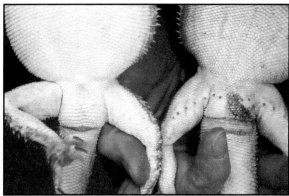

15.4 Bearded dragons. The female is on the left; the male is on the right.

- Male chameleons have larger casques and also have hemipenal bulges at the tail base.

Monitor lizards and skinks lack differences in secondary sexual characteristics. In these cases, other methods of sexing can be used. The inverted hemipenis can be probed in some species (but this is of little use in monitor lizards as they are too strong and there is a risk of damage). Popping of the hemipenis and hydrostatic eversion (saline injection) can be used, but both of these techniques require practice, and hydrostatic eversion should be performed under anaesthesia. Radiography can be used in some monitor lizard species as the hemibacula within the hemipenis can become calcified. Ultrasonography can also be used in expert hands. In addition, surgical sexing via endoscopy can be performed. Many owners rely on behavioural assessment of two individuals placed together. Many lizards are best housed alone to avoid conflict and attempts to defend a small territory. Aggression between captive lizards is common. The exception to this rule is where sexed pairs or trios are housed together (usually bearded dragons or leopard geckos).

Husbandry

Given the wide variety of lizards it is not possible to provide a comprehensive summary; however, categorizing species into groups can help the novice reptile veterinary surgeon evaluate the husbandry of an unfamiliar species prior to undertaking research (Figure 15.5). The references at the end of the chapter provide a good resource for such information.

- *Diurnal species*: These lizards rely on the sun to increase their body temperature and therefore benefit from an overhead basking site, mimicking solar radiation. They are also exposed to high levels of solar UV radiation in the wild, and many species cannot be kept in captivity successfully without an appropriate UV source.
- *Nocturnal species*: These lizards should not be exposed to high basking temperatures, but it should be noted that some species do still bask at dusk or dawn and so will benefit from exposure to UV radiation.

Species	Basking (°C)	Cold end (°C)	Overnight (°C)	UV-B required?	Dietary preferences	Water source and relative humidity	Furniture
Bearded dragons	40	25	21	Yes; a mercury vapour lamp or a fluorescent tube should be provided	Commercially raised invertebrates and leafy greens; greens should comprise 85% of the diet for adult	Large bowl with easy access in and out Humidity: 30–40%	Hides and low level branches and rocks to climb over; upright log for basking
Chinese water dragons	35	25	21	Yes; a mercury vapour lamp or a fluorescent tube should be provided	Commercially raised invertebrates with some whole prey (pinkie mice) for large animals	A very large bowl with easy access in and out; ideally a heated and filtered pool for swimming Humidity: 80–90%	Higher level branches to climb up to the basking site and UV source; real or plastic foliage can be used to provide some cover to reduce escape attempts
Veiled chameleons	40	25	21	Yes; a mercury vapour lamp or a fluorescent tube should be provided	Commercially raised invertebrates and leafy greens; greens should comprise 15% of the diet for adults	Will not recognize standing water, so water must be dripped from foliage into a reservoir or misting is required Humidity: 75–80%	Higher level branches to climb up to the basking site and UV source; real or plastic foliage can be used to provide some cover and facilitate providing 'moving' water; probably the hardiest of the chameleons, mostly captive-bred (USA)
Green iguanas	40	25	21	Yes; a mercury vapour lamp or a fluorescent tube should be provided	Totally herbivorous; diet should comprise 50% leafy greens, flowers and weeds, 25% legumes and vegetables and 25% fruit	A very large bowl with easy access in and out; ideally a heated and filtered pool for swimming Humidity: 75–100%	Higher level branches to climb up to the basking site and UV source; real or plastic foliage can be used to provide some cover
Dab lizards	40	25	21	Yes; a mercury vapour lamp or a fluorescent tube should be provided	Totally herbivorous; diet should consist of 50% leafy greens, flowers and weeds 40% legumes and vegetables and 10% fruit	Large bowl with easy access in and out Humidity: 25–50%	Hides and low level branches and rocks to climb over
Leopard geckos	30	25	21	No; however, studies have shown it to be beneficial and it is advised by the author	Commercially raised invertebrates	Large bowl with easy access in and out Humidity: 30–40%	Hides and low level branches and rocks to climb over; high humidity area critical when reproductively active or shedding
Bosc monitor lizards	40	25	21	No; however, studies have shown it to be beneficial and it is advised by the author	Commercially raised invertebrates with some whole prey (pinkie mice) for large animals	Large bowl with easy access in and out Humidity: 25–50%	Hides and low level branches and rocks to climb over

15.5 Species-specific husbandry recommendations.

- *Arboreal species*: These lizards require branches to climb and a vertically arranged environment. Many species will be exposed to higher levels of humidity in the wild and the captive environment should reflect this.
- *Terrestrial species*: These lizards require a horizontally arranged environment with a larger floor space. Hides should be provided to allow for visual security.
- *Desert species*: Many species are exposed to a dry environment and may require a low relative humidity; however, various species exploit microclimates and require areas of high humidity, so water should always be available.
- *Rainforest species*: These lizards are likely to require an environment with a high humidity to prevent chronic dehydration. Species found near water also require a large volume of water to bathe and swim in.
- *Herbivorous species*: A wide range of material can be offered, but for many species a large proportion of the diet will be foliage and green plant material. Providing sufficient calcium for these species is important.

- *Insectivorous species*: Invertebrate species commonly fed include brown crickets (*Acheta domesticus*), locusts (*Melanopus* spp.), waxworms (*Gallaeria mellonella*) and mealworms (*Tenebrio molitor*). These are all low in calcium so appropriate supplementation should be provided.
- *Omnivorous species*: These lizards can eat a wide variety of food items, but become more herbivorous with age. Dietary supplementation is also likely to be important.
- *Carnivorous species*: When young these lizards are insectivorous but take larger whole prey when older. Animals fed on whole prey are less likely to suffer from nutritional problems.

Housing

The enclosure (Figure 15.6) should meet all of the lizard's basic needs and mimic as closely as possible how this would be achieved in the wild.

Enclosure design

Enclosure design is important and many commercially available vivaria may not be suitable for the lizard in question. A vivarium should provide as much space as possible, but it is important for the lizard to be able to seek refuge. Provision of hides and logs (terrestrial species), substrates for burying (fossorial species), branches to climb on (arboreal species) and a pool area (aquatic species) are mandatory. Wooden or plastic vivaria are superior to glass tanks as they can be modified where required and provide visual security. In addition, lizards do not perceive glass as a barrier and can do significant damage to their rostrum as a result. This is particularly common in Asian water dragons. Wire mesh can also lead to facial trauma.

Heat source

At least two heat sources are required. The primary heat source is used to provide a basking site at the appropriate temperature. It is best if this site is available all day long to allow the lizard to bask at will.

However, many heat sources are quite potent (in order to achieve high basking temperatures), and in small poorly ventilated enclosures there is no way for the heat to dissipate. In these cases, the owner may have to either expand the enclosure or consider reducing the intensity (or regulate the heat output using a thermostat) of the basking site heat source to prevent over heating. It is important to measure the effectiveness of the basking site with either a maximum/minimum thermometer or a continuous recording device. This heat source should be left on during the day but turned off overnight. Typically, these heat sources can be placed on a time switch and activated/turned off at the same time as any lights. Large lizards will require more diffuse heat sources to allow them to increase their body temperature more evenly. For arboreal lizards, the basking site needs to be high in the environment and accessible via branches.

Background heat should be provided by a second heat source, which can be a tubular heater, heat tape, ceramic bulb or a radiator elevating the temperature of the vivarium or the background temperature of the room that houses the enclosure. The heat source should be thermostatically controlled and set at the minimum night time temperature. It is also important to measure and record the temperature of the cool end of the vivarium to ensure it is not overheating during the day and not dropping too cold at night. Underfloor heating, such as heat mats, can lead to burns when the lizard tries to cool down by burying in the substrate. Hot rocks can lead to burns as they provide focal areas of heat. All heat sources should be kept out of the lizards' way or guarded to prevent thermal burns; surface temperatures can exceed 150°C.

One of the main faults of husbandry is the failure to provide an adequate thermal environment for all or part of the daily routine, and this may lead to health problems or encourage the lizard to enter brumation (dormancy). Careful monitoring is required to enable a full evaluation of the thermal environment.

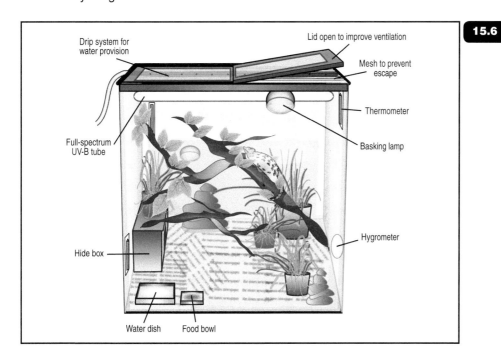

15.6 Suitable vivarium for an arboreal lizard.

Drip system for water provision

Lid open to improve ventilation

Mesh to prevent escape

Thermometer

Full-spectrum UV-B tube

Basking lamp

Hygrometer

Hide box

Water dish   Food bowl

Ultraviolet light

UV light is important to many species and there are a number of potential sources. Currently, mercury vapour lamps are favoured by many, particularly for diurnal basking species. These lamps also provide heat and can be used as a basking site heat source. However, they cannot be thermostatically controlled. Light sources should be on for 9–15 hours a day for most lizards. For nocturnal species a reverse lighting regime can be implemented. Nocturnal reptilian red lights are available and can be used during the reptile's 'night' so that the animal will be active and visible during the owner's waking hours.

For species that do not require such an intense basking site heat, there are a number of lamps available that produce UV-B light. Unfortunately, although many lamps on the market may be full spectrum and have a good colour rendering index, they produce no UV-B light. Other lamps may be full spectrum and produce UV-A light only. It is important to distinguish between the different types of lamp. UV-B light diminishes with distance according to the inverse square law. Glass and plastic filter 100% of UV-B rays and fine mesh can also lead to a substantial reduction in UV-B light. In addition, there is a progressive build-up of phosphor within the light, leading to reduced UV-B light output over time. Ideally, sources should be measured with a UV light meter to evaluate accurately the output and the amount the reptiles are exposed to; otherwise frequent changes are required, possibly as often as every 3 months. UV-B light sources should be placed close to heat sources as both UV-B light and heat are required for synthesis of cholecalciferol in the skin. It is useful and good practice to ask owners to bring their lights and any cage cover to the consultation so that the UV-B light output can be measured (the clinic should have a UV light meter). The owners can then be informed of the distance required for the lizard to be within the therapeutic range.

Ventilation

Ventilation is important for lizards, particularly chameleons. Vivaria can have ventilation holes made at the level of the lizard to allow a good throughput of air. Chameleons are best housed in mesh cages to allow for a rapid exchange of air.

Humidity

The lizards commonly seen in practice can come from markedly differing habitats or use different niches within one habitat, depending on species, age, physiological status and reproductive status. One aspect of the environment that changes as a result of this is the relative humidity. Unfortunately, providing good ventilation has the effect of reducing relative humidity and so greater attention has to be paid to maintaining the correct level. Drippers, misting devices, foggers, waterfalls and handheld sprayers can be used to increase relative humidity levels. Water bowls can be placed on heat mats to encourage evaporation or a damp substrate can be used. Elevated relative humidity is important for lizards that are about to shed their skin or reproduce.

Relative humidity can be monitored using a hygrometer or continuously monitored using electronic devices.

Substrate

The substrate used needs to be appropriate and should be non-toxic, digestible (or too large to be eaten) and non-abrasive; a natural substrate such as soil or leaf litter is preferable. Some commercially available substrates (e.g. wood chips, shavings, corncobs and walnut shells) have been reported to cause intestinal impactions in lizards. In the clinical situation, newspaper provides a suitable substrate as faecal and urinary output can be observed and hygiene maintained. However, this is not ideal for long-term maintenance as it does not provide an opportunity for digging.

Hygiene

Hygiene is very important and setting up a vivarium that is easily cleaned is important. Substrate selection is also important as expensive commercially available products are likely to be infrequently cleaned out.

Diet

Lizards use about 2–5% of the energy of a comparably sized mammal. Energy conservation is important and the life of a lizard is geared towards becoming metabolically active (which costs energy) to be able to forage and obtain food (which provides an energy source). This food source may be scarce and the cost of obtaining it against the benefits (in terms of energy) require consideration.

Herbivores

Herbivorous lizards will take a variety of vegetable food sources. A wide range of plants and leafy greens should make up a high percentage of the diet. Naturally grown weeds such as dandelion, grass, sow thistle, plantains, chickweed, milk thistle, sedum, honeysuckle, nasturtium flowers, hibiscus flowers or wild pansy are all exceptionally good food sources and are highly preferable to supermarket goods. However, in the absence of these, vegetables such as kale, spinach, broccoli, iceberg lettuce, romaine lettuce, cabbage, bok choi, turnip greens, endive, mange tout, spring greens, brussel sprouts, carrots, peppers, squash and tomatoes can be offered. A large variety of fruits such as apples, pears, strawberries and bananas, and higher protein foods such as beans, peas or pulses can be offered where appropriate, depending on the species and lifestage. Commercially available pelleted diets can comprise a small amount of the diet but should not be relied upon to provide a balanced diet. Supplementation with a vitamin and mineral powder with a high Ca:P ratio is required. Any uneaten food should be removed and discarded to reduce the risk of autoinfection with faecal parasites.

Omnivores

Omnivorous lizards may be 1–99% herbivorous and this must be taken into account. Most omnivores encountered will eat mostly invertebrate prey. Commercially available live food such as crickets, locusts, mealworms and waxworms are easily obtainable. Some owners also feed pinkie mice to these species. Items such as woodlice, millipedes and earthworms are far better than commercially available live food. Supplementation with a vitamin and mineral powder with a high Ca:P ratio is required. Gut loading the invertebrates with a high calcium diet (8% of the dry matter) is required for 48 hours prior to feeding. Many commercially available products fall far short of this requirement. Adding calcium carbonate to them can improve the calcium content of the invertebrate. Providing dark leafy greens for the invertebrates to eat prior to feeding to the lizard is also helpful. Invertebrates can get hungry if left in the vivarium and substantial damage to sleeping lizards is possible. To avoid this, all uneaten live food should be removed. Invertebrates are also an inadvertent vector of faecal parasites and infection if left in the vivarium too long.

Carnivores

Carnivorous lizards will usually be fed whole mammalian prey, and as a result vitamin and mineral deficiencies are rare. However, supplementation for monitors lizards is still advised as some prey items are obese and can lack sufficient vitamin E. Prolonged freezing of prey items can also lead to reduced nutritional value. As prey items get larger, the frequency of feeding can be reduced. Prey items should be thoroughly defrosted to blood temperature before feeding. Handling of the prey should be avoided so that there is no confusion between human scent and the prey item.

Water

Lizards require water for drinking, as well as for swimming in some cases (Figure 15.7). Aquatic or semi-aquatic species need a large area to swim in with a haul out area and basking lamp to allow them to dry thoroughly. The water should be heated and thermostatically controlled. All heaters should be well protected. Filtration of the water and feeding separately will reduce the frequency (and volume) of water changes required.

Protein breakdown and excretion of nitrogenous waste is one of the major factors influencing the amount of water lost by a lizard. Due to this, lizards are able to modify the protein breakdown products they utilize. Where water is limited (such as for terrestrial species from arid habitats), uric acid is the primary protein breakdown product, formed as insoluble urate salts in the bladder or coprodeum, and it exerts no osmotic effect. The bladder and coprodeum are used as water storage facilities. As the reptile dehydrates, it reabsorbs water from these organs to maintain its circulatory volume. In order to draw water into the circulation, the reptile must maintain an osmotic gradient. Many terrestrial lizards achieve this by increasing the sodium content of the blood, which in turn elevates the osmolarity.

Lizards drink by a variety of methods, from submerging the entire head underwater to licking droplets from foliage (chameleons). Fresh water should always be available and presented in an appropriate way. Bathing lizards weekly in a cat litter tray or a plastic box (under supervision) is a good idea to maintain hydration; the water temperature should be 25°C. Warm water bathing also serves as a stimulus for voiding urates and faecal material.

Breeding

- Owners may not wish to breed their lizards and are unprepared when even isolated individuals are stimulated into reproductive activity.
- Owners may wish to breed their lizards but find that incorrect husbandry prevents a sexually active female from successfully reproducing.

There is an increasing trend to provide seasonal changes within the vivarium, and in many cases the lizard is able to perceive the natural seasonality of the surrounding environment as well. This can act as a stimulus for reproductive activity. Many captive reptiles can reach a reproductive size far sooner than they would do in the wild; even very young males can stimulate a larger female to become sexually active.

Most commonly seen lizards are oviparous; however, some skinks are viviparous. Parthenogenesis is possible in some lizard species. The production of eggs or live young leads to anorexia in the female lizard due to a lack of space in the coelom for ingesta. This is natural and to be expected. Thus, lizards (in particular females) require additional calcium, UV-B light, protein and heat to reproduce successfully in captivity.

Lizards can be selective when it comes to laying; they need to be in familiar surroundings and all the environmental conditions need to be correct. Signs that a female wants to lay include increased roaming, sniffing and digging behaviour, and many of these are not noticed by an unsuspecting owner. Exposure to a male is not required for a female lizard to produce follicles or eggs. Food intake may be markedly reduced due to the coelomic cavity being filled. After laying, there is no maternal care of the eggs. Eggs can be removed for incubation, which lasts for 3–5 months. A mixture of 50:50 vermiculite and water is a suitable incubation substrate. Eggs should not be turned but incubated exactly as they are laid. Incubation temperatures of 26–30°C are required for most species.

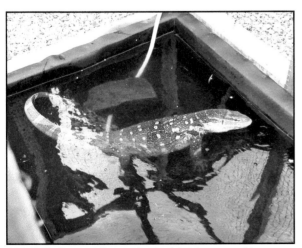

15.7 Ornate Nile monitor bathing in an outside enclosure.

Handling and restraint

Handling should be undertaken with care as many lizards can be fractious, and as a result may damage themselves whilst trying to escape (e.g. skin tearing in small geckos), autotomize the tail, or inflict injury on the handler.

- Small lizards should be weighed on accurate scales. Some species may need to be restrained in a plastic tank; this allows a thorough visual inspection prior to further handling. Geckos may reside on an open palm.
- Larger tame lizards may be allowed to move around the consulting room.
- Large or venomous lizards (*Heloderma* spp.) require an experienced handler.
- Aggressive or flighty lizards should be contained/ restrained at all times.

Control of the head to prevent biting is important and the tail should also be restrained to prevent whipping. This usually requires a two-hand hold (Figure 15.8). If possible, the limbs should be incorporated to reduce the risk of scratching. Large more aggressive individuals can be wrapped in a towel to facilitate handling. Covering the head of the lizard can have a calming effect. Chameleons benefit from having a twig to hold on to.

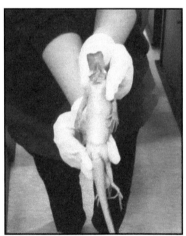

15.8

Handling a juvenile green iguana. (Reproduced from the *BSAVA Manual of Reptiles, 2nd edition*.)

The vasovagal reflex can be used to subdue an aggressive lizard; exerting pressure over the eyes leads to a parasympathetic reduction in heart rate and response to external stimuli. Placing a bandage over the head of the lizard with cotton wool pads over the eyes can enable quick procedures such as radiography to be undertaken. Lizards can revive themselves in response to noise or physical manipulation.

WARNING
Disposable gloves should be worn to handle lizards. This is to prevent the risk of disease transmission between the lizard and the handler, and also to reduce the risk of the handler being a vector for disease transmission between different species.

Diagnostic approach

History
A full history should be taken prior to performing a clinical examination. It is not within the scope of this chapter to discuss history-taking fully, but the reader should review the information on husbandry (see above) and ask questions in order to fully evaluate the lizard's care (for further details, see *BSAVA Manual of Reptiles, 2nd edition*). History-taking should take approximately 10–30 minutes, depending on the case.

Clinical examination
The lizard may be hypothermic when it arrives at the practice, and it is a good plan to place any reptile in a warmed environment prior to clinical examination. Observation or examination of a hypothermic lizard will yield confusing results and should not be attempted. Hospitalization for a period of observation after the lizard has warmed to its optimal body temperature is sometimes required. Alternatively, a warmed vivarium or brooder should be available in the consulting room.

Observation
The examination should begin by observing the lizard from a distance. Lizards should be bright and alert, able to lift their body off the ground and explore the environment. Monitor lizards should show increased tongue flicking; other lizards may lick surfaces and handlers. Body posture and movement should be critically assessed as abnormalities may suggest nutritional secondary hyperparathyroidism (metabolic bone disease) or neurological disease. Tremors or fasciculations can suggest hypocalcaemia.

Physical examination
A physical examination should be systematically performed in every case and mirror that conducted in more familiar species. Some lizards may require anaesthesia to facilitate examination.

The head should be completely examined, with particular attention paid to the tongue, eyes and ears. The oral cavity should be opened with a blunt tongue depressor and examined; trauma and stomatitis are common. Skin disease is frequently encountered in lizards and a complete examination for parasites, retained shed skin and injuries should be performed. Careful examination of the mucocutaneous junctions should be undertaken. Haemorrhage into the scales may suggest septicaemia or local trauma to the site. Clinically dehydrated lizards will have sunken eyes and skin folds.

Auscultation of the lung fields and heart is of limited use. The heart is best assessed using Doppler ultrasonography; respiration should be closely observed with the glottis checked to ascertain whether any noise is produced on exhalation. Swelling of the limbs can reflect trauma, nutritional secondary hyperparathyroidism or cellulitis. The coelomic cavity should be palpated gently for masses; caution is advised as female lizards with follicular disease can have very friable ovaries, which may rupture and cause peritonitis. Transillumination is possible in geckos with pale skin. This highlights the liver and the degree of fat within it can be assessed by coloration alone. Digital cloacal examination is possible in large lizards and the kidneys can be palpated dorsally within the pelvis via this method.

Imaging

Radiography
There are two standard radiographic views for lizards: dorsoventral (DV) and lateral. A DV view using a vertical beam is useful for evaluation of gastrointestinal tract disease, bladder calculi, eggs and bone abnormalities. Lizards may need to be anaesthetized for limb or head radiography. Lateral horizontal beam radiographs are required as lizards do not have a diaphragm and coelomic contents can move, compressing the lung fields (Figure 15.9). Barium studies are useful to assess gastrointestinal transit time. Barium contrast media equivalent to 1% of the lizard's bodyweight can be given by stomach tube.

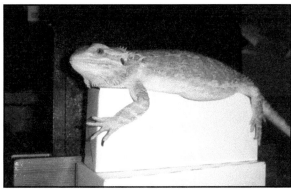

15.9 Positioning for a horizontal beam radiograph in a bearded dragon.

Ultrasonography
An ultrasound examination can be performed with a conscious patient in most instances. Probes with a small footprint are required. Examination of the coelomic cavity from the ventral aspect to assess the reproductive tract and liver is commonly performed. Examination of the heart is useful to determine whether pericardial fluid or any other abnormalities exist. Ultrasonography is also useful for checking swellings on the head of bearded dragons to rule out cerebral aneurysms. In cases of puncture wounds, ultrasonography can show haemorrhage or tissue damage. It is also useful to assess kidneys and renal blood flow.

Endoscopy
Rigid endoscopic examination is an under-utilized tool in reptile medicine. Endoscopic examination of the oesophagus, trachea and cloaca is possible. Examination of the coelomic cavity is possible in lizards and minimally invasive surgical techniques are reported.

The standard approach for coelomic assessment is from the left side in the sub-lumbar region, below the spine, in front of the hindleg and behind the

ribcage (Figure 15.10). Care should be taken in those species where the lungs can extend this far back (i.e. chameleons). The skin is incised and a blunt instrument can be used to puncture into the coelomic cavity. Tenting the skin up minimizes the risk of visceral puncture. Insufflation is ideal if available. A single horizontal mattress suture can be used to close the surgical wound. The ventral midline approach can be used for a more complete assessment of the liver. Typically, rigid endoscopes of 2.7 mm diameter are used for most lizards seen in practice.

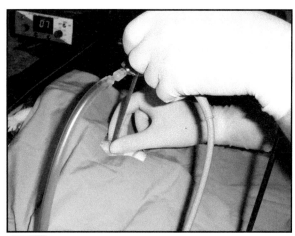

15.10 Endoscopic examination of a bearded dragon.

Sample collection
Most lizards are passive and stoical which enables a number of sampling procedures to be performed in the conscious animal. This can allow for at least a presumptive diagnosis prior to anaesthesia and more invasive procedures.

Blood
Venepuncture can be performed with the lizard conscious in most cases. Suitable sites are detailed in Figure 15.11. The maximum amount of blood that can be taken safely is approximately 0.5% of the patient's bodyweight.

Reptilian haematology is a specialized field and films should be examined by a haematologist with specialist knowledge. Blood samples submitted for haematological examination should be stored in heparin; although, recent reports demonstrate EDTA to be superior in some reptile species (Martinez-Jimenez *et al.*, 2007). However, it should be noted that haemolysis may occur in samples stored in EDTA. Heparin has the advantage of allowing both haematology and biochemistry to be performed on one sample. Reference ranges should be established in the laboratory. A suitable reference text (Campbell and Ellis, 2006) should be used to assist in the evaluation of blood films. Biochemical analysis should be performed after haematology. Selecting the correct biochemical profile is important and further advice should be sought if in-house testing is to be performed. It may be best to use a commercial exotic animal laboratory as the profiles will already be in use.

Vessel	Position	Technique	Comments
Ventral coccygeal vein	Dorsal recumbency or the tail can be hung over the edge of the table and accessed from below	Best site is a third of the way down the tail 1. Insert a fine-gauge needle at a 45 degree angle. 2. Advance the needle slowly, whilst applying negative pressure to the syringe. 3. Blood will enter the syringe. If there is no blood present, the vertebrae have been contacted, withdraw the needle slightly and reposition.	The vessel runs in the ventral midline of the tail and is larger closer to the cloaca. Care should be taken to avoid the hemipenes in males. First site to consider in most lizards. Caution is advised with geckos, which are best anaesthetized to reduce the risk of autotomy. A lateral approach just under the horizontal processes of the vertebrae can also be used. Catheterization has been reported
Jugular vein	Lateral recumbency with the side of the neck exposed	Raise vessel with pressure applied just in front of the shoulder	The vessel courses from the point of the shoulder to the angle of the jaw. The right jugular vein is larger than the left. Anaesthesia may be required. Suitable for catheterization
Ventral abdominal vein	Dorsal recumbency	Insert a fine-gauge needle in the midline at a 45 degree angle	The vessel courses along the ventral midline of the coelomic cavity, cranial to the umbilicus. Can be used when autotomy is a significant risk. It is impossible to control haemorrhage from this site and inadvertent puncture of coelomic organs is possible. For this reason, anaesthesia is indicated to facilitate correct needle placement
Cardiac puncture	Dorsal recumbency	Doppler ultrasonography can be used to locate the heart Insert a fine-gauge needle between the clavicles at the thoracic inlet	Location of the heart may vary in species (in monitor lizards the heart is in a more caudal position). There are risks with this procedure and anaesthesia is indicated prior to sampling. Last resort for venepuncture

15.11 Venepuncture sites in lizards.

Faeces

A faecal screen should be performed on every lizard presented to the veterinary surgeon. Many parasites have a direct lifecycle, and burdens can build up to critical levels over time. Some lizards can be heavily infected at the time of purchase. Food can quickly be contaminated with faecal material and, if ingested, can become a source of autoinfection. Parasitic infections can be reduced by using a substrate that can be easily and completely removed. Regular faecal screening is useful to identify whether any treatment is warranted. Ensuring lizards have a negative faecal sample prior to being placed on a particulate substrate is vital to limit pathogen build-up over time.

- Initially, a fresh wet preparation of faeces should be examined under the microscope; this will give an indication of parasite numbers and any motile organisms. Only a tiny amount of faecal material is needed; this can be diluted with warmed saline and examined immediately.
- Further testing should include a flotation and a concentration technique. A small amount of faeces is added to formalin and left overnight. The sample is then strained, suspended in ethyl acetate and centrifuged. The deposit is assessed for parasites. Quantitative testing is usually not indicated due to the small sample size. Iodine staining for parasitic cysts is not required as concentration techniques encourage protozoa to form cysts and thus are readily identified.

Obtaining a faecal sample can be difficult in some lizards if they have been chronically anorexic. Bathing can help (see below) or alternatively a cloacal flush can be performed. One percent of the lizard's bodyweight in warmed saline (i.e. 1 ml/100 g) can be infused into the cloaca/colon. In many cases, the insertion of the tube can induce voiding prior to infusion. This is preferred as the faeces are more concentrated. However, if infusion is required concentrating techniques can be used subsequently. Following infusion of the saline, the back end of the lizard is massaged and the watery contents aspirated.

Culture and sensitivity

Samples (including faeces) for culture and sensitivity testing can be taken from any appropriate site. Aerobic, anaerobic and fungal cultures should be performed. Most cultures will grow Gram-negative bacteria with multiple resistance patterns. This may be an incidental finding or the bacteria may be secondary opportunistic pathogens, but not the primary cause of disease. Thus, the significance of bacteria in a culture should always be questioned. Supportive evidence of an inflammatory response or suitable clinical signs are required to confirm the role of the bacteria in the disease process.

Cytology

Cytology is a useful tool in clinical practice and should be considered alongside culture. Samples can be taken from any lesion. Cytology can confirm the presence of an organism (including those which may be difficult to culture) and any associated inflammatory response, thus confirming its pathogenicity. Presumptive therapy can be started whilst waiting for culture results.

Tracheal wash and gastric lavage

If respiratory disease is suspected then a tracheal wash should be performed. One percent of the lizard's bodyweight of warmed saline is infused via an appropriately sized catheter into the trachea. The lizard is agitated and any fluid aspirated. The aspirated fluid should be submitted for cytology and culture.

Gastric lavage may also be useful. Stomach tubes (either metal or plastic) can be placed into the stomach (located approximately half way down the coelomic cavity). One percent of the patient's bodyweight of warmed saline is infused into the stomach. The lizard is then gently rocked from side to side, so that the fluid moves across the stomach lining. The stomach contents are then aspirated and should be submitted for cytology and culture.

Common conditions

There are a huge variety of diseases that may be seen in clinical practice. There is an ever increasing list of differential diagnoses, and keeping up to date with novel presentations and diseases is vital. It is intended to summarize only frequently seen conditions here. In addition, it may be impossible to obtain a definitive diagnosis in many patients due to financial constraints imposed by the owner. Most diseases are slow and progressive, and many owners present lizards either following a long clinical history or with acute clinical signs resulting from chronic disease.

Skin disease

Skin diseases are frequently presented. There are a number of specific infections that may be seen (such as fungal or viral lesions) but all skin lesions either become contaminated with opportunistic Gram-negative bacteria or are bacterial in origin. Anaerobic infections are probably underdiagnosed. Fungi are also possible wound contaminants.

Abscesses

Abscesses can result from bite wounds or trauma. A variety of Gram-negative and anaerobic bacteria are frequently isolated. Ocular infections can be seen in chameleons and result in swelling of the periorbital tissues. Infection of the temporal gland is also possible in chameleons, leading to swelling at the angle of the jaw. This can be debulked either via the commissure of the mouth passing lateral to the mandible, or in severe cases by a surgical approach. Although bacteria are usually implicated in abscessation, filarial worms, fungi and foreign bodies can also lead to subcutaneous swellings. Hypovitaminosis A has been implicated as a cause of chronic conjunctivitis and abscessation of the conjunctival sac in leopard geckos.

Burns

Burns are commonly seen in captive reptiles and result from contact with heat sources. Typically, burns on the dorsal aspect of the lizard result from heat lamps and burns on the ventral surface result from heat mats or hot rocks. Substantial damage and pain can occur with full thickness burns. Secondary infection with Gram-negative bacteria is common. Regular ecdysis allows the skin to heal over time. Substantial wounds can heal without surgical intervention, providing secondary complications are suitably controlled. Treatment involves fluid therapy, analgesics, systemic antibiotics and debridement under anaesthesia. Topical treatments such as silver sulfasalazine or silver sulfadiazine provide antimicrobial and anti-inflammatory/analgesic therapy.

Chrysosporium anamorph of *Nannizziopsis vriesii*

Chrysosporium anamorph of *Nannizziopsis vriesii* (CANV) is known as yellow fungus disease and is seen in bearded dragons (Pare and Jacobson, 2007) (Figure 15.12). This is a primary fungal infection that is fatal. Necrotic areas of skin occur and become secondarily infected with Gram-negative bacteria. Ulceration can be deep into tissues and many animals become terminally septic. Diagnosis is based on clinical presentation combined with histopathology, cytology or fungal culture. Current treatments have proven to be ineffective at controlling this pathogen and death is due to fluid loss and sepsis.

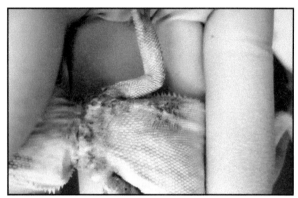

15.12 *Chrysosporium* anamorph of *Nannizziopsis vriesii* (yellow fungus disease) in a juvenile bearded dragon.

Dysecdysis

Low relative humidity is probably the most common cause of dysecdysis. Retained shed skin can lead to constriction of the digits and tail and obscure vision. Lizards can also suffer from dyspnoea if the shed skin obstructs the nares. Dysecdysis may also be due to skin infection, ectoparasites, trauma or general debility. Treatment involves addressing the husbandry and elevating humidity (see above). Bathing and topical ocular lubricants can be used to soften retained spectacles. Anaesthesia and gentle manipulation of retained skin or spectacles with forceps may be required to prevent loss of digits or vision.

Snake mites

Snake mites (*Ophionyssus natricis*) occasionally infest lizards (Figure 15.13), especially when they are housed in mixed collections. These are motile parasites, which lay eggs in the environment. The eggs

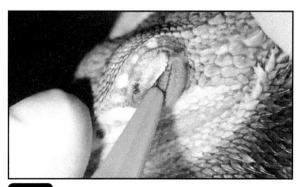

15.13 Snake mites on the eyelid of a bearded dragon.

hatch to produce nymphs, which then feed on the host prior to developing into adults. The lifecycle is 13–19 days, which allows numbers to increase dramatically in a short time. The mites like to hide in skin folds and a close inspection of the eyes, mouth, gular fold and cloaca is required. Snake mites are photophobic and examination of the environment in the dark with torch-light can give an indication of the level of infestation. Anaemia can develop in severe infestations.

Treatment involves environmental control and topical treatment of the lizard(s). Ivermectin in a spray form works well. Injectable ivermectin can also be given, depending on the species. Adverse reactions in chameleons and skinks have been reported. An alternative is to use fipronil as a wipe and a spray. Treatment every few days, until there are no mites, is recommended. Bathing regularly also helps. All disposable items should be burned and the vivarium simplified. Lizards should not be exposed to products containing dichlorvos, and organophosphate and pyrethroid toxicity have been reported. Any treated enclosure should be thoroughly washed prior to reintroduction of the lizard(s).

Trauma
Skin trauma can occur due to bite wounds from con-specifics or invertebrate prey. Trauma may also occur from other pets (dogs, cats, birds) in the household that can inflict puncture wounds. These puncture wounds can become infected with bacteria, and cellu-litis or abscessation (see above) is possible. Skin tears should be sutured under anaesthesia and antibiotic therapy instigated. Samples should be taken where possible and submitted for culture, and radiography may be needed to assess the underlying pathology.

Gastrointestinal disease

Salmonellosis
There has been much concern about *Salmonella* and reptiles. *Salmonella* rarely causes clinical disease in lizards but does remain a zoonotic risk. Owners should be made aware of the risks and use appropriate hygiene to minimize infection. There is no indication to treat a lizard with a positive *Salmonella* culture.

Protozoal diseases
There are a vast number of parasitic diseases that affect lizards, but only a few are commonly seen. Most infections are subclinical.

Coccidiosis: This is a common disease, particularly in bearded dragons and is caused in this species by *Isospora amphibolouri*. The cysts have two sporocysts, each containing four sporozoites. The lifecycle is direct; therefore, *I. amphibolouri* can be difficult to eliminate. Toltrazuril and sulphonamides are commonly used to treat this condition.

Cryptosporidiosis: *Cryptosporidium* is a common pathogen in some lizard species. Of importance to the practitioner is *Cryptosporidium saurophilum* in leopard geckos. This protozoal parasite resides in the small intestine and leads to anorexia, wasting and collapse. The diagnosis is confirmed via either Ziehl–Niessen staining of a faecal sample, or histo-pathology of an intestinal tract biopsy sample taken *post mortem*. Eighty percent of the oocysts re-infect the host without being shed. The remaining 20% are immediately infective upon being passed and are extremely resistant to most disinfectants. Heat (60°C for 5 minutes), formalin (10%, contact time of 18 hours) and ammonia (5%, contact time of 18 hours) are effective but impractical in most situations. Thus, to limit environmental contamination, meticulous attention to hygiene is required along with removal of all faecal material as soon as it is passed. Treatment is largely unrewarding. Hyperimmune bovine colos-trum has been shown to be effective in some species, but not in leopard geckos (Cranfield *et al.*, 1999).

Worms: Oxyurids are small worms up to 1 cm in length and are very common in lizards, in particular bearded dragons can have heavy burdens. The eggs are D-shaped with thin walls. The lifecycle is direct. Anorexia, intestinal obstruction and rectal prolapse are the clinical signs reported. Other roundworms such as *Capillaria* spp. and strongyles can also infect lizards. Fenbendazole is an effective treatment. Lower doses given over a few days are generally considered safer than one higher dose.

Other diseases
Other protozoa, yeasts and fungi may also be encountered and many of these are non-pathogenic. Fungal overgrowth is common after inappropriate or prolonged antibiotic therapy and can be fatal. Metronidazole and nystatin are suitable treatments for protozoa and yeasts.

Facial trauma
Flighty lizards (such as the Chinese water dragon) may sustain facial trauma from escape attempts, which can lead to the maxilla and mandible being exposed and subsequent osteomyelitis and stomatitis. In many cases, periodontal disease may also be present and contribute to the condition. Clinical signs include fracture of the mandibular symphysis and oral discharge. Treatment involves aggressive debridement of lesions under anaesthesia and systemic antibiotic therapy, including cover for anaerobic bacteria.

Periodontal disease
There are two different types of teeth found in lizards: acrodont and pleurodont. Acrodont teeth are found in agamids and chameleons. These are not replaced and sit on an exposed bony ridge. Pleurodont teeth are found in all other species. These sit on a ridge inside the jaw line and are replaced regularly. Periodontal disease is common in lizards with acrodont teeth and is frequently under- or misdiagnosed in water dragons and bearded dragons (Figure 15.14). Many of these cases will present as stomatitis ('mouth rot') and it is important to differentiate between the two conditions.

Patients with a mild case of periodontal disease have tooth loss, gingival recession and discoloration. Diagnosis and treatment involve radiography, dental scaling and improving the diet (giving harder, more chitinous invertebrates). Severe disease can result

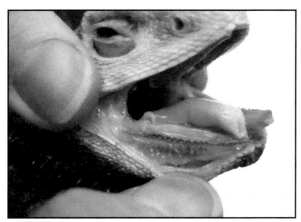

15.14 Severe periodontal disease in a bearded dragon.

in abscessation, osteomyelitis, gingival hyperplasia and bleeding. Systemic antibiotics are indicated in these cases.

Intestinal impaction
Lizards housed on an inappropriate substrate (such as wood chip or supposedly edible sand (to provide calcium)) or those allowed to roam unsupervised in the home can ingest foreign bodies. These foreign bodies can lead to impaction, which requires medical or surgical intervention. The diagnosis is based on clinical history and radiography. Medical treatment can include enemas to dislodge the impacted material over a few days. Should the lizard suffer a colonic prolapse, then anaesthesia is required to allow replacement of the prolapse. Renal enlargement may also lead to impaction.

Hepatic lipidosis
This is a common problem in captive reptiles, in particular in females that are reproductively active. This may in part relate to the anorexia associated with gravidity. In other animals it can be seen after a period of anorexia, and in many cases it is difficult to decide which came first. Obese reptiles seem especially prone to hepatic lipidosis. In leopard geckos, transillumination (Figure 15.15) can be used to evaluate the liver but in other species more invasive diagnostic techniques are required. Assisted feeding is required, and other therapeutics, such as anabolic steroids to encourage mobilization of fat stores, have been used.

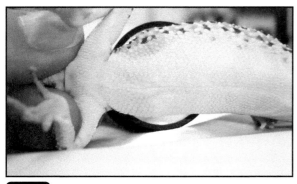

15.15 Transillumination of a healthy leopard gecko.

Musculoskeletal disease

Nutritional secondary hyperparathyroidism
Nutritional secondary hyperparathyroidism (NSHP, also known as metabolic bone disease) is very commonly seen in all species of juvenile lizard (Figure 15.16) and is due to inappropriate lighting, diet and heat.

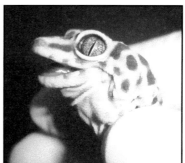

15.16 Leopard gecko suffering from severe nutritional secondary hyperparathyroidism.

Ultraviolet light: Many texts do not stipulate that nocturnal species require UV-B light. However, nocturnal species that feed on invertebrates, such as the leopard gecko, can and do suffer from NSHP commonly and present with the same clinical signs as diurnal lizards. This is due to a genuine dietary deficiency in calcium and vitamin D. Given the fact that UV light does no harm (in the levels considered here) and that nocturnal geckos do naturally bask and are highly efficient at skin production of vitamin D, it makes sense to offer UV-B light.

It has also been reported that carnivorous lizards (such as monitor lizards) are expected to obtain vitamin D from their prey; however, juveniles of these species are insectivorous and studies in the Komodo dragon have shown their capacity for vitamin D storage from prey items is limited. In addition, studies have shown that exposure to UV-B light enhances blood levels of vitamin D in the long term (Gymesi and Burns, 2002), hence monitor lizards can benefit from exposure to UV-B light.

Clinical signs: Deformities of the limbs, spine and jaw bones can occur and bones are able to deform under pressure. Fibrous osteodystrophy is seen as the fracture sites attempt to heal, with excessive fibrous tissue leading to swollen areas; alternatively, bone can be completely replaced with fibrous tissue. With continued growth, the bones can eventually ossify but leave marked deviations in anatomy. Other typical signs encountered include gastrointestinal tract stasis, cloacal organ prolapse and a lack of truncal lifting. In severe cases, hypocalcaemic tetany occurs. Reproductive problems can also be seen in females due to hypocalcaemia. Older animals remain distorted for the rest of their life and this can lead to future complications.

Diagnosis: This can be made using radiography, which can demonstrate gastrointestinal stasis, poor bone mineralization and, in cases with renal disease, articular gout. Blood ionized calcium levels can confirm the diagnosis in lizards suffering from hypocalcaemia.

Treatment: This consists of provision of UV-B light, oral or systemic calcium and thermal therapy. A number of species may not be able to use oral vitamin D (e.g. green iguanas) and those that can risk toxicity if overzealous supplementation is provided. Fractures should be stabilized by external coaptation, as in many cases the cortices are too weak to stabilize implants and further fracturing is possible. In small individuals, vivarium rest in a small enclosure may be preferable due to the relative weight of external coaptation. In addition, placement of an oesophagostomy tube and use of phosphate binders such as aluminium hydroxide may be necessary.

Osteomyelitis and septic arthritis
Osteomyelitis and septic arthritis are common in lizards and can result from local trauma or septicaemia. Swelling of the infected site is typically found. Radiography, cytology and culture should be performed to obtain a definitive diagnosis. Radiographically, there is loss of bone with minimal reaction. In green iguanas, septic spinal arthritis has been recently reported, and on radiographic examination there was evidence of proliferative spinal lesions. *Mycoplasma* spp. have been implicated as a cause of this condition in green iguanas (Westfall *et al.*, 2006). The inciting factor is assumed to be haematogenous spread. Treatment involves use of systemic and topical antibiotics over a period of weeks. Antibiotics effective against anaerobic bacteria are indicated.

Gout
Uric acid tophi can form in the joints of lizards and lead to swelling (Figure 15.17), which must be differentiated from infection. The radiographic appearance of gout can be similar to osteomyelitis, and cytology is required to distinguish between the two diseases. Blood biochemistry should be evaluated to assess the uric acid level. Allopurinol should be considered alongside flushing of the affected joints and analgesia, but the prognosis is poor.

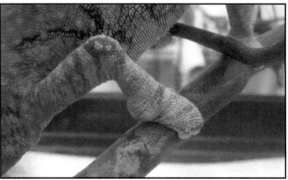

15.17 Swollen tarsal joint in a veiled chameleon suffering from articular gout.

Reproductive disease

Follicular stasis
Follicular stasis is common in isolated female lizards, which may lack the physiological cues to ovulate. Female lizards naturally go off their food when gravid due to the filling of the coelomic cavity with developing follicles. This places a huge demand on reserves, and metabolic problems associated with hypocalcaemia and loss of condition can be seen, leading to collapse. Infection and abscessation of the follicles is possible and they can rupture, leading to yolk coelomitis. Stasis (non-ovulation) of the follicles is also common. Diagnosis requires a good clinical history and radiography or ultrasonography. In many cases, surgical intervention is required to remove both ovaries. Typical species affected include veiled chameleons, bearded dragons, water dragons and iguanas. If the lizard is presented early, then medical management and aggressive supportive care can be attempted, in the hope that the female will resorb the follicles. However, many cases progress to collapse and if the lizard is not required for breeding then surgical intervention at this stage is thoroughly recommended and indicated (see Common surgical procedures).

Egg stasis
Egg stasis is also possible due to a lack of appropriate environmental stimuli, such as a suitable nesting site, temperature, heat or privacy. This can lead to the eggs being retained. If shelled eggs are present and there is no obvious reason for the stasis (i.e. it is behavioural not pathological), then giving calcium gluconate followed by oxytocin can lead to oviposition. However, if the egg quality appears poor on radiography or medical therapy is not successful, surgery is indicated. Dystocia can arise due to an obstruction (enlarged kidneys or bladder calculi) or be due to anatomical abnormalities as a consequence of NSHP as a juvenile. Many female lizards are capable of ovulating without exposure (or recent exposure) to a male. Dystocia in viviparous species (venomous lizards and some skinks) is very rare.

Hemipenile prolapse
Hemipenile prolapses can occur as a result of straining (e.g. intestinal impaction), after forced separation during mating, as a result of hypocalcaemia or due to foreign material becoming impacted in the sulcus. Radiography, blood biochemistry and cloacal endoscopy may be required to fully evaluate the problem. Male lizards have two hemipenes, which are used for mating only and not for excretion. Reduction of the prolapse is possible but not suitable in many cases due to engorgement or trauma. Amputation of a single hemipenis is possible without affecting reproductive activity, but amputation of both prevents copulation (see Common surgical procedures). However, as many owners do not wish to breed from their lizard, amputation is the most effective treatment for this condition as prolapse recurrence is impossible.

Urinary tract disease

Chronic renal disease
In chameleons and green iguanas, renal disease can result from chronic dehydration. Clinical signs of chronic renal disease can be non-specific and include anorexia, depression, weight loss and the presence of coelomic fluid. Hypocalcaemia can result from renal secondary hyperparathyroidism and lead

to muscle fasciculation. Renomegaly can result in colonic impaction. Renal disease can be diagnosed by blood biochemistry, radiography, ultrasonography and endoscopic or surgical biopsy samples submitted for histopathology. Biochemical changes include an inverted total Ca:P ratio and elevated uric acid levels. Renal function can be assessed by iohexol excretion to determine the glomerular filtration rate (GFR) by sequential blood analysis (Hernandez-Divers *et al.*, 2005b).

Bladder calculi

Bladder calculi are seen commonly in iguanas and other lizards that possess a bladder. The causes are multifactorial but high dietary protein and dehydration are believed to play a role. Clinical signs are variable and may be non-existent. Large calculi can inhibit egg laying and cause colonic impaction. They are typically composed of urate salts. Diagnosis can be made on physical examination combined with radiography. Bladder calculi are radiodense lamellar structures. Treatment involves surgical removal.

Respiratory disease

Respiratory diseases are rare in lizards. Clinical signs can include dyspnoea, open-mouth breathing, cyanosis or just depression and anorexia. A tracheal wash is indicated and the aspirated fluid should be submitted for culture and cytology. Mycobacterial, mycoplasmal, parasitic and viral infections (such as paramyxovirus, PMV) are possible in lizards and should be ruled out. Current PMV tests available include haemagglutination inhibition testing on heparinized blood. However, these tests are based on specific PMV isolates from snakes and are unlikely to be meaningful in lizards. Viral isolation, PCR and histopathology are likely to be required to confirm the diagnosis.

Neurological disease

Neurological disease is rarely presented in clinical practice. In female leopard geckos, neurological disease due to xanthomatosis is possible due to formation of fatty deposits within the central nervous system (CNS). Trauma from being dropped or inflicted by a cage mate can also lead to neurological signs. Hypocalcaemia can lead to tetanic spasms. A variety of clinical signs can be present with neurological disease and there are a number of references detailing neurological and cranial nerve assessment in reptiles (Mariani, 2007). Complex imaging studies such as magnetic resonance imaging (MRI) are available and can be used where finances permit.

Neoplastic disease

Neoplastic diseases are infrequently seen in lizards. Lymphoid neoplasia is the most common, and in bearded dragons leukaemia has been reported. Signs are of a systemically ill dragon with an abnormal haematological profile. Infiltrative cells can be found in multiple organs on post-mortem examination. The reader is referred to a recent review of neoplasia in reptiles for further information (Hernandez-Divers and Garner, 2003).

Other diseases

Many lizards present with anorexia or collapse as the presenting complaint. It is important that a work-up is performed (see above) to identify the underlying cause. The reader is referred to more detailed volumes should one of these presentations arise (Girling and Raiti, 2004; Mader, 2006).

Supportive care

Hospitalization

When a lizard is first presented to the clinic, it is important to elevate its body temperature to that which is optimal for the species, prior to consultation. Once the optimal body temperature has been reached, a complete clinical examination can be performed and drug uptake is more predictable.

Hospital facilities need to be functional, provide appropriate heat, light and humidity, and be easily cleaned out. Larger lizards or those requiring more specialized accommodation can be difficult to house appropriately in the clinic. Larger enclosures and more potent heat sources will be required. Collapsed lizards are unable to thermoregulate and it is important to be able to provide these animals with an even thermal environment. Thermal therapy is the most important part of supportive care for an ill lizard. Incubators, plant propagators and even avian brooders can all be used to good effect. The exact temperature required depends on species, but typically 28–30°C is acceptable.

High humidity is required for many lizards (e.g. those animals suffering from dysecdysis or renal disease) and this can be achieved by simply placing a cat litter tray of damp substrate within the tank. Having suitable UV-B light sources available is also important for clinicians wishing to treat lizards, both for maintenance of hospitalized animals and also to treat NSHP.

Drug administration

Antibiotic therapy may be indicated in a debilitated lizard. In the UK only one antibiotic, enrofloxacin, is authorized for use in lizards. This is bactericidal and effective against aerobic bacteria. It has good activity against many resistant Gram-negative bacteria. Pulse therapy works well, and efficacy is determined by obtaining a plasma level ≥eight times the minimum inhibitory concentration (MIC). Enrofloxacin has no effect against anaerobic bacteria. Ceftazidime is a third generation cephalosporin with excellent activity against Gram-negative bacteria. Its advantage is that it is effective against anaerobic as well as aerobic bacteria.

There have been concerns regarding the renal portal system in reptiles as this has the potential to allow drugs excreted by tubular secretion to bypass the systemic circulation. Practically, this has been found to have a minimal effect on pharmacokinetics in reptiles and there is no requirement to solely inject in the cranial end of a lizard. Common injection sites include the epaxial muscles and the limb musculature. Sites should be scrubbed with iodine solution prior to injection. Many animals demonstrate a pain response, and chameleons and water dragons can produce a black area in response to pain due to the excitement of melanophores. This should be explained to the owners prior to injection. This colour change is temporary.

Nebulization may also be considered as part of supportive care for lizards. This will elevate the relative humidity in the vivarium and provide some rehydration. A number of drugs can be nebulized and typically treatment is administered in a small environment for 20 minutes twice a day.

Fluid therapy

Fluid therapy is indicated in all sick reptiles. Lizards have a maintenance requirement of 30 ml/kg/day. This can be given via a number of routes:

- Bathing
- Stomach tube
- Parenteral administration.

Bathing

Bathing (either in water or a commercially available electrolyte solution) is effective for mildly debilitated lizards. A lizard should never be left unsupervised in a bath. The bath should be warmed and some lizards will tolerate a bath of 5 minutes. This can be performed in a small plastic tank (to prevent escape) or in a plant propagator as the water is then heated. Bathing may encourage the lizard to void faeces and if so they should be promptly removed and analysed where appropriate.

Stomach tube

Stomach tubing is easily performed and either rigid or flexible tubing is suitable. In many cases, a gag should be used to prevent trauma to the lizard and the tube. Caution is to be advised as lizards can bite hard on gags and trauma to the fragile teeth or even jaw fractures can occur. Gags should be padded to reduce this risk. Tongue depressors are ideal as they widen the load-bearing surface in the event of a bite. One percent of the lizard's bodyweight (i.e.1 ml/100 g) in fluid can be given by stomach tube up to four times daily. The tube should be passed down the oesophagus, avoiding the glottis, so that the tip reaches just behind the ribcage. Fluids should be warmed prior to administration and can be either tap water or a commercially available solution with additional electrolytes.

Parenteral administration

Parenteral fluids can be given at a rate of 1% of the lizard's bodyweight up to four times daily. Fluids used for mammalian species are acceptable as the sodium content of these fluids matches the level found in lizards. Most mammalian fluids have an osmolarity of 280–320 mOsm. All sites should be disinfected with an iodine-based scrub using a toothbrush prior to injection.

Intracoelomic fluids: These fluids are easy to give to lizards (Figure 15.18) but have the disadvantage of compressing the coelomic viscera, including the lung fields. Clotting and inflammatory factors are also diluted and may reduce wound healing. Many lizards present with coelomic effusions and intracoelomic

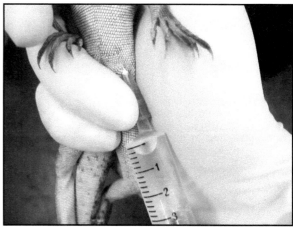

15.18 Intracoelomic fluids being administered in a Chinese water dragon.

fluids are of little benefit in these circumstances. The best site for injection is the caudal quarter of the coelomic cavity, off the midline, on the ventral aspect, with the lizard turned on its back.

Care should be taken to avoid the lung fields and this is of particular importance in chameleons. The author's preference is to give only one bolus of fluids in this manner as it is quick and can be performed as a solo procedure; subsequently, more technically demanding methods can be utilized when time is available. Should further doses be required, drawing back on the syringe can help determine whether there is any fluid left in the coelomic cavity from the last injection. If fluid is aspirated there is no point in injecting more into the cavity.

Intraosseous fluids: Intraosseous techniques are ideal for limbed lizards and are preferred to intracoelomic techniques. Many sites can be used, including the proximal femur, humerus and tibia. Many clinicians place intraosseous catheters under anaesthesia prior to surgical procedures.

1. Scrub the limb clean using iodine and surgical spirit.
2. Inject a small amount of local anaesthetic over the proximal end of the long bone.
3. Insert a spinal needle down the full length of the medullary cavity. Correct placement can be confirmed by drawing back on the syringe until blood is obtained (a small amount of saline may have to be injected first) or a test injection can be given. If there is swelling at the site then the fluid is going into soft tissue. Radiography can also be used to confirm correct placement.
4. Inject the fluid.

Intraosseous fluid therapy is painful if given at high speed and attachment to an infusion pump or syringe driver is best. There is also the risk of iatrogenic osteomyelitis, and providing antibiotic prophylaxis whilst the needle is in place is a sensible precaution.

Intravenous fluids: These are also an option for fluid therapy. The jugular and cephalic veins are the only sites readily available. The right jugular vein is preferred as it is a larger vessel in most lizards. To administer intravenous fluids via either the jugular or cephalic veins, a cut down technique is required. Anaesthesia is indicated in most patients. The jugular vein lies in a straight line from the angle of the jaw to the point of the shoulder. The cephalic veins run at an angle across the dorsal aspect of the forelimbs. The ventral abdominal and tail veins can also be catheterized, but with small individuals this is technically challenging. In extremely collapsed individuals it may be difficult to locate sites for catheter placement, and fluids can be given by injection via other routes to improve perfusion prior to catheter placement. Given the ease with which intraosseous fluid therapy can be administered, this is the most practical route to consider in the first instance.

Subcutaneous fluids: These have little use in reptilian medicine.

Nutritional support

Supportive nutrition is required, but is not so urgent as initially thought. A chronically anorexic lizard is deficient in fluids, electrolytes and energy. Cellular constituents are depleted in order to maintain plasma levels, which can prevent deficiencies being detected on a biochemical profile. Providing a glucose source encourages concurrent ion transport into cells, leading to the depletion of plasma potassium and phosphorus in particular, and is called the re-feeding syndrome. It is important to ensure that electrolytes are replaced prior to administering nutrition. For most patients, supportive fluids should be administered at a rate of 4% bodyweight daily until urination in achieved. Once this occurs, hydration has been successful and maintenance fluid therapy and nutrition can start.

The bodyweight of a lizard typically increases until rehydration is achieved, and should be maintained from this point onwards. Further dramatic weight gains will not occur. Energy requirements increase as the lizard's temperature elevates. The standard metabolic rate (SMR) of a reptile is defined as the maintenance requirement at a given temperature:

- SMR = (kJ/day) = 10 x bodyweight (kg)$^{0.75}$

This equates to the basal metabolic rate of endothermic animals. In general, maintenance energy requirements for a reptile are 1.5–2 times the SMR. This is about a twentieth of those for a comparable sized mammal; lizards do not need much to eat.

One percent of the lizard's bodyweight can be given at each feed by stomach tube (see above). Very weak lizards will require less than this. If there is any reflux, administration should be stopped and the feed quantity reduced accordingly. The lizard must be warm to be able to digest and assimilate the food. The lizard should be warmed slowly to its optimal temperature and be stable for at least 30 minutes prior to stomach tubing. The lizard should be kept warm for a number of hours following feeding. If capable, the lizard will seek warmer temperatures itself.

Stomach tubing is only a short-term solution and some recalcitrant individuals may be difficult. There are a number of commercially available preparations

that can be used with reptiles, both herbivorous and omnivorous species. Carnivorous species can be given diets intended for mammals; however, many of these diets contain high levels of purines which are metabolized to uric acid. This theoretically could lead to renal disease in debilitated uricotelic lizards. Pyramidine-based protein sources are safer. If the animal is appropriately rehydrated prior to feeding this should not prove to be a clinical problem. Progressive weight loss without supportive care is an indication that the reptile needs further nutritional and fluid support. Monitoring urine and faecal output is helpful. If long-term nutritional support is required then an oesophagostomy tube should be placed.

Anaesthesia and analgesia

Lesions that cause pain in mammals are also likely to cause pain in lizards. Clinical signs of pain tend to be limited but can include withdrawal of limbs, restlessness, aggression, increased respiratory rate and splinting of the region.

Analgesia

Non-steroidal anti-inflammatory drugs

Non-steroidal anti-inflammatory drugs (NSAIDs) should be used as routine. There have been two studies in the green iguana which evaluated the pharmacokinetics of meloxicam (Hernandez-Divers, 2004) and ketoprofen (Tuttle *et al.*, 2006), and provisional dosage regimes derived. These are the agents of choice until further studies are performed.

Opioids

Opioid analgesics are frequently used in lizards but their effectiveness is not certain. Recently, butorphanol has been shown to provide analgesia at set doses, but the report failed to demonstrate conclusively positive effects at all dosages used in the study (Greenacre *et al.*, 2006). Many veterinary surgeons feel that butorphanol does have a positive clinical effect.

Anaesthesia

Local anaesthetics

Local anaesthetics are underused. These can be sprayed on to wounds or injected into surgical fields. The maximum dose for lidocaine is 5 mg/kg. Dilution of local anaesthetics in saline may help to reduce overdosing in smaller species.

Gaseous anaesthetics

Gaseous induction of anaesthesia can be used for many species. This can be performed by directly intubating the conscious animal (possible in tractable animals of some species), using a facemask, using an induction chamber or using a plastic ziplock bag (Figure 15.19). Isoflurane (5%) in oxygen is a suitable induction agent. Although seveoflurane has been shown to reduce induction and recovery times, there are other far more important factors influencing recovery (see below).

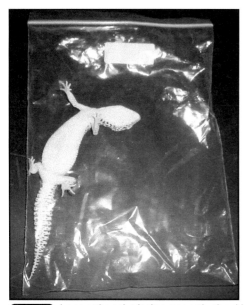

15.19 Leopard gecko being anaesthetized in a ziplock bag containing 5% isoflurane in oxygen.

Injectable anaesthetics
Injectable anaesthetic protocols vary and a variety of agents have been used. Propofol at 10 mg/kg given intravenously into the ventral coccygeal vein is commonly used, but alfaxalone (at 3–5 mg/kg) is currently increasing in popularity in the UK. Although top-up doses of intravenous agents can be used, intubation followed by gaseous anaesthesia for maintenance should be performed.

Intubation
Once the animal is sufficiently sedated (the exact depth required varies between individuals), intubation is possible. Small diameter endotracheal tubes are required and these should be of a suitable length, depending on the species. Customized tubes can be made from intravenous catheters. Endotracheal tubes as small as 1 mm in diameter are commercially available. It is relatively easy to achieve intubation by waiting for a breath and inserting the tube when the glottis is open.

Ventilation
A T-piece can be used for ventilation, but there is variation in both the tidal volume and the rate of respiration. Mechanical ventilation is superior. The respiratory rate should be 6 breaths per minute. Initially, higher ventilation rates can be used to deepen anaesthesia. Pressure cycling ventilators are widely available. Low flow rates are needed for animals requiring small endotracheal tubes.

Once the procedure has started, if there is no voluntary movement, then the percentage of isoflurane can be reduced to 2–3%. Generally, the maintenance anaesthetic agent can be withdrawn before surgery is complete. In many cases, the lizard can remain at a surgical plane of anaesthesia for ≥10 minutes.

Monitoring
Anaesthesia is best monitored using Doppler ultrasonography. The heart rate can be predicted by metabolic scaling (heart rate = 34 x bodyweight$^{-0.25}$). Most conscious reptiles at an optimal temperature have a heart rate of approximately 70 beats per minute. Anaesthetized lizards have a rate of 30–40 beats per minute. The Doppler probe is best placed at the thoracic inlet or over the carotid vessels. Reflexes such as the toe pinch, tail pinch, head withdrawal and jaw tone can be used to assess the depth of anaesthesia.

Recovery
Recovery can be protracted and therefore reptile anaesthetics should be performed early in the day. Many lizards can be given an intravenous bolus of an injectable anaesthetic agent for a short procedure and allowed to recover without any gaseous anaesthesia. Hypoxia elevates the respiratory rate and hypercapnia elevates both rate and depth of ventilation. Reducing oxygenation and allowing hypercapnia to occur should increase the recovery rate and has been shown to have a greater effect than sevoflurane (Hernandez-Divers *et al.*, 2005a). Maintaining the lizard at its optimal temperature will also speed recovery. The lizard will be unable to thermoregulate and should be kept at an even temperature initially until ambulatory. The lizard can be extubated when jaw tone increases and voluntary respiration occurs.

Common surgical procedures

Oesophagostomy tube placement
Tube feeding is only a short-term method for supportive care. Oesophagostomy tube placement allows for continued fluid and nutritional support and provides a route for oral drug therapy. Oesophagostomy tubes are placed mid-way down the neck and secured over the dorsal spine. The tube can be placed on the left or the right side. A pair of curved haemostats are introduced into the oesophagus and displaced laterally. Care should be taken to avoid the jugular vein and carotid artery. The skin tents and usually the vessels slip dorsally or ventrally.

The skin is cut (between scales) with a scalpel blade and the haemostats pushed through. The feeding tube is grasped and pulled through the incision and out of the mouth. It is best not to cut it to length at this stage (as it is easier to pull through the incision), but measuring and marking the tube before beginning surgery is wise. Once pulled out of the mouth, the tube is cut to an appropriate length and directed back down the oesophagus. The tube can be secured using surgical tape and sutured to the skin with horizontal mattress sutures. The tube should be flushed with a small amount of warmed water after each use. After removal the stoma is left to granulate.

Exploratory coeliotomy
There is a large ventral abdominal vein which arises from the confluence of the pelvic veins and passes in the ventral midline (on a short mesovasorum) to the liver. It passes through the liver, enters the hepatic vein and then on into the heart. Some authors recommend a midline incision, but most prefer a paramedian incision to avoid this vessel. The skin is cut with a scalpel blade directed dorsally to avoid traumatizing

the muscle. Blunt dissection through the muscle layer can be performed with scissors. In chameleons a flank incision between two ribs can be considered as an alternative. Closure of the muscle layer is preferable but the skin is the holding layer. Lizard skin should be sutured using a horizontal mattress pattern with a monofilament material such as polydioxanone (PDS). Skin staples have also been used.

Ovariectomy and salpingectomy

An ovariectomy may be required in female lizards suffering from follicular stasis or may be considered prophylactically to prevent reproduction. The ovaries are easy to discern at surgery. The follicles are very friable, and gentle manipulation is required. Haemostatic clips are required to ligate the vessels as the ovaries are closely associated with the caudal vena cava and adrenal glands.

In lizards with egg stasis the oviducts are easily visualized and they can either be incised, the eggs removed and then sutured closed with a fine monofilament suture material to allow for future reproduction, or removed. Removal of the oviduct down to the cloaca requires a circumferential monofilament suture to be placed at the junction. The oviduct has many vessels and these can be ligated with sutures or haemostatic clips, or radiosurgery can be used for coagulation. Both ovaries must be removed in order to prevent future egg yolk coelomitis. These are small and located dorsally. Oviduct prolapse can be seen and usually surgical exploration is required followed by salpingectomy (Figure 15.20).

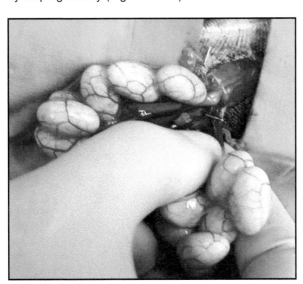

15.20 Salpingectomy of a veiled chameleon. Note the flank incision.

Hemipenile surgery

The hemipenis is the most common organ prolapsed through the cloaca. If the prolapsed hemipenis is viable then replacement is possible; however, if reproduction is not required then amputation should be performed. The hemipenis is extracted using tissue forceps. A haemostat can be clamped close to the cloacal mucosa. Horizontal mattress sutures using a monofilament material can be used to compress the main part of the stump. The tissue distal to the clamp

can then be removed. Abscessation of the site is also common and may require a surgical approach from the ventral aspect of the tail.

Castration

Castration is occasionally carried out in male lizards (e.g. green iguanas) to reduce aggression. The technique is the same as for ovariectomy (see above) (Figure 15.21).

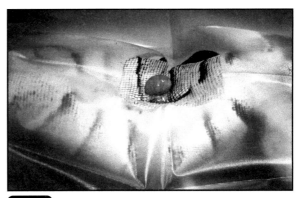

15.21 Castration of a sexually mature green iguana.

Cystotomy

The urinary bladder is thin-walled and transparent in normal lizards but can become thickened in response to chronic inflammation (e.g. from a bladder calculus). A longitudinal incision can be made in the ventral aspect of an avascular portion of the bladder. Stay sutures can be used to reduce coelomic contamination. Following calculus removal and flushing of the contents, closure using a simple interrupted pattern with a monofilament suture material should be performed.

Gastrointestinal surgery

Gastrotomy or enterotomy is indicated to remove foreign bodies. Colonopexy is indicated when a lizard is suffering from chronic colonic prolapse. The colon is sutured around the dorsal ribcage on the right-hand side. In a female lizard a unilateral right ovariectomy is indicated at the same time, as ovulation may be difficult following colonopexy.

Cloacal surgery

Colonic prolapses can occur for a variety of reasons (see above). Replacement of the prolapsed organ under anaesthesia is indicated and this may be possible without surgical intervention by performing a percutaneous colonopexy. However, if surgical intervention is required then a rib colonopexy should be performed. Resection and anastomosis has been successfully performed where the tissue is not viable.

Orthopaedic surgery

Tail and digit amputation may be indicated. In lizards that can regenerate their tails, the amputation site should be cleaned but not sutured to allow for regeneration. Suturing the tail stump will prevent re-growth. Amputated digits should be sutured so that the skin incision is brought dorsally over the toe. Limbs can be amputated at any point along their length as a stump may prove useful to a lizard in ambulation. Orthopaedic surgery can be performed when external coaptation is not indicated. Fractures can be difficult to repair surgically, particularly if they are pathological. Healing time takes 2 months in most cases. External fixation works well and should be placed in a craniocaudal direction.

Euthanasia

Humane euthanasia of lizards can be difficult as they have a high tolerance of hypoxia. It is theoretically possible for a lizard euthanased with pentobarbital to survive hypoxia due to cardiorespiratory system collapse for a prolonged period of time. This means that the CNS is capable of receiving noxious stimuli for some time after apparent death. Due to this, all lizards that have been euthanased or are believed to be dead should have their CNS destroyed. Decapitation is *not* suitable without destroying the brain.

Pentobarbital can be given via an intravenous (ideal) or intracardiac (collapsed lizards) route. Cardio-vascular collapse should be confirmed by using Doppler ultrasonography, and once the heart has stopped beating the lizard should be pithed via the roof of the mouth.

Post-mortem examination is advised in all cases, particularly if the reptile is from a group. This not only identifies a cause of death but is also useful to screen for underlying diseases. The CNS should not be pithed if it is required for histopathology, but should be removed and fixed as a priority.

Drug formulary

Most drugs used in reptiles are not authorized and most dosages are anecdotal based on experience and efficacy. Authorized products should be utilized first if suitable. Otherwise agents with pharmacokinetic studies in reptiles should be utilized next, followed by those products with anecdotal reports. Finally, agents that have been used in other species without specific data for reptiles should be used, but with caution (Figure 15.22).

Drug	Dose	Species	Source
Antimicrobial agents			
Amikacin	5 mg/kg i.m. then 2.5 mg/kg q3d	All	Pharmacokinetic study in snakes
Ceftazidime	20 mg/kg i.m. q3d	All	Pharmacokinetic study in snakes
Enrofloxacin	5 mg/kg i.m. q24h	Iguana	Pharmacokinetic study
	10 mg/kg i.m. q5d	Bosc monitor lizards	Pharmacokinetic study
F10	Nebulization: 1:250 dilution, for 30 minutes q12h	All	Anecdotal evidence
Marbofloxacin	10 mg/kg i.m./orally q48h	All	Pharmacokinetic study in royal pythons
Metronidazole	20 mg/kg orally q48h	All	Pharmacokinetic study in iguanas
Silver sulfadiazine	Topical q24h	All	Anecdotal evidence
Ticarcillin	50 mg/kg i.m. q24h	All	Pharmacokinetic study in sea turtles
Antifungal agents			
Itraconazole	23.5 mg/kg orally q24h for 3 days. Maintain level for 6 days	Spiny lizards	Pharmacokinetic study
	5 mg/kg orally q24h	All	Anecdotal evidence
Nystatin	100,000 IU/kg orally q24h	All	Anecdotal evidence
Antiparasitic agents			
Fenbendazole	50 mg/kg orally/*per cloaca* q24h for 3 days	All	Anecdotal evidence
Fipronil	Topical wipe once a week	All	Anecdotal evidence
Ivermectin	0.2 mg/kg i.m.; repeat after 2 weeks	Not skinks, caution if microfilaria suspected	Anecdotal evidence
	Environmental spray: 5 mg/l water. Mix ivermectin 50:50 with propylene glycol to facilitate mixing. Repeat weekly	Environmental treatment	Anecdotal evidence
Metronidazole	100 mg/kg orally; repeat after 2 weeks	All	Anecdotal evidence
Praziquantel	5–8 mg/kg orally/i.m.; repeat after 2 weeks	All	Anecdotal evidence

15.22 Drug formulary for lizards. (continues) ▶

Drug	Dose	Species	Source
Anaesthetics/analgesics			
Alfaxalone	2–5 mg/kg i.v. once	All	Anecdotal evidence
Ketamine	Up to 60 mg/kg i.m. once	All	Anecdotal evidence
Ketoprofen	2 mg/kg i.m./i.v. q36h	All	Pharmacokinetic study in iguanas
Meloxicam	0.2 mg/kg i.m. q48h	All	Pharmacokinetic study in iguanas
	0.2 mg/kg orally q24h for 5 days, then q48h	All	Pharmacokinetic study in iguanas
Propofol	10 mg/kg i.v. once	All	Anecdotal evidence
Miscellaneous			
Allopurinol	50 mg/kg orally q24h	All	Scientific evidence in iguanas
Calcium gluconate	100 mg/kg i.m. q6h	All	Anecdotal evidence
Furosemide	5 mg/kg i.m. q24h	All	Scientific evidence in chelonians
Oxytocin	2–10 IU/kg i.m. q2h	All	Anecdotal evidence
Povidone–iodine	Topical: 0.05% q12–24h	All	Anecdotal evidence

15.22 (continued) Drug formulary for lizards.

References and further reading

Campbell TW and Ellis CK (2006) *Avian and Exotic Animal Hematology, 3rd edn.* Wiley Blackwell, Iowa

Cranfield MR, Grazyk TK and Bostwick EF (1999) Therapeutic efficacy of hyperimmune bovine colostrums treatment against *Cryptosporidium* infections in leopard geckos (*Eublepharis macularius*) and savannah monitors (*Varanus exanthematicus*). In: *Proceedings of the Association of Reptilian and Amphibian Veterinarians*, ed. MW Willette, pp. 119–121. ARAV, Kansas

Girling S and Raiti P (2004) *BSAVA Manual of Reptiles, 2nd edn.* BSAVA Publications, Gloucester

Greenacre CB, Takle G, Schumacher JP, *et al.* (2006) Comparative antinociception of morphine, butorphanol and buprenorphine *versus* saline in the green iguana (*Iguana iguana*) using electrostimulation. *Journal of Herpetological Medicine and Surgery* **16(3)**, 88–92

Gymesi ZS and Burns RB (2002) Monitoring of plasma 25-hydroxyvitamin D concentrations in two komodo dragons (*Varanus komodoensis*): a case study. *Journal of Herpetological Medicine and Surgery* **12(2)** 4–9

Hernandez-Divers SJ (2004) Single-dose oral and intravenous pharmacokinetics of meloxicam in the green iguana (*Iguana iguana*). In: *Proceedings of the Association of Reptilian and Amphibian Veterinarians*, pp. 106–107. ARAV, Kansas

Hernandez-Divers SJ, Stahl SJ, Stedman NL, *et al.* (2005b) Renal evaluation in the healthy green iguana (*Iguana iguana*): assessment of plasma biochemistry, glomerular filtration rate and endoscopic biopsy. *Journal of Zoo and Wildlife Medicine* **36(2)**, 155–168

Hernandez-Divers SM and Garner MM (2003) Neoplasia of reptiles with an emphasis on lizards. *Veterinary Clinics of North America: Exotic Animal Practice* **(6)**, 251–273

Hernandez-Divers SM, Schumacher J, Stahl S, *et al.* (2005a) Comparison of isoflurane and sevoflurane following pre-medication with butorphanol in the green iguana (*Iguana iguana*). *Journal of Zoo and Wildlife Medicine* **36(2)**, 169–175

Jacobson ER (2007) *Infectious Diseases and Pathology of Reptiles.* CRC Press, Boca Raton, FL

Mader D (2006) *Reptile Medicine and Surgery, 2nd edn.* Saunders Elsevier, Missouri

Mariani CL (2007) The neurologic examination and neurodiagnostic techniques for reptiles. *Veterinary Clinics of North America: Exotic Animal Practice* **10(4)**, 855–891

Martinez-Jimenez D, Hernendez-Divers SJ, Bush S, *et al.* (2007) Comparison of the effects of dipotassium ethylenediaminetetraacetic acid and lithium heparin on hematologic values in yellow-blotched map turtles (*Graptemys flavimaculata*). *Journal of Herpetological Medicine and Surgery* **17(2)**, 36–41

Pare JA and Jacobson ER (2007) Mycotic diseases of reptiles. In: *Infectious Diseases and Pathology of Reptiles,* ed. ER Jacobson, pp. 527–570. CRC Press, Boca Raton, FL

Tuttle AD, Papich M, Lewbart GA, Christian S, Gunkel C and Harms CA (2006) Pharmacokinetics of ketoprofen in the green iguana (*Iguana iguana*) following single intravenous and intramuscular injections *Journal of Zoo and Wildlife Medicine* **37(4),** 567–570

Westfall ME, Democovitz DL, Plourde AA, *et al.* (2006) *In vitro* antibiotic susceptibility of *Mycoplasma iguanae* proposed sp. nov. isolated from vertebral lesions of green iguanas (*Iguana iguana*). *Journal of Zoo and Wildlife Medicine* **37(2)**, 206–208

Useful website

UV Guide UK (most current information regarding UV lighting)
www.uvguide.co.uk

16

Snakes

Paul Raiti

Introduction

There are approximately 2400 species of snake. The majority that are presented to veterinary surgeons belong to the families Boidae and Colubridae (Figure 16.1).

Biology

Biological data are summarized in Figure 16.2.

Sexing

Sexual dimorphism occurs among snakes. Physical differences are more obvious when conspecific members of each sex are examined together. Male Boidae generally have larger pelvic spurs than females. These structures are located dorsal to the vent and are used for tactile stimulation during copulation. Most female snakes are larger than conspecific males. This is due to the reproductive demands of carrying eggs or live offspring. Male snakes possess two copulatory organs

Family	Typical species	Family characteristics
Boidae (boas and pythons)	*Boa constrictor*, rainbow boa (*Epicrates cenchria*); royal python (*Python regius*); green tree python (*Morelia viridis*); blood python (*P. curtus*); Burmese python (*P. molurus*)	Primitive snakes, thought to have evolved from lizards; vestigial limbs called pelvic spurs (claw-like structures near base of tail); two lungs; diminutive caecum; linearly arranged depressions parallel to one or both lips (heat-sensitive organs enhancing ability to detect endothermic prey); boas have undivided ventral tail scales and are viviparous (bear live young); pythons have divided ventral tail scales and are oviparous (lay eggs)
Colubridae	Corn snake (*Elaphae guttata*); kingsnake (*Lampropeltis getulus*); garter snake (*Thamnophis* spp.); gopher snake (*Pituophis melanoleucus*)	Considered modern in evolutionary terms; right lung only; no caecum or pelvic spurs; venomous colubrids include the rear-fanged mangrove snake (*Boiga dendrophila*) and the hog-nosed snake (*Heterodon nasicus*)

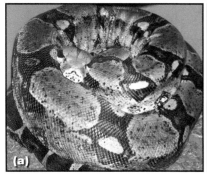 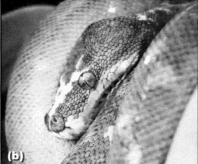 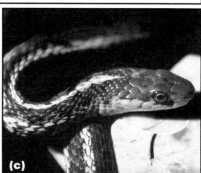

16.1 Commonly kept pet snakes. **(a)** Boa constrictor. **(b)** Green tree python. **(c)** Eastern garter snake. (Courtesy of J. Chuzi.)

	Boidae		Colubridae	
	Royal pythons	*Emerald tree boas*	*Kingsnakes/corn snakes*	*Garter snakes/water snakes*
Lifespan (years)	20–40	15–20	20–28	10–15
Reproduction	Egg bearers	Live bearers	Egg bearers	Live bearers
Clutch size	4–10 eggs	5–15 neonates	5–20 eggs	10–40 neonates
Incubation period	60–70 days	6 months until birth	60–65 days	4–6 months until birth
Preferred prey	Mice; rats	Mice; rats	Mice	Fish; insects; neonate mice

16.2 Biological data for Boidae and Colubridae.

(hemipenes) and have comparatively longer tails than females.

The most accurate method of gender identification is a technique known as 'probing', which is performed by gently inserting an appropriately sized blunt instrument into the base of the tail. Females can be probed to a depth of approximately 2–6 ventral scales; males can be probed to a depth of approximately 7–15 ventral scales because the probing instrument enters an inverted hemipenis (Figure 16.3).

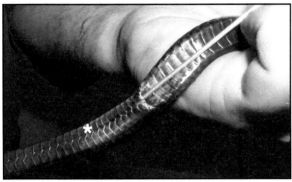

16.3 Probing depth in this male Asian ratsnake is 10 ventral scales (*).

Husbandry

Housing

As a general rule, snakes should be housed individually.

- Cage size should be adequate to permit normal behaviour for the particular species. As a rule of thumb, the diagonal of the enclosure should, as a minimum, approximate the length of the snake.
- Enclosures must be escape-proof and provide adequate ventilation.
- Glass or plastic aquaria are adequate for most colubrids and smaller boids. Secure lids, such as screen tops fastened with clamps, work well.
- Wooden cages should be well sealed with polyurethane to prevent deterioration and mould formation.

Environmental temperature

Despite being classified as poikilotherms, snakes have a preferred optimal temperature zone (POTZ) – a range of temperatures in which physiological processes such as immunogenics, digestion and reproduction occur.

- Most tropical snakes have a POTZ of between 27°C and 30°C.
- Temperate snakes have a POTZ of between 22°C and 28°C.

The high end of these ranges is provided by heat sources, such as heating pads or incandescent lights. The core temperature of larger snakes, such as boa constrictors and Burmese pythons, is best attained by regulating the room temperature to approximately 26°C and then providing focal hot spots. Night-time temperature drops of 2–5°C are recommended.

Enclosure design

Enclosure design can be broadly categorized into types that provide housing for fossorial (burrowing), ground-dwelling (Figure 16.4), semi-aquatic and arboreal species.

Fossorial, ground-dwelling and semi-aquatic species: Substrate or bedding material should be non-toxic if ingested, easy to remove from the cage, and resistant to microbial colonization.

- Burrowing snakes such as sand boas (*Eryx* spp.) that are found in dry desert habitats should be provided with several inches of fine-grain sand.

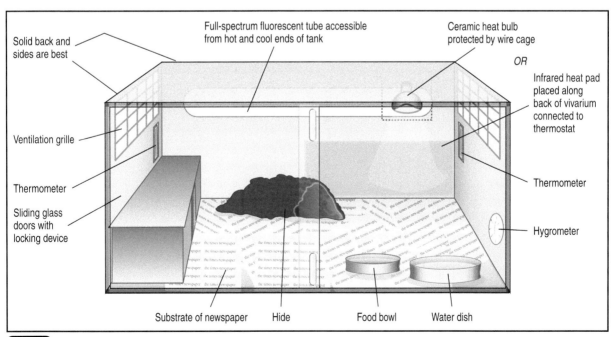

Solid back and sides are best

Full-spectrum fluorescent tube accessible from hot and cool ends of tank

Ceramic heat bulb protected by wire cage

OR

Infrared heat pad placed along back of vivarium connected to thermostat

Ventilation grille

Thermometer

Sliding glass doors with locking device

Thermometer

Hygrometer

Substrate of newspaper   Hide   Food bowl   Water dish

16.4 A vivarium suitable for a ground-dwelling snake.

- Newspaper or wood shavings (excluding cedar) are appropriate for ground-dwelling snakes such as boa constrictors, ball pythons and most colubrids.
- Other ground-dwelling boids that require higher humidity levels, such as the rubber boa (*Charina bottae*), rainbow boa (*Epicrates cenchria*) and viper boa (*Candoia asper*), should be provided with a shallow bowl containing damp sphagnum or peat moss.
- Semi-aquatic colubrids such as garter snakes (*Natrix* spp.) and water snakes (*Nerodia* spp.) should be kept on damp moss.

Arboreal species: Arboreal snakes, such as the green tree python (*Morelia viridis)* and the emerald tree boa (*Corallus caninus),* require climbing fixtures such as dowel or tree limbs, arranged horizontally at various levels. Higher humidity requirements are provided by a combination of sphagnum or peat moss as a substrate, live plants and daily misting. Appropriate ventilation (screen top and a fan that circulates room air) is important to counter the potentially deleterious effects of stagnant humid air.

Water bowls
All snakes should be provided with a shallow water bowl. Most species, with the exception of arboreal snakes, prefer to spend time immersed in water, particularly prior to ecdysis (shedding). Bowls should be replenished with fresh water every 48 hours and disinfected once a week with a suitable solution, such as chlorhexidine.

Hide boxes
Snakes should be provided with a shelter (hide box), which provides security and decreases stress. Snakes that have no place to hide commonly abrade the perinasal tissues, leading to infection and subsequent shedding problems. Arboreal snakes generally do not require hide boxes.

Ecdysis
Throughout their lives, all snakes periodically shed the entire epidermis. An abrasive surface is required for initiation of the shedding process. Ecdysis is controlled by the thyroid gland and occurs more frequently in juveniles than in adults. Approximately 2 weeks prior to shedding, lymph-like fluid is produced between the old and new layers of skin. The snake takes on an opaque hue, which is most visible over the eyes (Figure 16.5). Maintaining higher levels of

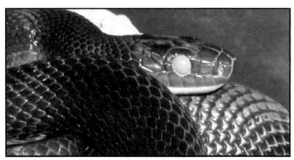

16.5 Normal appearance of spectacle prior to shedding in a Persian ratsnake.

humidity is critical in permitting removal of the epidermis. Ecdysis starts at the head and the shed skin should be a complete cast of the snake.

Diet
As a group, snakes consume a wide variety of prey, including mammals, birds, reptiles, amphibians, eggs, fish, molluscs, earthworms and insects.

- Most captive snakes are fed thawed rodents, such as mice or rats, of appropriate size. It should be noted that UK legislation *prohibits* the feeding of live vertebrate prey.
- Piscivorous snakes are fed live fish or thawed fish supplemented with thiamine (see Hypothiaminosis and Figure 16.35).

Boids have a slower metabolism than colubrids. As boids reach adulthood, the frequency of feeding should gradually decrease to one meal every 2–4 weeks, or a good rule of thumb is that defecation should occur after every third meal.

Quarantine
To maintain the long-term health of any reptile collection, it is imperative to place all new acquisitions in quarantine.

- A separate room with a closed door is strongly recommended.
- There should be no sharing of cage furniture, prey items or room air with the established collection.
- Gloves should be worn during physical contact with quarantined snakes.
- Haematology and biochemical analysis should be performed on wild-caught snakes. These animals are severely stressed from the time of capture to acquisition. Suboptimal ambient temperatures and dehydration cause a high incidence of respiratory and renal diseases.
- Snakes should be quarantined for a minimum of 6 months before being added to the main collection. During that time they should be stressed as little as possible and treated for parasitism, abscesses, etc.
- Snakes should begin to eat and defecate regularly during the quarantine period.

Breeding
All snakes require a period of physiological rest for the maintenance of long-term health. This usually occurs during changes in climatic conditions, such as decreases in temperature, rainfall and daylight hours. During this period, which may last several months, there is a 'priming' effect upon the hypothalamus–pituitary–gonadal axis.

- In captivity, this cycle is mimicked by decreasing the ambient temperature and lighting for 2–3 months.
- Temperate snakes are slowly cooled to 10–15°C; tropical snakes are provided with a daytime temperature of approximately 27°C and a night-time temperature of 21°C.
- Prior to this, snakes are fasted for 1 month to empty the gastrointestinal tract.

- Food is withheld and only water is provided during the cooling period.
- Water bowls should be cleaned and replenished with fresh water weekly.
- Animals should be checked weekly for any signs of illness, such as dehydration, dyspnoea or weight loss.

Toward the end of this dormancy stage, the ambient temperature and lighting are gradually increased. Feeding usually resumes intensely, particularly in females. The snakes are then paired for breeding.

- During copulation, one of the hemipenes is everted and inserted into the female's cloaca, where sperm is deposited.
- Ovulation occurs several weeks later, usually preceded by shedding.
- The caudal half of the female's body subsequently begins to swell as the fertilized ova develop.
- After the next shed, egg laying or parturition occurs.

Viviparous snakes require basking spots of relatively higher temperature during pregnancy. In captivity, eggs are usually transferred to an artificial incubator where the temperature is maintained at that required for the individual species (usually 27–29°C). Pythons under natural conditions, brood their eggs and are capable of raising their body temperature to 32°C to ensure proper development of the embryos.

Handling and restraint

Most snakes presented to the veterinary surgeon are relatively docile, but species such as tree boas (*Corallus* spp.), green tree pythons and reticulated pythons (*Python reticulates)*, can be aggressive. Each snake should be enclosed within an escape-proof container, such as a cloth bag tied with a knot. The bag should be placed within a secure box.

- Any snake more than 1.5 metres long (particularly boas and pythons) should be handled by two people.
- The snake should be approached from behind its head and grasped gently but firmly just caudal to the jaws.
- When lifted, the body should be supported in two places (Figure 16.6).
- Larger uncooperative pythons (e.g. Burmese, blood and reticulated) may require the use of chemical restraint in order to perform a detailed examination and diagnostic tests.
- It is not uncommon for frightened snakes to expel the contents of the cloaca and musk glands.

WARNING
Working with venomous snakes exposes personnel to potentially life-threatening situations. Legal liabilities for the veterinary clinic must also be considered. For a more detailed discussion, see *BSAVA Manual of Reptiles, 2nd edition.*

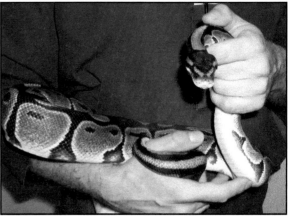

16.6 The preferred method for handling a snake is to control the head, whilst supporting its bodyweight.

Diagnostic approach

Initially, the snake should be weighed and a thorough case history obtained. The underlying cause of most diseases can be readily identified by obtaining a detailed history. Suggested husbandry modifications should be discussed, followed by a clinical examination.

Clinical examination

Observing the snake prior to handling enables the clinician to evaluate general appearance, state of nutrition, posture and locomotion.

- When lifted, the snake should possess good muscle tone and an awareness of the environment.
- Most snakes will actively flick the tongue when handled.
- There should be no retained pieces of epidermis on the body.
- Loose skin folds and prominent ribs are consistent with dehydration and malnourishment.
- The ventral scales should be checked for discoloration, swelling and ulceration.
- Indentations lateral to the dorsal spinous processes are due to fractured ribs; this is occasionally seen in wild-caught snakes.
- The vent should be clean and free of any matted excretions.

After assessing the snake's overall condition, the clinician may continue the examination in a more detailed fashion, commencing with the head.

- The mouth is opened by gently inserting a rubber spatula or an avian steel speculum between the jaws.
- The oral membranes are normally pale pink.
- The gingivae should be checked for swelling, haemorrhage, exudate and loose teeth.
- The teeth are curved, needle-like projections sheathed in the gums.
- The glottis is located on the floor of the oral cavity and opens to its maximum extent during inhalation. There should not be any exudate in the glottis.

- The lingual sheath is located under the glottis.
- The cranial portion of the oesophagus begins at the back of the oral cavity and may be pigmented with melanin.
- Each eye is covered by a single scale called the spectacle. Beneath the spectacle is the cornea. These structures are separated by the subspectacular space, which contains fluid produced by the nasolacrimal apparatus.
- Nocturnal snakes have vertical pupils; diurnal snakes have round pupils. Pupillary responses can be assessed using a bright light source.

Tractable snakes are palpated by using the index finger or thumb to press between the ventral processes of the ribs, beginning at the neck and continuing to the tail. Figure 16.7 lists the clinically important organs by location.

Organ	Comments
Heart	First palpable mass located in the cranial quarter of the body; its contractions are visible beneath the ventral scales except in large or obese snakes
Stomach	Located at the midway point of the body and is not palpable unless the snake has recently eaten or there is significant gastric pathology present
Liver	Located between the heart and the stomach
Lungs	Located dorsal to the liver; in colubrids only the right lung is significantly developed; boids possess two lungs; each lung terminates in an air sac
Gallbladder	Located just caudal to the stomach; it is occasionally palpable when there is biliary stasis secondary to anorexia or inflammation of the hepatobiliary system; closely associated with the spleen and pancreas which are only palpable when there is significant enlargement associated with inflammation/neoplasia
Ovaries	Paired linear organs located caudal to the gallbladder; can become visible as mid-body swellings during follicular development; shortly after ovulation, ova can be palpated in the caudal part of the body similar to 'marbles on a string'
Testes	Paired organs in the caudal third of the body just cranial to the kidneys; normally not palpable; gonads closely associated with adrenal glands
Kidneys	Paired organs located caudal to the gonads; pathological swelling of the caudal third of the snake's body may be due to constipation, renomegaly or retained products of conception
Cloaca	Terminal part of the gastrointestinal, urinary and reproductive systems
Vent	Ventral slit-like opening through which cloacal contents pass
Tail	Located caudal to the vent and is the terminal portion of the body; clinically significant structures contained within the tail are the paired musk glands, paired hemipenes (lateral to the musk glands) and the ventral coccygeal vein (venepuncture); pathological swelling of the base of the tail can be due to infection of the musk glands, inspissated semen or neoplasia

16.7 Clinically important organs of snakes by location.

Imaging

Diagnostic imaging techniques include radiography, ultrasonography and endoscopy. For a discussion of computed tomography (CT) and magnetic resonance imaging (MRI), see Raiti (2004).

Radiography

Optimal images are produced by radiographic machines that have the capacity to generate 300 milliamperes (mAs), exposure times of 1/60 second, and a kilovolt (kV) range of 40–100. Dorsoventral (DV) and horizontal lateral views are preferred for imaging snakes. The use of acrylic tubes for physical immobilization is strongly recommended (see Figure 16.16). Care should be taken to ensure that the tube is not too snug, thus preventing the snake from expanding its lungs. Larger snakes often require chemical immobilization.

Normal radiographic anatomy: Indications for radiography are evaluation of the skeletal, cardiopulmonary, gastrointestinal and reproductive systems. The skull and ribs are distinctly radiopaque with the latter extending to the tail. The trachea is visible on the lateral view, where it passes dorsal to heart and terminates in the lung(s). The lung is normally radiolucent and is visualized just caudal to the heart and gradually tapers before it terminates as an air sac (Figure 16.8). Inspiratory films are strongly recommended. The liver is located ventral to the lung. The gastrointestinal tract contains variable amounts of gas and ingesta depending upon the time of the last meal. The urogenital tract is normally not visible unless the snake is gravid or pregnant. Eggs occupy the caudal third of the body as a single row of poorly calcified oblong densities (Figure 16.9). Fetal skeletons are visible toward the latter third of gestation.

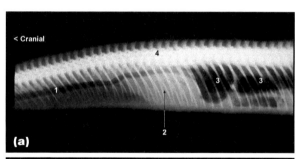

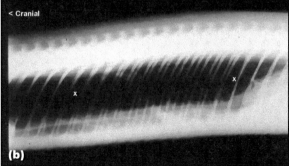

16.8 Right lateral radiographs of the cardiovascular and respiratory systems of a common boa.
(a) 1 = Trachea; 2 = Heart; 3 = Lung; 4 = Spine and ribs.
(b) X = Air sac. (Reproduced from *BSAVA Manual of Reptiles, 2nd edition.*)

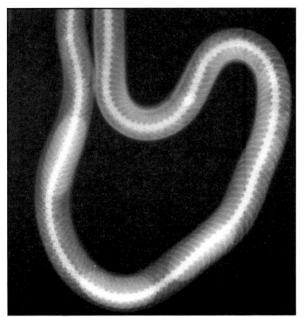

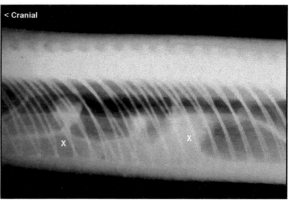

16.11 Right lateral radiograph of LRT disease in a Burmese python. X = Loculated pockets of exudates in the air sac. (Reproduced from *BSAVA Manual of Reptiles, 2nd edition.*)

16.9 DV radiograph of a gravid grey-banded kingsnake with three eggs.

Abnormal radiographic findings: Soft tissue swelling is associated with infection, inflammation and neoplasia. Osteomyelitis is characterized as a combination of lytic and proliferative bony changes (Figure 16.10). Cardiomegaly is occasionally seen and causes a mass effect on the trachea and proximal aspect of the lung. Lower respiratory tract (LRT) disease is characterized by the presence of opacities within the trachea, lung or air sac (Figure 16.11). Contrast studies of the gastrointestinal tract are indicated when inflammatory and/or obstructive conditions are suspected. Barium sulphate, ionic and non-ionic iodinated contrast agents have been used to aid in the diagnosis of foreign bodies, neoplasia, granulomas and intussusceptions (Figure 16.12).

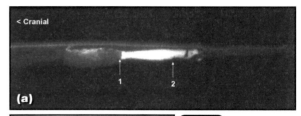

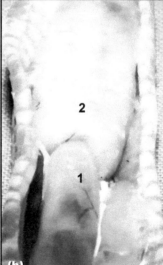

16.12

(a) Right lateral radiograph of a juvenile corn snake with an intussusception at the ileocolic junction (1) secondary to nematodiasis. Barium was administered in a retrograde fashion via the cloaca (2) and only a scant amount advanced beyond the obstruction. (Reproduced from *BSAVA Manual of Reptiles, 2nd edition.*) **(b)** Necropsy, demonstrating telescoping of the ileum (1) into colon (2).

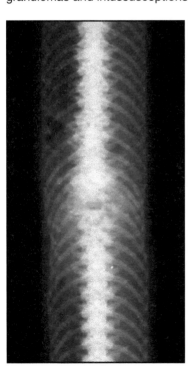

16.10

DV radiograph of vertebral osteomyelitis in a kingsnake. Note the combination of proliferative and osteolytic changes of the spine.

Ultrasonography

Ultrasonography is particularly helpful in visualizing the soft tissues, provided they are not surrounded by bone (brain) or contain air (lungs, gastrointestinal tract). In addition, any internal soft tissue swelling should be examined using ultrasonography whenever possible. Snakes with a diameter <5 cm require a stand-off pad to maximize tissue echogenicity. Snakes should not be examined using ultrasonography during ecdysis as the unshed skin interferes with beam penetration. Most ultrasound examinations are performed using a 7.5 MHz probe. Coupling gel should be applied at least 5 minutes before the examination to penetrate between the scales. The probe is placed either against the lateral body wall whilst the snake is in ventral recumbency, or against the ventral body wall whilst the snake is in dorsal recumbency. Sedation is rarely necessary, except for large or intractable snakes.

Organs commonly examined are the heart, liver, stomach, gallbladder, kidneys and reproductive tract (females). Structures should always be examined in both sagittal and transverse planes.

Normal ultrasonographic anatomy: The pulsating three-chambered heart is surrounded by the pericardial sac, within which is a small amount of anechoic pericardial fluid. The atria and ventricular chambers are visible as hypoechoic areas, whilst the cardiac muscle is strongly echogenic. Sagittal and transverse views permit visualization of the cardiac chambers, atrioventricular valves, pulmonic and aortic vessels (Figure 16.13). Cardiomyopathy, emboli and visceral gout have been identified with ultrasonography.

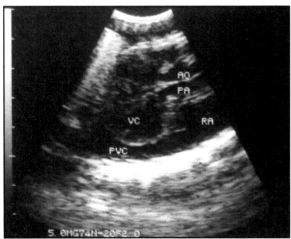

16.13 Echocardiogram (B-mode, right long-axis view) of a normal indigo snake. AO = Right aorta; PA = Pulmonary artery; PVC = Posterior vena cava; RA = Right atrium; VC = Ventricular chamber.

The single-lobed liver is uniformly homogenous in appearance and extends from the cardiac apex to the stomach. The hepatic vein is visible as an anechoic stripe traversing the length of the liver. The gallbladder is a hypoechoic sac located slightly more than half way along the length of the body. Just caudal to the gallbladder are the ovaries, which can be staged based upon their size and degree of echogenicity (Figure 16.14). Testes are normally not visible. The kidneys are

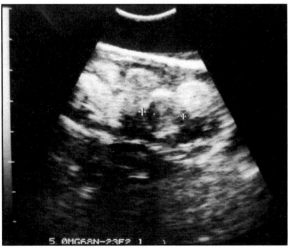

16.14 Ultrasonogram of developing follicles in a Solomon Island boa.

hyperechoic compared with the liver and possess a unique swirl-like parenchyma with vasculature; however, they are commonly obscured by fat deposits.

Endoscopy

Endoscopy is useful for direct visualization of the oral cavity, oesophagus, stomach, trachea, lungs, colon and cloaca. General anaesthesia is recommended. A rigid 2.7 mm telescope with a 30-degree oblique view and accompanying instrumentation (i.e. protective sheath, biopsy forceps, camera, light source, monitor) has been shown to be the most versatile system. Flexible endoscopes have been used for oesophagoscopy and gastroscopy. Small diameter (2.5 mm) flexible endoscopes are used for tracheal and pulmonic examinations in large snakes. When performing cloacoscopy, insufflation with warm saline dramatically increases visual acuity for examination and potential biopsy sites (Figure 16.15). Coelioscopy is rarely performed in snakes due to the linear anatomy, which precludes the ability to visualize all organs through one external entry site. Biopsy by coeliotomy is the most common method for harvesting tissue samples. A knowledge of regional anatomy is crucial when biopsying organs such as the liver or kidney. For a more complete discussion of endoscopy, see Hernandez-Divers (2004a).

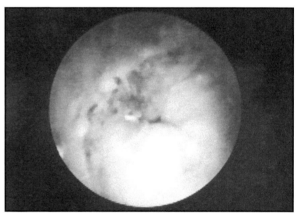

16.15 Cloacoscopy demonstrating appearance of coprodeum and junction with rectum in a green tree python after reduction of a prolapsed cloaca. Inflammatory debris is visible at the 10 o'clock position.

Sample collection

Blood

The indications for blood collection are the same as for other domestic animals.

- Physical restraint is usually adequate; however, large or intractable snakes can be restrained with transparent plastic tubes (Figure 16.16) or sedated with butorphanol (see Figure 16.35)
- Syringes should be heparinized prior to venepuncture.
- For most laboratories a minimum of 0.2–0.4 ml of whole blood is adequate for haematology and biochemical analysis, but it is advisable to check with the laboratory in advance.
- Blood smears should be made immediately after sampling.

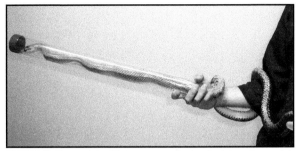

16.16 Restraint with transparent plastic tubes is useful for blood collection and radiography.

- The maximum volume of blood that can be safely taken from a reptile is calculated using the formula: weight (g) x 1% = ml blood.

The preferred method of blood collection in snakes is the ventral coccygeal vein (Figure 16.17). In small (≤0.2 kg) or dehydrated snakes, cardiocentesis may be necessary.

Ventral coccygeal venepuncture:

- After topical disinfection, venepuncture is performed by inserting a 22–24-gauge needle between the scales at an angle of 45 degrees, until it comes into contact with the coccygeal vertebrae.
- The needle is then withdrawn 1–2 mm and blood is gently aspirated.

Cardiocentesis:

- A bloodflow Doppler echocardiogram may be required to locate the heart.
- The needle is inserted between the ventral scales into the ventricle and gentle aspiration is performed.
- With each ventricular contraction, blood enters the syringe.
- If pericardial fluid is aspirated, the needle is withdrawn and venepuncture is performed again, using a new pre-heparinized syringe.

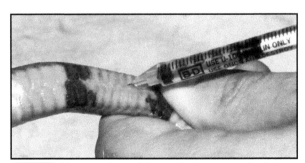

16.17 Venepuncture of the ventral coccygeal vein in a milk snake. (Reproduced from *BSAVA Manual of Reptiles, 2nd edition*.)

Normal haematological and biochemical data are summarized in Figure 16.18.

Urine

In snakes, uric acid rather than urea is the principal product of protein catabolism. Precipitates of uric acid

Parameter	Corn snakes	Royal python
Haematology		
RBC (x10¹²/l)	1.16 (0.62–1.86)	0.79 (0.36–1.31)
WBC (x10⁹/l)	9.221 (1.020–31.40)	9.448 (1.300–26.00)
Hb (g/l)	115 (97–135)	79 (67–101)
HCT	0.3120 (0.210–0.520)	0.230 (0.100–0.390)
Biochemistry		
Total protein (g/l)	66 (46–84)	67 (32–105)
Uric acid (μmol/l)	0.417 (0.077–1.184)	0.357 (0.042–1.369)
Urea (mmol/l)	0.7140 (0.0000–2.142)	0.7140 (0.0000–1.071)
Creatinine (μmol/l)	53 (18–177)	18 (0–44)
Glucose (mmol/l)	2.997 (1.721–4.884)	1.388 (0.2220–7.215)
Calcium (mmol/l)	3.95 (3.00–4.90)	4.00 (2.70–6.55)
Phosphorus (mmol/l)	1.23 (0.61–1.94)	1.16 (0.29–2.33)
LDH (IU/l)	173 (48–444)	263 (77–782)
GGT (IU/l)	10 (0–27)	3 (0–5)
ALP (IU/l)	64 (18–297)	49 (13–153)
AST (IU/l)	42 (9–224)	52 (5–153)
ALT (IU/l)	34 (4–62)	12 (1–26)
Triglycerides (mmol/l)	3.254 (0.5311–12.63)	0.3503 (0.3503–0.3503)
Cholesterol (mmol/l)	11.21 (8.133–14.81)	3.212 (0.5957–7.822)

16.18 Reference physiological values (mean, with range in parentheses) of the corn snake and royal python (International Species Inventory System, 2002).

are normally passed as hard concretions. Reptilian kidneys lack loops of Henle; hence, urine has a specific gravity (SG) of 1.002–1.015, regardless of hydration status. Snakes do not possess urinary bladders. Urine is stored in the distal ureters and cloaca, where it mixes with faeces. Evaluation of urine sediment should be interpreted in light of this fact.

Faeces

Cloacal excretions are a mixture of faeces and urates. Faecal material is brown and semi-formed to solid in consistency. Direct smears mixed with saline should be examined immediately for the presence of protozoa. A portion of faeces is suspended in a hypertonic solution (such as zinc sulphate), centrifuged and examined for parasitic ova and motile larvae. If a faecal specimen is not available, a colonic wash can be performed:

1. Infuse saline (approximately 10–20 ml/kg) into the cloaca through the vent, using a lubricated ball-tipped feeding needle.
2. Massage the caudal coelomic cavity.
3. Manually express the cloacal contents.

Lower respiratory tract

Harvesting cellular material from the LRT (trachea, lung) using a pulmonary wash technique for cytology, parasitology and microbiological culture and sensitivity is important for diagnostic and therapeutic reasons. Frequently, sedation is not required in debilitated snakes. Appropriately sized sterile feeding or tomcat urethral catheters work well:

1. Pass the catheter through the glottis.
2. Instil sterile saline (5–10 ml/kg) into the lung.

3. Coupage the snake's body to assist in loosening any pulmonary exudates.
4. Aspirate.
5. Make smears for cytological analysis and transfer fluid to test medium for aerobic, anaerobic and fungal cultures.

Common conditions

Common diseases are summarized in Figure 16.19.

Condition	Cause	Clinical signs	Diagnostics	Treatment
Cloacal prolapse	Obstruction; neurogenic; idiopathic	Prolapse of tissue from vent (cloaca, colon, oviduct)	Physical examination	Identify and reduce affected organs. Colopexy. Intestinal anastomosis. Salpingotomy. Salpingectomy
Constipation	Overfeeding; suboptimal temperature; dehydration; obstruction; neurogenic; idiopathic	Enlarged caudal part of the body; may have secondary cloacal prolapse	Palpation; radiography	Correct husbandry problems. Rehydrate or correct dehydration with parenteral fluids or soakings. Cholinergics. Enemas
Dermatitis (blister disease)	Poor husbandry with secondary bacterial infection; sepsis	Vesicles; necrosis of scales	History; physical examination; cytology and culture/sensitivity from lesions	Correct husbandry problems. Topical and systemic antibiotics. Maintain hydration status
Dysecdysis	Dehydration; lack of abrasive surfaces in cage; mites and ticks; systemic disease	Retained patches of epidermis	Physical examination	Identify underlying cause. Soak in shallow water for several hours to loosen skin
Dystocia	Lack of appropriate nest box; use of sub-adult or geriatric breeders; uterine infection; obstruction; idiopathic	Excessive cruising in cage; bulge(s) in caudal third of the body; only a portion of eggs or neonates passed within prior 48–72 hours	History; physical examination; radiography; ultrasonography	Check hydration. Provide nesting box. Administer oxytocin. Ovocentesis. Coeliotomy. Salpingotomy
Enteritis	Parasites; spoiled food; bacterial/fungal/viral infections; neoplasia	Diarrhoea (sometimes with mucus); blood	Faecal examination; contrast studies; endoscopy and biopsy	Appropriate drugs. Maintain hydration. If neoplastic mass impinging on gastrointestinal tract, consider surgical excision; if within the gastrointestinal tract prognosis grave
Musk gland adenitis	Poor husbandry; trauma; idiopathic; neoplasia	Swollen tail base (sometimes with a fistula)	Physical examination; culture/sensitivity; biopsy	Incise and flush gland. Topical and systemic antibiotics
Neurological	Trauma; hypothiaminosis; inclusion body disease (IBD); iatrogenic drug overdose; organophosphate toxicity; sepsis; parasites; idiopathic	Ataxia; tremors; paralysis; lack of righting reflex; anisocoria; opisthotonus; coma	History; physical examination; haematology; biochemistry; liver or kidney biopsy for IBD	Treat underlying cause if identified. Support with parenteral fluids. Atropine for organophosphate toxicity. Diazepam for seizures
Pneumonia	Hypothermia; inadequate ventilation; bacterial/viral/fungal/parasitic infection	Dyspnoea; puffy throat; oral exudate	Physical examination; radiography; pulmonary wash; cytology; culture/sensitivity of exudate	Increase ambient temperature. Antibiotics. Parenteral fluids. Bronchodilators. Coupage. Nebulization
Prolapsed hemipenis	Excessive breeding attempts; usually idiopathic	Protrusion of one or both copulatory organs from the vent	Physical examination	Amputation
Regurgitation	Extremes of ambient temperature; dehydration; excessive handling after eating; parasites (strongyles, cryptosporidosis)	Regurgitation of partially digested food several hours to days after eating	History; faecal examination; radiography; endoscopy; biopsy	Correct husbandry problems. Treatment based on underlying cause
Renal disease	Ambient temperature too cold; chronic dehydration; overfeeding; bacterial infection; misuse of aminoglycosides	Anorexia; dehydration; swollen caudal third of the body due to renomegaly	Haematology; biochemistry; biopsy	Parenteral fluids. Vitamins. Omega 3 fatty acids. Allopurinol. Anabolic steroids. Bone marrow stimulants. Antibiotics. Increase cage temperature

16.19 Common diseases of snakes. (continues) ▶

Condition	Cause	Clinical signs	Diagnostics	Treatment
Retained spectacle	Dysecdysis; dehydration; mites	Unshed spectacle(s); opaque appearance	History; physical examination	Increase cage humidity. Lift spectacle by edge and attempt to gently remove. Sometimes more prudent to wait until next shed and check snake/shed skin
Stomatitis	Stress; trauma; ambient temperature too cold; bacterial infection; neoplasia; gout	Reluctance to eat; gingivitis; oral exudate; swollen jaw	Direct smears for cytology; radiography to rule out osteomyelitis; microbiological culture/sensitivity; biopsy	Analgesics. Parenteral fluids. Oral debridement. Topical and systemic antibiotics
Subspectacular abscess	Ascending infection from oral cavity; sepsis; idiopathic	Hypopyon; swollen globe	Physical examination	Surgical drainage of subspectacle space
Thermal burns	Overexposure to heat sources	First-, second- or third-degree burns	History; physical examination	Analgesics. Parenteral fluids. Topical and systemic antibiotics

16.19 (continued) Common diseases of snakes.

Viral infections

Viral infections are usually suspected when an epizootic disease occurs after acquisition of a snake that has not been properly vetted and quarantined. Inclusion body disease (IBD) and paramyxovirus are the most well known viral diseases of snakes. For a more complete discussion of ophidian virology, see Marschang and Chitty (2004).

Inclusion body disease

IBD is caused by a retrovirus and primarily affects boids, although it has also been isolated from colubrids. Horizontal transmission is suspected to occur by blood-sucking arthropods such as the snake mite. Vertical transmission also occurs. In boas, IBD causes regurgitation. Affected snakes may slowly waste away or die acutely. After several months the clinical signs may progress to an encephalopathy, characterized by strabismus, head tilt, tremors, paralysis and opisthotonus (Figure 16.20). In pythons, the disease runs a much more acute course, characterized primarily by similar neurological clinical signs followed by death.

Diagnosis of IBD is based on histological identification of eosinophilic intracytoplasmic inclusions in tissues stained with haematoxylin and eosin. Biopsy samples from the oesophageal tonsils, liver, pancreas or kidney are the best sources for demonstrating viral inclusions. There is no effective treatment.

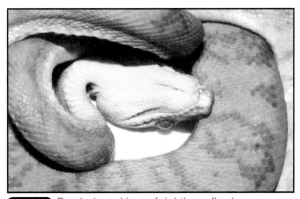

16.20 Paralysis and loss of righting reflex in an Amazon tree boa with IBD.

Paramyxovirus

Paramyxovirus affects the respiratory and central nervous systems and has been isolated from viperids, colubrids and boids. Signs range from flaccid paralysis and dyspnoea to sudden death without clinical signs. A presumptive ante-mortem diagnosis is reached by measuring haemagglutination inhibition titres (Schumacher, 1996). An increase of at least 2-fold in titres measured 2 weeks after resting titres is highly suggestive of the disease. Diagnosis is confirmed histologically by identifying eosinophilic inclusions in the lungs or brain. In zoological collections, clinically affected animals are permanently separated from healthy snakes. There is no treatment.

Bacterial infections

The majority of bacteria identified from infections in captive snakes are Gram-negative aerobes, including *Pseudomonas*, *Aeromonas*, *Klebsiella*, *Escherichia coli* and *Salmonella*. Examples of anaerobic bacteria are *Clostridium* and *Bacteroides*. Occasionally, Gram-positive bacteria such as coagulase-positive staphylococci are identified. Most of these bacteria are opportunistic pathogens; they are part of the normal flora that can cause disease during periods of immunosuppression. Sepsis occurs from haematogenous invasion from the integument, respiratory, gastrointestinal or lower urogenital tracts. The presence of petechiae or ecchymoses strongly suggests septicaemia.

Treatment

Identification and correction of inappropriate husbandry factors are essential. Particular emphasis should be placed upon temperature, humidity, quarantine practices and parasite identification. *Provision of adequate hydration and correct ambient temperature prior to systemic antibiotic therapy are mandatory.* Chronic abscessation requires a combination of surgical debridement, topical antibacterial preparations and systemic antibiotics. Healing time varies from weeks to months depending upon severity. Bactericidal drugs are generally preferred to bacteriostatics. The following important points should be considered when choosing an antibiotic:

- Penetrability of the targeted lesion
- Route of administration
- Hydration status
- Patient temperature.

If bacterial culturing and sensitivity cannot be undertaken, it is prudent to choose a combination of antibiotics that will provide activity against Gram-negative, Gram-positive, aerobic and anaerobic bacteria (e.g. ceftazidime and amikacin or enroflaxacin and metronidazole; see Figure 16.35).

Fungal infections

Fungal dermatitis is the most common manifestation of mycotic disease in snakes. Grossly, the lesions appear as discrete areas of wrinkled scales, which are often raised and discoloured and commonly develop on the ventrum due to contact with substrate. Most fungal organisms isolated from cases of dermatomycoses are saprophytes (*Geotrichum, Candida, Aspergillus, Penicillium* and *Trichosporon*) which populate the skin and gastrointestinal system via environmental exposure. There are usually multiple dermal lesions with potential invasion of the underlying musculature and bone.

To date, the *Chrysosporium* anamorph of *Nannizziopsis vriesii* (CANV) has been identified as the only primary fungal pathogen of snakes (Figure 16.21). Dermal lesions appear initially as vesicles, progressing to necrosis, and ultimately systemic invasion with a high mortality rate. There is no effective treatment.

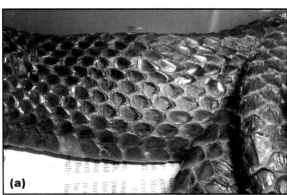

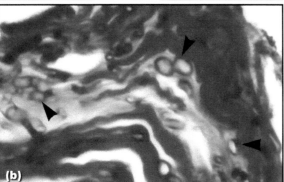

16.21 **(a)** Fungal dermatitis in an Asian ratsnake with CANV infection. **(b)** The section of skin has an overlying crust of cell debris, keratin and serum, supporting fungal hyphae (arrowheads). H&E stain; original magnification x40. (Courtesy of D. Reavill.)

Biopsy of suspicious dermal lesions and subsequent identification by microbiological culture is recommended. Treatment of fungal infections consists of a combination of topical and systemic antifungal drugs; however, long-term prognosis is usually poor. Fluconazole is recommended for yeast infections and itraconazole for filamentous fungal infections (see Figure 16.35).

Ectoparasites

The most common ectoparasite of snakes is the mite *Ophionyssus natricis*. Poor husbandry and an inadequate quarantine period for new acquisitions permit these haematophagous arthropods to reach very high populations before they are detected. Adult mites are black and nocturnal. The most common sites for mites to be identified are the edge of the spectacles and the ventral skin-fold caudal to the chin. Besides dysecdysis, mites cause anaemia and transmit bacteria and viruses. Treatment includes eradication of mites both in the environment and on the host. Cages and furnishings should be dismantled and washed with either hot water or diluted bleach solution (3%). The author has had success with diluted ivermectin applied as a spray (see Figure 16.35). Other acaricides used successfully in snakes are permethrins and fipronil.

Ticks of the genera *Amblyomma* and *Aponomma* commonly infest wild-caught snakes, particularly those of African origin. Ticks are capable of causing dysecdysis and anaemia, and of transmitting rickettsial diseases. Unlike mites, ticks are less mobile and prefer to stay embedded in the host's skin (Figure 16.22). Treatment is the same as for mites. Manual removal of ticks with forceps is performed several hours after topical treatment.

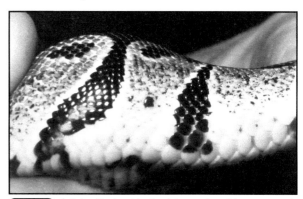

16.22 A tick attached to the interscalar skin on a royal python. (Reproduced from *BSAVA Manual of Reptiles, 2nd edition*.)

Endoparasites

Nematodes

The hookworm *Kalicephalus* is the most common nematode encountered in clinical practice (Figure 16.23a). Clinical signs include anorexia, regurgitation, diarrhoea and weight loss. Hookworms have a direct lifecycle and are capable of extensive tissue migration. Infection occurs through ingestion of embryonated ova or transcutaneous penetration by larvae. Subcutaneous nodules may contain hundreds of larvae. Ascarids, such as *Ophidascaris*, require intermediate hosts and

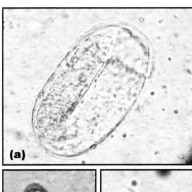

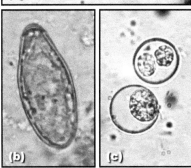

16.23

(a) Embryonated *Kalicephalus* ovum from an Asian ratsnake. **(b)** Trematode fluke egg from an Asian ratsnake. Note the single operculum. **(c)** *Isospora* oocysts from a green trinket snake.

Coccidiosis causes anorexia, weight loss and diarrhoea. Oocysts are readily identified on faecal flotation. *Eimeria* (four sporocysts) and *Isospora* (two sporocysts) (Figure 16.23c) are commonly seen in colubrids. *Caryospora* (single sporocyst) is approximately one-half the size of other Coccidia and is more common in boids. Ponazuril is the author's treatment of choice. The coccidian parasite *Cryptosporidium serpentis* produces two syndromes in snakes (Schumacher, 1996). The first is an acute form characterized by regurgitation within a few days after eating. The parasite colonizes the gastric crypts, causing an intense inflammatory reaction. Hypertrophy of the stomach is so severe that frequently a mid-body swelling becomes apparent. The chronic form is characterized by a gradual wasting away of the affected snake due to anorexia and diarrhoea. The parasite spreads by ingestion of infective oocysts by the host. Diagnosis is confirmed by a faecal fluorescent antibody test. Affected snakes should be permanently isolated from the main collection. Paromomycin has shown promise in preventing oocyst shedding; however, eradication of the parasite has yet to be documented.

are not as pathogenic as hookworms; however, they can cause intermittent regurgitation and weight loss. The lungworm *Rhabdias* has a direct lifecycle and causes LRT disease, which is often complicated by secondary bacterial pneumonia. Ova are detected when a pulmonary wash is performed. Treatment is with fenbendazole or ivermectin (see Figure 16.35).

Trematodes and cestodes

Flukes and tapeworms require one or more intermediate hosts, such as molluscs, fish or amphibians. Flukes inhabit the hepatobiliary system and cause cachexia and diarrhoea. The single operculated ova (Figure 16.23b) are commonly seen on examination of faecal samples from wild-caught snakes. Treatment is with praziquantel (see Figure 16.35). Adult tapeworms primarily inhabit the intestinal tract. Tapeworm larvae are capable of extensive tissue migration. Treatment is with praziquantel. *Spirometra* larvae commonly produce subcutaneous swellings and can be extracted after incising the skin.

Protozoa

Flagellates such as *Trichomonas* are commonly found in small numbers of clinically normal snakes. One type of flagellate, *Monocercomonas*, has been associated with nephritis and salpingitis. Large numbers of flagellates are commonly seen with nematodes during faecal examination. They should be eliminated with an appropriate antiprotozoal drug such as metronidazole (see Figure 16.35).

In snakes, *Entamoeba invadens* can burrow into the intestinal lining and cause haemorrhagic enteritis with associated high morbidity and mortality (Frank, 1984). This parasite also invades the bile duct and causes cholangiohepatitis. Quadrinucleated cysts or the motile trophozoites are visible upon direct faecal examination. This parasite is seen in stressed wild-caught snakes. Metronidazole is the treatment of choice.

Pentastomids

These are highly specialized arthropods with a zoonotic potential. Snakes acquire this parasite after ingesting an infected rodent. The larvae migrate to the lungs, where the adults either attach to the pulmonary epithelium or remain motile, sometimes migrating to the air sacs. The larvae, with four claw-like appendages, are identified in the faeces or pulmonary exudate. Extraction via pulmonoscopy has been reported. Ivermectin can decrease shedding of ova but is of questionable efficacy in eradicating adult stages.

Gastrointestinal disease

Stomatitis

Bacterial infections of the oral cavity, such as stomatitis (mouth rot), are common. Local infection due to trauma is the most common cause. Chronic stressors such as suboptimal ambient temperature play a role, especially in larger boas and pythons. Occasionally, stomatitis is secondary to a primary systemic process such as sepsis, renal failure, viral disease or neoplasia.

Haematology and biochemical analysis should be performed, in addition to direct smears of the infected tissues for cytology and microbiological culture and sensitivity testing. Radiography is recommended to rule out osteomyelitis (Figure 16.24). Treatment consists of analgesics, sedation, debridement, topical antibiotics, parenteral fluids and systemic antibiotics depending on severity. Re-check appointments are necessary to evaluate response to treatment.

Regurgitation

Regurgitation is the expulsion of partially digested food. In snakes this problem usually occurs within 72 hours following consumption of a meal. The most common causes are stress, parasitism, improper ambient temperature, consumption of too large a meal, viral diseases, foreign bodies, rancid prey items or excessive handling of the snake shortly after a

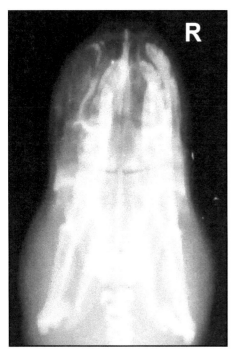

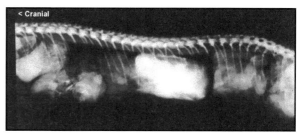

16.25 Right lateral radiograph of a constipated Burmese python that had been maintained at suboptimal temperatures. (Reproduced from *BSAVA Manual of Reptiles, 2nd edition.*)

16.24 DV radiograph of the skull of a boa constrictor with osteomyelitis of the rostral aspect of the left maxilla. Note the osteolysis and associated soft tissue swelling.

meal. Identification of inappropriate husbandry practices, faecal analysis, contrast radiography, endoscopy and gastric biopsy are required for diagnosis.

Enteritis

Parasitism is the leading cause of enteritis in snakes (see above). Treatment with appropriate parasiticides is usually effective (see Figure 16.35). Multiple treatments and re-testing of stools every 6 months are necessary to ensure parasite eradication, particularly in wild-caught animals. Enteritis can also be associated with enteroviruses, hepatic and renal diseases, and infiltrative bowel disease (parasitic migration, lymphoma).

Disruption of the normal enteric flora through the misuse of antibiotics has been incriminated as a cause of fungal overgrowth and subsequent diarrhoea. Administration of a fungicidal drug that is not absorbed from the gut, such as nystatin, is effective. Bacterial disease is an uncommon cause of diarrhoea in snakes. Intussusception is a potential consequence of enteritis and should be suspected when a soft tissue mass is palpated in the caudal half of the body of a snake exhibiting clinical signs.

Constipation

The most common causes of constipation are overfeeding, dehydration and suboptimal cage temperature (Figure 16.25). Green tree pythons and emerald tree boas are particularly prone to constipation due to their slow metabolic rate. Obstruction due to foreign bodies, granulomas, retained products of conception and neoplasia are less common causes, but should form part of the differential diagnoses list. Treatment of constipation is by soaking the snake in water for 24 hours to encourage defecation, enemas

with warmed water and administering cholinergics (e.g. metaclopramide or cisapride). If moderate to severe hydration is present, parenteral fluids may be necessary in addition to soaking. Coeliotomy may be required to remove retained eggs, mummified fetuses, foreign bodies and soft tissue masses. Constipation can also be neurological in origin. Snakes with congenital scoliosis or spinal trauma can have paralytic ileus, resulting in megacolon and subsequent cloacal prolapse.

Cloacal prolapse

Cloacal prolapse is the abnormal protrusion of tissue(s) through the vent (Figure 16.26). During defecation and oviposition, tissues normally protrude through the vent; however, they quickly retract. In addition to the cloaca, other organs that may prolapse through the vent in snakes include the colon and oviduct(s). Prolapse of any tissue from the vent should be considered an emergency. The owner should be instructed to keep the tissues clean and moist until presentation to the veterinary surgeon (see Common surgical procedures).

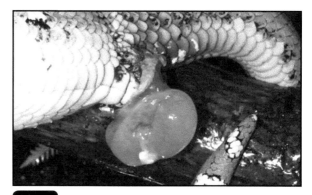

16.26 Cloacal prolapse in an emerald tree boa.

Nutritional disease

Obesity

Obesity, due to a combination of hyperalimentation and lack of exercise, is probably the most prevalent nutritional disease in snakes. It is best to compare captive animals with photographs of wild specimens. Obesity predisposes snakes to constipation, dystocia, atherosclerosis, hepatic lipidosis and visceral gout. Treatment consists of gradually reducing caloric intake and support of hepatic function (e.g. vitamins and parenteral fluids).

Hypothiaminosis

Hypothiaminosis (vitamin B1 deficiency) is seen in piscivores such as garter and water snakes, which are fed primarily frozen fish or fresh fish that have very high levels of thiaminase (sardines and whitefish). Freezing inactivates thiamine, which is necessary for proper functioning of the central nervous system (CNS). Unless the diet is supplemented with thiamine, or fish with high thiaminase levels are boiled, cerebrocortical degeneration and subsequent necrosis result. Clinical signs consist of tremors, paralysis and loss of the righting reflex. In the acute stages of the condition, response to treatment with injections of thiamine is often dramatic.

Ocular disease

Subspectacular abscess

Accumulation of purulent exudate between the spectacle and cornea can be due to sepsis, an ascending infection from the oral cavity via the nasolacrimal duct, or be idiopathic. The globe is not swollen unless panophthalmitis develops or there is a blockage of the nasolacrimal duct. Grossly the eye appears distinctly opaque (Figure 16.27a). Occasionally, a fluid line is visible in the subspectacular space. Treatment consists of surgically removing a small triangular piece of the spectacle between the 4 and 6 o'clock positions whilst the snake is anaesthetized. The subspectacular space is then flushed with 0.9% sterile saline solution infused through the surgical window (Figure 16.27b). Parenteral antibiotics based upon microbiological culture and sensitivity are administered for approximately 3 weeks. Healing is usually complete after the next shed.

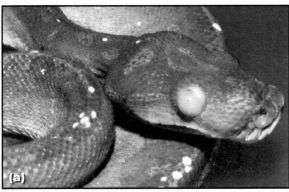

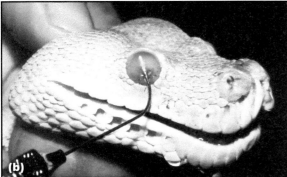

16.27 **(a)** Hypopyon and cellulitis in a green tree python. Note the opaque appearance of the spectacle. **(b)** Flushing of subspectacular space with sterile saline in an anaesthetized green tree python.

Respiratory disease

Stress and hypothermia are common causes of immunosuppression and subsequent LRT disease. The major clinical sign of LRT disease is dyspnoea, characterized by open-mouth breathing. A frothy or purulent exudate may be visualized in the glottis. Bacterial infections are the most frequently diagnosed; however, parasitism (lungworms, pentastomids) and viruses (paramyxovirus) should be included on the differential diagnoses list.

A pulmonary wash to harvest material for cytology and microbiological culture and sensitivity is recommended. *Pseudomonas*, *Aeromonas*, *Klebsiella* and *Escherichia coli* are commonly isolated. Radiographs demonstrate pulmonary infiltrates in the dependent portions of the lung(s) and air sac(s). Treatment consists of parenteral fluids, coupage, antibiotics and providing an ambient temperature at the upper end of the snake's POTZ to stimulate immunogenics. Due to the linear anatomy of the ophidian lung and air sac, the prognosis for LRT disease is guarded. In some cases nebulization has been shown to be effective.

Urogenital disease

Gout

Uric acid is produced in the liver and excreted by the renal tubules. Renal failure is the most common cause of gout in snakes. When blood levels of uric acid reach saturation point, uric acid crystals precipitate within the mucous membranes, pericardial sac, myocardium, liver and kidneys. Affected snakes are anorexic and dehydrated. Frequently, there is a diffuse swollen appearance to the caudal fourth of the snake's body due to renomegaly. The oral cavity should be examined for tophicaseous deposits.

Renal disease is caused by one or a combination of the following: suboptimal ambient temperature; chronic dehydration; infectious disease; or an overdose of nephrotoxic drugs such as aminoglycosides. Haematology and biochemistry commonly demonstrate haemoconcentration, increased total solids, leucocytosis, hypocalcaemia, hyperphosphataemia and hyperuricaemia. Renal biopsy provides valuable information as to aetiology, treatment options and prognosis. Although the prognosis is guarded at best, attempted treatment consists of intracoelomic fluids, allopurinol, erythropoietin, B complex vitamins and anabolic steroids.

Dystocia

Non-obstructive dystocia is the most common type in snakes. Frequently, the cause of uterine inertia is idiopathic; however, several risk factors have been implicated such as breeding animals of suboptimal size, lack of appropriate nesting sites, obesity, poor motor tone due to inactivity and the use of geriatric breeders. Non-obstructive causes of dystocia in viviparous snakes are early embryonic death due to suboptimal basking temperatures, and uterine infections. Obstructive causes are: abnormally large eggs; compressive injuries to the spine; coelomic masses; and retained products of conception from previous copulations.

Treatment of non-obstructive dystocia consists of correcting dehydration, supplying an appropriate nesting site and administration of oxytocin. Response to oxytocin is quite variable in snakes. Eggs that have not passed within 24 hours following passing of the first egg are not viable. Decompression of the distal egg(s) by transcutaneous aspiration (Figure 16.28), followed by warmed water soaks for several hours prior to oxytocin administration, significantly increases the likelihood of oviposition. If this is unsuccessful, gentle manipulation of each compressed egg toward the vent can be attempted whilst the snake is anaesthetized. The egg is then grasped with forceps and gently extracted. If extraction is not possible due to oviductal adhesions, the eggs should be removed via coeliotomy/salpingotomy (see Common surgical procedures).

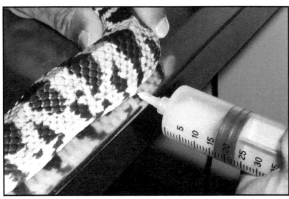

16.28 Transcutaneous aspiration of a retained egg in a pine snake.

Prolapsed hemipenis

Prolapse of a hemipenis (Figure 16.29) may occur after copulation. The aetiology is usually idiopathic. Application of gentle traction on the organ verifies its origin in the tail. Due to the fact that a prolapsed hemipenis quickly becomes swollen, desiccated and necrotic, amputation is the treatment of choice. Since male snakes possess two copulatory organs, amputation of one will not affect reproductive capability (see Common surgical procedures).

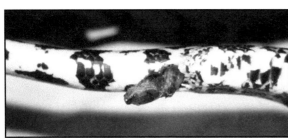

16.29 Prolapsed hemipenis in a boa constrictor. (Reproduced from *BSAVA Manual of Reptiles*, 2nd edition.)

Skin disease

Dermatitis

Bacterial infections of the skin, such as dermatitis (blister disease), are associated with poor husbandry. Prolonged contact with urine and faeces in a humid environment is conducive to bacterial and fungal

multiplication, with the potential for subsequent invasion of the dermis. Initially, lesions appear as vesicles on the ventral scales. Eventually, the blisters rupture, exposing the deeper tissues which subsequently become necrotic. Death can occur due to sepsis. Fluid from the vesicles should be examined for parasitic larvae (nematodes). Microbiological culture and sensitivity tests should also be performed. Treatment consists of correcting husbandry deficiencies, rehydration with parenteral fluids, and the use of topical and systemic antibiotics. Resolution can take weeks to months. Increased shedding frequency during the recuperative process facilitates healing.

Dysecdysis and retained spectacles

Suboptimal ambient humidity and acariasis are the most common causes of difficult shedding. Soaking the snake in a shallow water bath for several hours usually causes the skin to slough. It is recommended that owners always check a sloughed skin to make sure that the spectacles and nasal plugs (skin lining the nasal cavities) have shed. Identification of any underlying disease (renal failure, encephalopathy) is important.

Thermal burns

Most burns (Figure 16.30a) occur on the ventral scales due to snakes resting on heating stones. Occasionally, burns are seen on the dorsum of the body from overhead heating fixtures. Treatment consists of analgesics, topical antibiotics such as silver sulfadiazine, wet-to-dry bandages, parenteral fluids and systemic antibiotics. Increased shedding frequency contributes to the healing process (Figure 16.30b). Scars eventually become pigmented with melanin. Healing can take 6–8 months or longer.

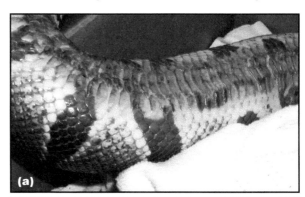

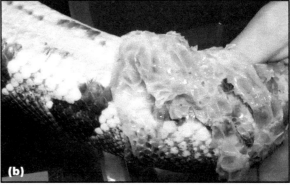

16.30 **(a)** Second-degree burns on a royal python. **(b)** The healing skin is visible during shedding.

Musk gland adenitis

Infection of the musk gland(s) (Figure 16.31) produces a swelling at the base of the tail. This condition is more common in snakes that are kept in unhygienic enclosures. Fistulation of the gland occasionally occurs. Treatment consists of analgesics, debridement, microbiological culture and sensitivity, and topical/parenteral antibiotics. Biopsy is recommended to rule out neoplasia.

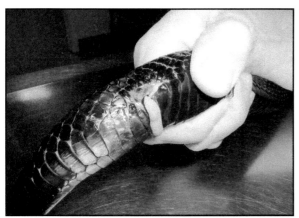

16.31 Drainage of exudate from an infected musk gland in an indigo snake. The tail is to the left.

Neurological disease

The most common causes of neurological disease in snakes are: overdose of drugs (metronidazole, ivermectin, miticides), trauma, IBD (boids), hypothiaminosis, hypothermia, sepsis and parasitic migration. Congenital encephalopathy has been observed in hatchling snakes that were maintained at extreme temperatures during embryonic development. Clinical signs include tremors, lack of righting reflex, anisocoria, ataxia, paralysis and opisthotonus. Diagnosis rests heavily upon a detailed case history. Many neurological diseases have a guarded prognosis. Early treatment of thiamine deficiency, organophosphate toxicity and metronidazole toxicosis offer the most promising outcomes.

Toxicoses

The most common toxicities seen in clinical practice are due to overdosing with acaricides and drugs. The use of organophosphates to treat mites is particularly dangerous to snakes. Impregnated strips containing dichlorvos have caused the most problems. Clinical signs are due to overstimulation of the nicotinic/cholinergic sites causing muscle fasciculations, tremors, spasms and muscular paralysis. Death is due to respiratory failure. Treatment consists of atropine, parenteral fluids and diazepam if seizures occur. Overdosing with ivermectin or metronidazole causes ataxia, tremors and paralysis. Treatment consists of parenteral fluids and diazepam. Permanent head tilt and strabismus have been seen associated with ivermectin toxicosis.

Neoplasia

A wide variety of neoplasms have been identified in snakes (Figure 16.32a). Most affect the integument,

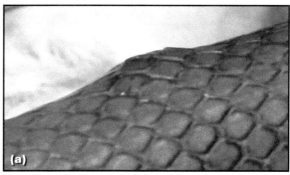

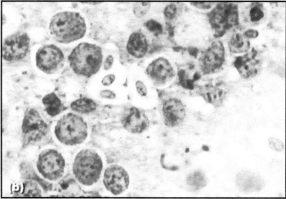

16.32 **(a)** Subcutaneous mass on a trinket snake. **(b)** Cytology of a needle aspirate demonstrating lymphoblasts. New methylene blue stain; original magnification x100 with oil immersion.

digestive tract and lymphoreticular system. Carcinomas and sarcomas are the most common malignant neoplasms of the integument and internal organs. Lymphoma is the most common malignancy of the haematopoietic system. Occasionally, extreme lymphocytosis of blast cells is identified in the haemogram of affected snakes. Neoplasia should be included in the differential diagnoses list when any mass or enlarged organ is identified. Examination of needle aspirates or tissue biopsy samples provides the diagnosis (Figure 16.32b). To date, wide surgical excision of discrete masses offers the best long-term results. Adjunctive chemotherapy has been attempted in a few cases with inconsistent results.

Congenital defects

Improper incubation temperature and inbreeding are the most common causes of congenital defects in snakes. Affected hatchlings possess spinal deformities. Neurological dysfunction such as loss of the righting reflex and ataxia has also been observed. Less common abnormalities are external herniations, anophthalmia and bicephalus.

Zoonoses

Examples of potentially zoonotic diseases of snakes are salmonellosis, mycobacteriosis and pentastomiasis. Personnel with compromised immune systems should not be permitted to handle snakes. Use of disinfectants, disposable gloves and good personal hygiene should be practised when handling ill snakes. Snakes diagnosed with zoonotic diseases should be humanely euthanased.

Supportive care

Drug administration
Intramuscular injections are administered in the long-issimus muscles parallel to the spine. As snakes possess a renal-portal system, antibiotics that undergo renal tubular excretion (penicillins) or that are nephrotoxic (aminoglycosides) should be administered in the front half of the body. Needle punctures should be made between the scales (interscaler skin). The subcutaneous route may also be used but some drugs, such as enrofloxacin and ketamine, are irritating and capable of causing sterile abscesses. The preferred site for intravenous injections is the ventral coccygeal vein.

Fluid therapy
Standard isotonic crystalloid fluids historically used in mammals work well for snakes. Examples include lactated Ringer's solution, Ringer's solution and 2.5% dextrose solution mixed with 0.45% saline solution. All surgical candidates should have parenteral fluids administered perioperatively. Warmed fluids can be administered to snakes by various routes:

- Soaking and bathing
- Oral
- Subcutaneous
- Intracoelomic.

Soaking and bathing
Warmed water or electrolyte/carbohydrate solutions are an effective method of replenishing body fluids in mildly dehydrated snakes. Depth should be no more than the diameter of the snake and soaks of up to 24 hours are beneficial. Weight gains of 5–10% are not uncommon.

Oral
Fluids and drugs can be administered via pre-lubricated rubber orogastric tubes, ball-tipped feeding needles or urethral catheters. The tube should be premeasured to make sure that fluids are administered into either the distal oesophagus or the stomach, which is located half way between the snout and the vent. The suggested maximum volume is 10–20 ml/kg/day.

Subcutaneous
Warmed fluids are administered at a rate of 5–10 ml/kg/day lateral to the dorsal spinous processes. When given properly, fluids can be seen moving in a cranial/caudal direction under the skin.

Intracoelomic
This route is recommended when larger volumes of fluids (10–25 ml/kg/day) are required for rehydration. Warmed fluids are administered in the caudal fourth of the body. Absorption is more rapid than via the subcutaneous route due to the large surface area of the coelomic membranes. The needle is inserted between the first two rows of lateral scales and directed cranially at an angle of 30 degrees to the long axis of the body. This route is not recommended if coelomic disease is present.

Anaesthesia and analgesia
For individual drug doses see Figure 16.35.

Analgesia
Pre-emptive analgesia is the administration of analgesics prior to a painful stimulus and is more effective than attempting to reduce pain that is already present. Pre-emptive analgesia should be a component of every surgical procedure, ranging from topical debridement to coeliotomy. Trauma and topical burns also require the use of analgesics. Signs of acute pain in snakes are excessive writhing movements or motor rigidity. Multimodal analgesia, which combines two or more analgesics with different mechanisms of action, is more effective than the administration of a single drug. Examples include use of a non-steroidal anti-inflammatory drug (NSAID, carprofen), an opioid (buprenorphine or butorphanol) and a local anaesthetic (bupivacaine) prior to coeliotomy.

Local anaesthesia
Lidocaine and bupivacaine have been effectively used in snakes for skin biopsy, topical debridement, line block for coeliotomy and topical burns. Lidocaine has a faster onset of action, whilst bupivacaine has a longer duration of action. Dilution with equal parts of sterile saline will increase accuracy of dose and reduce pain upon administration.

Injectable anaesthesia

Propofol
Propofol, an ultra short-acting anaesthetic, is useful for techniques such as radiography, skin biopsy and abscess debridement. Sedation/anaesthesia of 10–25 minutes duration is provided. Propofol can also be used to facilitate intubation and anaesthetic induction with inhalational agents for longer procedures (e.g. coeliotomy). Propofol must be administered as a slow intravenous infusion to prevent cardiopulmonary depression.

Ketamine and medetomidine
A combination of ketamine and medetomidine provides faster, smoother anaesthetic induction, improved muscle relaxation, more effective analgesia, and decreases the inhalation anaesthetic dosage required compared with ketamine alone. Additionally, medetomidine can be reversed with atipamezole at 5 times the medetomidine dose at the end of the surgical procedure. This is the author's injectable anaesthetic of choice. An NSAID (e.g. carprofen) is administered to provide pre-emptive analgesia. Recovery typically takes 45–70 minutes.

Tiletamine and zolazepam
Tiletamine and zolazepam have been used for physical restraint prior to intubation and induction with inhalation anaesthesia. Recovery is significantly longer than with ketamine and medetomidine. For this reason the author rarely uses this drug combination in reptiles.

Inhalation anaesthesia

Isoflurane is the gaseous anaesthetic of choice in snakes. Induction with isoflurane alone can be achieved at 4–5% and maintained at 1.5–2.5% with oxygen at 1 litre/minute; however, analgesia and muscle relaxation are minimal. Premedication with an opioid (butorphanol, buprenorphine) and ketamine, or ketamine and medetomidine followed by intubation work well. A surgical plane of anaesthesia is determined by the lack of various reflexes such as the righting reflex, tail-pinch reflex and tongue retraction reflex.

Maintaining the snake's core temperature at 28°C is critical during any procedure requiring sedation or anaesthesia. Circulating warm water pads are useful in preventing hypothermia. Cardiac monitoring with electrocardiography (ECG) or a bloodflow Doppler device at the level of the heart is strongly recommended. The normal pulse should be in the range of 20–40 beats/minute, depending on the size of the snake (smaller specimens have faster cardiac rates). Intermittent positive pressure ventilation (IPPV) using a mechanical ventilator (Figure 16.33) is required at the rate of one breath every 15 seconds. Adequate tidal volume is determined by observation of 'chest' expansion.

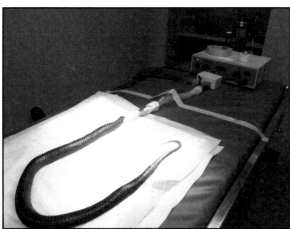

16.33 Intubated garter snake, connected to a mechanical ventilator which is utilizing isoflurane and oxygen. Note the circulating warm water pad beneath the snake.

Common surgical procedures

Skin biopsy

A local anaesthetic (bupivacaine or lidocaine) is administered subcutaneously at the target site. Disinfection of the skin is performed with 0.05% chlorhexidine, unless the integument is to be harvested for microbiological culture and sensitivity. Approximately 20 minutes following administration of the local anaesthetic, a number 11 scalpel blade is used to make a circumferential full-thickness incision in the interscalar skin, incorporating normal and abnormal scales. Due to the fact that the skin inverts when incised, horizontal mattress sutures are used for closure.

Hemipenis amputation

An injectable anaesthetic (propofol, ketamine/medetomidine, ketamine/butorphanol or buprenorphine) is administered preoperatively. After infusion of a local anaesthetic into the base of the prolapsed hemipenis and double ligation with an absorbable monofilament such as polyglycolic acid, the hemipenis is amputated.

Colopexy

The cloaca is the most common organ to prolapse through the vent. Arboreal boids are particularly prone to this problem. Prolapse commonly occurs secondary to constipation. Occasionally, gravid snakes prolapse an oviduct. Sometimes an egg can be visualized within the prolapsed oviduct. Cloacal prolapses do not respond to simple reduction and sutures around the vent; the best results are obtained when either external or internal colopexy is performed.

External colopexy

With the snake under general anaesthesia:

1. Use a pre-lubricated blunt probe to gently push the prolapsed tissue in an antegrade direction, making sure that the telescoped portion has been completely reduced inside the vent.
2. Place external colopexy sutures at the junction of the ventral and lateral scales, cranial to the vent.
3. After penetrating the skin, allow the suture needle to bounce off the probe before pushing it out through the skin.
4. Place several sutures bilaterally in a linear pattern, using an absorbable monofilament material such as polyglycolic acid or polydioxanone. The sutures are removed approximately 2 months later, or can be left *in situ* and allowed to slough.

Internal colopexy

Internal colopexy is indicated either when the cloaca is too swollen to reduce or there is a recurrence of prolapse from previous procedures. With the snake under general anaesthesia:

1. Make a coeliotomy incision (see below) at the junction of the ventral and lateral scales, several centimetres cranial to the vent.
2. Use traction to reduce the prolapse. Once reduced, anchor the colon around several ribs using polydioxanone.
3. Close as for coeliotomy.

Small meals can be offered 2–3 weeks following the procedure. If the prolapsed colonic tissue is necrotic, then resection and anastomosis must be performed. Treatment of a prolapsed oviduct consists of coeliotomy and salpingotomy, or removal of the devitalized oviduct (salpingectomy).

Coeliotomy and salpingotomy

The indications for coeliotomy are: to remove retained eggs (salpingotomy); to obtain incisional biopsy samples (internal organs); to obtain excisional biopsy samples (granulomas, tumours); to remove foreign bodies; and to facilitate intestinal resection and anastomosis.

1. After disinfection of the skin with 0.05% chlorhexidine, perform a line block with lidocaine or bupivacaine.
2. Make an incision between the first and second row of lateral scales above the retained egg(s).
3. Penetrate the muscle layer and coelomic membrane with the tip of a number 11 scalpel blade and continue incising with iris scissors.
4. Exteriorize the portion of the oviduct with the retained egg(s) and place stay sutures at each end of the intended incision.
5. Incise the oviduct and remove the egg(s) (Figure 16.34).
6. Close the oviduct with 1.5 metric (4/0 USP) polyglycolic acid suture material, using a simple continuous pattern.
7. Close the coelom by suturing the thin coelomic musculature and subcutaneous tissues with absorbable suture material, such as polydioxanone, in a simple continuous pattern.
8. Suture the skin with horizontal mattress sutures.
9. Keep the incision dry for 2 weeks. Remove the sutures after 4 weeks.

The snake should be allowed to rest for a year before being bred again.

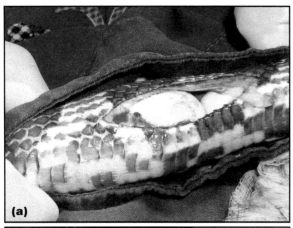

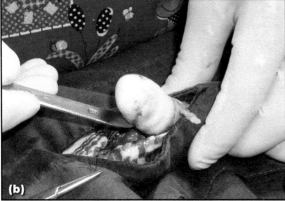

16.34 **(a)** A carbon dioxide laser has been used to incise the skin, muscle and oviduct to expose the retained eggs in a 100 flower ratsnake. Note the absence of haemorrhage when using the laser. **(b)** An exposed egg is gently lifted from the oviduct.

Euthanasia

It is the veterinary surgeon's responsibility to ensure that euthanasia of any pet is as painless as possible. Snakes are usually euthanased to terminate suffering due to acute physical injury or chronic disease. Most snakes presented to the veterinary surgeon are privately owned; accordingly, compassion and empathy must be communicated to the pet owner by the entire veterinary staff.

All snakes should be initially sedated with either ketamine or a combination of teletamine and zolazepam administered intramuscularly or intracoelomically. Thirty minutes later, euthanasia is achieved using pentobarbital sodium administered by an intravenous, intracardiac, intramuscular or intracoelomic route (see Figure 16.35). The latter two routes are effective but have a slower onset of action. Sedation of moribund snakes is usually not necessary. As all reptiles can tolerate prolonged periods of hypoxia, it can be difficult to determine the exact time of death. Accordingly, owners who are present at the time of euthanasia must be advised of this. For those clients who request the return of their pet following euthanasia, it is strongly recommended that the euthanased snake be kept an additional 24 hours at the hospital, whereupon the carcass is frozen after an ECG confirms cardiac arrest.

Necropsy

A knowledge of normal ophidian internal anatomy and gross appearance of organs is essential to performing a necropsy. The author recommends maintaining a series of gross photographs that can be referred to for reference. It should be noted that there are normal variations among taxa, such as degree of coelomic melanosis and proximity of the gallbladder, spleen and pancreas to each other. Reptiles, when cooled immediately after death to a temperature of 4°C, can be necropsied up to 5 days later.

To begin a necropsy, the snake is positioned in dorsal recumbency. Scissors are used to cut the body wall, beginning at one of the temporomandibular junctions and continuing caudally to the vent. In larger snakes, dissection through the extensive coelomic membranes can be a time-consuming process, which must be completed prior to visualization of the parenchymal organs. The next step is a systematic evaluation by organ system, accompanied by written observations and photographs. Tissue samples are then harvested for histopathology. Ribs can be submitted for bone marrow examination. Additional tissue samples should be stored in formalin. The carcass should be frozen until the laboratory results are known. If needed, additional testing such as immunohistochemistry can be undertaken using frozen tissue. Disposal of carcasses should comply with local legislation.

Drug formulary

A basic drug formulary for snakes is given in Figure 16.35.

Drug	Dose	Comments
Antimicrobial agents		
Amikacin	5 mg/kg i.m. loading dose then 2.5 mg i.m. q3d Ball python: 3.48 mg/kg i.m. once	Should be administered in front half of body due to nephrotoxicity; reptile must be properly hydrated; refrain from use in sedated animals due to neuroblocking effects
Amoxicillin	22 mg/kg orally q12–24h 10 mg/kg i.m. q24h	Can be used with aminoglycosides
Carbenicillin	200–400 mg/kg i.m. q24h	Good efficacy against *Pseudomonas* and anaerobes; should be administered in front half of body due to renal tubular excretion
Ceftazidime	20 mg/kg i.m. q3d	Good efficacy against *Pseudomonas* and anaerobes; can be used with aminoglycosides
Cefuroxime	100 mg/kg i.m. q24h	Good efficacy against *Pseudomonas* and anaerobes; can be used with aminoglycosides
Enrofloxacin	5–10 mg/kg i.m./orally q24h	May cause muscle necrosis due to high alkalinity
Metronidazole	Flagellated protozoa/amoebas: 100 mg/kg orally q2wks until negative for parasites Anaerobic bacteria: 20 mg/kg orally q48h	
Paromomycin	100 mg/kg orally q24h for 7 treatments; then twice weekly for 3 months	*Cryptosporidium* (long-term cure not proven); amoebas
Piperacillin	100 mg/kg i.m. q48h	Gram-negative, Gram-positive, aerobic and anaerobic bacteria
Silver sulfadiazine cream	Apply topically daily	Skin infections, third-degree burns
Antifungal agents		
Clotrimazole	Apply topically q24h	Fungal dermatopathy
Fluconazole	5 mg/kg orally q24h	Dermatophytosis
Itraconazole	5 mg/kg orally q24h	Systemic fungal infections
Ketoconazole	25 mg/kg orally q24h	Systemic fungal infections
Nystatin	100,000 IU/kg orally q24h for 7 treatments	Enteric fungal overgrowth
Antiparasitic agents		
Fenbendazole	100 mg/kg orally q2wks until negative faecal examination; better efficacy with same dosage divided over 3 days	Nematodes; cestodes; flagellates
Fipronil	0.29% topical spray Spray reptile; wipe with dampened gauze; wash off with water after 5 minutes; can be repeated in 7 days	Mites; ticks
Ivermectin	Nematodes/microfilariae: 200 µg/kg i.m. q2wks until negative for parasites Mites/ticks: 5 mg/0.95 l of water sprayed topically q1wk on snakes and enclosure for 8 treatments Ticks: 200 µg/kg i.m. once followed by manual removal of tick 24 hours later	Use with caution in indigo snakes (*Drymarchon* spp.)
Levamisole	10 mg/kg i.m. q2wks until negative for parasites	Nematodes; microfilariae; narrow margin of safety
Permethrin (10%)	Dilute to 1% in tap water; apply topically in well ventilated room. Repeat in 10 days if necessary	Mites
Ponazuril	30 mg/kg orally Repeat in 48 hours	Coccidians
Praziquantel	10 mg/kg orally/i.m. q2wks	Cestodes; trematodes
Sulfadimethoxine	90 mg/kg orally first dose; 45 mg/kg orally q24h for 1 week	Coccidians

16.35 Drug formulary for snakes. (continues) ▶

Drug	Dose	Comments
Analgesics/anaesthetics/sedatives		
Bupivacaine	1–2 mg/kg local infiltration q4–12h	Longer duration than lidocaine
Buprenorphine	0.02–0.20 mg/kg s.c./i.m. q12–24h	Opiod analgesic more potent than butorphanol
Butorphanol	0.5–1.0 mg/kg i.m./i.v. q12–24h	Opioid analgesic
Carprofen	1–5 mg/kg i.m./i.v./orally q24h	NSAID analgesic; proper hydration necessary
Isoflurane	Induction: 4–5% Maintenance: 1.5–2.5%	Mechanical ventilation is mandatory
Ketamine + Buprenorphine	10 mg/kg K + 0.02–0.20 mg/kg B i.m.	Mild sedation; facilitates intubation for gaseous anaesthesia
Ketamine + Butorphanol	10 mg/kg K + 0.5–1.0 mg/kg Bt i.m.	Mild sedation; facilitates intubation for gaseous anaesthesia
Ketamine + Medetomidine	5 mg/kg K + 100 µg/kg M in one syringe i.m	Light general anaesthetic; facilitates intubation for gaseous anaesthesia; reverse with atipamezole i.m. at 5 times the medetomidine dose
Lidocaine (2%)	5 mg/kg infiltration s.c.	Local anaesthetic
Meloxicam	0.1–0.2 mg/kg i.m./orally q24h	NSAID; analgesic
Propofol	5–10 mg/kg i.v./intracardiac	Short-acting anaesthetic; cardiopulmonary depression if injected too quickly
Tiletamine/Zolazepam	2–4 mg/kg i.m.	Induction of anaesthesia; facilitates intubation
Miscellaneous		
Adrenaline	0.02 ml/kg of 1:1000 concentration intracardiac/i.v.	Asystole
Allopurinol	20 mg/kg orally q24h	Gout (decreases uric acid production)
Aminophylline	2–4 mg/kg i.m. once	Bronchodilator
Atropine sulphate	0.1–0.2 mg/kg i.m. q24h	Organophosphate toxicity; bradycardia
Barium sulphate suspension	5 ml/kg orally	Gastrointestinal tract contrast study
Cimetidine	5 mg/kg i.m. q12h	Antacid; decreases phosphorus levels associated with renal disease
Cisapride	1 mg/kg orally q24h	Stimulates gastric motility
Dexamethasone	0.5–1 mg/kg i.m. q24h for up to 3 days	Anti-inflammatory
Diazepam	2.5 mg/kg i.m.	To control seizures
Doxapram	5–10 mg/kg i.v./i.m.	Respiratory stimulant
Erythropoietin	100 IU/kg i.m. q1wk	Bone marrow stimulant
Lactated Ringer's solution	10–25 ml/kg intracoelomic/s.c. q12–24h	Corrects dehydration
Metoclopramide	0.05 mg/kg orally q24h	Stimulates gastric motility
Oxytocin	20–40 IU/kg i.m./i.v. q12–24h	Oviductal stimulant for non-obstructive dystocia
Pentobarbital sodium	150 mg/kg i.v./intracardiac/i.m./intracoelomic	Euthanasia
Stanozolol	5 mg/kg i.m./orally q1wk	Anabolic steroid
Vitamin B complex	0.5 ml/kg i.m. q48h	Appetite stimulant; anaemia; liver disease
Vitamin B1 (thiamine)	25 mg/kg i.m. q24h 30 g/kg in food q24h	Thiamine deficiency; to offset diet high in thiaminase
Vitamin K1	0.5 mg/kg i.m. q24h	Liver disease; warfarin toxicity

16.35 (continued) Drug formulary for snakes.

References and further reading

Calvert I (2004) Nutritional problems. In: *BSAVA Manual of Reptiles, 2nd edn*, ed. SJ Girling and P Raiti, pp. 289–308. BSAVA, Gloucester

Cooper JE (2004) Humane euthanasia and post-mortem examination. In: *BSAVA Manual of Reptiles, 2nd edn*, ed. SJ Girling and P Raiti, pp. 168–183. BSAVA, Gloucester

Cranfield MR and Graczyk TK (2006) Cryptosporidiosis. In: *Reptile Medicine and Surgery*, ed. DR Mader, pp. 756–762. Saunders Elsevier, St. Louis

DeNardo D (2006) Dystocias. In: *Reptile Medicine and Surgery*, ed. DR Mader, pp. 787–792. Saunders Elsevier, St. Louis

Frank W (1984) Non-hemoparasitic protozoans. In: *Diseases of Amphibians and Reptiles*, ed. GL Hoff, FL Frye and ER Jacobson, pp. 259–384. Plenum Press, New York

Frye FL (1981) Parasitology. In: *Biomedical and Surgical Aspects of Captive Reptile Husbandry*, ed. FL Frye, pp. 305–312. Krieger Publishing Co. Inc., Malabar

Funk RS and Diethelm G (2006) Reptile formulary. In: *Reptile Medicine and Surgery*, ed. DR Mader, pp. 1119–1146. Saunders Elsevier, St. Louis

Garner MM (2006) Overview of biopsy and necropsy techniques. In: *Reptile Medicine and Surgery*, ed. DR Mader, pp. 569–580. Saunders Elsevier, St. Louis

Girling SJ and Raiti P (2004) *BSAVA Manual of Reptiles, 2nd edn*. BSAVA Publications, Gloucester

Heard D, Harr K and Wellehan J (2004) Diagnostic sampling and laboratory tests. In: *BSAVA Manual of Reptiles, 2nd edn*, ed. SJ Girling and P Raiti, pp. 71–86. BSAVA, Gloucester

Hernandez-Divers SJ (2004a) Diagnostic and surgical endoscopy. In: *BSAVA Manual of Reptiles, 2nd edn*, ed. SJ Girling and P Raiti, pp. 103–114. BSAVA, Gloucester

Hernandez-Divers SJ (2004b) Surgery: principles and techniques. In: *BSAVA Manual of Reptiles, 2nd edn*, ed. SJ Girling and P Raiti, pp. 147–167. BSAVA, Gloucester

International Species Information System (2002) *Reference physiological values of the corn snake and royal python*. Apple Valley, Minnesota

Jacobson ER, Gaskin JM, Wells S, *et al.* (1992) Epizootic of ophidian paramyxovirus in a zoological collection: pathological, microbiological and serological findings. *Journal of Zoo and Wildlife Medicine* **23**, 318–327

Jacobson ER (2007) *Infectious Disease and Pathology of Reptiles*. CRC Press Taylor & Francis Group, Boca Raton,

Keeble E (2004) Neurology. In: *BSAVA Manual of Reptiles, 2nd edn*, ed. SJ Girling and P Raiti, pp. 289–308. BSAVA, Gloucester

Mader DR (2006) Acariasis. In: *Reptile Medicine and Surgery*, ed. DR Mader, pp. 720–738. Saunders Elsevier, St. Louis

Mader DR (2006) Euthanasia. In: *Reptile Medicine and Surgery*, ed. DR Mader, pp. 564–568. Saunders Elsevier, St. Louis

Marschang RE and Chitty J (2004) Infectious diseases. In: *BSAVA Manual of Reptiles, 2nd edn*, ed. SJ Girling and P Raiti, pp. 330–345. BSAVA, Gloucester

Mattison C (1990) *A–Z of Snake Keeping*. Sterling Publishing Co. Inc., New York

Micinilio J (1996) Ivermectin for the treatment of pentastomids in a tokay gecko (*Gekko gecko*). *Bulletin of the Association of Reptilian and Amphibian Veterinarians* **6**(2), 4

Raftery A (2004) Clinical examination. In: *BSAVA Manual of Reptiles, 2nd edn*, ed. SJ Girling and P Raiti, pp. 51–62. BSAVA, Gloucester

Raiti P (2002) Snakes In: *BSAVA Manual of Exotic Pets, 4th edn*, ed. A Meredith and S Redrobe, pp. 241–256. BSAVA, Gloucester

Raiti P (2004) Non-invasive imaging. In: *BSAVA Manual of Reptiles, 2nd edn*, ed. SJ Girling and P Raiti, pp. 87–102. BSAVA, Gloucester

Redrobe S (2004) Anaesthesia and analgesia. In: *BSAVA Manual of Reptiles, 2nd edn*, ed. SJ Girling and P Raiti, pp. 131–146. BSAVA, Gloucester

Schumacher J (1996) Viral diseases. In: *Reptile Medicine and Surgery*, ed. DR Mader, pp. 224–234. Saunders Elsevier, St. Louis

Schumacher J, Jacobson ER, Homer BL, *et al.* (1994) Inclusion body disease in boid snakes. *Journal of Zoo and Wildlife Medicine* **25**, 511–524

Schumacher J and Yelen T (2006) Anesthesia and analgesia. In: *Reptile Medicine and Surgery*, ed. DR Mader, pp. 442–452. Saunders Elsevier, St. Louis

Varga M (2004) Captive maintenance and welfare. In: *BSAVA Manual of Reptiles, 2nd edn*, ed. SJ Girling and P Raiti, pp. 6–17. BSAVA, Gloucester

17

Frogs and toads

Tracy D. Bennett

Introduction

Frogs and toads constitute the Order Anura, which is the largest order of the Class Amphibia and comprises over 4000 species. The designation of 'frog' or 'toad' is somewhat artificial and, in general, only members of the family Bufonidae are correctly referred to as toads. However, the designation 'toad' is usually applied to those species perceived to have thick or textured skin. Anurans are distinguished anatomically from other amphibians by the absence of a tail and the presence of long back legs designed for jumping. All anurans secrete substances from their skin which are potentially toxic or irritating, though toxicity varies greatly from species to species. Frogs and toads are popular in the pet trade and also important from an ecological perspective. Amphibians have been recognized as an important environmental indicator and their numbers are declining worldwide. Species commonly kept as pets are illustrated in Figure 17.1.

Biology

Amphibians are ectothermic, and thus biological parameters are difficult to define for most species.

Amphibians in general need to be kept within their preferred optimal temperature zone (POTZ) (see Figure 17.2). Animals kept at temperatures above their POTZ may show inappetence, weight loss, immunosuppression, agitation and changes to skin colour. Those kept below the POTZ may show lethargy and inappetence, may become immunocompromised, and may develop abdominal bloating due to bacterial overgrowth from poorly digested food within the gastrointestinal tract. They will also have poor growth rates.

Frogs and toads develop via metamorphosis from egg to larvae (tadpole) to adult. Most adults live in terrestrial habitats but return to the water to mate and lay their eggs. Some frogs lay eggs in moist terrestrial sites where the larval stages develop in the egg and the young emerge fully formed; this direct development circumvents the free-living tadpole (larval) stage.

Anatomy and physiology

Anurans, like all amphibians, can absorb water and other aqueous substances through their permeable non-keratinized skin. The permeability of their skin is a major factor affecting their husbandry and

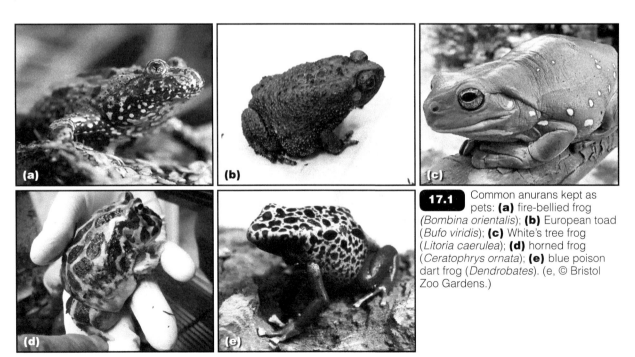

17.1 Common anurans kept as pets: **(a)** fire-bellied frog (*Bombina orientalis*); **(b)** European toad (*Bufo viridis*); **(c)** White's tree frog (*Litoria caerulea*); **(d)** horned frog (*Ceratophrys ornata*); **(e)** blue poison dart frog (*Dendrobates*). (e, © Bristol Zoo Gardens.)

also their susceptibility to pollutants in the wild. Fluid absorbed through the skin can flow directly into the lymphatic system. Lymph is circulated via a variable number of 'lymph hearts', and flows independently of the cardiovascular system. Frogs and toads have a three-chambered heart, with one common ventricle.

Anurans can utilize three different forms of respiration: cutaneous; buccopharyngeal; and pulmonic. The extent to which each system is used depends on the species. Anurans are carnivorous and possess a short gastrointestinal tract. The urinary system in some species has become adapted to aquatic environments and nitrogenous wastes are excreted directly into the water; more terrestrial species have urea or uric acid as their major metabolic waste product.

Sexing

Sexual dimorphism is common in anurans but specific characteristics vary widely between species (see Figure 17.2). One commonly observed feature is the presence of 'nuptial pads' on the feet and forearms of males while they are in breeding condition. Vocalization and size can also be an indicator of gender. In many species the male will 'call' in an attempt to attract a mate.

Husbandry

Figure 17.2 summarizes the lifestyle, housing and dietary requirements for the commonly kept pet species.

Species	Preferred optimal temperature zone (POTZ) (°C)	Adult size/ weight	Lifestyle and housing requirements	Diet	Gender determination	Comments
White's tree frog (*Litoria caerulea*)	24–29	100 mm	Nocturnal and arboreal, and require access to shallow water in a moist terrarium	Crickets (gut-loaded) and other invertebrates 2–3 times per week	Males have 'nuptial pads' on forelimbs and call during breeding season. Males smaller than females	Wide variation in coloration from green to rust-coloured, bluish or brown
Horned frog (Pacman frog, *Ceratophrys ornata*)	23–30	Males: 10 cm Females: 14 cm Both species prone to obesity	Tropical. Require leaf litter and hide areas for cover, with access to shallow water in a moist terrarium	Crickets (gut-loaded), earthworms, silkworms and other invertebrates as primary diet. Fish or small pre-killed rodents once a month	Males often have dark pigment over ventral cervical area. Males smaller than females and call during breeding season	Voracious feeders, sometimes mistaking caregiver's finger for food. Will eat inappropriate objects
Leopard frog (*Rana pipiens*), Bullfrog (*R. catesbiana*), European common frog (*R. temporaria*) and other *Rana* species	20–25	Leopard frog: males 25–42 g; females 25–46 g Bullfrog: 225–306 g	Arboreal and require access to shallow water in moist terrarium. Leopard frog native to North America; does well at lower temperature range	Crickets (gut-loaded) and other invertebrates	Females larger than males	European common frog inhabits temperate climes and hibernates during the winter
Poison dart frogs (*Dendrobates* spp.)	22–28	15–75 mm snout to vent	Tropical. Arboreal and diurnal, requiring access to shallow water. Humidity 70–100%. Can be housed as 1 male to 1–2 females	Gut-loaded small crickets, wingless fruit flies, springtails and other invertebrates	Male exhibits calling behaviour	May live 6–10 years in captivity. May be illegal to own in some localities. **Handle with gloves;** poison only dangerous if ingested or introduced into the bloodstream
African clawed frog (*Xenopus laevis*)	20–22	10 cm	Tropical. Fully aquatic, requiring water 10–20 cm deep. Also require a platform in shallow water to rest	Commercial aquatic frog diets, brine shrimp, *Tubifex* worms, bloodworms and other invertebrates. Commercial diets are not complete and should only constitute a portion of the diet. Usually fed twice a week. Tadpoles will feed on suspended food particles	Black nuptial pads on males while in breeding condition. Females much larger, with developed anal papillae	Do not possess a tongue or eyelids

17.2 Biological data and husbandry information for commonly kept pet species. (continues) ▶

Species	Preferred optimal temperature zone (POTZ) (°C)	Adult size/ weight	Lifestyle and housing requirements	Diet	Gender determination	Comments
True toads (*Bufo* spp.)	Varies with species. *Bufo bufo* (European common toad): 20–23)	Varies with species	Nocturnal. Temperate to tropical, depending on species. Terrestrial but require access to shallow water. Most need large vivarium, deep leaf litter, high humidity. Breeding pair of *B. bufo* and offspring need at least a 100 litre vivarium	Gut-loaded crickets and other invertebrates	Black nuptial pads on first three fingers of males. Croak only exhibited by males	Do not have teeth. Secrete bufotoxin
Fire-bellied frog (*Bombina orientalis*)	18–24	Approximately 5 cm	Temperate and diurnal. Require access to shallow water in moist terrarium	Crickets (gut-loaded) and other invertebrates 2–3 times per week	Males have small bumps on first two digits. Males call and are smaller than females	Brightly coloured, with red ventrum. Secrete irritating and toxic substance and should not be handled directly. Breeds readily in captivity

17.2 (continued) Biological data and husbandry information for commonly kept pet species.

Housing

Most pets are kept as solitary animals, as size differences may prevent smaller animals from feeding. In breeding situations, males and females need to be housed together, although adults should then be removed from the tank where the eggs were laid. Different species should not be housed together at any time.

Semi-aquatic species

A vivarium can be constructed using a glass or plastic aquarium. The tank should be smooth and easily cleaned and free of toxic glues or other chemicals. A tight-fitting screened lid prevents escape and allows ventilation. Coconut fibre is a good substrate for many species and orchid bark can be mixed in to improve drainage. Placing a layer of smooth stones below the mulch layer will also improve drainage but care must be taken to avoid objects that are small enough to be ingested.

A dish of water large enough for whole body immersion should always be available. The water needs to be shallow enough to allow the head to be held easily above the waterline.

Hide areas are important for all anurans. Arboreal species prefer tree branches and leaves for camouflage; ground-dwelling species need leaf litter or sphagnum moss to allow camouflage on the cage floor. All species need hide boxes that are easy to clean and lightweight (to prevent damage to the animal should the cage contents shift). Living non-toxic plants enhance the terrarium but must be placed in small pots for easy removal during cage cleaning (Figure 17.3).

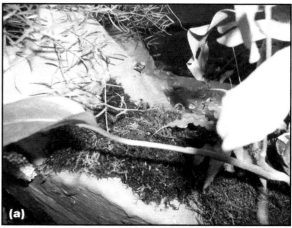

(a)

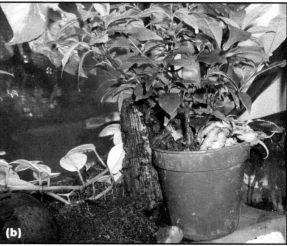

(b)

17.3 Enclosures for small anurans. (© Bristol Zoo Gardens.)

Aquatic species

A water-filled tank should be provided, with a layer of gravel large enough to prevent ingestion. Shallow areas are essential to allow extension of the head or nares above the water. Hide areas are also required in fully aquatic enclosures. Water plants can be included but care must be taken to avoid introduction of snails or parasites that may be present on the plant. Most commonly kept species prefer stagnant water and become stressed if the water has any current.

Water quality

All anurans must have constant provision of water. Care must be taken to ensure that clean, natural water is used: de-ionized or distilled water should not be used as these can disturb the osmotic balance of the animal. The usual method of water preparation is to aerate tap water for 24–48 hours to remove added chlorine prior to introduction into the tank. Spring water can also be used. Water filters are not recommended. **Water 'conditioners' and other water additives used for fish are often toxic to anurans.**

Water provided in a bowl should be changed daily. For fully aquatic individuals the water needs to be changed two or three times a week.

Heat and lighting

A temperature gradient is necessary for all ectotherms and is specific to each species (see Figure 17.2). For a terrarium a ceramic heat emitter should be placed above the screen top at one end of the enclosure. The heat emitter needs to be far enough away from the highest basking site in the cage to prevent thermal burns. Aquatic frogs must have a water heater in the tank, which should be protected so that the frog cannot directly come in contact with it. Direct contact with any heating devise can cause thermal burns. At least two thermometers need to be present to measure the temperature gradient between the warmest and coolest portions of the enclosure.

A hygrometer is also essential to ensure that humidity stays in the recommended range. A minimum relative humidity (RH) of 70% is required for most species. A full-spectrum ultraviolet (UV) lamp that includes UV-B is generally recommended to provide a regular photoperiod and allow vitamin D production in the skin. The lamp must produce an adequate amount of UV-B radiation (280–320 nm) and should be placed within 45 cm of the primary resting place of the anuran. Additionally, UV-B lamps need to be replaced every 3–6 months as the UV-B emitted declines over time.

Most anurans do well with a 12-hour day/night photoperiod. Nocturnal animals should have a 'night light' to allow feeding and ambulation during their active period.

Diet

Adults

All adult anurans are insectivorous, with some species also adapted to ingesting vertebrate prey (see Figure 17.2). Crickets are the most widely available invertebrate feed in the pet trade. Crickets should be gut-loaded with a mineral and vitamin supplement prior to being fed to the anuran, as they contain an inverse Ca:P ratio and are fairly nutrient-poor. A comparative study of commercial gut-loading formulas found only one brand provided adequate calcium content (Finke *et al.*, 2005). Prey items with a naturally high calcium content are phoenix worms (*Hermetia illucens*) and silkworms (*Bombyx mori*). Other acceptable invertebrate prey includes springtails (Collembola), wingless fruit flies (*Drosophila*), earthworms and redworms (*Eisenia foetida*). More carnivorous anurans, such as horned frogs (*Ceratophrys* spp.) and cane toads (*Bufo marinus*), can be offered occasional vertebrate prey such as rodents and fish; frozen fish should be supplemented with thiamine if offered on a regular basis as they contain thiaminase and can cause thiamine deficiency. Aquatic frogs do well on a combination of invertebrates and commercial turtle foods, consumed in the water.

Tadpoles

Many tadpoles will feed on the filamentous algae that grow 'spontaneously' in a tub of dechlorinated fresh water left in the sunlight. Boiled dark greens may be substituted for algae in the short term. Vitamin C is essential in tadpole diets, and should be adequate unless fed a dried, commercial diet. Thirty percent (dry weight) protein will give optimal weight gain. Tadpoles should be fed several times a day or they may cannibalize each other. Feeding is stopped as the legs emerge and the mouth widens during metamorphosis.

Breeding

Female receptivity is induced by male courtship glands on the chin (mental glands) or side of the head (genial glands). They are highly vocal during courtship. Anurans fertilize their eggs externally, with males ejaculating on eggs extruded from the females. The male will clasp the female during mating, a process known as amplexus.

In most species, the eggs hatch into larvae (tadpoles) which then metamorphose into adults: the tail is lost gradually as the body shortens and limbs grow and lengthen. The external gills are resorbed and lungs develop internally.

Handling and restraint

Anurans are easily stressed and should be handled very carefully to avoid damaging their sensitive skin. Handling time should be minimized and observations recorded prior to restraint as much as possible. Non-powdered gloves moistened with dechlorinated or spring water prevent introduction of contaminants from human skin. Small anurans can be picked up initially using cupped hands to remove them from their container. For restraint during direct examination, the patient can be held gently with two fingers behind the ramus of the lower mandible, anterior to the forelimbs with the body cupped in the palm of the hand. This method allows easy examination of the ventrum and caudal portion of the body. To examine the dorsum and cervical area the patient can be grasped around the hindlimbs, restricting forward movement (Figure 17.4).

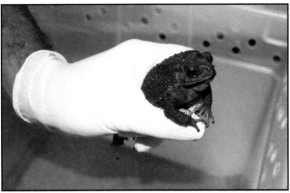

17.4 Restraint of a toad with the rear legs immobilized. Note the rinsed latex gloves used for handling.

Diagnostic approach

- Ask the client to bring some of the water from the tank or terrarium. A water test kit should be available to test this sample. Water test kits suitable for home aquaria are adequate.
- Have spring water or physiological saline available to rinse instruments prior to use.
- A heat pad should be available for sick or chilled patients.
- Clean gloves should be worn that have been rinsed in dechlorinated or spring water.
- The skin of frogs can dry out quickly, so a spray bottle filled with chlorine-free water should be available for frequent misting.
- Most anurans are slippery and agile, so the examination room should be checked for any small holes (heater vents, etc.) from which they might escape.
- A gram scale with an accuracy of 1 g or less is essential. Weights are most easily obtained by weighing the patient in its container and then weighing the empty container while the patient is being physically examined, subtracting the second weight from the first.
- If gentle digital pressure is unsuccessful, a soft rubber spatula can be used gently to examine the mouth (Figure 17.5).
- A 7.5–8 MHz Doppler probe with water-soluble gel should be on hand to evaluate the heart.

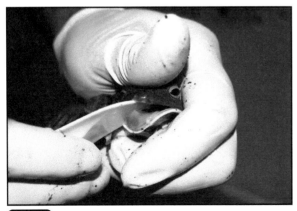

17.5 Oral examination using a soft rubber spatula.

History

A thorough history is very important, including all husbandry practices.

Clinical examination

Figure 17.6 outlines the components of a thorough anuran physical examination.

Neurological considerations
Is the animal alert and aware of its surroundings? Normal posture is upright with legs folded naturally under the body Rapid withdrawal of limbs when extended manually Menace response
Skin
In most frogs the skin should appear uniformly moist No ulcerations, erythema or areas of haemorrhage should be evident Pigmentation is roughly symmetrical and typical of the species
Musculoskeletal system
Good muscle tone should be exhibited The long bones and jaw should be firm and symmetrical The pelvic and other bones should be well fleshed and not protruding
Oral cavity
The oral cavity and tongue (where present) should be evaluated for colour and presence of swellings, ulcerations or foreign bodies
Eyes
Use an ophthalmoscope or transilluminator to reveal any corneal or lenticular opacities Pupillary light reflex is unreliable, as iris contains skeletal muscle and is under voluntary control Examine the globes for buphthalmus and asymmetry Semi-aquatic frogs and toads have eyelids that should be clear and free of swellings or erythema (aquatic frogs lack eyelids)
Cardiovascular system
The mucous membranes of the mouth should be moist and pink in species with non-pigmented oral tissues A Doppler probe can be placed under the sternum to evaluate heart sounds and rate The heart beat can sometimes be observed in the area of the xiphoid process
Respiratory system
Respiration is primarily evaluated by observing movement in the submandibular space Breathing is often rapid but should be regular, with the mouth closed Nares should be open and clear
Urogenital system
Many anurans will urinate when handled, allowing sample collection and visual inspection of the urine The bladder can sometimes be palpated in the caudal coelom Sexually dimorphic characteristics should be noted, such as the presence of nuptial pads The cloaca should be examined for erythema, swelling, discharge or prolapse

17.6 Physical examination.

Imaging

Radiography

Many anurans are small, with indistinct internal structures necessitating high-detail radiography. Rare earth screens along with mammography film provide excellent detail and fast exposure times. A small focal spot improves radiographic quality in these patients and a dental machine with a mobile tube is ideal for this purpose. The patient can be placed in a clear container such as a plastic bag or box to minimize restraint (Figure 17.7ab).

- Many anurans will briefly sit directly on the film cassette without restraint to give a dorsoventral (DV) view.
- If the X-ray machine is mobile, the patient can be placed on a table with the cassette behind the lateral aspect of the body and the beam centred on the area of interest in the horizontal plane.
- A mobile X-ray machine allows other views such as anterioposterior (AP) to be taken with little restraint.
- If the X-ray machine is fixed, and the patient is not overly stressed, it may be laid on the plate with limbs extended using gauze bandage material looped over the wrists and ankles, and taped to the plate to achieve a lateral view. Tape should not be applied directly to the anuran's skin. If manual restraint (Figure 17.7c) is required, the Ionising Radiation Regulations 1999 should be followed. Alternatively, the anuran can be sedated for this view.

The lungs and skeletal structure are well visualized (Figure 17.8). The coelom exhibits poor detail and radiography is most useful to rule out foreign bodies or large masses.

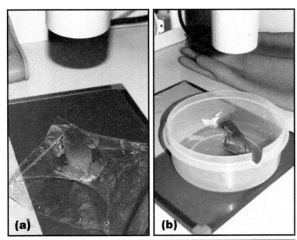

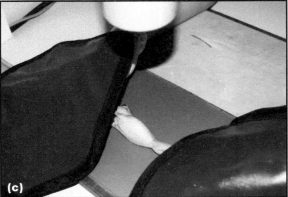

17.7 Radiography of anurans. A transparent plastic bag **(a)** or container **(b)** can be used for minimal restraint. **(c)** Positioning for a lateral view.

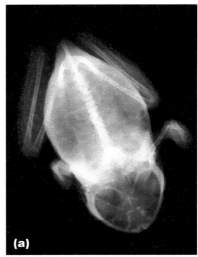

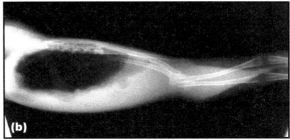

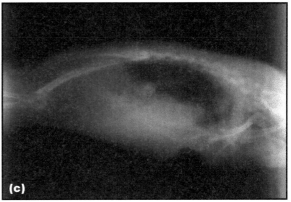

17.8 **(a)** DV view of a normal anuran obtained with a dental machine. **(b)** Lateral view of a normal White's tree frog. **(c)** Pneumonia in a bullfrog. (c, Courtesy of B. Levine.)

Ultrasonography

Given the difficulty of visualizing the coelom with radiography, ultrasonography is very useful for imaging anurans. Sound waves easily penetrate the moist skin and the patient can be placed into shallow water during the procedure to further improve the image. A high-frequency probe is ideal, in the range 7.5–8 MHz. Either microconvex (Figure 17.9a) or linear transducers are effective. Water-based coupling gel can be used and there are no reported toxicities. Amphibians do not have a compartmentalized coelomic cavity and do not possess a diaphragm. Patients are usually placed in dorsal recumbency, which simplifies imaging but can be stressful to the patient. For a debilitated or stressed patient imaging can be accomplished in a plastic container with a small amount of water (Figure 17.9b). The probe can be placed on the bottom of the container with coupling gel and imaging accomplished without restraint of the patient (Schildger and Triet, 2001). Anechoic fluid is sometime visible in the coelomic cavity and represents a normal finding that assists imaging.

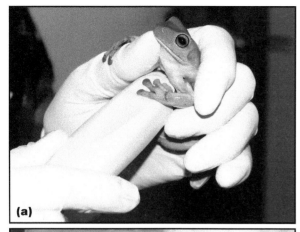

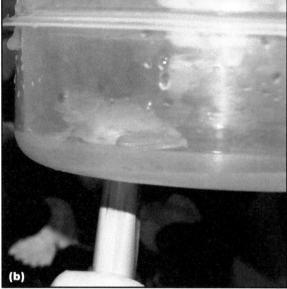

17.9 Ultrasonography of anurans. **(a)** Using a 5 MHz convex probe on a White's tree frog will show the beating heart and the presence of eggs, but a higher frequency probe (e.g. 7.5–8 MHz) will give far better diagnostic detail. **(b)** A transparent container with a small amount of gel for the anuran to sit on, as well as gel on the probe on the other side of the container, allows minimal restraint for stressed or debilitated patients for a quick assessment of the coelomic cavity.

- The midline vein over the ventral coelom is often visible and can be accessed with a small-gauge needle.

Using either of these sites the clinician can attempt to collect blood into a syringe or, with the syringe removed, directly from the hub of the needle into a microhaematocrit tube. In both cases pressure should be applied after venepuncture with a sterile swab.

If blood collection is essential and other methods unavailable, the patient can be sedated and blood drawn directly from the ventricle of the heart. If this method is chosen, visualization can be improved by ultrasonography, passing a light source, such as an endoscope, into the stomach or by using an ophthalmic transilluminator. The needle is inserted into the distal aspect of the ventricle and allowed to fill with the natural beat of the heart.

Slides of whole blood should be made prior to placement in the collection tube. Blood samples should be placed in lithium heparin for analysis, as EDTA causes lysis of amphibian red blood cells. The interpretation of amphibian blood values must be undertaken with care, as many factors are known to affect results. Such factors include the time of year, the gender and reproductive status of the animal, the sampling method and the health status of the patient, as well as body temperature. Very few normal values have been validated (Figure 17.10).

Cytology and histology
One of the most useful diagnostic methods in amphibian medicine is cytology or histology of dermal lesions. Since dermatoses are common, and metabolic disease often manifests dermatologically, sampling skin lesions is very rewarding. Cytology can be performed on impression or swab smears. Wright's–Giemsa, Ziehl–Neelson and Gram stains are most commonly used.

Culture and sensitivity testing
This is another useful, relatively non-invasive, technique that often achieves good results due to the prevalence of bacterial infections in amphibians. Aerobic, anaerobic and fungal culture should be considered. Sensitivity testing allows the clinician to choose appropriate antibiotic therapy. A sterile mini-tip culturette swab is used to take samples from lesions.

Faecal examination
Many parasites are easily detected by direct microscopic examination of a faecal wet mount. Faecal flotation should also be performed.

Blood sampling
Blood collection can be difficult as many patients are very small. A volume of 1% of the patient's bodyweight can be removed safely from a healthy animal.

- In some patients the most accessible route of blood collection is the **venous** sinus just ventral to the tongue.

Parameter	Leopard frogs	Bullfrogs	European common frogs	*Xenopus* sp.
PCV (%)	16–52	39–52	No data	No data
RBC (x10³/μl)	174–701	450	461	566
Hb (g/dl)	2.7–14.6	9.3–9.7	14.34	14.9
WBC (x10³/μl)	2.8–25.9	No data	14.4	8.2

17.10 Haematological reference ranges for selected species. Values vary with sex, season and stage of development, as well as body temperature.

Common conditions

Figure 17.11 outlines common clinical presentations in anurans, their possible causes, diagnostics and treatment.

Infectious diseases

Viral infections

Iridoviruses of the genus *Ranavirus* have been extensively studied as a cause of disease in wild populations of anurans. They are associated with high mortality, particularly in tadpoles and individuals undergoing metamorphosis. Adults can act as asymptomatic carriers. Diagnosis is accomplished through histology, electron microscopy and PCR. An oncogenic herpesvirus has been documented in leopard frogs (*Rana pipiens*).

Bacterial infections

Many bacteria are part of the normal flora but can become pathogenic if immunosuppression or injury occurs. Immunosuppression generally results from poor husbandry and diet. Examples of potentially pathogenic bacteria include *Aeromonas, Pseudomonas* and *Escherichia coli. Aeromonas* is an organism that thrives in an aquatic environment and is frequently cultured in high numbers from sick anurans. The classic appearance of an anuran suffering from bacterial septicaemia is ventral erythema and petechial haemorrhage, commonly called 'red-leg' (Figure 17.13). Many other clinical signs may be associated with bacterial disease such as anorexia, lethargy, ataxia and coelomic effusion. *Chlamydophila* and *Mycobacterium* are also sometimes identified on histology. *Chlamydophila* causes clinical signs similar to other bacterial pathogens and can be treated with doxycycline; PCR tests are available to detect the organism. *Mycobacterium* spp. usually cause granulomatous disease similar to that in other species and is considered **zoonotic**.

Fungal infections

The most significant fungal pathogen of anurans is *Batrachochytrium dendrobatidis,* the causative agent of chytridiomycosis. This organism is not only a

Clinical presentation	Possible causes	Diagnostics	Treatment
Cloacal/intestinal prolapse	Parasitism; foreign body; coelomic mass; bacterial enteritis	Faecal flotation and direct smear; culture; cytology; biopsy; radiography/ ultrasonography	Reduce prolapse. Antiparasitics. Antibiotics. Endoscopic surgery
Coelomic distension	Renal disease; cardiac or lymphatic disease; liver disease; retained ovum; neoplasia; bacterial coelomitis	Palpation; fluid aspirate and cytology; culture and sensitivity; ultrasonography/ radiology; haematology; endoscopy	Antimicrobials. Surgical removal of mass. Supportive care for organ failure
Corneal disease (Figure 17.12)	Excessive dietary fat; trauma; infection	Fluorescein staining; cytology; culture; serum cholesterol; biopsy	Topical antibiotics. Dietary adjustment
Dermatitis	Chytrid fungus (*Batrachochytrium dendrobatidis*); bacteria (*Mycobacterium, Chlamydophila*); parasites; toxins; trauma	Wet mount of skin scrape; Gram stain of impression smears; culture; exploration of any dermal swellings, pustules or nodules; biopsy	Antifungals. Antibiotics. Manual removal of external parasites. Husbandry correction
'Red-leg': dermal erythema or ulcerations (see Figure 17.13)	Bacteria (e.g. *Aeromonas, Pseudomonas*); chytridiomycosis; trauma (chemical or thermal burns); enviromental (over-oxygenation)	History; culture; skin cytology and wet mount	Antibiotics. Antifungals. Improve water quality. Correct husbandry

17.11 Common medical conditions of anuran amphibians, based on clinical appearance.

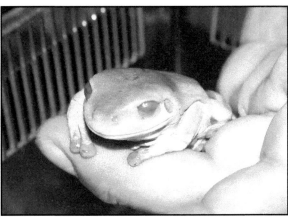

17.12 Corneal oedema in a White's tree frog. The cause was determined to be bacterial and the patient responded to topical antibiotics.

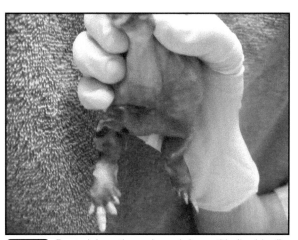

17.13 Bacterial septicaemia and dermatitis ('red-leg') in a frog. (Courtesy of A. Lennox.)

concern for pet anurans but is a major pathogen of wild amphibians. It appears to be a primary pathogen capable of infecting otherwise healthy individuals. Transmission occurs by contact with infected individuals, contaminated water, or through human or mechanical vectors. Clinical signs include dermal erythema, ulcerations and sloughing of the skin. Systemic signs, such as lethargy, anorexia, oedema and ataxia, are also common. The fungus can also lead to secondary bacterial infections and should be considered in cases of 'red-leg'. Diagnosis in severe infection can sometimes be made by microscopic examination of sloughed skin or skin scrapings, the organism appearing as a flagellated zoospore on a wet mount. More often diagnosis is made with histology or PCR. Treatment is possible with a 0.01% solution of itraconazole used as a daily bath for 11 days (Wright, 2005a).

Other fungal infections, such as chromomycosis and basidiobolomycosis, can cause dermatological lesions and high mortality. Saprolegniasis, caused by water moulds, is an opportunistic infection in susceptible individuals and appears as a cottony white substance over dermal ulcerations; the characteristic appearance and microscopic detection of hyphae are diagnostic. Treatment with malachite green, benzalkonium chloride and sea salt baths have been reported to be successful (Pessier, 2005).

Parasites

A wide variety of parasites is found in anurans, and parasitism is extremely common. In all cases, isolation and hygiene are required to prevent re-infection. Antiparasitic drugs may be oral or topical, depending on the parasite in question.

Ciliate protozoans are often part of the normal flora but if the patient is clinically ill or very high numbers are present treatment is suggested with tetracycline or paromomycin. *Entamoeba ranarum* is a significant pathogen of anurans and causes general unthriftiness. Differentiation from commensal amoeba species is difficult. Treatment with metronidazole is suggested when faecal amoebiasis is present in conjunction with clinical signs.

Nematodes of all types are present in anurans. A significant nematode pathogen is the lungworm *Rhabdias,* which can cause significant pathology to the respiratory tract; ante-mortem diagnosis is by observation of larvae or embryonated ova in a faecal or oral smear.

Cutaneous nematodes, trematodes, protozoans and cestodes have been reported. Dermal cysts may contain worms (Figure 17.14), which can be removed through a small incision.

Nutritional disease

Hypovitaminosis A and nutritional secondary hyperparathyroidism (NSHP; Figure 17.15) are the most common nutritional disorders recognized in amphibians. The cause of NSHP in amphibians is thought to be a lack of total calcium in the diet, and diets containing an inverse Ca:P ratio. The lack of UV-B (280–320 nm) radiation is thought to play a part, since hypovitaminosis D can then develop, preventing

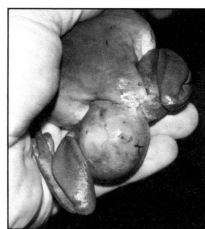

17.14 Tapeworm cysts in a White's tree frog. (Courtesy of B. Levine.)

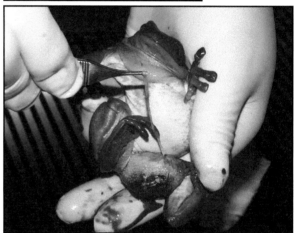

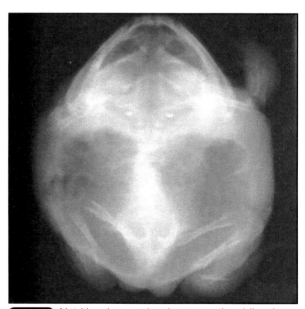

17.15 Nutritional secondary hyperparathyroidism in a horned frog. Note the deformities of the cortices of the long bones, including the pathological fracture in the extended forelimb. There is poor definition of the pelvis. (Courtesy of M. Conn.)

absorption of calcium from the gut. Clinical signs are similar to those seen in lizards, i.e. tetany, and deformity of the long bones and jaw. Pathological fractures are common. Treatment involves dietary correction and calcium supplementation.

Hypovitaminosis A has been recently identified as a significant problem in captive anurans. Squamous metaplasia of the lingual mucous glands prevents affected individuals from feeding, as the tongue cannot adhere to the prey item. Other signs such as conjunctival swellings, immunosuppression and gastrointestinal bloat have been reported. Successful treatment with a liquid vitamin A supplement administered topically every 3 days has been described (Fleming and Valdes, 2008).

Neoplasia

Many neoplasms have been reported in anurans, with most occurring in the coelom or cutaneously (Figure 17.16). Masses in the coelomic cavity often cause coelomic effusion and can be confused with other causes of this sign. Cutaneous masses can be removed surgically but internal neoplasms usually carry a poor prognosis.

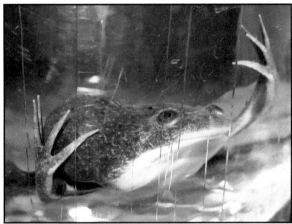

17.16 Neoplastic mass in an African clawed frog. (Courtesy of M. Kramer.)

Supportive care

Many anurans are presented to the clinician with long-standing and advanced illness. In cases where hospitalization is necessary, supportive care is essential to stabilize the patient until diagnostics can be performed.

Hospital accommodation

The patient should be placed in a temperature- and humidity-controlled enclosure suitable for the species and the condition of the patient: a plastic or glass aquarium tank, with an attached thermometer and hygrometer, works well for this purpose. Ill patients should be kept at their POTZ. Moist paper towels are generally used to ensure that the patient does not desiccate. The tank should be designed so that it can be connected to a continuous flow of humidified oxygen if the patient is in shock or respiratory distress. The tank can be heated with an under-tank heating pad or can be placed in a temperature-controlled room if it achieves adequate temperatures. Many incubators with heaters and temperature gauges built in are commercially available.

Drug administration

Medicines can be given by a variety of routes:

- Oral: the mouth can be gently opened with a rubber spatula (see Figure 17.5), plastic card or mouth speculum
- Topical: drugs are delivered in a bath filled to a level where the patient can hold its head easily above the water
- Subcutaneous: anurans have loose skin that allows easy administration into the dorsal area over the shoulders. Caution must be used not to tear the fragile skin
- Intramuscular: injections can be made into the limbs. If the musculature allows, the front limb is preferred (Figure 17.17a), as the effect of the renal portal system is unknown
- Intracoelomic: using the caudal lateral space just cranial to the hindlimbs (Figure 17.17b)
- Intravenous: catheterization is difficult but can be performed through the femoral or midline abdominal vein in large species
- Intralymphatic: medication can be introduced via injection into the dorsal lymph sacs (Figure 17.17c) with good results.

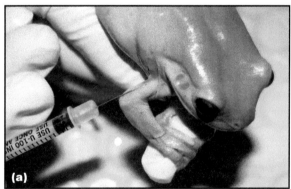

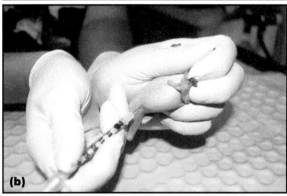

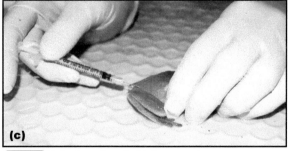

17.17 Injection sites. **(a)** Intramuscular. **(b)** Intracoelomic. **(c)** Dorsal lymph sac.

Assisted feeding

Many ill frogs and toads will eat a prey item if it is placed in the mouth. Invertebrates with potential for harming a debilitated patient (crickets, mealworms) should be decapitated and vertebrate prey should be killed prior to feeding. If the patient will not swallow items given in this way, a liquid diet may be given using a red rubber tube passed into the stomach. Anurans have a very short oesophagus; care should be taken not to advance the tube past the level of the stomach to avoid gastric rupture. In most species the stomach lies at the level of the clavicle. Formulas made for debilitated carnivores can be used for tube feeding. Alternatively, meat baby food supplemented with a multivitamin can be used.

Fluid therapy

Many compromised anurans are dehydrated on presentation. Hydration can be restored in several ways. Amphibians, like reptiles, clear lactate slowly, so non-lactated fluids should be used whenever possible.

- The patient can be placed in a shallow electrolyte solution to increase uptake of fluid through the permeable skin. Amphibian Ringer's solution can be formulated as follows:
  - 1 litre dechlorinated water
  - Sodium chloride 6.6 g
  - Potassium chloride 1.5 g
  - Calcium chloride 1.5 g
  - Sodium bicarbonate 2 g

Alternatively, a solution of 800 ml Ringer's solution plus 200 ml of 5% dextrose can be used (Crawshaw,1998).

- The humidity in the tank should be kept at a maximum level, and the patient misted frequently.
- If the condition and size of the patient allows, sterile fluids can be given intracoelomically.

Anaesthesia and analgesia

The preferred method of anaesthesia is with a bath of buffered (pH 7.0–7.4) tricaine methane sulphonate (MS-222). The patient is placed in a 1 g/l solution (adults) for approximately 30 minutes or until the desired plane of anaesthesia is established. The water level should be in contact with the ventral portion of the body but still allow the head and neck to be above water (Figure 17.18). The solution can be applied to the dorsal body with a syringe. The bath should be oxygenated with 100% oxygen during anaesthesia. The patient can be recovered using pure dechlorinated water. If the anaesthetic plane becomes too deep the MS-222 can be alternated with dechlorinated water during surgery. A Doppler audio probe should be used for surgical monitoring.

Anaesthesia can be induced by alternative methods, such as isoflurane administered by induction chamber or by topical administration. Intubation is possible but difficult due to the small glottis. Isoflurane and other inhalant gases appear to have significantly longer recovery times than MS-222.

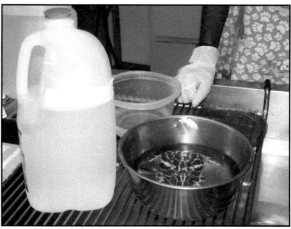

17.18 Anaesthetizing a horned frog with MS-222. (Courtesy of B. Levine.)

Analgesia

If surgery is to be performed, it is recommended that a pre-emptive analgesic is used (e.g. butorphanol at 0.2–0.4 mg/kg i.m. or buprenorphine at 20–38 mg/kg s.c.), although the dosages for most species have not been determined. It is assumed that the analgesic dose and action will be similar to those in mammals. Topical and local anaesthetics such as lidocaine 1–2% become systemic and should be used only with extreme caution. Postoperative analgesia should follow guidelines in mammals for the procedure and estimated amount of pain involved.

Common surgical procedures

The disinfectant of choice in amphibians is chlorhexidine, as others such as povidone–iodine can be toxic. **The patient's skin should not be scrubbed, as this will cause serious abrasions.** Gauze soaked in chlorhexidine solution can be applied to the area 10 minutes before surgery or anaesthesia.

For most surgical procedures, postoperative antibiotics are recommended due to the increased risk of infection to the damaged skin. MS-222 has been shown to have antibacterial properties and provides some protection during surgery.

Anuran skin is constantly wet after surgery and this is the most important consideration when choosing a suture material and pattern. A non-absorbable monofilament suture of appropriate size (usually 0.7–3 metric (2/0–6/0 USP)) is recommended, with an interrupted suture pattern to prevent suture line dehiscence. Skin glue (surgical cyanoacrylate) works well, aids haemostasis and provides a waterproof coating.

Foreign body retrieval/coeliotomy

Foreign body ingestion is not uncommon, particularly in species that are voracious feeders. If the object is large it often remains in the stomach and can be retrieved with a rigid small-diameter endoscope. If an endoscope is unavailable, the short oesophagus allows manual removal in some patients with the aid of an otoscope for visualization. If the foreign body has moved into the intestine and medical therapy is unrewarding, a coeliotomy may be necessary. A paramedian incision is made to avoid the midline abdominal vein. Closure of the gut allows only one layer, as the gut wall is very thin.

Limb amputation

Traumatic injury to the limbs is not uncommon in pet anurans. In general, captive amphibians adapt well to limb removal. It has been suggested that in the powerful hindlimbs the entire bone should be removed at the level of the joint to prevent abrasion of the stump (Wright, 2001).

Fracture repair

Fracture healing can be protracted in amphibians and any fixation method must be compatible with a long recovery in an aquatic environment. Complete calcification of the bone can take months. Intramedullary pins have been used with acceptable results but the patient must be strictly confined, as the pin provides no rotational stability. A successful repair of bilateral tibial fractures using type 1 external fixation devices has been reported in an American bullfrog (Johnson, 2003; Figure 17.19).

Euthanasia

Euthanasia is usually accomplished with an overdose of an anaesthetic agent. MS-222 is the most common agent used. This method also offers the advantage of minimal stress to the patient. As for anaesthesia, the patient is immersed in the agent for a prolonged period – until there is all cessation of movement and no response to toe pinching. If desired, once the patient is anaesthetized an intracardiac injection of pentobarbital can be administered. Humane euthanasia is usually defined as methods that depress or eliminate brain function prior to death. Freezing patients is common in the pet trade but is unacceptable as it causes considerable damage to the patient prior to cessation of brain function; it also requires pithing to ensure death.

Drug formulary

A drug formulary for anuran amphibians is given in Figure 17.20.

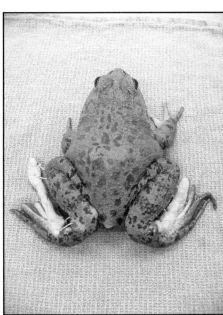
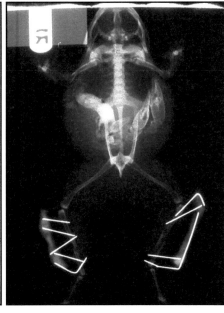

17.19 Successful repair of bilateral tibial fractures in an American bullfrog, using an external fixation device. (Courtesy of D. Johnson.)

Drug	Dose	Use/Reference
Antibacterial agents		
Amikacin	5 mg/kg i.m. q24–48h for 5–14 treatments	Wright and Whitaker (2001)
Carbenicillin	100 mg/kg s.c./i.m. q72h	Crawshaw (1998)
	200 mg/kg s.c./i.m./intracoelomically q24h	Wright (2005b)
Chloramphenicol	50 mg/kg s.c./i.m./intracoelomically q12–24h	Wright (2005b)
	20 mg per litre as a bath	
Ciprofloxacin	10 mg/kg orally q24–48h for 7 days minimum	Wright and Whitaker (2001)
	500–750 mg per 75 litres as a bath for 6–8 hours q24h	
Doxycycline	10–50 mg/kg orally q24h	

17.20 Drug formulary for anuran amphibians. (continues) ▶

Drug	Dose	Use/Reference
Antibacterial agents continued		
Enrofloxacin	5–10 mg/kg i.m. q24h for 7 treatments	Wright (2005b)
	5–10 mg/kg s.c./orally/intracoelomically for 7 days minimum	Wright and Whitaker (2001)
Gentamicin	3 mg/kg i.m. q24h at 22.2°C	Wright (2005b)
	2–4 mg/kg i.m. q72h for 4 treatments	Wright (2005b)
	1 mg/ml solution as an 8-hour bath q24–48h	Wright and Whitaker (2001)
	2 mg/ml dilution topically for ocular disease	Wright (2005b)
Metronidazole	50 mg/kg orally q24h for 3 days	Anaerobic infections: Wright and Whitaker (2001)
	50 mg per litre as a bath for up to 24 hours	
Piperacillin	100 mg/kg i.m./s.c. q24h	Wright (1996)
Rifampin	25 mg per litre as a 24-hour bath	Wright (2005b)
Sulfamethazine	1 g per litre as a bath to effect; made fresh daily	Crawshaw (1992)
Tetracycline	50 mg/kg orally q24h	Wright (2005b)
	10 µg/ml in 0.5% saline as a 24-hour bath; made fresh daily	Wright (2005b)
Trimethoprim/ Sulfadiazine	15–20 mg/kg i.m. q48h for 5–7 treatments	
Trimethoprim/ Sulfamethoxazole	15 mg/kg orally q24h for up to 21 days	Wright and Whitaker (2001)
	20 µg/ml in 0.5% saline or 80 µg/ml in 0.15% saline as a 24-hour bath; made fresh daily	Wright (2005b)
Trimethoprim/ Sulphonamide	3 mg/kg s.c./orally q24h	Crawshaw (1992)
Antifungal agents		
Amphotericin B	1 mg/kg intracoelomically q24h for 14–28 treatments	Internal mycoses: Wright and Whitaker (2001)
Benzalkonium chloride	2 mg per litre as a 1-hour bath q24h	Saprolegniasis: Wright and Whitaker (2001)
	0.25 mg per litre as a bath for 72 hours	Saprolegniasis: Crawshaw (1992)
Copper sulphate	500 mg per litre for 2 minutes as a bath q24h for 5 days; then q7d until healed	Saprolegniasis: Wright and Whitaker (2001). **NB Copper may be toxic to some amphibians**
Itraconazole	10–20 mg/kg orally q24h for 14–28 days (liquid formulation)	Chytridiomycosis: Wright (1996)
	10 mg/ml of a 0.01% solution in 0.6% saline as a soak for 5 minutes q24h for 11 days	Wright (2005b)
Ketoconazole	10 mg/kg orally q24h	Crawshaw (1992)
	10–20 mg/kg orally q24h for 14–28 days	Wright (1996)
Malachite green	0.2 mg per litre as a bath for 1 hour q24h	Saprolegniasis: Wright (2005b)
Methylene blue	50 mg/ml as a 10-second dip (tadpoles: do not exceed 2 mg/ml)	Saprolegniasis: Wright (2005b)
	3 mg per litre as a continuous bath for up to 5 days	Saprolegniasis: Wright (2005b)
Miconazole	5 mg/kg intracoelomically q24h for 14–28 days	Wright (2005b)
Sodium chloride	10–25 g per litre as a bath for 5–30 minutes	Saprolegniasis: Wright (2005b)
Antiparasitic agents		
Copper sulphate	0.0001 mg per litre as a continuous bath to effect	External protozoans: Wright (2005b). **Copper may be toxic to some amphibians**
Fenbendazole	100 mg/kg orally q10–21d	Nematodes: Wright (2005b)
Ivermectin	2 mg/kg cutaneously	Nematodes, arthropods: Wright and Whitaker (2001)
	0.2–0.4 mg/kg i.m./orally q14d	

17.20 (continued) Drug formulary for anuran amphibians. (continues) ▶

Drug	Dose	Use/Reference
Antiparasitic agents continued		
Levamisole	8–10 mg/kg intracoelomically or topically q14–21d	Nematodes: Wright (2005b)
	10 mg/kg i.m. q14d	Nematodes: Wright (2005b)
	100–300 mg per litre as a bath for 72 hours; made fresh daily q14–21d for a minimum of 3 treatments	Nematodes: Wright and Whitaker (2001)
Metronidazole	10 mg/kg orally q24h for 5–10 days	Flagellates: Wright (2005b)
	50 mg/kg orally q24h for 3–5 days	Amoebiasis, high levels of flagellates: Wright (2005b)
	50 mg per litre as a bath for up to 24 hours	
Paramomycin	50–75 mg/kg orally q24h	Amoebiasis: Wright (2005b)
Praziquantel	8–24 mg/kg orally/s.c./intracoelomically/cutaneously q7–21d	Trematodes, cestodes: Wright (2005b)
Sodium chloride	6 g per litre as a 24-hour bath for 3–5 days	External protozoans: Wright (2005b)
Sulfamethazine	1 g per litre as a bath for 24 hours daily to effect; made fresh daily	Potentially useful for coccidiosis: Wright and Whitaker (2001)
Tiabendazole	50–100 mg/kg orally q2wk	Cutaneous nematodes: Wright (2005b)
Anaesthetics/analgesics		
Buprenorphine	38 mg/kg s.c.	Analgesic: Wright (2005b)
Butorphanol	0.2–0.4 mg/kg i.m.	Analgesic: Wright (2005b)
Codeine	53 mg/kg s.c. (leopard frog)	Analgesic: effective dose for 4 hours: Wright (2005b)
Fentanyl	0.5 mg/kg s.c. (leopard frog)	Analgesic: effective dose for 4 hours: Wright (2005b)
Isoflurane	0.28 ml per 100 ml bath	Anaesthesia: Wright (2005b)
Ketamine + Diazepam	20–40 mg/kg K + 0.2–0.4 mg/kg D i.m.	Anaesthesia, muscle relaxant: Wright (2005b)
Lidocaine 1%, 2%	Local infiltration: volume as in mammals per area to be anaesthetized	**Use with caution as it becomes systemic**
Meperidine	49 mg/kg s.c. (leopard frog)	Analgesic: effective dose for 4 hours: Wright (2005b)
Morphine	38–42 mg/kg s.c.	Analgesic: Wright (2005b)
Nalorphine	122 mg/kg s.c.	Analgesic: Wright (2005b)
Naloxone	10 mg/kg s.c. to effect	Opioid reversal: Machin (1999)
Pentobarbital	60 mg/kg intracoelomically/i.v.	Euthanasia: Wright (2005b)
Propofol	60–100 mg/kg intracoelomically	Euthanasia: Wright (2005b)
Tricaine methane sulphonate (MS-222)	0.5–2 g per litre as a bath in a buffered solution; to effect	Anaesthetic of choice: Crawshaw (1993)
Miscellaneous		
Allopurinol	10 mg/kg orally q24h	Gout: Wright and Whitaker (2001)
Atropine	0.1 mg/kg s.c./i.m. as needed	Organophosphate toxicity: Wright and Whitaker (2001)
Calcium glubionate	1 ml/kg orally q24h	Nutritional secondary hyperparathyroidism: Wright and Whitaker (2001)
Dexamethasone	1.5 mg/kg s.c./i.m.	Williams (1994)
Flunixin meglumine	1 mg/kg s.c./i.m. q24h	Analgesic and septicaemia: Wright and Whitaker (2001)
Prednisolone sodium succinate	5–10 mg/kg i.m./i.v.	Shock: Wright and Whitaker (2001)
Vitamin B1	25 mg/kg in feeder fish	Thiaminase deficiency: Wright (2005b)
Vitamin D3	2–3 IU/ml in a continuous bath with 2.3% calcium gluconate	For nutritional secondary hyperparathyroidism
	100–400 IU/kg orally q24h	Wright and Whitaker (2001)
Vitamin E	1 mg/kg i.m./orally q7d	Steatitis: Wright and Whitaker (2001)

17.20 (continued) Drug formulary for anuran amphibians.

References and further reading

Crawshaw GJ (1992) Amphibian medicine. In: *Kirk's Current Veterinary Therapy XI Small Animal Practice*, ed. RW Kirk and JD Bonagura, pp. 1219–1230. WB Saunders, Philadelphia

Crawshaw GJ (1993) Amphibian medicine. In: *Zoo and Wild Animal Medicine: Current Therapy 3*, ed. ME Fowler, pp. 131–139. WB Saunders, Philadelphia

Crawshaw GJ (1998) Amphibian emergency and critical care. *Veterinary Clinics of North America: Exotic Animal Practice* **1**(1), 212

Downes H (1995) Tricaine anesthesia in Amphibia: a review. *Bulletin of the Association of Reptile and Amphibian Veterinarians* **5**(2), 11–16

Fedewa LA and Lindell A (2005) Inhibition of growth for select Gram-negative bacteria by tricaine methane sulfonate (MS-222). *Journal of Herpetological Medicine and Surgery* **15**(1), 13–17

Finke MD, Dunham SU and Kwabi CA (2005) Evaluation of four dry commercial gut loading products for improving the calcium content of crickets, *Acheta domesticus*. *Journal of Herpetological Medicine and Surgery* **15**(1), 7–12

Fleming GJ and Valdes EV (2008) Hypovitaminosis A in a captive collection of Amphibians. *Proceedings, Association of Reptile and Amphibian Veterinarians* pp.6–8

Johnson D (2003) External fixation of bilateral tibial fractures in an American Bullfrog. *Exotic DVM* **5**(2), 27–30

Johnson-Delaney CA (1997) Amphibians. In: *Exotic Companion Medicine Handbook for Veterinarians, Amphibian section*, pp.1–16. Zoological Education Network, Lake Worth, FL

Machin KL (1999) Amphibian pain and analgesia. *Journal of Zoo and Wildlife Medicine* **30**, 2–10

Pessier AP (2005) Amphibian chytridiomycosis. *Journal of Herpetological Medicine and Surgery* **15(3)**, 32–41

Schildger B and Triet H (2001) Ultrasonography in amphibians. *Seminars in Avian and Exotic Pet Medicine* **10**(4), 169–173

Williams DL and Whitaker BR (1994) The amphibian eye: a clinical review. *Journal of Zoo and Wild Animal Medicine* **25**, 18–28

Wright K (2001) Surgical techniques. In: *Amphibian Medicine and Captive Husbandry*, ed. Wright K and Whitaker B, pp. 273–283. Krieger, Malabar, FL

Wright K and Whitaker B (2001) *Amphibian Medicine and Captive Husbandry*. Krieger, Malabar, FL

Wright KM (1996) Amphibian husbandry and medicine. In: *Reptile Medicine and Surgery*, ed. DR Mader, pp. 436–459. WB Saunders, Philadelphia

Wright KM (2005a) Overview of amphibian medicine. In: *Reptile Medicine and Surgery*, ed. DR Mader, pp. 953–954. Saunders/Elsevier, St. Louis

Wright KM (2005b) Amphibians. In: *Exotic Animal Formulary, 3rd edn*, ed. JW Carpenter, pp. 33–54. Saunders/Elsevier, St. Louis

18

Salamanders, axolotls and caecilians

Peter Scott

Introduction

Salamanders and axolotls

Caudate amphibians belong to the Order Caudata, which contains approximately 375 species. These include:

- Sirenidae: the sirens
- Hynobiidae: Asian salamanders
- Cryptobranchidae: including hellbenders and giant salamanders
- Proteidae: neotenic salamanders such as the mudpuppy
- Amphiumidae: three limbless species
- Salamandridae
- Ambystomatidae: mole salamanders, including the Mexican axolotl
- Plethodontidae.

Popular terminology for this group is somewhat messy, as the term 'salamander' tends to be used for all the limbed caudates. The term 'newt' is simply a familiar name, used for the species that spend a lot of time on land. In some parts of the world the gilled neotenous/larval forms are all 'sirens', in others they are all referred to as 'axolotls'. The true axolotl is only one species, the Mexican axolotl *Ambystoma mexicanum* (Figure 18.1). The word 'axolotl' derives from the Aztec 'nahuatl' which, in theory, means water dog.

Caecilians

Caecilians belong to the Order Gymnophiona – the limbless amphibians – of which there are almost 180 known species (it is expected there are others to find):

- Beaked caecilians (Rhinatrematidae) – 2 genera, 9 species
- Fish caecilians (Ichthyophiidae) – 2 genera, 39 species
- Indian caecilians (Uraeotyphlidae) – 1 genus, 5 species
- Tropical caecilians (Scolecomorphidae) – 2 genera, 6 species
- Aquatic caecilians (Typhlonectidae) – 5 genera, 13 species
- Common caecilians (Caeciliidae) – 26 genera, 99 species.

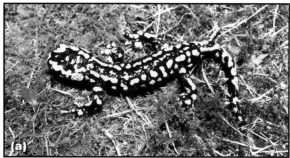
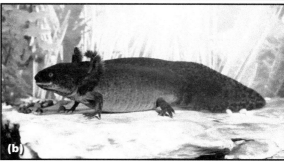

18.1 Common caudate amphibians. **(a)** Salamander (*Salamandra s. terrestris*). (Courtesy of C. Newman.) **(b)** An axolotl on a large stone 'slab' on which it can be hand-fed to avoid picking up substrate.

Biology

Salamanders and axolotls

Most salamanders are nocturnal. The group includes aquatic species, semi-aquatic and terrestrial species. Water plays an important part in the lives of all of them, and all the species spend larval stages in water.

Amphibians are highly adapted to their environment. Their skin is unlike that of fish, despite the similarities in environment. They are scaleless but the outwardly appearing soft skin is surprisingly tough, despite the minimal or absent keratinization of the stratum corneum. This is partly due to the surface layers but also to desmosomal attachments. Amphibian skin produces considerable quantities of mucus, which includes antibacterial and a variety of toxic/irritant components to protect the animal. In addition there is a mucoid layer within the skin. The mucus is believed to act as an ion trap, possibly functioning with flask cells which are involved in salt regulation. Their skins also contain Merkel cells, which have a tactile function. The stratum corneum is shed regularly, and quite often eaten.

The layout of internal organs is much as expected. All adults, being carnivorous, have a short and relatively simple gastrointestinal tract. Although natural diets have not been studied, they seem to take everything from beetles to lizards and snakes, depending on size.

Aquatic amphibians excrete ammonia as their nitrogenous waste; in most terrestrial species this is converted in the liver to urea.

All Caudata are oviparous (Figure 18.2). The axolotl is neotenous, as are all members of the four families of salamander. They remain as a larval form, not completing metamorphosis, yet grow to adult size and are capable of breeding. There are other species, such as the Tiger salamander (*Ambystoma tigrinum*), in which neoteny is facultative, metamorphosis occurring if their aquatic habitat becomes uninhabitable.

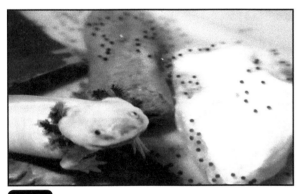

18.2 Female axolotl with egg strings.

Caecilians

Caecilians are generally secretive, living in soil, leaf mould, etc. There are also partially and fully aquatic species. Some of the terrestrial species are only known to science from single specimens.

The Caecilians are limbless: the small species resemble earthworms, whilst the larger ones resemble snakes. In general, their tail is short. The skin is smooth and, in most species, quite dark, containing small calcite scales. There are also toxic 'glands' in the skin. The eyes are small and covered in skin for protection. Their vision is limited to light and dark perception. All species have two small 'tentacles' which are believed to have an olfactory function. Apart from one species, all caecilians have lungs (usually the right lung is reduced in size), although young aquatic species have beautiful feathery gills. Caecilians may be oviparous or viviparous.

Husbandry

Housing

As for fish, a major aspect of the successful keeping of amphibians is water management. Whilst many of them live in muddy environments in the wild, and indeed some caecilians have been found in essentially raw sewage, this is not recommended. The permeability of amphibian skin makes them susceptible to water-borne toxins and in general good hygiene is vital to maintaining captive health.

Standard aquarium and specialist reptile and amphibian 'kit' is now available: tanks; vivaria with sliding fronts and/or secure lids; under-tank heaters (always leave a section unheated for safety); mosses, plants; and moulded pools. There are a variety of devices available for generating mist in closed tanks; initially these were the preserve of zoos but they are now more widely available. For the more 'clinical' environments maintained by enthusiasts, there are foam substrates that hold water and raise humidity.

Good ventilation is important; the humid environments needed conflict somewhat with this need but poor ventilation will encourage fungal and bacterial growth.

The three habitat types are:

- **Aquatic habitats:** Sturdy plants are needed to survive with larger animals blundering around. Large pea gravel is a popular substrate but care needs to be taken when feeding to avoid ingestion. Worn slate works well as a substrate.
- **Semi-aquatic vivaria:** Standard aquarium and reptile technology makes setting up a vivarium relatively easy. Semi-aquatic species in general thrive in a humid environment, and using small aquarium filter pumps to provide moving water is a good way of achieving this. Some extremely attractive and rich environments can be created using easily available equipment (Figure 18.3); sterile potting soil is a good substrate for parts, on top of sand or gravel.
- **Terrestrial vivaria/terraria:** Well landscaped rich environments can be built, but they must still be humid.

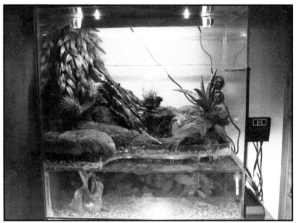

18.3 An enriched semi-aquatic environment suitable for a salamander.

Semi-aquatic and terrestrial species need hides; they are thigmotaxic (tend to stay close to or in contact with objects and to avoid open areas) and prefer to be surrounded, so some thought should be given to appropriate provision of such spaces.

In general amphibians are quite sensitive to noise and vibration, so these should be kept to a minimum. Appropriate siting of vivaria is important. It is essential to research the species being kept thoroughly; whilst they are amazingly 'forgiving', there is no excuse for ignoring their specific needs with regard to husbandry and welfare.

Light

Lighting is not a major issue as most species, except for the aquatic ones, are nocturnal. Some consideration of photoperiod is still important, however, and plants require good lighting if natural systems are used. Lights need guards to keep animals away from them. Caution is needed with regard to UV-B emitting bulbs as amphibians are highly sensitive to excessive UV-B radiation. The increased use of more 'efficient' UV-B emitting bulbs in reptile keeping will need to be monitored with regard to amphibian husbandry.

Temperature

Temperate species do not need any supplementary heat. Under-tank heaters are safer than in-tank heaters, which can cause burns to inhabitants that 'snuggle' them. Heat lamps are unsuitable as they cause too much drying.

Temperate species will often try to hibernate; this is believed to be physiologically important to them, so providing a hide at the cool end of a vivarium is sensible. Dimming lights and dropping the temperature to 8–10°C is usually sufficient, and they can be kept in a state of relative torpor for 3–4 months. Many such species actually have a blood 'antifreeze' system and can freeze and thaw safely – this is to be avoided where possible as not all individuals will do this successfully. Frostbite is also seen. The cold tolerance of amphibians is also used in the process of 'fridging' (see later).

Humidity

Water uptake is through the skin, and amphibians do not drink. Therefore, maintaining a suitable humidity is vital. Relative humidity above 70% will suit most amphibians.

Diet

Little is known about the natural diets of many amphibians in their various habitats and life stages, especially the caecilians. However, it is pretty clear that they are primarily carnivorous, taking insects and invertebrates found in their respective habitats. Larger species will take small fish, or other amphibians. Many have a staple diet of earthworms and take in a considerable amount of general organic and inorganic debris with them. As noted above, aquatic species kept on gravel may ingest gravel intentionally or accidentally, so it is safer to hand-feed or feed them on a solid slab (see Figure 18.1) rather than simply put food on the floor of the tank.

All of these animals are attracted to moving prey. Encouraging hand feeding using long forceps is good but not always possible. Smaller timid species are reluctant. A variety of insects, crickets, locusts, earthworms and even strips of heart muscle are used. Larvae enjoy tubificid worms, daphnia, and small mealworms. Species with very small larvae will even accept brine shrimp. Supervised daily feeding is preferred. Larvae of salamanders are cannibalistic so complex habitats with 'hides' are vital. Use of vitamin/mineral supplements is recommended as metabolic bone disease is not uncommon. Dusting powders and loading diets are useful.

Preventive healthcare

Because of the threat from introduction of chytridiomycosis (*Batrachochytrium dendrobatidis*) (see Chapter 17) in particular, there is considerable interest in developing systems for quarantine. Key elements for proper biosecurity are:

- All animals receive a veterinary examination: any lesions are sampled and losses investigated thoroughly
- Separation, of both animals and systems. Individual filtration is needed
- 60 days minimum quarantine time on an all-in, all-out basis
- Use of gloves between animals and any tank servicing
- Disinfection of all shoes, equipment, surfaces, etc.
- Disinfection of waste water by adding bleach and waiting for at least 10 minutes before disposal. This is important to avoid risks to indigenous wildlife.

Handling and restraint

None of these animals is suitable for handling or petting. Their skins are sensitive to the oils in human skin, and some produce skin toxins of their own as a protection against predators. If they must be handled for examination or transfer, then well washed and rinsed hands are preferred, although some use latex gloves. Prolonged handling is best avoided, and some brands of glove have been known to cause skin problems in amphibians. Fine fish nets can be used to manoeuvre animals carefully. The larger species, such as hellbenders, may need sedation using tricaine methane sulphonate (MS-222) (see Anaesthesia) to make handling safe.

Amphibians do not show autotomy (tail shedding) as a defence, but some do have an equally strange ability. Axolotls in particular have an alarmingly useful 'gift' of being able to regrow lost body parts. Unfortunately, they are not always entirely accurate, so reduced limbs or duplicate limbs are seen.

Diagnostic approach

The diagnostic approach to an amphibian is not significantly different from that applied to any species:

1. Take a history:
   - What is the current problem?
   - How long in current ownership? Level of experience of the owner?
   - How is the animal kept, what sort of housing and food?
   - How is water filtered, humidity maintained, etc.?
2. Observe the animal without handling. Look for:
   - Asymmetry
   - Visible lesions
   - Obvious respiratory effort
   - Ability to make coordinated movements.

3. Physical examination. Check for:
   - Asymmetries
   - Fractures or other injuries
   - Fluid accumulation.
4. Consider what diagnostic samples might be useful/possible to obtain.
   - Blood – peripheral vessels or cardiac puncture (the latter is a course of last resort).
   - Faeces – usefully examined fresh for parasites.
   - Swabs of lesions, cloaca, mouth, etc.
   - Scrapings for fresh examination.
   - Needle aspirates of retained fluid.
   - Biopsy.
5. Diagnostic imaging.
   - Radiography – high definition imaging is most useful.
   - Ultrasonography.

6. Other approaches.
   - Surgical investigation: laparotomy/laparoscopy.

Common conditions

Amphibians are extremely good 'indicators' of environmental quality. Despite the very poor conditions in which some caecilians are found, in general they are highly susceptible to toxic effects of the environment and so environmental management is important in captivity. Certainly in the wild, man's impact in terms of chemical spillage and contamination has had a terrible effect on populations. Common presentations in salamanders, axolotls and caecilians are discussed in Figure 18.4.

Clinical presentation	Comments
Anorexia	Most commonly due to poor husbandry, e.g. incorrect temperature, humidity, types of food offered
Found dead	Investigation is often unrewarding, but a good post-mortem examination, with histopathology if animals are fresh enough, is worthwhile
Loss of gills or death in neotenous species	It is thought that neoteny is based around a very slow hypothalamus–pituitary–thyroid axis. Neotenous species such as axolotls have been known to metamorphose partially or completely when exposed to iodine. Some 'races' cannot complete metamorphosis and may die if attempts are made to force the transition by administration of thyroid hormone
Metabolic bone disease (Figure 18.5)	Salamanders, axolotls and caecilians have all been seen with problems. The origin is likely to be dietary in the majority, but it is believed that certain species of salamander living naturally in moist limestone crevices may absorb calcium via the skin. Avoided using appropriate supplements
Oedema (anasarca, ascites)	Common. Seen with septicaemia, heart failure, kidney (Figure 18.6) or liver disease, and hypocalcaemia. General mineral deficiency and osmotic failure
Septicaemia	Water-borne pathogens, especially *Aeromonas hydrophila*. Red lesions or ecchymotic haemorrhages are seen (Figure 18.7)
Skin diseases (Figure 18.8)	Ectoparasitic and, especially, fungal diseases are relatively common. Gentle skin scrapings examined immediately as wet mounts will often reveal parasites or fungi. Bacterial infections with hyperaemia, discoloration or ulceration are seen. The term 'red-leg' is used for aggressive *Aeromonas*-type bacterial infections of the skin, which often become systemic. Dysecdysis, with or without increased mucus production, is seen in a range of systemic or skin conditions. These animals do suffer from chytridiomycosis (*Batrachochytrium dendrobatidis*) (see Chapter 17)
Visceral nodules at post-mortem examination	Parasitic cysts, mycobacteriosis, fungal infection

18.4 Common presentations in salamanders, axolotls and caecilians.

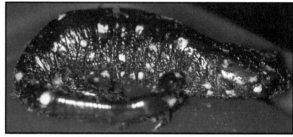

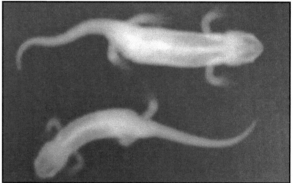

18.5 Metabolic bone disease in a salamander (*Salamandra iberica*). Note the weak legs. The radiograph shows very poor bone density in two specimens.

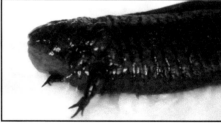

18.6 An oedematous axolotl with kidney failure.

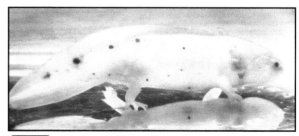

18.7 An axolotl with septicaemia-related petechiation.

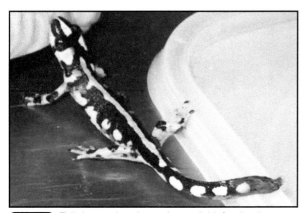

18.8 Tail tip erosion due to bacterial infection in a newt.

Supportive care

Drug treatment

- Topical treatment, either by percutaneous application or via baths, is the most common route and has the advantage of being non-invasive.
- Medication can be given orally, administered in a food item or by gavage using a soft tube or pipette.
- Parenteral routes include intramuscular, intracoelomic and lymph sac injection. In caudates and caecilians the subcutaneous space is not present. Intravenous injections are difficult and generally not practical.

As might be anticipated, the high permeability of the skin, and the presence of gills in some species, make these amphibians susceptible to the presence of chlorine in the water. Adopting a principle that they may well be affected even more than fish of similar size by water-borne toxicants is a good startpoint. There have been few pharmacokinetic studies in amphibians, so some of the work in fish and reptiles has been extrapolated. Doses for antibiotics and anthelmintics are given in Figure 18.9.

Antiseptics

- Benzalkonium chloride is a very well used and widely recommended topical antiseptic and antifungal agent for amphibians.
- In recent years F10 has been used in a similar way, although as yet there are no published safety data.
- There is conflicting evidence and may be intraspecific differences in relation to the use of iodine. Iodine disinfection and inadequate removal of the trace iodine has led to suspected toxicity; yet iodine deficiency has been implicated in spindly legs in frogs. A number of authors (including this one) have used povidone–iodine widely without any concerns, other than one instance of triggering metamorphosis in an axolotl having a wound treated repeatedly. It was suggested in Wright and Whitaker (2001) that, in addition to differing amphibian species susceptibility, toxicity may vary with the salt/type of iodine.

Fluid therapy

Bathing in isotonic or near isotonic electrolyte solutions is valuable for sick animals (0.6–0.8% saline or more specialized solutions).

Cooling

'Fridging' is used commonly. Animals are accommodated in small plastic ventilated containers, amongst moist towelling or foam, and placed in the salad section of a domestic refrigerator for a few days. This area is usually set slightly warmer than the rest of the fridge, closer to a recommended 8–10°C. This is a common hobbyist 'treatment', which slows down metabolism at times of stress, and has been used to slow down infectious processes whilst healing continues.

Anaesthesia and analgesia

Agents

Tricaine methane sulphonate (MS-222)

MS-222 is currently the only anaesthetic authorized for use in fish in the UK; it also has the benefit of being water-soluble. It is well used in amphibians at similar doses to those in fish, from 10–100 mg/l depending on depth of anaesthesia required.

Depth of anaesthesia needs to be monitored carefully and the animal removed when the desired plane is reached. There is always continued deepening of anaesthesia after removal, due to circulating drug, so in practice removal of animals at a lighter stage than actually required is worthwhile.

Recovery is achieved by placing animals in fresh water of the same temperature or slightly warmer than that in which they are normally kept. The MS-222 is lost through the skin, resulting in a slow recovery. The water should be aerated and, ideally, for the most rapid recovery, the animal or water should be moving to maximize skin exposure.

Ketamine

Ketamine has reportedly been used successfully in a number of species, but the dose ranges used and the results obtained appear widely varied. A figure of 70–100 mg/kg was reported in Wright and Whitaker (2001) as being suitable for surgical procedures in *Ambystoma* species; recovery took up to 12 hours.

Analgesia

Analgesia is probably not used sufficiently and this area would benefit greatly from further investigation. Amphibians must be regarded as being capable of feeling pain. Opioid mechanisms have been demonstrated and appropriate neural pathways exist. 'Fridging' (see above) is used by many keepers to slow animals down metabolically, but this should not be regarded as in any way analgesic. A report by Mitchell *et al.* (2009) examined the use of clove oil and propofol in urodeles and reviewed the relevant literature regarding anaesthesia of amphibians: clove oil (eugenol) was found to be effective, whilst propofol was variable.

Common surgical procedures

Amphibians are, in general, good surgical patents, provided some straightforward preparation is carried out.

- See above for notes on anaesthesia and analgesia. For long surgeries, using a recirculation system with background MS-222 and aeration is perfectly viable.
- If the surgery is elective rather than emergency, the animal should be fasted for 2–7 days, depending on size and diet.
- Ensure proper hydration:
  - For semi-aquatic and terrestrial species this will mean simply putting them in shallow water or having very wet moss packed around them for an hour or so before commencing
  - **Do not smear animals with K–Y jelly as a moisturiser as it is suggested that this may interfere with cutaneous respiration**
  - Surgical boards with foam, similar to those used for fish, are useful to retain contact with moisture.
- Provide antibiotic cover. Accept that achieving a sterile field is unlikely/impossible. Work quickly, cleanly and minimally. Postoperative infection is relatively unusual.
- Skin preparation can be achieved using dilute povidone–iodine (but see Antiseptics, above, for note on iodine toxity), and benzalkonium chloride 2 ppm.
- Basic plastic drapes are used, without adhesives. Cloth drapes are unsuitable due to wicking moisture away from the skin.
- Various suture materials have been used. Non-absorbable monofilaments are most suited for skin closure; absorbables are not recommended.

Slightly everting suture patterns help the necessary watertight seal to develop quickly. Because of the environment in which the animals live, secondary use of surgical tissue adhesives is very valuable.

- Biopsy samples are easily taken, and electrosurgery is very useful for controlling bleeding.
- Laparoscopy is straightforward, and insufflation using sterile air or oxygen may help with visibility.

Common procedures include biopsy and removal of cutaneous masses. Fracture repair is possible in larger specimens using standard orthopaedic techniques. Coeliotomy can be performed via a paramedian incision to avoid the ventral midline blood vessel; the presence of fat bodies and ovaries in females can make visualization of organs difficult.

Euthanasia

An overdose of MS-222 is a simple, low-stress means of euthanasia. It also provides a simple means of restraint should intracardiac or intracoelomic injection of barbiturates be preferred; these latter routes may affect the quality of any subsequent post-mortem histopathology, however. Freezing using a standard home freezer is an *unacceptable* means of euthanasia as it takes far too long. Cooling animals in a refrigerator sufficiently to allow non-stressful intracoelomic barbiturates is acceptable.

Drug formulary

A formulary for salamanders and axolotls is given in Figure 18.9.

Drug	Dose	Use/comments
Antibiotic agents		
Ciprofloxacin	10 mg/l as a bath for 6–8 hours q24h for 7 days	
Enrofloxacin	2 mg/l q24h immersion or 5–10 mg/kg orally/parenterally	
Itraconazole	2–10 mg/kg (topical 0.01%) as a bath for 5 minutes q24h	
Oxytetracycline	100 mg/l as a bath for 1 hour q24h	
Anthelmintic agents		
Ivermectin	10 mg/l as a bath for 60 minutes, repeated for 7 days	Used in a range of species
Levamisole	100–300 mg/l as a bath for 24 hours, 3 times, q7–14d	
	Species of caecilian have shown toxicity to that dose; 50–100 mg/l as a bath for 1–8 hours q7d have been used in these	Toxicity leads to paralysis and drowning
Praziquantel	10 mg/l as a bath for 3 hours	Internal or external trematode infections
Miscellaneous		
Benzalkonium chloride	2 mg/l for 30 minute dips	
Salt	10–15 g/l for 5–15 minute dips	

18.9 Drug formulary for axolotls and salamanders.

References and further reading

Davidson EW, Parris M, Collins JP *et al.* (2003) Pathogenicity and transmission of chytridiomycosis in Tiger Salamanders (*Ambystoma tigrinum*). *Copeia* **3,** 601–607

Duellman WE and Trueb L (1986) *Biology of Amphibians.* Johns Hopkins University Press, London

Machin KL (2001) Fish, amphibian, and reptile analgesia. *Veterinary Clinics of North America: Exotic Animal Practice* **4(1)**, 19–33

Mitchell MA, Riggs SM, Singleton CB, *et al.* (2009) Evaluating the clinical and cardiopulmonary effects of clove oil and propofol in Tiger Salamanders (*Ambystoma tigrinum*). *Journal of Exotic Pet Medicine* **18**(1), 50–56

Pessier AP (2003) Practical gross necropsy of amphibians. *Seminars in Avian and Exotic Pet Medicine* **12**(2), 81–88

Whitear M (1977) A functional comparison between the epidermis of fish and amphibians. *Symposia of the Zoological Society of London* **39,** 291–313

Wright KM and Whitaker BR (2001) *Amphibian Medicine and Captive Husbandry.* Krieger, Malabar, FL

Useful websites

Spear, R. Amphibian diseases Home Page: http://www.jcu.edu.au/school/phtm/PHTM/frogs/ampdis.htm

19

Freshwater ornamental fish

Helen E. Roberts

Introduction

Keeping fish as a hobby dates back many centuries. Modern aquarists have thousands of species and a variety of life support equipment essentials to choose from to help maintain their collections. While the diversity of possible aquatic patients may seem overwhelming, the information and techniques described here will be readily applicable to most freshwater ornamental fish presented to the veterinary practice.

Freshwater fish are the most common group kept by aquarists and may be kept in a range of containers, from small bowls to aquaria or ponds with elaborate and expensive set-ups. Goldfish (*Carassius auratus*), koi (*Cyprinus carpio*) and bettas (*Betta splendens*) are the most common species presented in the private practice setting (Figure 19.1). Fish kept exclusively in outdoor ponds (koi and goldfish) are more often presented during the warmer months, when their owners are feeding and interacting with their fish on a regular basis.

Biology

Anatomy and physiology

Fish are poikilothermic, and each species has its own preferred optimal temperature zone (POTZ). Appropriate water temperatures are needed for proper metabolism, immune function and disease resistance; physiological stress, sometimes fatal, occurs when water temperatures fall outside this range.

Fish are covered with a layer of mucus, secreted by goblet cells in the epidermis, that contains lysozyme (and other enzymes), antibodies, and reactive proteins to protect against pathogens. The mucus layer will thicken with irritation if there is poor water quality, parasites or noxious chemicals in the water. The cuticle and epidermis form the waterproof, external layer of the skin. Scales develop in pockets located in the dermis and are covered by the epidermis. Scaleless fish have a thicker epidermis.

The gills are the site of respiration (oxygen/carbon dioxide exchange), ammonia excretion (by diffusion), acid–base balance, and osmoregulation (fluid balance). They are very thin; typically one cell layer separates the fish from its environment. Gills are susceptible to injury due to poor water quality, ectoparasites, infectious disease and other irritants. Hyperplasia is the most common finding, resulting in impaired gill function.

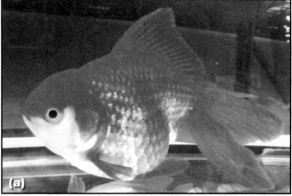

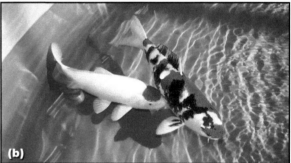

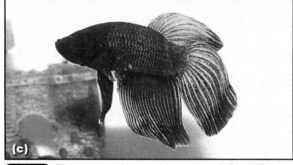

19.1 Fish commonly seen in practice: **(a)** goldfish (*Carassius auratus*); **(b)** koi (*Cyprinus carpio*); **(c)** betta (*Betta splendens*).

The swim bladder, important for buoyancy and maintenance of position in the water column, is present in most pet fish and is located in the dorsal aspect of the coelomic cavity. It is described by the connection, or lack of, to the digestive system: physostomous fish have a direct connection; physoclistous fish do not. Koi and goldfish have a bilobed swim bladder, with a cranial and a caudal lobe. Buoyancy disorders are common in varieties of goldfish with short round bodies, such as orandas.

Several variations exist in the digestive system; for example, koi do not have a true stomach. Herbivores have a longer gastrointestinal tract than carnivores.

The anterior ('head') kidney, located dorsocranially, performs haemopoietic and lymphoid functions. The posterior ('tail') kidney performs osmoregulatory, mineral balance and minor excretory functions. It is located dorsal to the swim bladder, in the retroperitoneal space.

Osmoregulation

Freshwater fish live in an environment that is hypo-osmotic relative to their internal fluids. These fish constantly expend energy to maintain homeostasis and prevent overhydration and salt depletion. Passive osmotic intake of water occurs over the gill epithelium at a constant rate. To compensate, freshwater fish drink very little, or not at all, and excrete large volumes of dilute hypotonic urine (2–4 ml/kg/h).

Persistent acute stress may cause an increase in diuresis and ion depletion that can be life-threatening. Pathology of the gills, kidney or skin can also result in osmotic imbalance. Adding sodium chloride to the water of debilitated fish can reduce the energy expenditure required to maintain osmotic balance. Salt is commonly added to transport water to lower the osmotic gradient, reducing stress and increasing survival rates.

Sexing

Some species are sexually dimorphic. In others of sufficient size, sex can sometimes be determined by gently applying pressure to the caudal aspect of the coelomic cavity towards the vent. Milt or eggs may be seen. This technique works well on koi and goldfish but should always be performed **very cautiously.** It is not recommended in cases of suspected egg binding or internal masses, where rupture could have fatal consequences.

Husbandry

Housing

Materials and décor

Modern ornamental ponds use a range of construction materials, such as plastics (preformed or as liners), concrete (e.g. Gunite™) and fibreglass. Each has its own advantages and disadvantages. Materials may have tendencies to leak (especially liners), may be easily chewed or gnawed on by rodents, may crack (concrete, Gunite™) with earth movement or may be dislodged (preformed ponds) and generally deteriorate over time due to constant exposure to the elements.

Most fish ponds are water gardens with aquatic plants, fountains and decorations in addition to the fish. Aquatic plants can aid in the removal of nitrates, although water changes will still be necessary. Plants can also serve as 'environmental enrichment' for koi and goldfish. All decorations and fountains should be checked for sharp edges and toxic materials. Copper-based statuary or fountains with copper tubing do not belong in an aquatic garden containing fish.

Stocking densities

Most ponds will, over time, develop high stocking densities, the owners either acquiring too many fish or purchasing fish that grow larger than they anticipated. Some strains or lines of koi can grow to over a metre in length. Goldfish tend to breed frequently; it is not unusual to start with half a dozen and end up with several hundred in a year or less. Fish can be kept at high densities for short times, such as in commercial aquaculture systems, but owners may not adapt their equipment to meet the high demands of large populations. Many pond owners who build a small pond initially go on to build a larger pond, or two. Large fish, such as koi, seem to be healthier in ponds with larger volumes and depth. The author recommends a conservative minimum of 1000 US gallons (*c.* 3800 litres) for a koi pond, and 500–1000 US gallons (*c.*1400–3800 litres) *per koi* to pond owners.

Aquarium stocking densities depend on owner experience, species of fish, volume of the aquarium, and life-support equipment used to maintain the aquarium. One of two general rules can be used: one inch (*c.* 2.5 cm) of total body length of fish per 5–10 US gallons (*c.* 19–38 litres); or one inch (*c.* 2.5 cm) of body length of fish for every square foot (*c.* 900 cm^2) of surface area in the aquarium.

Outdoor ponds

Typically, ponds are placed where the homeowner can enjoy them most – usually close to the house, near a viewing window or next to (or incorporated into) a deck design. The site should be assessed for potential rainwater runoff, predator access, amount of sunlight and shade, and possibility for falling debris, leaves, etc. into the water. The author has seen cases where ornamental copper flashing on a roof created copper toxicity after a period of heavy rains, causing fish deaths. Long-term (25–50 year) roofing shingles can contain a copper-based algicide that can also contribute to water toxicity. Treated lumber and paint or stain may contain toxic additives that can leach into the water, and pond owners should be advised to use extreme caution when repainting or restaining a fence adjacent to the pond. Trees can provide excessive shade in northern climates, preventing full growth of aquatic plants. Leaf debris and pine needles will easily clog a mechanical filter if not removed by the pond owner on a regular basis. The electrical supply for pumps, filters and air hoses must be safe. An area where water changes or drainage can be carried out without potential flooding is invaluable; most pond designs do not include this.

The margins of the pond should be evaluated for ease of predator access. Ornamental ponds are seen as a 'buffet' by many predators. Stone 'beaches' are very appealing but make the pond inhabitants an easy meal for wading birds of prey such as herons. Mink, raccoons and domestic cats may also prey on the fish. Heron decoys, pond netting (Figure 19.2) or motion-activated water sprinklers may reduce or eliminate predator access. Hiding areas of rock, PVC and other materials can be useful to the fish when evading predators, though they will also hinder fish capture.

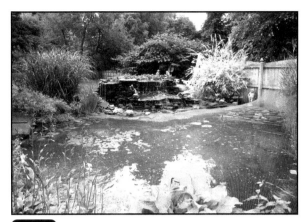

Pond netting may deter predators.

Indoor ponds

Some owners, in colder climates or those with shallow ponds, take their pets indoors for the winter. Indoor ponds are not usually as large as those built outdoors, so care must be taken to monitor water quality. Limiting feeding can be beneficial. Indoor ponds also do not usually provide adequate (natural) photoperiods for fish. This may contribute to reproductive problems, such as egg binding.

Life-support systems

Most ponds and aquaria the practitioner will encounter have some sort of life-support equipment that attempts to maintain water parameters within the optimal range. Recognizing the main types of equipment used in ponds and aquaria lends the aquatic practitioner some credibility when dealing with experienced hobbyists. Despite the knowledge of fish diagnostics, disease and treatments, failure to recognize a 'trickle system' or 'bead filter' may lead to compliance issues on the part of the owner. The most common types of equipment seen are filters (external, internal or combination), heaters (especially in tropical fish tanks), specialized lighting and pumps (Figure 19.3). A novice practitioner should 'follow the water' when evaluating life-support systems. In most systems, water flows into an intake pipe or skimmer from the pond or tank, through a series of tubing or pipes, into the main filtration system, then returns to the tank or pond. Most filters perform several functions, including removal of solid waste and debris (mechanical filtration), detoxification of harmful waste products to a less toxic form (biological filtration; see below), and removal of potentially harmful organic compounds (chemical filtration). All filter systems require some form of maintenance.

Water quality

Most systems, ponds and aquaria that maintain captive pet fish are closed recirculating systems. Water is not continually refreshed as in natural systems, and steps must be taken to replace lost critical components and remove potentially toxic compounds. The most common cause of stress in pet fish is poor water quality. This predisposes the fish to disease outbreaks. Clients will often have the water tested at local pet shops and are told that 'levels are fine', but numerical results are preferable. Measurement of water quality parameters is done with specialized test kits; reagents may need to be replaced regularly. Test kits can vary in the reliability of results, depending on the type used. Professional grade, multiparameter test kits are available at a reasonable cost. 'Alkalinity' (concentration of bicarbonate ions) measures the buffering capacity of the water. 'Hardness' is a measure of levels of the divalent metal cations in water, primarily calcium and magnesium. Water quality is much easier to maintain in a larger volume of water (>400 litres) compared with a small volume, provided the carrying capacity (stocking density) is not overwhelmed. Figure 19.4 summarizes water quality parameters, problems and corrective measures.

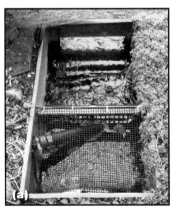
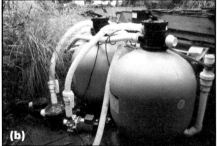
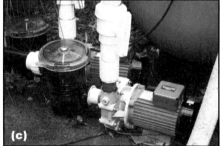

19.3 Example components of a life-support system for an ornamental fish pond: **(a)** skimmer with submersible pump; **(b)** bead filter system; **(c)** external pump.

Parameter	Acceptable levels	Clinical signs of toxicity	Corrective measures	Comments
Ammonia	0 ppm	Lethargy; anorexia; increased opercular beat rate; convulsions/coma; gill hyperplasia; death	Frequent water changes; reduce or stop feeding; reduce stocking density; add ammonia-binding compounds. Monitor	Ammonia is more toxic at higher pH and higher water temperatures. Ammonia levels in new systems should always be monitored ('new tank syndrome'). Chemicals and drugs that adversely affect biofiltration bacteria can lead to elevations in ammonia

19.4 Water quality parameters, signs of problems and corrective measures. (continues) ▶

Parameter	Acceptable levels	Clinical signs of toxicity	Corrective measures	Comments
Nitrite	0 ppm	Gasping/piping; opercular flaring; increased respiratory rate; lethargy; dyspnoea; pale/tan gills; death	Frequent water changes; add 0.1–0.2% sodium chloride. Monitor by frequent testing	Also seen in newly established systems. Nitrite binds to haemoglobin (Hb), forming methoxyhaemoglobin. 'Brown blood' will not be apparent until 40% of Hb is bound. Chloride competitively inhibits nitrite uptake across the gills
Nitrate	<50 ppm	Chronic stress; growth suppression; may contribute to or cause immunosuppression and/or buoyancy disorders	Water changes; add plants	Algal blooms may occur with increased nitrate levels
pH	6.5–8.5	Low pH: tremors; hyperactivity; increased mucus production; stress; sudden death	Low pH: water changes; add buffering agents; increase filtration capacity if needed. **Measure ammonia before changing pH acutely**	Acceptable pH can vary with species. Small changes are less stressful than large, rapid changes. Most fish can adapt to a stable pH. Optimal pH ranges vary within species
		High pH: skin and gill cloudiness; acute and chronic stress	High pH: water changes; add buffering agents. In ponds and heavily planted aquaria: remove excess vegetation (plant photosynthesis consumes CO_2, raising pH)	
Dissolved oxygen (DO)	6–10 ppm	Dyspnoea; increased opercular beat rate, gasping, piping; lethargy; death	Identify cause(s). Add aeration or pure oxygen; decrease feeding, stocking density; reduce temperature if possible; 3% hydrogen peroxide (0.5 ml/l) can be added to water carefully in emergency situations	Lowest levels measurable at dawn (before photosynthesis starts in plants). Large fish will succumb first (higher oxygen requirement). Medication such as formalin can reduce DO. Biofilter requires adequate oxygen to function: monitor ammonia after DO returns to normal
Alkalinity (bicarbonate)	>100 ppm		Water changes; baking soda can raise alkalinity in a low pH crisis	Alkalinity (bicarbonate) levels decrease before there is a decrease in pH
Chlorine	0 ppm	Hypoxia/dyspnoea; gill necrosis; haemolytic anaemia; acute mortalities	Immediate water changes with dechlorinated water; lower water temperature to reduce oxygen demand; add oxygenated water or bubble pure oxygen	Dechlorinate all water with water changes. Methods include: use of commercial dechlorinators containing sodium thiosulphate (3.5–10 mg/l) or vigorous aeration for 24 hours
Hydrogen sulphide	0 ppm	Dyspnoea/gasping; lethargy/anorexia; acute death	Massive water changes; remove decaying material from pond; vigorous aeration of water; reduce water temperature; elevate pH to more alkaline levels	Biofilter failure: H_2S produced by anaerobic bacterial metabolism. Characteristic 'rotten egg' smell may be noted. Common in poorly maintained systems with large amount of detritus on bottom. Toxicity increases at higher water temperatures and low pH

19.4 (continued) Water quality parameters, signs of problems and corrective measures.

The nitrogen cycle: The bacterial oxidation of toxic ammonia first to nitrite and ultimately to a less toxic form (nitrate) is often called the nitrogen cycle or nitrification. Biological oxidation occurs throughout the system but is concentrated primarily in biological filters. Biofilters are designed to support high numbers of bacteria by using filter media, floss, plastic balls and mesh to provide a large surface area for the bacteria to colonize. Water is directed over the media at a controlled flow rate.

Important facts to consider include:

- Ammonia is the primary waste product produced by fish
- Total ammonia nitrogen (TAN) measured in a system is a combination of the NH_4^+ ion (ionized ammonia) and NH_3 (un-ionized ammonia). Un-ionized ammonia is the more toxic form. Toxicity of ammonia is higher at high pH levels and high temperatures
- Ammonia toxicity is common in new systems
- Toxicity is also seen when filters have been adversely affected by added products (therapeutic agents in particular) or a low level of dissolved oxygen is present
- Toxicity of ammonia and nitrite varies depending on species' tolerance and level accumulated
- Biological filters take several weeks to become 'mature' and fully efficient
- Biofilters require adequate oxygen to function efficiently

- Biological filtration releases acids as a byproduct of the nitrogen cycle. Naturally occurring pH buffers in the water help control drastic pH changes for a certain amount of time. When buffers are consumed, the pH can fall dramatically. This is called a 'pH crash', often seen in mature tanks ('old tank syndrome') that have not been maintained well. The pH crash is preceded by a drop in 'alkalinity' (bicarbonate concentration).

Temperature

Fish are poikilothermic. Optimal temperatures vary between fish species and within general groups: tropical (warmwater) or temperate (coldwater). Changes in the water temperature affect a fish's ability to respond to stress, mount an immune response and maintain vital metabolic functions. Water temperature also affects the ability to metabolize drugs and can affect the overall response to treatment. Disease outbreaks are common in outdoor ponds in the spring and autumn when temperatures are fluctuating. In aquaria, heater failures can predispose fish to disease outbreaks. Most fish can tolerate a rapid drop in water temperature better than a rapid rise. Water at high temperatures contains less dissolved oxygen, making the fish more susceptible to the toxic effects of ammonia. When the water temperature is high, it is best to limit or stop feeding, minimize fish stress, and add extra aeration. Commercial chillers, in addition to heaters, are available for aquaria.

Diet

A variety of commercial food exists for pet fish, with several for specific groups (e.g. cichlid foods) or feeding types (herbivores, omnivores, carnivores). Food may be formulated as pellets, flakes, freeze-dried, frozen or gel; or live prey, such as *Artemia salina* (brine shrimp), rotifers, small fish and some species of worms, can be fed.

- Food should be offered in small quantities several times daily in an amount that fish will consume in 3–5 minutes.
- Sinking pellets are best for fancy goldfish varieties prone to buoyancy disorders.
- Commercial food should be purchased in small quantities and rotated among brands for optimal nutrition.
- Food should be stored adequately to preserve freshness. Rancid or mouldy food should not be fed. Discard food after 6–8 months.
- Outdoor pond fish should not be fed when water temperatures are <6°C.
- Live food should be quarantined or raised to prevent the introduction of parasites and other pathogens.

Preventive healthcare

All new introductions to an established system should undergo a quarantine procedure. Failure to do this is a leading cause of the introduction of infectious disease. During quarantine, new fish can be observed for clinical signs of disease. Prophylactic treatments for common disorders, such as monogenean fluke infestations, can be instituted. Quarantine systems can also function later as hospital tanks.

With koi, the water temperature should be raised to permissive temperatures for viral diseases, specifically koi herpesvirus (KHV). The length of quarantine is determined by the function of the fish (wholesale, retail, home aquaria or pond), fish species, and use of prophylactic treatments or diagnostic testing. The author recommends a very conservative quarantine period of 6–12 months for koi by hobbyists prior to introduction into a closed population. Retailers should hold fish for at least 30 days, although 60 days would be preferable.

Handling and restraint

Fish are very susceptible to stress, and all interactions should have preparations made to reduce capture stress whenever possible. Capture should be done as efficiently as possible, with minimal time spent chasing fish. Removal of aquarium décor may improve capture time in tanks. If capture is not possible with minimal stress, fish can be sedated *in situ* (see below).

Nets are notorious for damaging delicate fins, other appendages and the mucus layer, and abrading the thin fish epithelium. Nets should be made of a fine material to minimize potential damage. The use of seine and sock nets in outdoor ponds can facilitate capture of specific individuals. Large fish should be afforded extra care, as their skeletal system does not provide adequate support out of the water. For the capture of koi, a 'bowling' technique can be used. A bowl of suitable size is floated in the pond. With a large net, the koi can be gently guided into the bowl or into a sock net and then placed into the bowl (Figure 19.5). The lidded bowl containing the koi is then removed from the water.

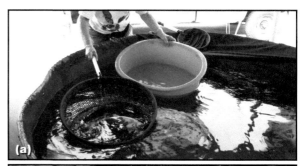
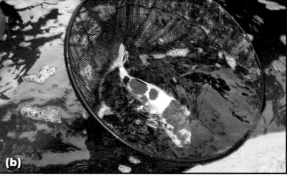

19.5 Capture techniques of koi: **(a)** netting the fish; **(b)** using a round net prior to transfer of the koi to a bowl. (continues)

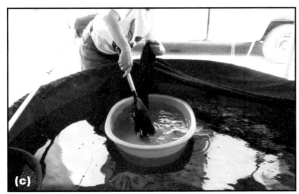

19.5 (continued) Capture techniques of koi: **(c)** the koi is transferred to a bowl using a sock net.

Most fish are restrained by chemical means for examination and diagnostic testing. It is possible to handle very small or debilitated fish carefully without using sedation but for a more comprehensive evaluation, sedation or anaesthesia will be necessary (see below). Unpowdered gloves should be used whenever handling fish to minimize damage to the protective mucus layer and to minimize exposure to zoonotic pathogens such as *Mycobacterium*.

Transport

When it is not possible to make a site visit, clients can transport their fish to the veterinary hospital. Insulated containers with enough water to cover the fish are ideal for short trips. Longer trips may require supplemental aeration and containment of the fish in plastic bags. Oxygen can also be added to the transport bag. If the visit is scheduled in advance, it may be beneficial to withhold food for at least 24 hours prior to the trip. All clients should be asked to bring separate containers of water from the fish's tank or pond; this will be used for water quality testing, for anaesthesia induction and recovery.

Diagnostic approach

The first contact a fish practitioner has with a client is usually a frantic phone call with a description of the problem. Many clients will only want advice regarding a 'miracle' tablet or liquid that can be added to the tank or pond to 'cure' the problem. After careful questioning, a presumptive diagnosis may be apparent but only tests can provide a definitive diagnosis in most cases. Pathognomonic lesions are very rare in pet fish medicine.

History

The importance of an accurate and complete history cannot be overemphasized. A differential diagnosis list can then be prepared. A trained veterinary nurse or technician can assist the practitioner by obtaining a complete history (Figure 19.6). A common cause of poor water quality is failure to maintain the life-support equipment as needed. It is important when evaluating sick fish, particularly when several fish are affected, to evaluate the filtration system, supporting equipment, and maintenance practices. When a visit to the site is

Tank/pond life-support systems
Age of tank/pond Volume Lighting/photoperiod Pumps (including gallons/litres per hour) Biofilter type Aeration Bottom substrate/thickness Pond lining Tank/pond décor Plants Location Nets/other equipment
Water
Source Temperature Water change schedule and amount changed Date of last water change Water treatments including UV filters (wattage), ozone, protein skimmers and chemicals added Last test results Type and age of test kit used
Husbandry
Schedule Equipment maintenance Water changes
Inhabitants
Species and numbers Compatibility Recent introductions? When? Previous problems?
Quarantine protocols
Length of time Treatments routinely used Any abnormalities noted? Plants quarantined or treated?
Food
Type Quantity/frequency Source of live food
Clinical signs observed
Number of fish affected Description of clinical signs Length or duration of signs Deaths? Medications or treatments used: dosage, duration and result
Miscellaneous
Use of chemicals near pond/tank? Predator activity (ponds)? Anything unusual?

19.6 Elements of a clinical history.

not feasible, the client should be instructed to bring pictures or video images of the set-up and equipment and of any abnormal behaviours noted.

Home visit

It is advisable to recommend that the client isolate the affected fish prior to a home visit. Equipment such as nets and bowls should be restricted for use to one system only to minimize spread of disease.

Practitioners should carry a disinfecting solution to clean and disinfect their own equipment when working with different aquaria and ponds.

Observation

The patient should be observed from a distance initially to assess behaviour, body condition, symmetry and respiratory effort. It is preferable to observe the fish in its home environment (tank or pond) with minimal interference.

Abnormal behaviours include:

- Flashing: fish with pruritus due to external parasites may rub vigorously on surfaces and expose the ventrum, a 'flash' of pale colour
- Gasping/'piping': open-mouth breathing at the water's surface
- Congregation at areas of increased aeration (increased dissolved oxygen) such as waterfalls
- Exaggerated opercular excursions
- Clamping: fins held close to the body instead of outward
- Isolation, hiding or staying near the bottom of the pond or tank when food is presented.

The patient should also be assessed for the presence of buoyancy problems, clinical signs and external lesions.

Clinical examination

Sedation can facilitate a complete physical examination. Supplies needed for examination, anaesthesia and diagnostic testing should be gathered in advance in order to minimize the time the patient is under anaesthesia and to streamline the process. Supplies include:

- Induction/holding container with known volume of water
- Water from patient's aquarium or pond
- Anaesthetic agent (tricaine methone sulphonate, MS-222) and sodium bicarbonate
- Gram scale to weigh patient
- Instruments, materials (slides, etc.) for procedures
- Recovery tank and supplemental aeration if needed.

A systematic approach, 'nose to caudal fin', should be used. Skin disease may present as flashing, scale loss and epidermal ulcers. The ventral aspect can 'hide' cutaneous ulceration that may not be easily observed without sedation. Fluorescein dye strips can be used not only to evaluate corneal integrity (Figure 19.7) but also to evaluate epidermal integrity.

Gills should appear uniformly red and 'meaty', with no ragged edges or focal colour changes suggesting infection, inflammation or necrosis. Behavioural signs of gill pathology include gasping/piping, increased opercular rate, opercular flaring, and congregation at highly aerated areas (waterfalls, etc.). Diagnostic examination is done by wet mount cytology of a gill biopsy or a gill scrape (see below).

The oral cavity can be internally examined with an otoscope and cone for foreign bodies (gravel, décor) or ulcers. Goldfish and koi frequently ingest tank or

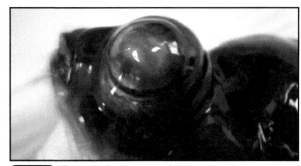

19.7 Corneal damage can be shown using fluorescein dye.

pond substrate as they scavenge for food. Diagnostic techniques for the gastrointestinal tract include wet mount examination of fresh faeces, cytology of cloacal washes and squash preparations of gastrointestinal organs made at necropsy.

The kidney can be sampled aseptically for bacterial culture in cases of suspected septicaemia. The cloaca (vent) should be examined for swelling or protrusion of internal parasites.

Fish presenting with abdominal distension and buoyancy disorders should be carefully palpated for the presence of firm masses, gas distension and fluid distension.

Water quality evaluation

If a site visit is not possible, the client should be instructed to bring a water sample, separate from the transport water, that is kept cool in transit. In addition, the client should be questioned as to the appearance of the water in the system: cloudiness, turbidity, colour, odour (if any). Water temperature, ammonia, nitrite, nitrate, pH and alkalinity levels are the minimum parameters evaluated. In addition, other parameters such as dissolved oxygen (measured early in the morning if possible), salinity, chlorine levels, and copper (if added as a therapeutic agent or is suspected as a contaminant) may need to be measured. Figure 19.4 summarizes desired levels and the effects of abnormalities.

Imaging

Radiography

Radiography is the most common technique used in pet fish. As with other procedures, materials and equipment should be prepared in advance. Sedated fish can be radiographed in a typical small animal hospital using tabletop techniques or through a plastic container filled with water. The tabletop technique yields higher quality images. The fish is briefly placed on the cassette for the image to be taken. As long as the fish is moist, it will be able to breathe; most fish are anaesthetized for the procedure. Sponge, foam or sandbags can be used as positioning devices and should be protected by plastic bags. The cassette should also be protected by a plastic bag. A minimum of two views should be taken for proper evaluation. When radiographing novel species, it is beneficial to have a 'normal' member of the species available to use as a reference. Cases that benefit from radiographic imaging include buoyancy disorders, skeletal disorders, enteric diseases, and coelomic masses (Figure 19.8).

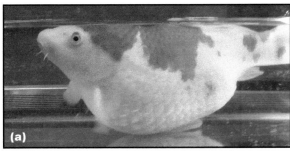

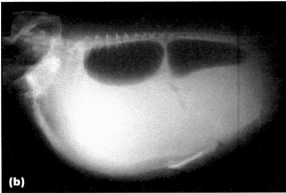

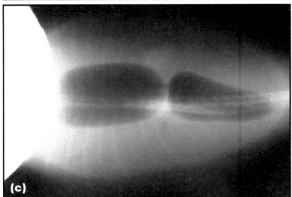

19.8 **(a)** This koi (kohaku) has a coelomic mass, which was investigated using radiography. **(b)** Lateral view. **(c)** Dorsoventral view.

Orally or rectally administered barium or water-soluble iodinated contrast media can enhance viewing of soft tissue structures and identify gastrointestinal involvement in suspected masses.

Ultrasonography
Ultrasonography is useful for evaluating soft tissue structures and possible masses in the coelomic cavity. Reproductive evaluation is especially well suited to the use of ultrasonography. In addition, fine-needle aspiration of internal organs and suspected masses can be performed more accurately in conjunction with ultrasound guidance. Ultrasonography can be performed with the patient in the water, sometimes making general anaesthesia unnecessary.

Other
Advanced imaging techniques such as magnetic resonance imaging (MRI) and computed tomography (CT) are more frequently available at large institutions and referral hospitals. These techniques have been used in fish medicine and their use is likely to increase in the future.

Sample collection

Blood
Venepuncture is best carried out using the caudal vein on a sedated or anaesthetized fish. A 25-gauge (1 ml) needle and syringe can be used on fish as small as 30 g. The client should be advised that bruising may occur, though this can be minimized by applying digital pressure at the site. Spinal injury is possible, although rare. Haemolysis may occur if excessive pressure is used when collecting the sample. Unless serum is required for a specific test, heparinizing the needle and syringe can prevent coagulation, which occurs rapidly in most fish species.

- Ventral approach:

1. Enter on the ventral midline at the level of the tail between the anal fin and the tail.
2. Advance the needle dorsally from the ventral surface of the tail, towards the spinal column, applying gentle negative pressure.

- Lateral approach (Figure 19.9)

1. Insert the needle slightly below, and parallel to, the lateral line.
2. Advance the needle in a craniomedial direction until the needle hits bone. Withdraw slightly and apply gentle negative pressure.

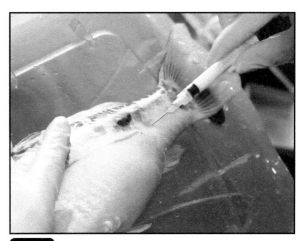

19.9 Venepuncture in a koi, lateral approach.

There is an increasing amount of published information on the use of haematology, serum chemistry and serology, but reference values have not been established for all species a practitioner may encounter. Blood sampling techniques, age, season, water temperatures, water quality, and reproductive status can affect haematological and biochemical values. It is important to note these factors when interpreting results. A recent article by Palmeiro *et al.* (2007) describes use of an in-house analyser for koi plasma chemistry values. Sick or debilitated fish may show anaemia, leucocytosis, hypoglycaemia, hypoprotein-aemia, and an elevation in liver enzyme values. Further information can be found in the References and further reading.

A blood smear can be evaluated for the presence of blood pathogens, parasites and changes in haematological parameters.

Samples for cytology

Cytology is one of the essential diagnostic tools employed for disease diagnosis in ornamental fish. Samples include skin (mucus) scrapes, gill scrapes and biopsy samples, fin biopsy, faeces, and squash preparations of organs at necropsy. Aspirates of external masses and coelomic fluid can also be obtained and fluid accumulations collected and submitted for both cytology and bacteriology. Acid-fast staining should also be performed on samples to check for the presence of *Mycobacterium* spp.

Advance preparation of material and supplies is suggested prior to obtaining samples, with or without sedation. Supplies needed include: glass slides, latex gloves (unpowdered), cover slips (plastic or glass), microscope, and sedation/holding container for the patient.

Severely debilitated fish should be approached with caution due to the added stress of handling, with or without sedation.

Skin: A skin scrape can be obtained and examined for parasites. This should not be attempted for small fish unless extreme care is taken **not to remove** most of the surface mucus layer. Applying excessive pressure and performing numerous scrapes can cause loss of scales and create entry points for bacteria. The procedure has also been described using the end of a glass slide or a scalpel blade.

1. Place a drop of water from the patient's tank or pond on a slide.
2. **Gently** scrape a cover slip at a 45-degree angle over a small area of skin of the fish, in a cranial to caudal direction (Figure 19.10). Suggested sites include the leading edges of lesions, under the mandible and just caudal to the fins.
3. Place the cover slip with the sample face down on the drop of water.
4. Starting with the lowest power objective, immediately examine the tissue microscopically for parasites, looking for characteristic movement, shape and size.

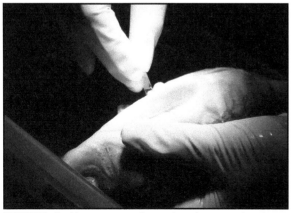

19.10 A skin scrape performed on the ventral surface of a koi.

Gills: Fish should be sufficiently calmed or sedated prior to performing a gill biopsy or scrape. Some bleeding may occur when excessive pressure is applied during a scrape; this is most often seen in large mature female koi. Bleeding can increase the risk of fatality in anaemic fish.

1. Place a drop of water from the patient's tank or pond on a slide.
2. Gently lift the operculum.
3. Biopsy: with small, sharp scissors remove a tiny piece of tissue from the end of the gills
   OR
   Scrape: using a glass or plastic coverslip, **gently** scrape a small section of the distal end of the gills.
4. Place the sample on the prepared slide and examine for pathogens and secondary lamellar pathology (e.g. hyperplasia, hypertrophy, necrosis, lamellar fusion).

Faeces/cloacal wash: Fish will often defecate when sedated or anaesthetized, or gentle pressure on the vent may yield a small faecal sample. The fish should be placed in a clean container to obtain a **fresh** sample; a plastic pipette can be used to remove this from the water. Wet mount cytology in a sample of the patient's water should be performed on the fresh sample, which can also be examined for parasites or their eggs.

If no stool is available, a cloacal wash can be performed:

1. Sedate or anaesthetize the fish.
2. Using a lubricated cannula/feeding tube/catheter, enter the vent and gently instil a small volume of sterile saline solution.
3. Gently aspirate some fluid and place on a slide for microscopic examination. Additional fluid can be collected into a sterile container for further examination.

It should be remembered that colonic tissue is very thin and can be ruptured if rough technique is used. The sample may be non-diagnostic if the fish has been chronically anorexic.

Microbiology

Virology: Diseases with a viral aetiology can be diagnosed with a variety of methods, including histopathology, tissue culture, cytology, serology, PCR, ELISA and electron microscopy.

Bacterial culture: Koi often present with cutaneous ulcers; these should be cultured using good technique, due to the possibility of contamination by surface and environmental bacteria. Debris and tissue should be debrided from the surface and the culture sample taken from the exposed deeper tissues. Alternatively, a biopsy sample can be submitted for culture.

In cases of suspected septicaemia a blood sample can be drawn from an affected fish and incubated in brain–heart infusion broth medium for 24 hours, then plated on to a culture dish. If culture is to be done *post mortem*, samples should be taken aseptically from the posterior kidney at the beginning of a necropsy to reduce the possibility of contamination.

Samples should be sent to a diagnostic laboratory that is familiar with fish pathogen identification. Most samples should be incubated at room temperature instead of the higher temperatures used for mammalian samples. Results should be interpreted with care, as some isolates may be environmental contaminants. Occasionally human enteric pathogens are cultured from fish lesions, usually in aquaria. These pathogens are not part of the normal flora of fish, and infections should be treated in line with sensitivity testing; they are most likely introduced to the tank from people with inadequate hygiene.

Necropsy

A complete history and water quality evaluation can lead the clinician to several differential diagnoses that can be confirmed by a prompt necropsy examination. In order to acquire diagnostic samples in a case affecting multiple fish, it is best to choose a freshly dead fish; it may be necessary to euthanase a moribund individual. Clients are often disappointed that no relevant data can be acquired from dead fish they present to the veterinary surgeon. Fish tissues undergo autolysis very quickly after death, so it is essential to perform a necropsy immediately. Knowing the anatomy of a normal fish (of the same species) makes recognition of abnormal anatomy much easier. Detailed notes should be taken during the procedure and kept as part of the complete medical record, with a copy submitted with the necropsy samples to the pathology laboratory. Digital images can also be included with the submission. Small fish, such as neon tetras, can be sent whole in formalin.

1. Record the weight and length of the fish.
2. Document all external abnormalities, including number, size and location. Lesions can be sampled for possible parasites and other pathogens.
3. Carefully examine the gills (grossly and microscopically), the inside of the oral cavity, the vent and fins for any lesions. The gills and associated structures can be examined in more detail by removing the operculum.
4. Place the body in lateral recumbency.
5. Start an opening on the ventrum with a scalpel blade or sterile sharp scissors at the level of the pectoral fins and extend to the caudal aspect of the coelomic cavity, then dorsally. At the cranial border, extend the opening dorsally towards the spine. This creates a flap in the body wall that can be reflected, allowing access to the coelomic cavity. **Avoid contaminating or cutting into any organs.**
6. Reflect the swim bladder to expose the posterior kidney and use aseptic technique to take renal samples for culture.
7. Take samples from other organs; place in formalin or use for squash preparations for immediate on-site evaluation. Incising the coelomic cavity along the ventral aspect in small fish helps with fixation of the specimen.

Common conditions

Common conditions seen in pet freshwater fish, their causes, characteristics and diagnostic tests are listed in Figure 19.11 and illustrated in Figures 19.12 to 19.16.

Condition or agent	Clinical signs	Predisposing factors	Diagnostics	Comments
Viral infections				
Carp pox (cyprinid herpesvirus 1, CyHV-1)	White to grey slightly raised smooth plaques; resemble 'melted candle wax'		Gross appearance: classic pale, waxy lesions; histopathology	May regress with time or in warmer water
Goldfish herpesvirus (cyprinid herpesvirus 2, CyHV-2)	High mortalities (80%+); lethargy; anaemia; anorexia; pale patches on skin and gills; enlarged spleen and kidney with white nodules	Water temperatures >15°C	PCR is test of choice: can detect active and carrier infections	
KHV (koi herpesvirus) (cyprinid herpesvirus 3, CyHV-3)	Acute mortalities (90%+); focal gill necrosis (Figure 19.12); enophthalmia; cutaneous ulcers	Water temperatures 16–28°C for optimal viral growth. Often associated with failure to quarantine new fish	Clinical signs; seasonality; high mortality; gross lesions. PCR is test of choice for active infections (submit kidney, spleen, gill tissue)	Goldfish may serve as vectors or carriers once exposed. Fomites may also transmit the virus. Serological test available to determine prior exposure (identify latent carriers)
Lymphocystis (iridovirus)	White/grey/tan masses on skin; hypertrophy of epidermis; lesions can be anywhere	Associated with stress. The Ornamental Aquatic Trade Association (OATA) specifically does not recommend dyeing or painting fish due to an increased susceptibility to lymphocystis	Wet mount cytology/ histopathology (showing dermal fibroblasts)	Can resolve with correction of environmental stressors; usually self-limiting. Surgical excision required when interferes with eating

19.11 Common conditions seen in pet freshwater fish. (continues) ▶

Condition or agent	Clinical signs	Predisposing factors	Diagnostics	Comments
Bacterial infections				
Columnaris disease (*Flavobacterium*, formerly *Flexibacter*)	Cutaneous erosions, erythema. Lesions can appear fluffy, white ('cotton wool disease'). 'Mouth rot' (oral lesions); 'fin and tail rot' (fin/tail lesions); 'saddleback disease' (lesions over dorsum)	Poor water quality; stress; high temperatures; overcrowding	Lesion cytology shows classic 'haystack' appearance of bacteria	Common in live bearers (guppies, sword tails, mollies)
'Dropsy' (Figure 19.13)	Coelomic distension with cutaneous oedema causing scales to protrude ('pinecone disease'); ascites; death			Multiple causes, including septicaemia, renal/osmoregulatory failure
Mycobacteriosis (*Mycobacterium* spp.)	Chronic, wasting disease: emaciation, sunken abdomen; ascites/dropsy; fin rot; exophthalmia; granulomas in many organs	Older fish. Common in *Betta splendens*	Acid-fast rod bacteria	Long incubation period; history of chronic low level mortalities. No effective treatment. **Zoonotic**
Septicaemia (Figure 19.14)	Lethargy; anorexia; colour changes; petechiae/ecchymosis; erosion; red appearance to fin and tails ('rot'); cutaneous oedema; 'dropsy'; exophthalmia; death		Blood culture	Add NaCl to reduce osmotic gradient. Improve water quality and management practices. Poor prognosis
Ulcerative dermatitis (Figure 19.15)	Superficial to deep ulceration of the skin; single or multiple lesions. Can be progressive: if body cavity penetrated, ulcer can be fatal due to loss of osmoregulation	External parasites; poor water quality; poor husbandry; septicaemia; loss of epithelial integrity. Bacterial invasion secondary or primary	Culture of blood or lesion samples	
Fungal infections				
Branchiomycosis ('gill rot')	High mortalities (50%+); haemorrhage, congestion and necrosis of gills; dyspnoea/gasping	Poor water quality; overcrowding; other stressors	Wet mount cytology; histopathology; fungal culture	
Saprolegnia	White, tan, green, red or brown cottony mass. Disease can progress to osmoregulatory compromise and death	Usually secondary to acute or chronic stress. Often seen in cooler weather. May be associated with immune suppression	Cytology reveals non-septate hyphae (differentiates from *Flavobacterium* and *Epistylis*)	Ubiquitous in environment
Ectoparasites				
Protozoa				
Chilodinella spp.	Excess mucus (gills and skin irritant); flashing; can be fatal	Can be seen in cooler water temperatures (5–10°C)	Wet mount cytology: skin scrapes and gill biopsy. Microsocopy: heart- or onion-shaped	
Ichthyobodo spp. (*Costia*)	Excessive mucus; flashing. Debilitating; can be fatal		Wet mount cytology: skin scrapes and gill biopsy. Smallest protozoan parasite on skin scrapes. Can be identified by 'flickering', corkscrew motion on slide	
Ichthyophthirius multifiliis ('Ich', 'Ick', 'whitespot disease')	Small circular raised white nodules; severe infection causes depression, acute death		Skin scrape: large, slow-moving organisms on wet mount	Obligate parasite with direct lifecycle. Only free-swimming life stages are affected by treatments
Tetrahymena spp. ('Guppy disease')	Excess mucus production; patchy epithelial damage and necrotic lesions. Can be cutaneous surface contaminant on bottom-dwelling fish; can invade and progress to internal infection, causing exophthalmia, periocular lesions, muscle swelling and systemic disease		Pyriform or cylindrical	Usually found in organic debris on bottom of tank and pond

19.11 (continued) Common conditions seen in pet freshwater fish. (continues) ▶

Condition or agent	Clinical signs	Predisposing factors	Diagnostics	Comments
Ectoparasites continued				
Protozoa continued				
Trichodina spp.	Pruritus; flashing; skin lesions; anorexia. Secondary bacterial infections. Chronic low level mortalities	Common in pond fish; often associated with poor water quality	Wet mount cytology: skin scrapes and gill biopsy. Microscopy: round; rapid movement; characteristic denticulate ring	
Flukes				
Dactylogyrus spp.	Flashing; epithelial integrity compromised; secondary ulcers/erosions	Often found on fancy goldfish	Wet mount cytology: skin scrapes and gill biopsy. Microscopy: oviparous; four anterior 'eye spots'	Require multiple treatments
Gyrodactylus spp.	Flashing; epithelial integrity compromised; secondary ulcers/erosions		Wet mount cytology: skin scrapes and gill biopsy. Microscopy: viviparous larvae can be seen inside female; no 'eye spots'	
Crustaceans				
Argulus spp.	Skin lesions; flashing/irritation. Secondary infections possible		Visible on examination with naked eye, though may not be obvious due to small size. Motile	Can act as vectors for infectious diseases
Lernaea spp.	Flashing/irritation; inflamed wounds at site of attachment. Secondary infections possible		Visible with the naked eye; owner may mistake them for 'sticks' adhering to fish	Often respond to chitin inhibitors. Can be carefully removed manually
Miscellaneous				
Buoyancy disorders	Positive ('floaters') or negative ('sinkers') buoyancy	May be secondary to trauma/neurological disease, mass causing compression of swim bladder. Swim bladder disorders common in globoid fancy goldfish	Radiography; FNA if fluid-filled (culture, cytology, acid-fast staining)	Treatment is not always successful
Cutaneous neoplasia	Raised growth on epidermis: smooth or rough; yellow, brown, red, blue-black, white; benign or malignant; locally or systemically aggressive	Fibromas/fibrosarcomas common on goldfish, angelfish (oral)	FNA or biopsy. Differentiate from lymphocystis, carp pox, trauma, and other causes of nodular disease	
Coelomic cavity swollen (egg binding, ascites, mass, buoyancy disorders, granulomatous disease)	Distension of coelomic cavity		Radiography/ultrasonography; FNA if fluid suspected	Prognosis determined by aetiology
Head and lateral line erosion (HLLE, 'hole-in-the-head' disease) (Figure 19.16)	Cutaneous depressions with colour change (usually pale): localized to head and lateral line but can spread to other areas. Ulcerations can infiltrate dermis and underlying cartilage	Chronic stress: poor water quality, nutritional disorders, parasitism, immunosuppression. Often seen in older fish		Not completely understood; multiple aetiologies. Multiple treatment regimens have been reported
Ophthalmic diseases	Corneal abrasions/inflammation; neoplasia; uveitis; lens luxation; trauma	Fish with prominent eyes (e.g. bubble-eye goldfish) more susceptible to trauma		Treatment depends on aetiology
Sunburn		Shallow ponds with minimal shade; light coloured fish		
Trauma (predation attempts (see Figure 19.18), inter/intraspecies aggression, iatrogenic, external parasites, lightning strike/stray voltage)	Dorsal lesions: range from petechiae and ecchymosis to superficial ulcerative dermatitis and necrosis. Secondary bacterial infection		Radiography for suspected skeletal lesions	Wounds may require surgical debridement. Treat for secondary infections. Eliminate cause if possible

19.11 (continued) Common conditions seen in pet freshwater fish.

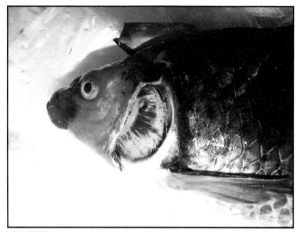

19.12 Typical gill lesions associated with koi herpesvirus infection.

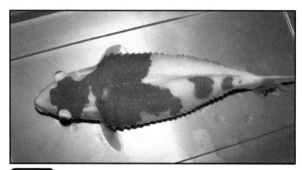

19.13 'Dropsy' in a koi.

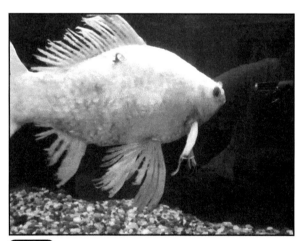

19.14 Septicaemia in a goldfish.

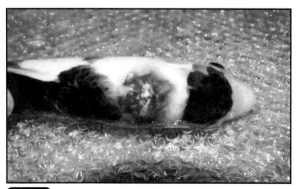

19.15 Cutaneous ulcer in a koi.

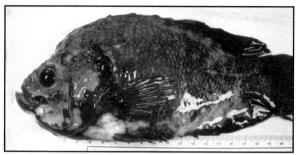

19.16 Severe head and lateral line erosion in an oscar (*Astronotus ocellatus*).

The role of stress

Stress is the most common factor involved in fish disease, with poor water quality being the most common stressor. Initially the stress response is beneficial but it leads to further problems when it becomes chronic. The generalized stress response is characterized by the initial response to a stressor, followed by a period of adaptation or resistance, including the release of the chemical mediators of stress – catecholamines and cortisol. External or visible signs of catecholamine and cortisol release include random swimming behaviour (ataxia), increased respiratory rate and colour change. Both mediators affect ion transport at the gill level, causing temporary changes in gill permeability. Several physiological changes also occur internally, including measurable alterations in heart rate, blood parameters and metabolic effects. Cortisol release can continue for weeks or months, depending on the severity of the stress. Fish can and do adapt to stress over time but the initial effects may still be seen. The long-term effects of chronic stress include increased susceptibility to disease, poor growth and reproductive failures.

It makes sense to prevent or reduce the amount of stress whenever possible. This can be achieved by the following:

- Adding sodium chloride to the water to reduce the osmotic gradient, reducing energy expenditure
- Reducing stocking density or bioload
- Using sedation or anaesthesia when handling or transporting
- Withholding food prior to handling or transporting
- Pre-planning any involved procedure (e.g. surgery, examination), evaluating logistics of the procedure, and gathering all materials in advance.

Supportive care

Medication alone will usually not treat or prevent a recurrence of disease unless management changes are implemented. There are several contributory factors and stressors to any disease outbreak situation in fish and it is important to identify these. Supportive care is also vital to the overall success of treatment. Supportive care in fish involves management and husbandry changes, medical or surgical intervention, and providing for adequate nutrition. Supportive care needs to be accomplished with a minimum of stress to the patient.

First aid

When clients make initial contact with one or multiple health problems in their fish and are unable to travel to the veterinary hospital, some general recommendations for first aid can be given. Clients should stop the use of any unknown or proprietary over-the-counter treatments, measure the basic water quality parameters, and perform several water changes. Clients should reduce feeding and isolate affected fish if the problem is not widespread.

Sodium chloride (non-iodized and without additives) can be added as a general stress-reducing aid at the rate of 1–3 g/l (1–3 parts per thousand). Fish that may be 'salt-sensitive' should be monitored for adverse effects. Some plants cannot tolerate elevated salinity in ponds and should be removed.

General guidelines for treatment of fish and their systems include:

- Clean the pond or tank (e.g. for heavy levels of organic materials, detritus, debris, etc.) and perform water changes as needed
- Clean biofilters for maximum efficiency
- Remove carbon and charcoal filters; increase aeration
- Treat any pathogen or disease situation affecting gills first
- Reduce population if possible
- Reduce or stop feeding if treatment allows
- Monitor for adverse reactions
- Perform a biotest when using new treatments
- Monitor water quality, including ammonia, nitrite, dissolved oxygen and pH levels
- In general, antimicrobial treatment should be administered for a minimum of 2 weeks if a positive response to therapy is seen, regardless of route of administration
- Double check all calculations.

Hospitalization

Hospitalizing fish does not occur often in private practice. Post-surgical monitoring may be the only time a fish needs to stay at the veterinary hospital for any length of time. The client should provide most, if not all, of the water for the duration of the patient's stay. In social species such as koi and goldfish, a conspecific should be provided to reduce stress and provide companionship. The client should also provide food if indicated.

Facilities for hospitalization do not need to be extravagant, but the following should be provided:

- A cover or lid to prevent accidental death due to jumping
- Container of adequate size for the species
- Separate nets and other equipment for each container or tank
- Daily monitoring of water quality and daily water changes
- Aeration equipment (air stones, air pumps, bubblers, etc.)
- Heating equipment when required by species
- Education of the staff with regards to monitoring, management, and husbandry of the patient
- For long-term stays, biofiltration systems.

Drug administration

Medications can be administered to fish by several routes. When developing a treatment plan for fish, several factors must be considered:

- Number of fish requiring treatment and number of treatments required
- Cost of treating entire system and population
- Ease of capture of fish and stress involved
- Effect of treatment on non-target species.

Water treatment

Water treatment, baths, dips or prolonged immersion regimens are convenient and can be carried out by the owner in most situations. Bath and dip treatments in small containers are sometimes less expensive that prolonged immersion, which requires the medication to be added to a larger volume of water. Gram scales should be used to measure medications accurately.

- A dip is a water treatment that can be measured in seconds or minutes. Most dips require removal of the fish at the first sign of stress.
- Bath treatments are longer, lasting up to 24 hours.
- Treatments requiring prolonged immersion can last indefinitely or for several days. When choosing a prolonged immersion treatment, it is essential to know the correct volume of water.

The following formulae are useful when calculating dose rates:

- Ponds:
  - Average depth (metres) x average width (metres) x average length (metres) x 1000 = volume in litres
  - Average depth (feet) x average width (feet) x average length (feet) x 7.5 = volume in US gallons.
- Aquaria:
  - Length (cm) x width (cm) x depth (cm) ÷ 1000 = volume in litres
  - Length (inches) x width (inches) x depth (inches) ÷ 231 = volume in US gallons.
- 1 part per million (ppm) = 1 mg/l = 1 microlitre (µl) per litre
- 1 part per thousand (ppt) = 1 g/l = 0.1% = 1 ml/l.

A biotest should be performed when administering drugs to a novel species. Idiosyncratic or hypersensitivity reactions can occur. In general, species without scales tend to be more sensitive to added drugs. It is important to remind the client to remove carbon or activated charcoal in the filters, mix medication according to directions, and disperse the drugs in the water column. Antibacterial medication will not only affect target microbes on the fish but also the nitrifying bacteria; monitoring ammonia and nitrite levels is recommended during and following the use of antimicrobials.

Freshwater fish drink very little or no water, so medications added to water for internal disorders are seldom effective. They are best suited for external pathogens and gill pathogens. Water temperature and pH can affect the efficacy or potential toxicity of water treatments. Water temperatures need to be within the optimal range for metabolism of the drug and pH must be measured prior to starting treatment. High levels of organic debris and detritus can reduce the effectiveness of some products. Finally, discharge of the contaminated water needs to be done within local guidelines.

Topical applications

Wound management, including traumatic injuries, cutaneous ulcers and surgical incisions, can include the use of topical medications in addition to systemic treatments. In cases involving superficial small wounds, topical treatment alone may suffice. Medications should be applied to a clean or freshly debrided wound; drying the area by careful use of gauze squares or sterile cotton swabs before application may facilitate adherence.

In-feed medication

Administering medication in feed is much less stressful than any other method of treatment and is also more cost-effective when treating many fish in one habitat. A number of techniques are used, including: top dressing existing feed; feeding commercial formulas; mixing medication into a gelatin-based homemade preparation; and adding medication into food substances by injection or soaking. Fish will eat between 1 and 6% of their bodyweight in food, depending on health status, water temperature, growth stage and other variables. It is best to calculate the amount ingested at 0.5–1.0% bodyweight when feeding medicated food to sick, non-anorectic fish. Consumption of any oral medication can be enhanced when fish are fasted temporarily for 12–24 hours prior to use of the medicated food. Disadvantages of in-feed administration include improper dosing, leaching of medication into the water, and the labour-intensive effort involved in preparation.

Injection sites

Injectable medications are the most effective way to dose fish accurately, but administering injections can be very stressful to the patient. Two main techniques are used in private practice: intracoelomic and intramuscular. Intravenous administration is primarily done in research situations. Despite initial hesitation, most clients can be taught to administer intramuscular injections to their fish when multiple treatments are recommended.

Intramuscular injection:

- Can be accomplished through a net or plastic bag without anaesthesia or sedation
- Best given in the epaxial musculature parallel to the dorsal fin and above the lateral line (Figure 19.17)
- At a 45 degree angle, bury the needle under a scale and enter the muscle. Inject the medication, withdraw the needle and apply digital pressure to minimize leakage
- Warn owner a bruise may develop at the site of injection. Sterile injection site reactions have been reported
- Alternate sides when giving multiple or a series of injections.

Intracoelomic injection:

- Inject just off the ventral midline, midway between the pectoral and pelvic fin, cranial to the vent. Holding the fish (sedated or anaesthetized) in dorsal recumbency facilitates injection
- Use as short a needle as possible
- Try to insert needle under a scale in scaled fish to minimize leakage
- Can also be done through netting or a plastic bag but the risk of internal injury is higher without sedation or anaesthesia
- Fasting the fish for 12–24 hours prior to injection reduces the risk of injecting an organ
- There is a risk of an internal reaction or hypersensitivity to the material injected.

Anaesthesia and analgesia

Unless a patient is fragile, moribund or extremely debilitated, sedation or anaesthesia will be required to obtain diagnostic samples. Sedation and anaesthesia are also helpful to reduce the stress of handling and transport. Most fish can be transferred to a water-filled anaesthetic chamber or container.

In situations requiring sedation or anaesthesia of large fish that cannot be removed from their original tank or pond, sedation and anaesthesia must take place *in situ*. Two options are available for this: either applying a very concentrated solution of anaesthetic to the gills with a spray bottle or similar and extracting

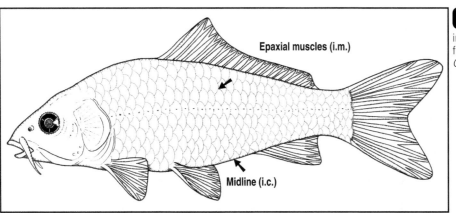

19.17 Intramuscular and intracoelomic injection sites. (Reproduced from *BSAVA Manual of Ornamental Fish, 2nd edition.*)

Epaxial muscles (i.m.)

Midline (i.c.)

the sedated fish; or reducing the tank volume to a practical level and adding the anaesthetic directly to the tank. The presence of other tank inhabitants, décor and equipment must be considered. There can also be a significant cost factor with the amount of anaesthetic, time and labour involved.

MS-222

Currently, the only anaesthetic authorized for use in finfish in the USA and European Union (including the UK) is tricaine methane sulphonate, also known as TMS or MS-222. This is a white crystalline powder that is mixed with the (patient's own) water. Sodium bicarbonate is used to buffer an otherwise acidic solution that can have harmful effects on the fish, including corneal and epidermal damage. The ratio varies depending on the local water supply characteristics, but in most cases, 2 parts of sodium bicarbonate to 1 part of MS-222 is effective. The anaesthetic powder and sodium bicarbonate should be weighed on a gram scale for accurate dosing. A working stock solution of 10 g/l MS-222 can be prepared in advance and stored for several months (must be protected from light). The calculated amount can then be added to a known volume of water when needed.

Most fish can be sedated with a 50–100 ppm (mg/l) solution in 3–5 minutes. Some finfish species may require a higher dose. The initial concentration should be decreased for sick or stressed, debilitated fish. Novel species should always be approached with care when anaesthetizing for the first time: it is always better to start with a lower dose and increase if needed. Cooler water will result in a longer induction time.

MS-222 at a concentration of 1 g/l has also been directly applied to gills as a spray for faster induction of anaesthesia in larger species.

> **WARNING**
> **Gloves should always be worn when handling MS-222 to reduce the potential for mucous membrane irritation. Retinal toxicity has been reported as a potential sequel of long-term exposure, so protective goggles are recommended during handling of the powdered form. Idiosyncratic inflammatory reactions can also occur and possible carcinogenicity has been reported in a few studies.**

Other agents

Benzocaine is sometimes used, although it is not currently authorized for use in fish. It is insoluble in water and must be prepared with acetone or ethanol prior to use. A stock solution of 100 g/l can be made in advance and, if protected from light exposure, may be kept for up to a year. The margin of safety is reported as being reduced in higher water temperatures.

Isoeugenol is licensed for use in New Zealand, Australia, Chile, Korea and Costa Rica but is not authorized for use in the UK or the USA. It is used for humane harvesting and transport of fish. Several countries are currently investigating this drug for approval. Recently a National Toxicology Program (NTP) exposure study found evidence of carcinogenicity in isoeugenol and currently all investigational use studies have ceased in the United States.

Metomidate is a water-soluble anaesthetic compound that has been used in aquaculture. It has a rapid induction and recovery compared with MS-222. Colour changes and transient muscle twitches may be observed in some species. In June 2009, the United States Food and Drug Administration (FDA) added metomidate to the Index of Legally Marketed Unapproved New Animal Drugs for use as a sedative and anaesthetic in ornamental finfish.

Clove oil is often used by koi and goldfish hobbyists to sedate their own fish. Dispersion in water can be improved by initially mixing with warm water and shaking the solution prior to adding to an anaesthesia container. Clove oil is not approved for use in fish but is widely available without a prescription. It has several disadvantages: it is poorly soluble in water, has a rapid induction rate, a prolonged recovery rate, a narrower margin of safety, and is a potential carcinogen. In addition, clove oil has fewer analgesic properties than MS-222 and the concentration of active ingredient can vary between lots. However, clove oil does seem to have a measurable benefit in reducing short-term stress compared with MS-222.

Stages of anaesthesia

- Stage 0: Normal.
- Stage 1: Light sedation – will react to external stimuli; normal equilibrium (adequate for handling and transport in most species).
- Stage 2: Deeper sedation – less reactive to stimuli; normal equilibrium.
- Stage 3: Light anaesthesia – some analgesia; partial loss of equilibrium.
- Stage 4: Moderate anaesthesia – loss of equilibrium; slight reaction to strong stimuli.
- Stage 5: Deep anaesthesia (surgical anaesthesia) – no reaction to any external stimuli.
- Stage 6: Respiration ceases, cardiac arrest, death.

Some group the above into stages and planes of anaesthesia but the progression is the same.

Analgesia

Several compounds have been used to provide analgesia in fish. These include ketoprofen, carprofen, morphine, butorphanol and buprenorphine. These compounds are often administered as a single injection preoperatively or postoperatively, but could also be used in treating traumatic injuries that do not require complicated surgical procedures.

Common surgical procedures

Most pet fish species make excellent surgical candidates. They tend to be fairly hardy and most are of sufficient size to undergo and recover from surgical intervention. Many procedures can be performed on site at the client's home or pondside.

Surgical 'tables' will vary greatly depending on the patient size and procedure required. Simple, quick procedures can be performed on a flat surface, protected from water damage and covered by a chamois cloth. Delivery of the anaesthetic can be accomplished via syringe or a water pump set to the appropriate flow rate. More extensive procedures require positioning devices, a constant delivery of anaesthesia, and the ability to aerate the anaesthetic solution if needed. Most anaesthetic units are recirculating systems that will collect and redeliver the liquid anaesthetic solution.

Suture material should be non-absorbable, minimally reactive, monofilament and of appropriate size. Suture material with swaged-on cutting needles works best on the tough skin of fish. Suture removal should be done 3–6 weeks postoperatively. Surgical tissue adhesive has been known to cause reactions in fish skin and is best avoided.

Wound management

There are many causes of wounds, including environmental factors such as sharp objects in the pond/tank, iatrogenic practices such as rough handling, abnormal fish behaviours such as jumping or 'flashing' secondary to poor water quality or external parasites, and inter- and intraspecies aggression or attempted predation (Figure 19.18). Early intervention and wound management can effect a positive outcome in many cases.

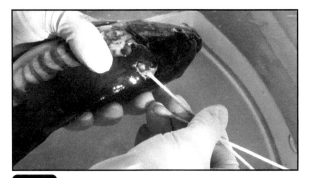

19.18 Assessing the severity of a heron injury in a koi.

Most fish require anaesthesia to evaluate and treat their injuries fully. All wounds should have samples taken for culture prior to treatment. Defects are then rinsed with dilute povidone–iodine, chlorhexidine or sterile saline. Debris should be gently removed with sterile gauze. Further surgical debridement of necrotic tissue, damaged scales and abnormal tissue can be done. Measures such as the use of sterile transparent drapes can be taken to protect the undamaged mucus layer and skin of the patient and to retain moisture. Sterile ophthalmic lubricant should be applied and the eyes covered by a moistened cloth.

Most injuries are left open to heal, but loose skin flaps where circulation has not been compromised should be sutured back into place to provide a barrier against osmotic disruption. Topical medications or waterproof pastes can be applied to the open wounds; adherence is improved by gently drying the defect with gauze prior to application. Parenteral injections of analgesics and antimicrobials can be given if indicated.

The patient is returned to the tank or pond if the injury is not too severe and does not need frequent monitoring or repeated injections. Seriously injured fish should be placed in a hospital tank or container and monitored. Sodium chloride is added to reduce osmotic stress and aid in healing, and the water temperature raised to the upper limit of the optimal range for the species. Strict attention to water quality and stress reduction is important during recovery.

External masses

External masses are a frequent client complaint in fish practice and can occur anywhere on a fish.

Masses can be removed under anaesthesia using good surgical technique (Figure 19.19). If the mass cannot be entirely removed, debulking and submitting tissue for histopathology is recommended. Most surgical sites cannot be closed and are left open to heal by second intention. Luckily, given good water quality, fish heal very quickly when compared with their terrestrial counterparts. Histopathology should be performed on all masses to give the owner a definitive diagnosis and offer a future prognosis on recurrence.

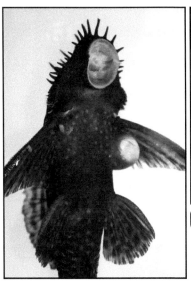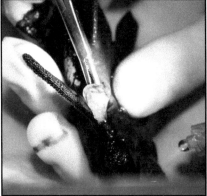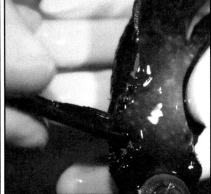

19.19 Surgical removal of a mass from a bristlenose plecostomus (*Ancistrus* spp.).

Ophthalmic surgery

Ophthalmic problems requiring surgical intervention are common in pet fish, most often affecting goldfish. Fish with prominent eyes or elaborate tissue growth near and around the eyes are more susceptible to injury, especially when housed in outdoor ponds. Enucleation (Figure 19.20) is the most common procedure performed; conditions requiring enucleation range from traumatic injuries and infections to neoplasia. Most patients recover uneventfully. Careful, direct pressure is usually sufficient for haemostasis. Healing is very rapid and the fish readily adapts to manoeuvering in its environment and acquiring food.

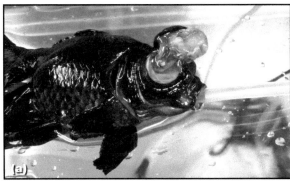

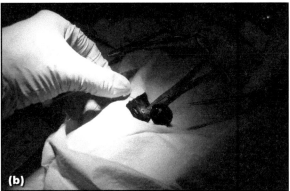

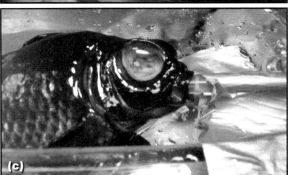

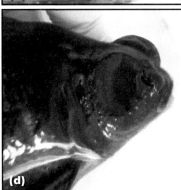

19.20

(a) Traumatic eye injury.
(b) Enucleation.
(c) Immediate postoperative appearance.
(d) Two weeks after operation.

Exploratory coeliotomy

Indications for surgical exploration of the coelomic cavity include the presence of intracoelomic masses, organ biopsy, elective gonadectomy, buoyancy disorders and research procedures. Knowledge of the internal anatomy of the affected species is essential.

1. Place the patient in dorsal recumbency.
2. Gently lavage the ventral midline with sterile saline or dilute povidone–iodine or chlorhexidine.
3. Scales can be removed to facilitate entry in large fish.
4. Use sterile, clear plastic drapes to retain moisture and minimize contamination of the surgical field.
5. Make a skin incision caudal to the pectoral fins, extending just past the pelvic fins.
6. Fish body walls are inflexible and tissue retractors can be used to improve visualization of the surgical field. Koi and goldfish may have multiple intracoelomic tissue adhesions; this is common.
7. Closure can be accomplished in one or two layers (body wall or muscle and body wall) using an appropriate suture material.
8. Sutures should be removed after 3–6 weeks. Fish held postoperatively in water of their preferred optimal temperature will heal faster compared with those kept in cooler water.

Euthanasia

Any method of euthanasia should be humane and efficient as well as safe to the person administering it. Several methods have been recommended. Physical methods include decapitation or pithing, and cranial concussion but most clients would find these unacceptable for their pets. In addition, it may be difficult for practitioners to administer physical euthanasia adequately without regret. Anaesthetic overdose and chemical euthanasia provide acceptable alternatives. Chemical methods (excluding anaesthetic overdose) should not be used in food fish.

Euthanasia for the fish patient in the hospital:

- Overdose of MS-222 (5–10 times the anaesthetic dose) or other immersion-type anaesthetics
- OR intracoelomic administration of barbiturates
- OR intracardiac injection of barbiturates (in larger fish).

Euthanasia that can be performed by owners at home:

1. Add 10–20 drops of clove oil to a small amount of warm (21°C) or hot (32°C) water.
2. Add to 1 litre of water and vigorously agitate to disperse the oil.
3. Add the fish.
4. Wait a minimum of 30 minutes following loss of consciousness.
5. Place the dead fish in a plastic bag and then in a freezer. If the patient is to be necropsied, immediate refrigeration or transport to the veterinary facility is preferred to freezing.

Drug formulary

Few drugs are authorized for use in pet fish practice, although the number is slowly growing. Many drugs are used 'off-label'; drug doses are often extrapolated from other species and the potential for effectiveness and adverse effects has not been fully evaluated in all species. Pharmacokinetic studies of readily available drugs are limited for fish and may describe results from only a limited number of species. Proprietary formulations available to the general consumer do not always list active ingredients or concentrations. It is worthwhile to ask the owner to bring in the containers of any medications used. Drugs added to the patients' tanks or ponds have the potential to adversely affect the environment and other inhabitants. For example: biofiltration failure is a frequent sequel of antimicrobials given as a prolonged immersion treatment; formalin can reduce dissolved oxygen levels; copper can be toxic to invertebrates and sensitive species; and organophosphates can be fatal to non-target species.

A drug formulary for freshwater ornamental fish is presented in Figure 19.21. This formulary is not meant to be complete nor to be an exhaustive list of available treatments. Some treatments and regimens have been excluded due to the potential for toxicity in the patient and the practitioner. For more detailed information on fish medicine see the *BSAVA Manual of Ornamental Fish*, 2nd edition.

Drug	Dose	Uses	Comments
Anaesthetics			
Benzocaine	25–50 mg/l for immersion		Insoluble in water. 100 g/l stock solution can be prepared with ethanol or acetone
Clove oil	25–100 mg/l for immersion		Used by hobbyists. Potentially carcinogenic. Not approved for use in UK or USA
Isoeugenol	10–25 mg/l for immersion (doses vary by species)		Not approved for use in UK or USA. Carcinogenic
Ketamine	66–88 mg/kg i.m.		Recovery can be prolonged
Metomidate	2.5–5 mg/l for immersion (effective dosage varies by species)		Muscle tremors and colour changes noted. Inhibits cortisol synthesis
Tricaine methane sulphonate (MS-222)	Koi, goldfish: Sedation: 10–50 mg/l Induction: 50–150 mg/l Maintenance: 25–75 mg/l Buffer with two parts sodium bicarbonate to one part MS-222 Some species may require higher dose Large fish: 1 g/l directly sprayed on gills		Can prepare 10 g/l stock solution. Protect from light. Effective for 1–3 months. Start with lower dose in novel species or debilitated animals. Recovery prolonged in cooler water, with older, gravid or obese fish
Analgesics			
Butorphanol	0.1–0.4 mg/kg i.m.	Surgery. Deep ulcers and other wounds	Unknown effectiveness in many species
Carprofen	2–4 mg/kg i.m.		Long-term effects unpredictable
Flunixin meglumine	0.25–0.5 mg/kg i.m.		Long-term effects unpredictable
Ketoprofen	2 mg/kg i.m.		Long-term effects unpredictable
Meloxicam	0.1–0.2 mg/kg i.m.		Long-term effects unpredictable
Morphine	0.3 mg/kg i.m.		Not widely used in private fish practice
Antifungal agents			
Itraconazole	1–5 mg/kg/day in feed for up to 7 days	Systemic mycoses	
Ketoconazole	2.5–10 mg/kg i.m. or daily in feed for 7–10 days	Systemic mycoses	
Antimicrobial agents			
Amikacin	5 mg/kg i.m. q12h	Sepsis. Ulcerative dermatitis. Other bacterial infections	Can be very toxic. Layperson use at inappropriate dosages very common
Aztreonam	100 mg/kg i.m/intracoelomically q48h	Sepsis. Ulcerative dermatitis. Other bacterial infections	Often used by US koi hobbyists

19.21 Drug formulary for freshwater ornamental fish. (continues) ▶

Drug	Dose	Uses	Comments
Antimicrobial agents continued			
Ceftazidime	20–30 mg/kg i.m. q72h	Sepsis. Ulcerative dermatitis. Other bacterial infections	Use by hobbyists uncommon. Must be frozen in aliquots once reconstituted
Enrofloxacin	5–20 mg/kg i.m/intracoelomically q48–72h or 2–5 mg/l bath treatment for 2–5h q24–48h or 1% in feed daily for 14–21 days	Sepsis. Ulcerative dermatitis. Other bacterial infections	Resistance not uncommon
Erythromycin			Common over-the-counter immersion treatment: toxic to biofilter. **NOT RECOMMENDED**
Florfenicol	25–30 mg/kg i.m. q12–24h or 30–50 mg/kg in feed q12–24h for 14 days (dosage and frequency may vary depending on species)	Sepsis. Ulcerative dermatitis. Other bacterial infections	
Oxolinic acid	25 mg/l as a bath for 15 minutes q12h for 3 days or 1 mg/l for prolonged immersion or 10 mg/kg in feed for 10 days	Bacterial infections	Over-the-counter product. Resistance common
Oxytetracycline	7–25 mg/kg i.m. q24h or 10–50 mg/l as a bath for 1 h or 5–10 mg per g of food for 7–10 days or 50 mg/kg bodyweight in feed for 10 days	Bacterial infections	Over-the-counter product. Resistance common. Toxic to biofilter. Light-sensitive
Sulfadimethoxine/ Ormetoprim	50 mg/kg bodyweight in feed daily for 5 days	Bacterial infections	Resistance common
Trimethoprim/ Sulphonamide	20 mg/l as a bath for 6 h q24h for 7 days or 0.2% in feed daily for 10–14 days	Bacterial infections	
Tris-EDTA and Tris-EDTA/Neomycin	Spray affected area or dip daily or as needed	Ulcerative dermatitis	Mix in spray bottle to extend usage. Dip must be discarded after use. **Do not add to tank or pond.** Medications can be added to Tri-cide as per package directions
Antiparasitic agents			
Diflubenzuron	0.4 mg/l for prolonged immersion	Crustacean ectoparasites	Chitin inhibitor. May affect non-target invertebrates
Fenbendazole	25–50 mg/kg in feed for 3–5 days; repeat after 14 days or 2 mg/l for prolonged immersion q7d for 3 treatments	Intestinal nematodes	Biotest with novel species. Potentially fatal toxicities can occur. **Change 50% water between each treatment**
Formalin (37% formaldehyde)	0.125–0.25 ml/l as a bath for up to 60 minutes daily for 2–3 days or 0.015–0.025 ml/l (15–25 ppm) for prolonged immersion q2–3d (change 50% water on non-treatment days)	Protozoal parasites. Crustacean ectoparasites	**Carcinogenic.** Depletes oxygen; additional aeration required. Some fish very sensitive. **Not for use in stressed fish.** Do not use if white precipitate forms. **Contraindicated >27°C**
Levamisole	1–2 mg/l as a bath for up to 24 h	Intestinal nematodes	
Lufenuron	0.1–0.2 mg/l prolonged immersion	Crustacean ectoparasites	Chitin inhibitor. May affect non-target invertebrates
Metronidazole	7–15 mg/l for prolonged immersion q24–48h for 5–10 days (change 50% water between treatments) or 25–50 mg/kg (0.25% in feed at 1% bodyweight/day) for 3 days	Some protozoal parasites including *Hexamita*, *Spironucleus*	Not very water-soluble. One in-feed treatment may be as effective as three water treatments
Praziquantel	Flukes: 2–10 mg/l as a bath for 2–4h or for prolonged immersion Dactylogyrids: q7d for 4–6wk Gyrodactylids: q7d for 2–4wk Cestodes: 50 mg/kg single oral dose q24h		Add aeration. Powders not very water-soluble. Can be expensive in large systems. Re-check wet mount cytology should be performed after treatment

19.21 (continued) Drug formulary for freshwater ornamental fish. (continues) ▶

Drug	Dose	Uses	Comments
Topical medications		Postoperative incisions. Cutaneous ulcers	Most require a dry surface for better adherence
Betadine (povidone–iodine) ointment	q12h		
Orabase (2-octyl-cyanoacrylate) bioadhesive paste	Once		Waterproof paste
Panolog (nystatin, neomycin, thiostrepton, triamcinolone) ointment	q12–24h		Unknown whether chronic use inhibits healing
Regranex (becaplermin)-recombinant platelet derived growth factor	q24h	Promotes angiogenesis	Has been used to treat chronic wounds and head/lateral line erosion. Expensive
Silver sulfadiazine	q12 h		
Triple antibiotic ointment	q12h		
Miscellaneous			
Chlorhexidine	Dilute to 10% solution	Wound, ulcer, surgical site irrigation	Avoid scrub formulation
Hydrogen peroxide 3%	0.25–5 ml/l in water	Hypoxia	Emergency treatment of water
Potassium permanganate	2 mg/l for prolonged immersion or 5–20 mg/l as a bath for 1 h Bath disinfectant for new plants: 5 mg/l for 1–24h	External infections. Ectoparasites. Fungal infections	Inactivated by organic compounds in water. Caustic. Toxic in high-pH water. Stains hands/clothing. Can be toxic to some fish species, such as orfe and closely related species. A biotest should be performed when in doubt or with use in a novel species. Can cause blindness (powder) in humans. Watch for signs of stress with use. **Better products are available**
Povidone–iodine	Dilute to 10% solution	Wound, ulcer, surgical site irrigation	Avoid scrub formulation
Sodium bicarbonate	To effect	Low pH ('pH crash')	
Sodium chloride	1–3 g/l for prolonged immersion Osmotic stress reduction: 3–6 g/l for prolonged immersion For protozoan parasites: 10–30 g/l dip (for minutes until fish shows signs of stress)	Transport stress. Loss of epidermal integrity. Post-surgical recovery. Nitrite toxicity	Monitor for adverse effects in scaleless fish and other potential salt-sensitive species. Can be toxic to some plants. Dip is often used in quarantine
Sodium thiosulfate	10 mg/l		Widely available in many preparations. Also available as crystals (more cost-effective for large systems). Dechlorinates municipal water. Requires water changes
Virkon S	1–2 ppm	Water disinfectant	Has been used with some aquatic species remaining in the system. A biotest is recommended when using a product on a novel species

19.21 (continued) Drug formulary for freshwater ornamental fish.

References and further reading

Boyd CE (1990) *Water Quality in Ponds for Aquaculture.* Birmingham Publishing, Birmingham, AL

Ferguson HW (2006) *Systemic Pathology of Fish, 2nd edn.* Scotian Press, London

Fontenot DK and Neiffer DL (2004) Wound management in teleost fish: biology of the healing process, evaluation, and treatment. *Veterinary Clinics of North America: Exotic Animal Practice* **7**, 57–86

Greenwell MG, Sherrill J and Clayton LA (2003) Osmoregulation in fish: mechanism and clinical implications. *Veterinary Clinics of North America: Exotic Animal Practice* **6**, 169–189

Hrubec TC and Smith AT (2000) Haematology of Fish. In: *Schalm's Veterinary Haematology, 5th edn,* ed B Fieldman and JG Zinkl, pp. 1120–1125. Lippincott, Williams and Wilkins, Baltimore, MD

Klinger RE, Francis-Floyd R, Riggs A *et al.* (2003) Use of blood culture as a nonlethal method for isolating bacteria from fish. *Journal of Zoo and Wildlife Medicine* **34-2**, 206–207

Lewbart GA (1998) Clinical nutrition of ornamental fish. *Seminars in Avian and Exotic Pet Medicine* **3**, 154–158

Lewbart GA (2006) *Invertebrate Medicine.* Blackwell Publishing, Ames, IA

Love NE and Lewbart GA (1997) Pet fish radiography: technique and case history reports. *Veterinary Radiology and Ultrasound* **38-1**, 24–29

Noga EJ (1996) *Fish Disease: Diagnosis and Treatment.* Mosby, St. Louis

Palmeiro BS, Rosenthal KL, Lewbart GA *et al.* (2007) Plasma biochemical reference intervals for koi. *Journal of the American Veterinary Medical Association* **230**, 708–712

Reavill D and Roberts H (2007) Diagnostic cytology of fish. *Veterinary Clinics of North America: Exotic Animal Practice* **10**, 207–234

Roberts HE (in press) *Fundamentals of Ornamental Fish Health.* Wiley-Blackwell, Ames, IA

Roberts RJ (2001) *Fish Pathology, 3rd edn.* WB Saunders, Philadelphia

Ross LG and Ross B (2008) *Anaesthetic and Sedative Techniques for Aquatic Animals, 3rd edn.* Blackwell Publishing, Oxford

Stoskopf M (1993) *Fish Medicine.* Saunders, Philadelphia

Weber ES (2007) Piscine patients: basic diagnostics. *Compendium on Continuing Education for the Practicing Veterinarian* **5**, 276–288

Wildgoose W (2001) *BSAVA Manual of Ornamental Fish, 2nd edn.* BSAVA Publications, Gloucester

Yanong RPE (1999) Nutrition of ornamental fish. *Veterinary Clinics of North America: Exotic Animal Practice* **2**, 19–42

Yanong RPE (2003) Fungal diseases of fish. *Veterinary Clinics of North America: Exotic Animal Practice* **6**, 377–400

20

Marine fish

Ruth Francis-Floyd and B. Denise Petty

Introduction

Aquarium-keeping is increasing as a hobby. A consideration for veterinary surgeons interested in developing clientèle with marine aquaria is that in addition to providing a service to pet owners, it may be beneficial to work with the non-veterinary professionals in the field who are responsible for many of the larger and more complex, and hence more valuable, aquarium systems. The aquarist may have more expertise in water quality systems, design, and even biology and husbandry of fish, whereas the veterinary surgeon has the ability to provide diagnostic services, assess a case, and develop a rational management strategy.

There are many species of marine fish sold through the pet trade. The most common specimens come from five broad groups: damselfish (Pomacentridae) (Figure 20.1a); surgeonfish (Acanthuridae) (Figure 20.1b); wrasses (Labridae) (Figure 20.1c); gobies (Gobidae); and marine angelfish (Pomacanthidae) (Figure 20.1d). Most cultured marine fish are anenomefish or clownfish (*Amphiprion*) (Figure 20.1e), which are part of the Pomacentridae. Although statistically not one of the most common marine fish, the seahorse family (Syngnathidae) (Figure 20.1f) are among the most popular in zoological collections and medical care is often provided to these animals.

Biology

It is important to research available information on life history and husbandry on a case-by-case basis when working with marine fish. Maintaining a quick book for reference in the office and accessing information available on the internet can be very helpful. Information on a few select species will be presented here, beginning with a brief overview of each of the families listed above.

Damselfish and anemonefish

The damselfish (Figure 20.1a) and anemonefish are members of the family Pomacentridae, and represent the largest group (42%) of marine aquarium fish. Damselfish are hardy and often brightly coloured, making them especially appealing to hobbyists setting up their first marine tank. They are also notoriously

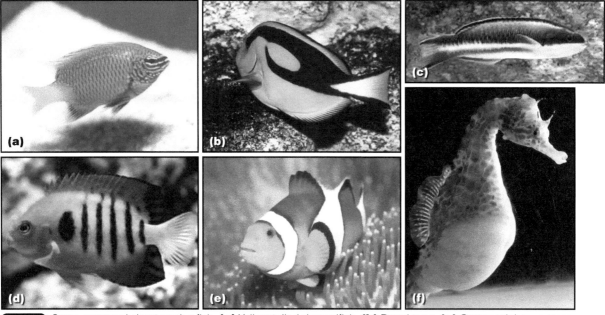

20.1 Some commonly kept marine fish. **(a)** Yellow-tailed damselfish. **(b)** Regal tang. **(c)** Cortez rainbow wrasse. **(d)** Flame angelfish. **(e)** Common clownfish. **(f)** Seahorse. (a,e Courtesy of WH Wildgoose; reproduced from *BSAVA Manual of Ornamental Fish, 2nd edition*.) (b,f © Bristol Zoo Gardens.) (c,d Courtesy of Segrest Farms Inc.)

aggressive and therefore the furnishings within the aquarium should be designed so that individual fish can establish their own space within the tank. Failure to supply adequate habitat may result in fighting, which in turn can lead to primary or opportunistic (i.e. stress-related) bacterial infections.

The other important members of this group are the anemonefish, members of the subfamily Amphiprioninae, and include the many species of clownfish (Figure 20.1e). Members of this group are relatively easy to culture, and several species are reared on a commercial scale. On the reef, these fish live with an anemone, creating one of nature's most recognized examples of symbiosis. In aquaria, the fish can be maintained successfully without anemones. They are protandrous: when paired, the loss of a female can result in the transition of the remaining male into a functional female who will then attract a new mate. This transition is non-reversible. Clownfish can be bred in home aquaria and some hobbyists are able to raise and sell enough young fish to create some significant supplemental income.

Surgeonfish
The surgeonfish, or acanthurids, are also extremely popular in marine aquaria. There are more than 80 species; most are from the Indo-Pacific but a few occur in the Atlantic and Caribbean basin. In general, surgeonfish are herbivorous and graze shallow reefs in large schools. Anatomically, there seem to be two different approaches to gastric digestion of plant material. Some species, such as the blue (regal) tang (*Acanthurus coeruleus*) (Figure 20.1b), have a thin-walled stomach; it is hypothesized that they rely on acidic secretions to break down plant material for digestion. Other species, such as the ocean surgeonfish (*A. bahianus*), have a thick gizzard-like stomach wall and may rely on mechanical disruption of ingested material to aid digestion. Availability of sandy substrate may be important in these latter species; wild ocean surgeonfish have been observed routinely ingesting sand, where as the blue tang does not seem to (Tilghman *et al.*, 2001).

Wrasses
Wrasses represent the family Labridae (Figure 20.1c); with 68 genera, it is the third largest family of marine fish. Most are found in tropical waters around the world, though a few reside in subtropical or temperate water. In addition to their beauty, their behaviour is fascinating. Their feeding behaviour is specially diverse. Some wrasses (*Labroides*) perform a parasite cleaning service for other fishes, although it is important to note that they feed on large parasites such as monogeneans and crustaceans, and not on protistan parasites. Some species feed on zooplankton, some on coral polyps, and some are piscivorous. Some have teeth adapted to crush the shells of large invertebrates. Most species may be a threat to invertebrates in a reef aquarium. All wrasses have sharp conical teeth to grasp prey items, and all are protogynous hermaphrodites. Some genera (*Coris*, *Halichoeres*, *Macropharyngodon*, subfamily Novaculini) require a fine sand substrate, and may bury themselves at night.

Gobies
The gobies, family Gobiidae, comprise the largest family of marine fish. They are found primarily in tropical and subtropical waters around the world. While many are marine or from brackish waters, some live in fresh water but spawn in sea water (catadromous). Their pelvic fins are fused to form an adhesive disc, similar to a suction cup; this is more developed in fish found in fast-flowing water. Gobies are carnivorous, primarily feeding on small invertebrates.

Dragonets
The dragonets, which include the mandarinfish (*Synchiropus splendidus*) and the psychedelic fish (*S. picturatus*) are commonly called gobies, but they are not related. Though popular due to their bright coloration, they are not appropriate for any but the most advanced aquarists. Like seahorses, they do best in a reef aquarium or a live rock tank in which there is adequate growth of small crustaceans to serve as a food source. They should not be kept with aggressive hunting fishes, as they cannot compete with them for food items.

Angelfish
The marine angelfishes (family Pomacanthidae) (Figure 20.1d) are strikingly beautiful. Some exhibit sexual dimorphism, and all have preopercle spines. Many feed on algae and sessile invertebrates, though some (e.g. *Genicanthus*) specialize on zooplankton. Some, such as the rock beauty (*Holacanthus tricolor*) feed mostly on sponges; others feed on plants and animals; and some are detritivores. Most species are bold and aggressive, and they may 'terrorize' tankmates. Some are very large (e.g. *Pomacanthus*), while others are small and do well in species-only tanks as small as 20 US gallons (e.g. *Centropyge*).

Seahorses
The sygnathids (seahorses, pipefish and sea dragons) are incredibly popular display animals in public aquaria, but maintaining them can be challenging because of the need to feed live foods. Dedicated aquarists maintain and breed seahorses (Figure 20.1f), and are often extremely enthusiastic about their hobby. Many aquaria maintain seahorse exhibits, and exhibits of sea dragons are among the most prized of any fish for commercial display. Seahorses have a long tubular mouth, a prehensile tail, and are covered with bony 'armour'. They have unique reproductive biology, characterized by parental care provided by the male seahorse which holds eggs and fry in a brood pouch.

Husbandry

Keeping marine fish healthy can be challenging, especially for the novice, as water quality and life support are more complex than in freshwater systems. The fish themselves can be prone to a number of infectious diseases, which may be exacerbated by less than optimal husbandry, and in many cases less information is available to assess disease progression and management.

Housing

Husbandry of marine fish is species-specific to some degree but the major variables are water quality and feeding.

Water quality

Water quality parameters for marine aquaria are summarized in Figure 20.2.

Parameter	Desirable range
Dissolved oxygen	Saturation (always >5.0 mg/l)
Carbon dioxide	<20 mg/l
pH	7.8–8.4
Total ammonia nitrogen	<0.5 mg/l
Un-ionized ammonia nitrogen [a]	<0.05 mg/l
Nitrite	0.0 mg/l
Nitrate	<100 mg/l
Chlorine (free and total)	0.0 mg/l
Salinity	up to 34 g/l
Total alkalinity [HCO_3^-]	>175 mg/l
Total hardness	Not applicable [b]
Temperature	22–28°C

20.2 Water quality parameters for marine aquaria. [a] Un-ionized ammonia nitrogen concentrations must be calculated using the measured total ammonia nitrogen concentration, pH and temperature. [b] Total hardness may be >6000 mg/l in a marine tank.

Temperature: Species-specific water quality requirement relates largely to temperature. Most other parameters have an optimum range that will be favourable for most commonly kept marine aquarium species. Most marine aquarium fish are from tropical climes and therefore temperatures in the range of 22–28°C are often ideal.

Oxygenation: Oxygen concentration should be very close to saturation in any aquarium system. Salt water typically holds less oxygen in solution than does fresh water. A quick and easy way to assess saturation is to use the online Aquaculture Network Information Center (http://www.aquanic.org/); with information on temperature, salinity and altitude the programme will immediately provide the concentration of oxygen that should be present if the system were saturated. If oxygen levels cannot be maintained at or near saturation, one of two processes is out of balance: either insufficient oxygen is being introduced to the system; or something is using up the oxygen that is present. Common causes of this are overstocking, overfeeding, inadequate aeration, or an accumulation of organic debris in the system. Often a thorough cleaning, especially the removal of debris from beneath an undergravel filter, will solve the problem. If setting up a water quality testing protocol with a client it may be appropriate to ask them to record oxygen levels as both actual concentration (i.e. mg/l) and percentage saturation. Oxygen and other gases (nitrogen, carbon dioxide) can cause 'gas bubble disease' if supersaturation develops (see below).

Nitrogen compounds: Ammonia and nitrogenous waste products (nitrites and nitrates) can be problematic in marine tanks. Fish foods tend to be high in protein and fish excrete ammonia directly across the gill into the water. Ammonia is more toxic at higher pH, which is typical of marine tanks. If a biofilter is not functioning, for whatever reason, or if an excessive amount of ammonia is suddenly introduced to the tank, ammonia toxicity may be seen (see below).

If a biofilter is only partially functioning, ammonia may be oxidized to nitrite but not further oxidized to nitrate, resulting in an accumulation of nitrite in the water column. Fish exposed to nitrite develop methaemoglobinaemia. Sensitivity to nitrite seems to be somewhat species-specific; surgeonfish appear to be quite sensitive. Accumulation of nitrite in a marine system can be associated with a biofilter's failure to cycle or the use of copper as a therapeutic. Total alkalinity (bicarbonate) should be checked and if low (<175 mg/l), calcium carbonate should be added to the system. Nitrite levels will often begin to fall a few days after this is done. Acute nitrite exposure may result in fish showing signs of hypoxia, and mortality. Water changes can be used to control nitrite concentration in small systems until biofilter function improves and concentrations fall.

Nitrate can accumulate in marine systems if water changes are limited. Nitrate is naturally eliminated by anaerobic metabolism in sediments, something that should not be happening in display aquaria. Some large commercial exhibits may have separate side-stream filters set up to convert nitrate anaerobically to nitrogen gas, but these systems are expensive and not routinely used. Nitrate can also be removed from a system by plants, but these are not typically maintained in marine aquaria. Nitrate is harmful to corals and invertebrates so is very undesirable in a living reef tank.

Alkalinity, hardness and pH: Total alkalinity, total hardness and pH are all related. In a marine tank, pH should be in the range of 7.8–8.4. A significant deviation from this range is problematic, and an acidic pH is often indicative of system problems, most commonly 'old tank syndrome'. A sudden drop in pH can occur when water changes are insufficient to remove accumulated organic acids from the aquarium. Over time, the carbonates present in the buffering system are used up, resulting in a loss of alkalinity, and then the pH will begin to fall. If not corrected, the pH will eventually plummet into a very acidic range (i.e. <5). This may result in biofilter failure and morbidity or mortality of the resident fish. If pH is out of the desired 7.8–8.4 range, alkalinity should be checked at once. In marine systems, alkalinity should be >175 mg/l. Any time total alkalinity (bicarbonate concentration) falls *below* 175 mg/l in a marine system, corrective action should be taken; this usually consists of adding dolomite, aragonite, crushed coral, baking soda or some other form of soluble carbonate.

Although total hardness is separate from total alkalinity, they are related, and both are reported as mg/l of calcium carbonate. Total hardness measures the minerals in water, which are typically dominated by calcium, magnesium and manganese, and should be >6000 mg/l in a marine tank. Low total hardness rarely occurs if a good sea salt mix is used, but a deficit can be corrected by adding crushed coral, dolomite or agricultural limestone to the system.

Chlorine: If mains water is used for the aquarium, aquarists need to be diligent about dechlorination. City water is typically treated with chlorine, chloramine or some combination of the two, and each municipal water supply is unique. Even experienced aquarists can have health problems in their collections caused by sublethal or transient concentrations of chlorine in the water. Any detectable free or total chlorine is problematical. Test kits are readily available, very inexpensive and quick to run. Routine monitoring for chlorine should be done with any case presented for which the water source is municipal water, and aquarists should be educated to test water for chlorine after every water change. Use of dechlorinators does not eliminate all chlorine-related problems. Routine testing is very important.

Toxins: There are several endogenous or exogenous toxins that can cause problems if they get into a tank. Hydrogen sulphide, which has a distinctive rotten egg smell, is highly toxic to fish, and any detected is significant. Some well water supplies may contain it. If contaminated water is used as source water for an aquarium, it is important that the water is well aerated before it goes into the aquarium. Hydrogen sulphide can also form in a tank if anaerobic conditions are allowed to develop due to poor sanitation. In this situation, there may be a history of acute catastrophic mortality, often associated with disruption of bottom sediment. Diagnosis can only be confirmed if a water sample is taken at the time the event occurs, as hydrogen sulphide is extremely volatile.

Other sources of toxins may include the use of household chemicals or cleaning products around the tank, pesticides, and nicotine. Heavy metals can be a problem in older buildings with copper pipes. Galvanized metal is a source of zinc toxicity. If a problem is identified, correction will include preventing exposure to the chemical of concern. In the case of metal pipes, the installation of an activated carbon filter for water to pass through before entering the aquarium may be very useful. For maximum protection, filter media need to be changed on a regular basis. Some pumps have internal parts made of copper or brass, which may be a source of heavy metal ions.

Diet

A diet similar to that which the fish would consume in its natural environment should be fed. However, feeding marine fish can be challenging and pet owners should be cautioned that some prepared diets may not be adequate for marine fish maintained in the home aquarium. Feeding small amounts twice a day may be preferable to feeding larger amounts once a day, but either strategy is acceptable.

Complete diets which have vitamin supplements, including vitamin C should be fed. Flake diets can create a tremendous amount of debris in a tank if fed in sufficient quantity to maintain body condition (often

3–7% bodyweight per day, depending on species). Complete pelleted diets may be a better option as nutrients are present in a denser form and therefore there is less impact on water quality. When feeding complete pelleted diets, it is important to feed a variety of different diets.

Herbivorous fish can be fed on commercially available seaweed (e.g. nori) as well as part boiled or blanched fresh vegetables (e.g. courgette/zucchini, broccoli). Commercial diets that contain spirulina are also available. Herbivorous species should be offered a complete diet in addition to the vegetables or seaweed provided. Some fish may require live foods, including brine shrimp, mysid shrimp and other invertebrates. Many of these are available in a frozen form. Seafood for human consumption (e.g. live muscles, shrimps and fish) may be used. Live marine baitfish may introduce pathogens, so quarantine is necessary. Feeding live goldfish is **not recommended** as these may be a source of disease introduction; *Mycobacterium* is easily introduced in food items.

Under-feeding is usually more of a problem with marine fish than over-feeding, and owners should be advised on how to monitor body condition. Fish presented for veterinary examination can be weighed and, if desired, microchipped so that weight and medical records can be logged for each individual fish in the collection.

Identification

In commercial exhibits it may be useful to mark specific animals so that they can be identified and medical records maintained on individual animals. This is rarely done for privately owned pet fish. One of the best methods for individual identification is injection of a PIT tag (microchip) into the dorsal musculature, which can then be scanned to identify the fish. The disadvantage of this system is that the individual cannot be visually identified and therefore must be caught, handled and scanned for proper identification. In many exhibits, aquarists are able to recognize individual animals visually with accuracy. Few externally visible tagging systems are appropriate for identification of fish on display in private or public collections.

Preventive healthcare

Most (>98%) of marine fish in collections are wild-caught. The clinical importance of this is that a great deal of disease occurs in newly acquired fish, which may be immunosuppressed due to transport and handling; these fish may come in with overwhelming loads of parasites and (often opportunistic) bacteria. Establishing baseline diagnostic testing services for clients, and educating them about prevention of common diseases, can make a huge difference in their level of satisfaction, or financial success, within the hobby.

Handling and restraint

When catching fish, nets should be soft. Choice of net size is somewhat species-specific but many small marine fish are best caught using nets with very small mesh so as to minimize scale loss and the possibility of eye trauma (Figure 20.3). Eye trauma should not be overlooked as a cause of unilateral exophthalmia, ulceration or other obvious eye lesions.

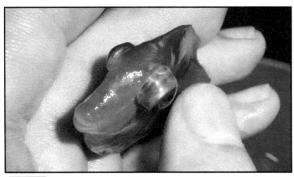

20.3 Eye trauma in a juvenile surgeonfish, believed to have been caused by improper netting. (Courtesy of GC Tilghman.)

Some species, especially those with prickly fins, may be easier (and safer) to handle in nets with larger mesh. Other concerns include scale loss or blunt trauma if a fish hits the side of a tank or jumps out of a bucket. Various slings and other modifications of a typical net are commercially available and can be explored for possible application to ease handling and minimize trauma when manipulating fish.

When using physical restraint alone, the minimal amount of pressure should be used. If possible, the fish should be handled in water and kept immersed as much as possible, especially the gill and opercular area. Some handlers feel that covering the eyes results in decreased struggling by the fish, facilitating handling and manipulation. Keeping the area darkened and quiet may also help.

If fish are restrained or moved in a cooler, suddenly opening the lid will result in an immediate flash of light hitting the fish, which may cause a strong evasive reaction. It may be easier to prop the lid of the cooler partially open to minimize sudden changes in light intensity during the handling process (Figure 20.4). The propped lid also allows easier direct monitoring of the patient, as well as maintaining patent air lines, and monitoring with a dissolved oxygen meter, if one is available. Closing the cooler during transport is appropriate, though air lines need to remain patent.

Most handling of marine fish will involve sedation or anaesthesia (see below).

Diagnostic approach

Handling fish for a diagnostic work-up should be fairly straightforward. After biopsy samples have been collected, the fish can be sedated or anesthetized for the remainder of the examination (see below). If the fish is large enough to be difficult to handle, or will not settle down to allow biopsy specimens to be collected safely, it should be sedated earlier in the examination process. Since prolonged anaesthesia (>15–30 minutes) can result in hypoxaemia, the fish should be carefully monitored to ensure safe recovery and a good outcome.

Other common diagnostic techniques may include radiography, ultrasonography and endoscopy, but it is not necessary or appropriate to use these for routine examinations.

Sample collection

Tissue samples

Biopsy samples should be collected **before** the fish is exposed to chemical restraint if possible. An easy way to accomplish this is to restrain the animal manually at the side of the tank or transport unit. A handler can gently expose the back of the fish and the veterinary surgeon can carefully remove a few scales and some mucus by gently running a glass coverslip along the back of the fish for a short distance, minimizing damage to the external surface.

Gill tissue can be exposed by an assistant, tilting the fish and lifting the opercular flap (Figure 20.5). Covering the eyes seems to decrease struggling by the restrained fish. The practitioner can then gently cut the tips off a few gill filaments (three or four) for examination with a light microscope. Tank water should be used to make wet mounts, as matching the salinity of the wet mount is important to keep parasites alive long enough for an identification to be made. Wet mounts should be examined immediately with a light microscope as parasites die rapidly once the preparation starts to dry.

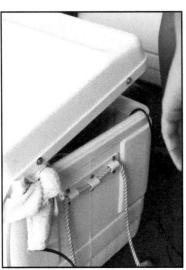

20.4 A large cooler used as a holding tank for anaesthesia and clinical handling of small bamboo sharks. The lid is propped open to: keep the air line patent; allow for passive observation of the animal; and minimize sudden changes in light intensity. This also allows easy monitoring with a dissolved oxygen meter.

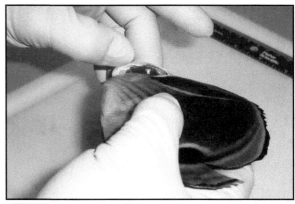

20.5 Exposure of gill tissue prior to sampling in a raccoon butterflyfish (*Chaetodon lunula*).

Faeces

A faecal sample can be collected by gently expressing the abdomen, but in many cases the fish will defecate as it succumbs to anaesthesia. Old faecal samples collected from the bottom of a tank can be misleading, but a fresh sample collected during induction is fine. A direct smear of the sample can be examined with a light microscope for the presence of parasites or eggs.

Blood

- The caudal vessels are usually the site of choice. The caudal vein runs ventral to the vertebral column, and the best landmark is the lateral line in the proximal peduncle. A ventral (Figure 20.6) or lateral approach can be used; the lateral approach is often easier for small finfish.
- For very small fish (<20–25 g), a lethal approach (for herd health; not routinely used) using the severed caudal peduncle may be employed. It is important to note for clinical chemistry that blood obtained from the caudal peduncle is often composed of both arterial and venous blood plus fluid from adjacent tissues.
- In fishes more than 10 cm long, the cardiac approach may be achieved with relative ease. However, care must be exercised not to damage the heart with multiple needle sticks.
- In fish with large mouths, the dorsal aorta may be used.
- The duct of Cuvier (common cardinal vein) is preferred if multiple samples are required.

Lithium heparin is the anticoagulant most suitable for most fish work, and the plasma can be used for biochemical tests if desired.

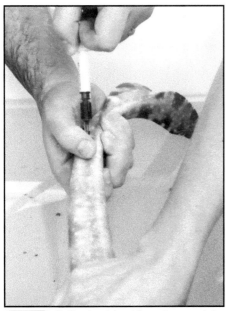

20.6 Collecting blood from the caudal vein of a bamboo shark.

Common conditions

'Gas bubble disease'

Oxygen and other gases (nitrogen, carbon dioxide) can cause 'gas bubble disease' if supersaturation develops. Clinical signs may include acute mortality or malaise. Examination of fish may reveal tiny sub-epithelial gas bubbles, often most easily seen on fins or in the cornea. Definitive diagnosis may be achieved by observing gas bubbles within gill capillaries, something easily seen on wet mounts. Treatment of gas bubble disease involves locating the source of supersaturation and correcting it. Increased aeration will usually help blow excess gas out of the water fairly quickly, resolving the clinical condition, but the underlying problem must be corrected to prevent recurrence.

Ammonia toxicity

Acute ammonia toxicity is typically manifest by neurological changes: fish tend to be disoriented and may swim in spirals, or even appear convulsive. Diagnosis is easily made by testing the water. Water quality testing equipment will provide the total ammonia nitrogen (TAN) concentration; to assess ammonia toxicity, the un-ionized ammonia nitrogen (UIA) concentration should be calculated (Figure 20.7). Un-ionized ammonia concentrations >0.05 mg/l are considered toxic to fish, although behavioural signs and death may not be observed until levels approach or exceed 1 mg/l.

To calculate the amount of un-ionized ammonia present in an aqueous solution, the total ammonia nitrogen (TAN) should be multiplied by the appropriate fraction in the table below, based on the pH and temperature measurements of the water sample, as determined using conventional testing kits.

Example: TAN = 2 mg/l
pH = 8.2
Water temperature = 28°C

Using the pH and temperature values, determine the fraction of un-ionized ammonia – in this case the fraction is 0.0998.

Multiply TAN by the un-ionized ammonia fraction:
2 x 0.0998 = 0.1996 rounded up to 0.2 mg/l

This amount of un-ionized ammonia is high enough to cause changes to gill tissue (particularly hyperplasia), but should not cause mortality in most species of marine fish.

pH	Temperature (°C)					
	22	24	26	28	30	32
7.8	0.0281	0.0322	0.0370	0.0423	0.0482	0.0572
8.0	0.0438	0.0502	0.0574	0.0654	0.0743	0.0877
8.2	0.0676	0.0772	0.0880	0.0998	0.1129	0.1322
8.4	0.1031	0.1171	0.1326	0.1495	0.1678	0.1948
8.6	0.1541	0.1737	0.1950	0.2178	0.2422	0.2768

20.7 Fraction of un-ionized ammonia in aqueous solution at different pH values and temperatures. (Calculated from data in Emerson *et al.*, 1975.)

Signs of chronic exposure to lower concentrations of ammonia can be more subtle and may not be readily detected: affected fish may have swollen gills, may appear darkened and exhibit a non-specific malaise.

Infectious diseases

- Damselfish are susceptible to the protistan parasites, including *Cryptocaryon irritans, Amyloodinium oscellata* and *Brooklynella hostilis.*
- Clownfish are susceptible to protistan parasites such as *C. irritans, A. ocellatum,* and *B. hostilis.* They are also susceptible to a bacterial disease similar to freshwater columnaris disease.
- In addition to the protistan parasites listed above for damselfishes and clownfishes, surgeonfishes are susceptible to *Uronema marinum.*
- Surgeonfishes and the marine angelfishes may display head and lateral line erosion.
- Wrasses are susceptible to infections with *C. irritans* and *A. ocellatum.*
- Marine angelfishes are susceptible to parasitism by *C. irritans* and *A. ocellatum.* They also appear to be susceptible to the effects of the capsalid monogeneans. In addition, they are more likely to exhibit characteristic lesions when lymphocystivirus is introduced into a mixed species tank.
- New seahorses should be carefully examined for infection with microsporidians, usually *Glugea* spp. In addition, seahorses seem to be more susceptible to mycobacterial infections.

Protozoan parasites

Cryptocaryon irritans: *Cryptocaryon irritans* is a ciliated protozoan that is an obligate parasite of marine fish. It can be devastating because it penetrates the epithelium of skin, fin and gill. Infested fish usually succumb to osmoregulatory failure. Although the lifecycle of *C. irritans* is direct, it is complex. The trophont stage is grossly visible on the fish, appearing as if the fish were salted or dusted. As the trophont is subepithelial it cannot be harmed at this stage. Trophonts actively feed on cell debris and fluid. Depending on water temperature, trophonts emerge from the host after 3–7 days, usually in the pre-dawn hours. Eight to twelve hours after emergence, they encyst on the substrate; at this stage they are called tomonts. Within the cyst, the tomont divides into multiple daughter cells (tomites). When the tomites leave the cyst, they are the infective stage, or theronts. The theronts actively swim, seeking a fish. When contact with a fish is made, the theront can penetrate the epithelium within 5 minutes.

Diagnosis is made easily on wet mounts of skin, fin and gill tissue (Figure 20.8), as the trophont stage is large (60–450 µm) and moves constantly.

Treatment may be approached by several methods: copper, formalin, chloroquine, or hyposalinity. It is important to note that regardless of treatment method, failure to eliminate the parasite is not uncommon. The trophont and tomont stages are impervious to treatment, which means the window for treating the susceptible theront stage is small.

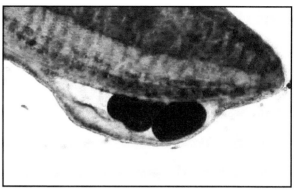

20.8 Subepithelial trophonts of *Cryptocaryon irritans* in gill tissue. Original magnification x100.

Amyloodinium ocellatum: *Amyloodinium ocellatum,* a dinoflagellate, is another common and potentially devastating protistan parasite of marine fish. An obligate fish parasite, it has a complex lifecycle somewhat similar to that of *C. irritans.* The teardrop-shaped trophont stage attaches to the gills or skin with rhizoids. After feeding on the host, the rhizoids retract and the trophont leaves the fish and encysts (tomont). Within the tomont, it divides into multiple dinospores. When released from the tomont, the free-swimming dinospores are the infective stage. Heavy infestations can impact respiration and osmo-regulation. Affected fishes may congregate at the surface or near aeration devices. In some fishes, the surface of the skin may appear to be dusted with fine gold particles.

Examination of wet mounts of skin, gill and fin tissue will reveal trophonts approximately 150 µm in size (Figure 20.9).

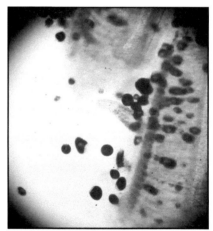

20.9 *Amyloodinium ocellatum* trophonts in gill tissue from a pinfish (*Lagodon rhomboides).* Also visible is a single monogenean, most likely of the genus *Ancyrocephalus.* Original magnification x100.

Chloroquine phosphate at 10 mg/l is the drug of choice, but *A. ocellatum* is difficult to eliminate completely. Copper and formalin at standard dosages have also been used, with limited success.

Others: Several other protistan parasites are commonly found on marine fish, including *Brooklynella, Uronema,* and a marine form of *Trichodina.* Parasites that dig into epithelial tissue or skeletal muscle, including *Brooklynella* and especially *Uronema*, may be more refractory to treatment. Improvements in sanitation are always an excellent accompaniment to chemical control.

Treatment:

- Copper maintained at 0.18–0.2 mg/l for 3 weeks has been the standard treatment for external protistan infestations of marine aquarium fish for many years. However, copper is lethal to most invertebrates and has the potential to cause heavy metal toxicity in sensitive fish species. Daily use of a good copper test kit is critical, as copper levels may fluctuate.
- Formalin (37% formaldehyde in aqueous solution) used at 25 mg/l every other day for 3 weeks has also been useful. Formalin is a potent respiratory poison and carcinogen, and removes oxygen from the water, so these factors must be kept in mind.
- Most recently, chloroquine at 10–15 mg/l has shown promise for treatment of *Cryptocaryon*. Repeat treatment after one week (10 mg/l) is recommended.
- Hyposalinity may have the most value in control of *Cryptocaryon*, as long as the salinity change is rapid. Decreasing the salinity by 50% (or to 16–18 g/l) within 30 minutes, and maintaining it there for 3 hours, is very effective. The salinity should be increased slowly over a period of days (Hemdal, 2006). In addition, hyposalinity aids fish struggling to maintain osmoregulation.

Flatworms

Monogeneans are very common flatworms of marine fishes. Most are ectoparasitic, though a few are found internally. Their lifecycle is direct. Most groups are egg-layers, though one family, the Gyrodactylidae, gives birth to live young. These worms are characterized by a haptor, an organ on one end with holdfasts, which varies depending on species. All the families common to freshwater fish can also be found on marine fish; however, the Capsalidae, which are found only on brackish and marine fish, are of more importance due to the extensive damage they inflict. In addition, capsalids are more likely to have a wider range of hosts than other monogeneans. Capsalids are frequently large enough to be observed on gross examination.

Monogeneans feed on epithelial cells, and move around easily and quickly on the surface of the fish. Their feeding usually results in extensive skin, eye or gill lesions, which may be colonized by opportunistic bacteria. If presented with a fish with severe eye damage (typically corneal oedema), unilateral or bilateral, the presence of capsalids should be suspected. As the capsalids are often not found in association with the eye at the time of examination, other fish with normal-appearing eyes should also be examined. The eggs of capsalids (Figure 20.10) are very sticky and thus may be found on almost any surface in a tank. This makes eradication extremely difficult, even when using the drug of choice, praziquantel.

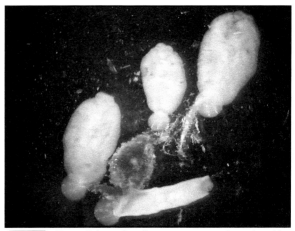

20.10 Capsalids and amber egg masses from the skin of a lookdown (*Selene vomer*) as they appear under a dissecting microscope. Original magnification x20.

Turbellarians are occasionally observed on surgeonfish and others. Some may be easily seen as small irregular dark spots on light-coloured fish, or they may appear similar to *Cryptocaryon irritans*. Turbellarian flatworms are unique in that they are ciliated. This feature is easily seen on a wet mount, though they are fragile and can be damaged by pressure from a coverslip. If turbellarians are suspected, the coverslip used to gently scrape the affected area should be placed on the slide upside-down and viewed under low power. Praziquantel, formalin and organophosphate compounds are used to control them.

Viral infections

Lymphocystis is caused by an iridovirus that is ubiquitous. Interestingly, certain fish (e.g. pomacanthids) appear to be more susceptible. Infected fish usually exhibit pale grey rough masses on the fins or on the body. Histological examination of a skin scraping will reveal greatly hypertrophied fibroblasts (Figure 20.11). This viral infection rarely results in death, unless masses around the mouth interfere with feeding. Some juvenile fishes (e.g. redfish, *Sciaenops ocellatus*), have internal infections that result in high mortality. There is no treatment for this virus, but it is very important to minimize stressors such as poor water quality or aggression from tankmates.

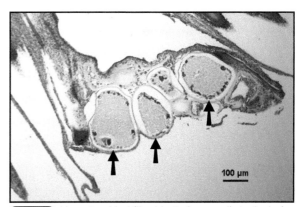

20.11 Hypertrophied fibroblasts (arrowed), typical of lymphocystis, in the anal fin of an infected juvenile clownfish (*Amphiprion*). H&E stain; original magnification x100.

Infections with betanodavirus have been described more frequently in the last decade. Many infections have been reported in cultured marine food fishes in Asia, Europe and Canada, and subclinical infections in marine aquarium fishes have also been reported. Betanodavirus is the causative agent of viral nervous necrosis (VNN). A typical clinical sign of infection is abnormal body posture and swimming. Diagnosis is made through virus isolation or PCR.

Bacterial infections

Opportunistic bacterial infections are not uncommon in marine fishes. *Vibrio* spp. are the most commonly encountered opportunists in marine water, as many *Vibrio* species are halophiles. This makes culture media selection critical for bacterial isolation, especially for any fish with external lesions. For such conditions, marine agar or blood agar with 3% sea salt added should be used in addition to standard blood agar. Another bacterial pathogen of concern is *Photobacterium damselae* subspecies. *piscicida* (formerly *Pasteurella piscicida*); infection can result in bacterial granulomas in the posterior kidney and other organs.

Skin and gill infections with bacteria similar to *Flavobacterium columnare* in fresh water have been observed in clownfishes and pompano (*Trachinotus carolinus*). Affected fish displayed thick skin mucus and a cream-coloured exudate on the gills. Long thin bacteria in haystack formations were observed on wet mount preparations of gill and skin tissue, though attempts to culture and isolate the bacterium were not successful. The clownfishes readily consumed feed containing oxytetracycline and subsequently improved in appearance.

Non-tuberculous (atypical) *Mycobacterium* species reported in marine fish include *M. chelonae*, *M. fortuitum*, *M. marinum* in wild rabbitfish (*Siganus rivulatus*) and captive frogfish (*Antennarius striatus*), and *M. montefiorense* in green moray eel (*Gymnothorax fenebris*). Chronic infections with mycobacteria frequently present as granulomatous disease, but a more acute histiocytic response is not uncommon. The bacteria preferentially infect macrophages, resulting in insidious disease that responds poorly to antimicrobial therapy. Management is critical and depends on the type of system, display or broodfish tank. In a display tank, animals that show clinical signs of disease should be removed because they may shed mycobacteria into the water. In contrast, all animals in an infected broodfish tank should be humanely euthanased and the tank or system, including life support, completely disinfected. Disinfection begins with application of sodium hypochlorite bleach to all surfaces. This is then neutralized and the tank and equipment allowed to dry. After drying is complete, all equipment is thoroughly sprayed with 70% isopropyl alcohol. Mycobacteria can be detected using acid-fast staining. Granulomas may show few rods, so examination should include oil immersion (1000X). These bacteria can be difficult to culture; specialized media are required and incubation temperature and time are both important.

Fungal infections

Fungal diseases are uncommon in marine fish. *Fusarium solani* has been reported from a diverse group of both freshwater and marine fish, and clinical disease in sphyrnid sharks has been associated with housing at water temperatures <27°C (Yanong, 2003). Infected fish may present with what appear to be skin ulcerations; however, otherwise healthy appearing tissue may also be affected. Extensive dermatitis, myositis and cellulitis may result in death. Fungal hyphae can be observed in tissues with Grocott's or Gomori methenamine silver (GMS) stain. There is no effective treatment at this time, but proper environmental management is important. Suboptimal water temperature may predispose susceptible fish to infection.

Though not a true fungus, the oomycete *Aphanomyces invadans* is a pathogen of fish residing in water of low salinity (≤15 g/l). Estuarine fish may be susceptible when an influx of freshwater occurs. The Aquatic Animal Health Code 2009 lists epizootic ulcer disease, caused by *A. invadans* as a notifiable disease.

Microsporidiosis

Microsporidia are intracellular parasites closely allied with the true fungi. Over 100 species have been reported to infect fish. Important genera that infect marine fish include *Glugea* and *Kudoa*. Spores are ingested by fish, where they infect host cells. Infected cells are first filled with the multinucleated stage, and eventually filled with spores. Some microsporidians result in hypertrophy of the host cell; this form is called a xenoma. In severe infections, normal organ function is compromised. Depending on species, spores range from 2 to 12 μm, and usually may be observed in tissue squashes under light microscopy. The spores stain positive with period acid–Schiff (PAS) and mature spores are acid-fast positive. There is no effective treatment. Since microsporidians are transmitted directly from fish to fish, removal of infected fish is recommended.

Supportive care

Often, the most important consideration in providing support to an ill fish is maintaining good water quality (see above).

Drug administration

In feed

Antibiotics can be administered to marine fish in medicated foods or by injection. Medicated foods can be prepared by adding the medication to flake food, using a cooking spray as a binder; or the drug can be added to a gel food. When making gel foods it is important that drugs, especially oxytetracycline, are not added until the mixture is cool to the touch, as heat will break down some active ingredients. In the case of piscivores, it may be possible to inject prey items with the desired dose of antibiotics.

Oral medication may also be delivered via a gastric tube (see below).

Injection sites

Injectable drugs can be administered either intra-muscularly or intracoelomically. Intravenous injections into the caudal vein are possible, but are less commonly used.

Landmarks for an intramuscular injection are fairly straightforward. The needle should be placed lateral to the posterior insertion of the dorsal fin, and should be directed into the muscle mass and not into the posterior kidney and abdominal cavity, which are located just ventral to the lateral line.

Intracoelomic injections can be given by rolling the fish into dorsal recumbency. The needle should be directed cranially, and can be inserted just under the ventral musculature, and anterior to the pelvic fins. The angle of the needle should be as shallow as possible to minimize the chance of damaging viscera or puncturing the intestinal tract.

Nutritional support

It is important to try and get sick or stressed fish to eat, as long as water quality parameters are acceptable. When otherwise apparently healthy fish refuse to eat it may be possible to stimulate the appetite by force-feeding. Passing a gastric tube can be used as a means of delivering oral medication or nutrition in an anorectic animal. The tube needs to be small enough to pass through the mouth and oesophagus; tomcat catheters can be used in small fish. There is no concern about aspiration, as the fish do not have a trachea or lungs. The tube should be marked before being passed to the perceived level of the stomach, given the anatomy of the species. Once in place, a slurry of food or medication can be gently pushed into the stomach using a syringe. Volume should be appropriate for the size of the animal. Use of significant volumes of fresh water to tube-feed marine species should be approached with caution, as ingestion of fresh water is not something these animals would naturally experience. It is not unusual for a fish to begin feeding after being force-fed once or twice.

Anaesthesia and analgesia

For some of the small marine aquarium fish it may not be necessary to sedate them for simple handling, and collection of tissue samples. If it is possible to collect gill and skin samples prior to exposing fish to tricaine methane sulphonate (MS-222) or other chemical agents in the water, the chance of observing parasites may be improved. In many cases, however, handling fish is challenging, especially when they are removed from the water, and sedation can make the process safer for the patient and the examiner, and more aesthetically acceptable to the owner.

Agents

Tricaine methane sulphonate (MS-222)

MS-222, a benzocaine derivative, is the most commonly used fish anaesthetic, and in many countries is approved for use in food fish as long as appropriate withdrawal times are honoured. If unfamiliar with the effect of MS-222 on a species of fish, an initial dose of 50 mg/l is a conservative place to start. Because the drug is acidic, it should be buffered: sodium bicarbonate should be added to the solution at a rate of two times the amount of MS-222 by weight. An induction dose of 100 mg/l or more may be needed but once the desired plane of anaesthesia has been reached, the required maintenance dose may be lower, often in the range of 50–75 mg/l. When anaesthetizing fish, the water should always be well aerated and the fish should be watched closely for regular respiratory movement at the opercular flap.

Other

Other water-borne drugs that have been used to anaesthetize fish include eugenol, clove oil and related derivatives metomidate and quinaldine. Eugenol and clove oil are not approved for use in fish in the USA or Canada and therefore should not be used in these countries. Aqui-S is a eugenol derivative, isoeugenol, that is authorized for use in fish (with no withdrawal period) in a number of countries including Australia, Chile, Finland and New Zealand. Drugs in this group are effective, and Aqui-S seems to be the most effective, but they have been shown to have a lower safety margin when compared with MS-222 (Sladkey *et al.*, 2001).

Metomidate has been approved in Canada as an anaesthetic of non-food fish. It is most useful for sedation (0.25–1.0 mg/l) but may also be used as an anaesthetic (5–10 mg/l). The manufacturer cautions against use on fish in an acidic environment, and on air-breathing species; neither of these contraindications should impact on use in marine fish. Metomidate is often considered an excellent choice for use in transport, although recent work with freshwater fish suggests that species-specific responses to the drug may be highly variable. It may be safer for use in some marine species than MS-222.

Injectable anaesthetics are being used more commonly in public aquaria to facilitate handling of very large and valuable fish. Information on dosages is scant and seems unreliable, possibly due to significant species-specific differences, as well as other variables. For most practitioners working with fish in privately owned collections, MS-222 will be very adequate for routine anaesthesia and sedation.

Monitoring

Monitoring during anaesthesia should include oxygen concentrations in the water with a dissolved oxygen meter, if possible recording both total concentration of dissolved oxygen (mg/l) and percentage saturation. If using oxygen tanks, as opposed to room air and an airstone, oxygen concentrations can become supersaturated very quickly. Equally, oxygen levels in a small container drop very quickly, emphasizing the need for careful monitoring.

Other parameters that can be used to monitor fish during an anaesthetic procedure include: respiratory rate, which is easily visualized; heart rate, which can be measured using a Doppler unit (Figure 20.12); and blood gases, using a point-of-care analyser. Veterinary blood analysers have not been validated for use in fish and so results must be interpreted with caution.

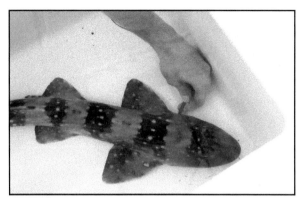

20.12 Use of a Doppler device to monitor heart rate in an anaesthetized bamboo shark.

Due to the anatomy of the fish circulatory system, blood samples collected for blood gas analysis are likely to be mixed venous/arterial samples.

Analgesia

Little work has been done on the use of analgesics in the clinical management of marine fish.

Common surgical procedures

Use of surgery to manage health problems in fish is becoming more common, although the small size of many pet fish can be a constraint against surgical intervention. Examples of surgical procedures that could be performed in marine fish include:

- Wound care with debridement
- Swim bladder repair
- Enucleation of a diseased eye
- Gonadectomy in an eggbound fish
- Removal of a mass.

Once the fish is anaesthetized, surgical manipulations are quite similar to those used in other species. A few special considerations apply.

A simple set-up for fish surgery requires an aquarium tank (filled with aerated water and appropriate concentration of anaesthetic) and a perforated cover (glass or plastic cookware works well) on which the fish will be positioned, usually by use of foam pads. Aerated water containing the anaesthetic solution is pumped out of the aquarium and over the fish's gills using a small tube or catheter placed in the fish's mouth. Holes are drilled in the aquarium cover so that water passes back into the aquarium when it leaves the fish. The fish's body can be positioned using foam pads, which are easily cut from a commercially purchased piece of foam bedding.

Once anaesthetized and positioned, scales can be plucked from the incision site and the area swabbed or rinsed with sterile saline. **The use of surface disinfectants to prepare a surgical site on a fish is contraindicated.** The surgical site can be covered with a sterile plastic (avian) drape and proper sterile technique should always be followed.

Choice of suture materials may be more limited than in terrestrial species. Monofilament sutures are preferable, as they are less likely to 'wick' material from the aquatic environment into the surgical site. In addition, absorbable sutures may not be absorbed as well as would be expected in fish patients. Harms (2003) mentions that the use of tissue adhesive to close incisions may be problematical in some species, particularly marine angelfish. He also recommends use of povidone–iodine ointment on the incision site after closure.

Use of postoperative analgesia has not been well assessed for fish patients. Keeping water clean is very important for healing, and modifying salinity (1–3 g/l) has been used in freshwater fish to decrease osmotic stress during recovery. Marine fish are not always as tolerant of modifications in salinity as their freshwater counterparts, but many reef species can be maintained in a hyposaline environment (16–18 g/l) during treatment of some parasitic diseases; therefore, decreasing the salinity in a marine fish recovering from surgery may be worth trying.

Euthanasia

In clinical practice buffered MS-222 (1000 mg/l) is most frequently used to euthanase pet fish. MS-222 is not authorized as an agent for euthanasia, but it is considered safe and effective in fish not intended for human consumption. If MS-222 is to be used, it is important to buffer it with sodium bicarbonate. This is easily done by calculating the amount of MS-222 required (grams), and then weighing out double that amount of sodium bicarbonate. These can be added together to create the euthanasia solution in which the fish will be immersed.

Rapid freezing is specifically mentioned as 'not a humane method' in the current AVMA Guidelines on Euthanasia (AVMA, 2007) unless the fish is anaesthetized prior to being frozen. Clients calling a clinic to enquire about euthanasia of a pet fish are most likely to want to freeze the animal. Recommending that the fish be brought into the clinic for euthanasia is an appropriate professional response to such a request for information.

There are several other options for euthanasia of fish (Figure 20.13).

Agent	Dose	Precautions	Comments
Benzocaine	>250 mg/l	None specified	
Carbon dioxide	None specified	Fish tolerant of high CO_2. Hazardous to personnel	

20.13 Agents that may be used to euthanase non-food fish (AVMA, 2007). None of these agents is FDA-approved for euthanasia of fish. For all agents listed, fish should be left in the euthanasia solution for at least 10 minutes following cessation of opercular movement. [a] The authors recommend 1000 mg/l buffered MS-222. (continues) ▶

Agent	Dose	Precautions	Comments
Carbon monoxide	None specified	Hazardous to personnel	
Inhalant (halothane preferred)	None specified	Hazardous to personnel	
MS-222	>250 mg/l [a]	Buffer with sodium bicarbonate	Expensive. Carcass contamination
2-Phenoxyethanol	0.5–0.6 ml/l or 0.3–0.4 mg/l	None specified	
Sodium pentobarbital	60–100 mg/kg i.v./intracoelomically	DEA controlled substances May take >30 minutes	Carcass contamination

20.13 Agents that may be used to euthanase non-food fish (AVMA, 2007). None of these agents is FDA-approved for euthanasia of fish. For all agents listed, fish should be left in the euthanasia solution for at least 10 minutes following cessation of opercular movement. [a] The authors recommend 1000 mg/l buffered MS-222.

Drug formulary

The medications listed in Figure 20.14 provide a basic formulary for the veterinary practitioner specifically caring for marine aquarium fish. Several excellent reviews of the use of drugs in fish have been presented (Stoskopf, 1993; Noga, 1996; Wildgoose and Lewbart, 2001).

A few special considerations should be kept in mind when treating marine fish:

- Bath treatments work differently from freshwater fish. Unlike freshwater fish, marine fish drink water but do not typically absorb ions across the gills. Many medications, especially antibiotics, will not therefore be absorbed from a bath treatment in the way they are in freshwater fish.
- Oxytetracycline chelates in the marine environment and therefore is not effective as a bath treatment for marine species, even though it works well in freshwater fish.
- Potassium permanganate (often used as a parasiticide and antibacterial agent in freshwater fish) is contraindicated in marine fish due to damage to gill epithelium that increases as salinity increases (Marecaux, 2006).
- Organophosphates are often used in marine systems at higher concentrations than in freshwater systems, due to the decrease in efficacy as pH increases. As a precaution some veterinary surgeons feed atropine to marine fish prior to giving them an organophosphate bath.

Drug	Dose	Indication	Comments
Antimicrobial agents			
Amikacin [a]	5 mg/kg i.m. q3d	Bacterial infection	Nephrotoxic. Avoid in fish exposed to ammonia
Enrofloxacin [a]	5–10 mg/kg i.m. q3d (for higher dose)	Bacterial infection	Use small animal preparation (i.e. 22.7 mg/ml)
Florfenicol (*Aquaflor*)	10 mg/kg orally q24h for 10 days	Bacterial infection	For use only as Veterinary Feed Directive
Ormetoprim/ Sulfadimethoxine	50 mg/kg orally q24h for 5 days	Bacterial infection	
Oxytetracycline	88 mg/kg orally q24h for 10 days	Bacterial infection	Heat labile
Antiparasitic agents			
Chloroquine [a]	10 mg/l prolonged bath 15 mg/l for 7 days, followed by 10 mg/l prolonged bath	*Amyloodinium* *Cryptocaryon*	Accompany with hyposalinity (16–18 parts per thousand) when possible for *Cryptocaryon*. May need to treat after 21 days. Excellent efficacy with *Amyloodinium*; less information for *Cryptocaryon*. Toxic to algae and some invertebrates
Copper ion [a]	0.18–0.2 mg/l prolonged bath	External protists	Monitor copper ion daily. Maintain for 3 weeks. Highly toxic to invertebrates and plants; some fish are sensitive. May impact biofilter
Diflubenzuron [a]	0.03 mg/l prolonged bath	Crustacean parasites	Long half-life; water must be retained for days. Chitin synthesis inhibitor, so toxic to all crustaceans
Formalin	25 mg/l bath q2d for *Cryptocaryon*, *Brooklynella* and *Uronema*	External protists	Good aeration is essential. Impact on biofilter is minimal
Organophosphates (trichlorfon) [a]	0.50–1.0 mg/l bath	Capsalids and other monogeneans; leeches	High pH, temperature, aeration and light decrease half-life. Protective equipment should be worn. **Do not use more than once a week**. Pre-treat fish with atropine medicated feed
Praziquantel [a]	2 mg/l once prolonged bath	Capsalids and other monogeneans	Monitor for eggs and recurrence. Avoid large particle sizes (gill damage)
	50 mg/kg orally once	Intestinal trematodes	

20.14 Drug formulary for marine fish. [a] Not currently approved for use in food fish in the USA. (continues) ▶

Drug	Dose	Indication	Comments
Miscellaneous			
Atropine [a]	0.1 mg/kg	Counteract effect of organophosphate	In feed prior to treatment with organophosphates
Dexamethasone [a]	1–2 mg/kg i.m./i.p.	Shock, trauma, stress	

20.14 (continued) Drug formulary for marine fish. [a] Not currently approved for use in food fish in the USA.

References and further reading

American Veterinary Medical Association (AVMA) (2007) *AVMA Guidelines on Euthanasia.* http://www.avma.org/issues_welfare/euthanasia.pdf

Cato J and Brown C (2003) *Marine Ornamental Species: Collection, Culture and Conservation* Iowa State Press, Ames, IA

Clauss TM, Dove ADM and Arnold JE (2008) Hematological disorders of fish. *Veterinary Clinics of North America: Exotic Animal Practice* **11**, 445–462

DiMaggio MA (2008) *Parasitological and Osmoregulatory Evaluations of the Seminole Killifish, Fundulus seminolis, a Candidate Species for Marine Baitfish Aquaculture.* MSc thesis, University of Florida

Emerson K, Russo RC, Lund RE and Thurston RV (1975) Aqueous ammonia equilibrium calculations: effects of pH and temperature. *Journal of the Fisheries Research Board of Canada* **32**, 2379–2383

Francis-Floyd R and Watson C (1996) *Ammonia.* Florida Cooperative Extension Service Fact Sheet No.FA-16. (http://edis.ifas.ufl.edu)

Gomez DK, Lim DJ, Baeck GW, *et al.* (2006) Detection of betanodaviruses in apparently healthy aquarium fishes and invertebrates. *Journal of Veterinary Science* **7**, 369–374

Harms C (2003) Fish. In: *Zoo and Wildlife Medicine, 5th edn,* ed. ME Fowler and RE Miller, pp. 2–20. Saunders/Elsevier, St Louis

Harrenstien LA, Tornquist SJ, Miller-Morgan TJ, Fodness BG and Clifford KE (2005) Evaluation of a point-of-care blood analyzer and determination of reference ranges for blood parameters in rockfish. *Journal of the American Veterinary Medical Association* **226**, 255–265

Hartman KH (2006) Fish. In: *Guidelines for Euthanasia of Non-domestic Animals,* ed. CK Baer, pp.111. American Association of Zoo Veterinarians, Yulee, FL

Hemdal JF (2006) *Advanced Marine Aquarium Techniques.* TFH Publications Inc., Neptune City, NJ

Hoff FH (1996) *Conditioning, Spawning and Rearing of Marine Clownfish.* Aquaculture Consultants Inc., Dade City, FL

Kiryu Y, Shields JD, Vogelbein WK, Kator H and Blazer VS (2003) Infectivity and pathogenicity of the oomycete *Aphanomyces invadans* in Atlantic menhaden *Brevoortia tyrannus. Diseases of Aquatic Organisms* **54**, 135–146

Mainous ME and Smith SA (2005) Efficacy of common disinfectants against

Mycobacterium marinum. Journal of Aquatic Animal Health **17**, 284–288

Marecaux E (2006) *Effects of Potassium Permanganate on the Sailfin Molly Poecilia latippinna at varying Salinity Levels.* MSc thesis, University of Florida

Michael S (1998) *Reef Fishes. Vol. 1.* Microscosm Press, Shelburne, VA

Michael S (2004) *Angelfishes and Butterflyfishes.* TFH Publications, Neptune City, NJ

Michael S (2009) *Wrasses and Parrotfishes.* TFH Publications, Neptune City, NJ

Neiffer DL (2007) Bony fish (lungfish, sturgeon and teleosts). In: *Zoo Animal and Wildlife Immobilization and Anesthesia,* ed. G. West *et al.,* pp.159–196. Blackwell Publishing, Ames, IA

Noga EJ (1996) *Fish Disease: Diagnosis and Treatment.* Mosby, St Louis

Sladkey KK, Swanson CR, Stoskopf MK, *et al.* (2001) Comparative efficacy of tricaine methane sulfonate and clove oil for use as anesthetics in red pacu (*Piaractus brachypomus*). *American Journal of Veterinary Research* **62**(3), 337–342

Spotte S (1992) *Captive SeaWater Fishes: Science and Technology.* Wiley, New York

Stoskopf MK (1993) *Fish Medicine.* WB Saunders, Philadelphia

Tilghman GC, Francis-Floyd R and Klinger-Bowen R (2001) Feeding electivity indices of surgeonfish (Acanthuridae) of the Florida Keys. *Aquarium Sciences and Conservation* **3**, 198–205

Whittington ID and Chisholm LA (2008) Diseases caused by monogenea. In: *Fish Diseases,* ed. J Eiras *et al.,* pp. 683–816. Science Publishers, Enfield, NH

Wildgoose WH (2001) *BSAVA Manual of Ornamental Fish, 2nd edn.* BSAVA Publications, Gloucester

Wildgoose WH and Lewbart GA (2001) Therapeutics. In: *BSAVA Manual of Ornamental Fish, 2nd edn,* ed. WH Wildgoose, pp. 237–258. BSAVA Publications, Gloucester

Yanong RPE (2003) Fungal diseases of fish. *Veterinary Clinics of North America: Exotic Animal Practice* **6**, 377–400

Yanong RPE, Hartman KH, Watson CA, *et al.* (2008) Fish slaughter, killing and euthanasia: a review of major published U.S. guidance documents and general consideration of methods. *EDIS Circulars no.1525.* http://edis.ifas.ufl.edu/FA150

21

Invertebrates

Romain Pizzi

Introduction

Pet invertebrates are occasionally presented to veterinary surgeons and can be an interesting change from the more routine cases seen in exotic animal practice. While over 1 million invertebrate species have currently been described, most sources estimate the true number is likely to be between 6 and 10 million, and some estimate that it may be as high as 80 million. Despite this large number of species, only a handful are ever presented to veterinary surgeons dealing with exotic pets. This chapter will concentrate on a small number of common terrestrial species, and will aim to provide practical and useful information as a starting point for pet invertebrates. For a more comprehensive review of invertebrate medicine readers are referred to Lewbart (2006). Commonly kept species include Giant African land snails, land hermit crabs, tarantulas and scorpions (Figure 21.1).

Giant African land snails

There are over 200 species of Achatinidae in sub-Saharan Africa. Giant African land (GAL) snails are among the most commonly and easily kept pet invertebrates. Owners may be unaware that there are several common species, which can have different husbandry requirements.

The most common pet species is the East African GAL snail (*Achatina fulica;* Figure 21.1a) from Kenya and Tanzania. These have become an introduced agricultural pest and are hence illegal in some countries. Adults average 10 cm in length, although individuals may be as long as 20 cm. Dextral (right-handed) shells

are most common. The snails reach adult size within about 6 months and live approximately 5 years.

The largest species is *A. achatina*, the West African or Tiger snail, also called the giant Ghana snail. These are not as common as *A. fulica*, but are prized for their large size and striped appearance.

Land hermit crabs

The two most commonly kept semi-terrestrial land hermit crabs are the Caribbean or purple claw hermit crab (*Coenobita clypeaus*) and the Ecuadorian hermit crab (*C. compressus*). These decapod crustaceans live up to 15 years in captivity, with occasional reports of individuals living past 20 years of age.

Spiders

There are approximately 900 species of Theraphosidae (tarantula) spider, with more than 100 species available in the pet trade from time to time. Specialist keepers may also keep more unusual araneomorph species such as *Argiope* or *Nephila* orb web spiders free in a room, as they remain in their webs.

Some of the most commonly kept theraphosids include the terrestrial Mexican redknee tarantula (*Brachypelma smithi;* Figure 21.1b), Chilean rose tarantula (*Grammostola rosea*), Goliath birdeater (*Theraphosa blondi*) and curly hair tarantula (*Brachypelma albopilosum*), as well as arboreal species such as the pink-toe tarantula (*Avicularia avicularia*) from the Americas, and the Asian ornamental tarantulas (*Poecilotheria* spp.). Terrestrial African 'baboon' spiders (e.g. *Ceratogyrus, Pterinochilus, Hysterocrates*) are less popular but are kept, despite their more

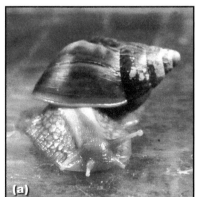
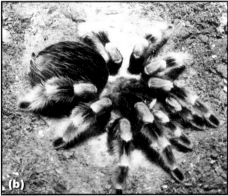
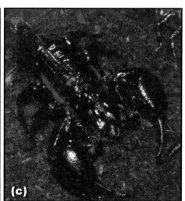

21.1 Some commonly kept invertebrates. **(a)** GAL snail. **(b)** Mexican redknee tarantula. **(c)** Imperial scorpion. (a,b Courtesy of DL Williams.)

aggressive nature. *Brachypelma* species, including *B. smithi* (Mexican redknee tarantula), are currently listed in Appendix II of CITES, which has increased their financial value. Serious hobbyists may keep several hundred or even thousand spiders belonging to a large number of species.

There is an unfortunate tendency among pet shops and traders to make up imaginative names for tarantulas, so reliance should never be placed on common names, and owners may not be aware what species they in fact possess. There have been a large number of taxonomic revisions that further complicate literature searches. For example: the Mexican redknee and other *Brachypelma* species were previously referred to as *Euthalus* spp.; the Chilean rose (*Grammostola rosea*, previously *Phrixotrichus spatulata*, previously *Grammostola spatulata*) is often still referred to by its previous names in current publications.

Adult female spiders can be extraordinarily long-lived; reports vary from 6–12 years in some African theraphosids to over 30 years in some New World terrestrial tarantulas, such as *Brachypelma* spp. Only females are long-lived, with males having a terminal instar once they moult to maturity. For this reason females are more desirable as pets.

Scorpions

The most commonly kept pet scorpion is the imperial or emperor scorpion (*Pandinus imperator*; Figure 21.1c), which originates from North Africa. One of the largest scorpion species, adults commonly reach over 20 cm in length. Despite their impressive appearance imperial scorpions have weak venom and are relatively timid and reclusive in nature, hence their popularity as pets. Individuals can live up to 8 years in captivity. Exhibits often include an ultraviolet (UV) light source to demonstrate their blue-green fluorescence; only adults have cuticles that fluoresce.

Biology

Sexing

Some pet invertebrates show sexual dimorphism, e.g. male Macleay's spectres (*Extatosoma tiaratum*) have wings while the females do not. Many insects have distinct differences, such as an ovipositor or genital claspers.

Adult males of many of the common pet tarantula species, such as Chilean rose tarantulas, have hooked spurs on the tibial section of the first pair of legs, which are used to secure the female's fangs during mating (Figure 21.2), and can be used to differentiate adult males. Subadult tarantulas can be sexed by microscopic examination of the epygial region of shed cuticle for presence or absence of spermathecae.

Husbandry

Invertebrates are poikilothermic and hence highly dependent on environmental factors, such as temperature range and humidity, for normal physiological

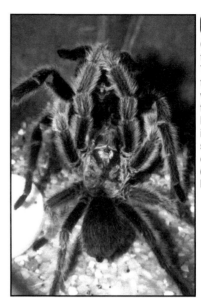

21.2

Chilean rose tarantulas mating. The male catches the female's fangs with tibial hooks on the first pair of his legs and inseminates her with sperm stored in the distal pedipalps. (© Zoological Medicine Ltd.)

functioning. Infectious and non-infectious diseases are often a reflection of underlying environmental deficits, and some health problems will resolve simply with husbandry changes, while more severe conditions will not respond to attempts at veterinary treatment unless the captive environment is optimized. Pet invertebrates are commonly kept by herpetologists and may therefore be treated by veterinary surgeons more accustomed to treating reptiles; for this reason several erroneous husbandry requirements based on herpetology have been reported in the literature.

Housing

General considerations

- Land hermit crabs are gregarious and can be kept in large tanks if sufficient space and spare shells of various sizes are provided to prevent fighting and shell stealing.
- Tarantulas need to be housed individually, or they will predate each other.
- Imperial scorpions can be kept communally, especially if youngsters are reared together or kept with their parents. Scorpions raised in isolation are more likely to try and predate each other, particularly if overcrowded or food is scarce.

Size

Size is an important consideration. If enclosures are too small, Indian stick insects (*Carausius morostus*) and some other phasmids will suffer from dysecdysis, and so enclosures should be at least twice their maximum body length in size in all dimensions.

In contrast, provision of overly large enclosures can be a problem in large terrestrial tarantulas such as the Goliath birdeater. An awkward fall from as little as 30 cm can cause fatal opisthosoma trauma in heavy-bodied individuals. Flat tanks under 30 cm in height are therefore advisable. Mesh-top tanks are not preferred for terrestrial tarantulas as they have fine hooks on their feet, which may become stuck in the mesh and lead to injury or limb autotomy. Arboreal species, such as Indian ornamental (*Poecilotheria regalis*) and pink-toe tarantulas, can be provided with high but narrow enclosures.

Lighting

A fallacy to be found in some literature is that scorpions or other arthropods need a source of UV light. Adult scorpions fluoresce blue-green under UV lighting, but UV light is not actually needed for any normal physiological process. Scorpions are nocturnal, and tarantulas are photophobic, and excessive lighting may just lead to stress and anorexia.

Heating

In many arthropods temperature stability appears to be more important than the provision of a precise temperature gradient. Many specimens can be safely kept at fairly cool temperatures once accustomed to these, but sudden temperature drops from a heated environment to that same lower temperature can cause mortalities due to 'cold stress'. On post-mortem histology these specimens may show pathology of structures such as the Malphigian tubules.

Additional heating is required in colder climates, but unfortunately there is little precise information on optimum temperatures for most common terrestrial pet invertebrate species. A minimum/maximum thermometer is useful for monitoring environmental temperature stability. Small heat mats beneath part of the enclosures are often best, as some species are photophobic or nocturnal. The heat mat should not be inside the enclosure as some species will instinctively burrow into the substrate if too warm. Temperatures in the range of 20–30°C for tarantulas are recommended by most authors for normal growth and ecdysis rates, and in practical terms mean that room temperatures are sufficient in many localities without additional heating.

Humidity and water provision

Arthropods need lower humidity than gastropods. High humidity also means enclosures need much more frequent cleaning to prevent food residue rotting and causing proliferation of Gram-negative bacteria that may cause disease.

GAL snails, particularly *A. achatina,* will aestivate by sealing themselves into the shell with a dried mucus film if conditions are too hot, or if humidity is insufficient. Light misting is helpful for all species, and especially important for *A. achatina.*

While some literature recommends misting tarantulas daily, this is not advisable. Tarantulas locate prey by detecting air current movements via their highly innervated and sensitive hairs. Blowing on these hairs, or misting, causes irritation and stress. Humidity is better provided by moistening the substrate, providing a water bowl and reducing enclosure ventilation for species requiring higher humidity. The common *Brachypelma* species and Chilean rose tarantulas do well at relatively low humidity and so are low maintenance in terms of husbandry and cleaning.

Water is best offered to arthropods such as spiders and insects in a shallow dish. A ramp or small pebble will also allow prey insects such as crickets to escape rather than drowning and rotting in the dish. Wet cottonwool balls are not recommended as they quickly

become soiled and can harbour heavy Gram-negative bacterial growth. Fibres can also become entangled on limbs.

Substrate and hides

Sufficiently deep sand should be provided for hermit crabs to burrow into for ecdysis. Occasionally an individual will moult on the surface; a simple separator made from a ring of a plastic bottle can be a useful barrier to prevent injury from other crabs without risking damage by handling and moving the moulting crab itself.

Retreats and hides should be provided in most arthropod enclosures. Imperial scorpions, despite their appearance, are reclusive in nature due to their weak venom. This species hides in burrows in termite mounds when not hunting and it is important to provide hides to limit stress. If a captive scorpion is frequently raising its tail in threat displays, this may indicate environmental stress due to lack of a hide, ground vibrations, or bright lighting.

Diet

Snails

Herbivores such as GAL snails should be offered a variety of fresh leafy vegetables, which should be thoroughly washed to ensure no pesticides are fed inadvertently. Shelled gastropod molluscs such as GAL snails need a dietary source of calcium, easily provided by cuttlefish bone; otherwise they will rasp other snails' shells with the radula to obtain the calcium they need for continued shell growth.

GAL snails do not readily accept powdered calcium on their food.

Arthropods

Tarantulas are normally fed live invertebrates such as crickets and locusts, depending on their size. Anorexic spiders may be tempted with waxworms. Some tarantulas will accept small pieces of raw meat or chicken, or whole killed vertebrates such as mice, and although breeders may claim faster growth rates with these diets, an entirely invertebrate-based diet is perfectly adequate.

Scorpions will accept freshly killed prey, although they prefer live invertebrates, and two or more scorpions may feed collaboratively on the same prey item. Imperial scorpions are reported to prey mainly on termites in the wild, and in captivity are commonly fed crickets, cockroaches and mealworms. These scorpions are often fed killed small mice in captivity, but these are not part of their natural diet in the wild.

Invertebrates as food items

When crickets and locusts are used as food items, it is important to provide them with food and water for 48 hours before being offered as food. If starved, they will rapidly metabolize their adipose bodies and will then hold little nutritional value for the tarantula or scorpion consuming them. Provision of dry bran is not sufficient, as these insects will also metabolize their adipose bodies to liberate water if they become dehydrated.

Calcium supplementation

The need for calcium supplementation in all invertebrates is a common fallacy, even in peer-reviewed literature. The majority of arthropods, such as pet scorpions and tarantulas, do not need calcium supplementation. The arthropod exoskeleton consists of a combination of chitin, a long-chain polymer of N-acetylglucosamine, and hence a polysaccharide carbohydrate, which is embedded in a mix of various proteins. Differing proportions of chitin lead to differences in rigidity and flexibility between species, as well as anatomical regions, and even between the layers of the cuticle. The hardening or scleritization after ecdysis is mediated by hydrophobic phenolics. Only some crustaceans and myriapods (millipedes) will incorporate minerals, predominately calcium carbonate, into their exoskeletons. Other arthropods do not. In fact, forced calcium supplementation of food in some insects will cause decreased survival and fecundity, due to abrasive damage to the gastrointestinal tract. While many invertebrates will form noncalcified eggs, there are exceptions, such as some large beetles and GAL snails, which produce eggs with a mineralized shell.

Breeding

Uncontrolled breeding of snails, phasmids and insects can be a serious problem in captivity and culling may be needed to keep numbers manageable.

Snails

GAL snails are hermaphrodites, containing both ovaries and testes; sperm can be stored viably for over a year. They can produce up to 200 eggs five times a year. The eggs are large (3–5 mm in length) with a calcified shell and are buried in the substrate. Care should always be taken when changing the substrate, as this may contain eggs.

Arthropods

The Indian stick insect is parthenogenetic, that is it will produce fertile eggs without a male being present.

Male tarantulas are only briefly introduced into the female's enclosure for breeding attempts (see Figure 21.2) and swiftly removed after this has occurred. It is recommended that tarantulas be housed individually as cannibalism can occur. Although some arboreal species (*Avicularia* and *Poecilotheria*) have been kept together in large communal enclosures, cannibalism does still occur and thus is not advised. Spiderlings are commonly left together after hatching for the first few moults, and the stronger spiderlings will predate the weaker ones.

All scorpions give birth to live young. Newly emerged scorpions are vulnerable and unable to fend for themselves, and are cared for by the mother, sometimes for several months. The mother will defend them and will be more aggressive to handling attempts during this period. They will ride on their mother's back (Figure 21.3) and she will kill prey for them. The youngsters venture off their mother's back as they grow, eventually dispersing and becoming independent.

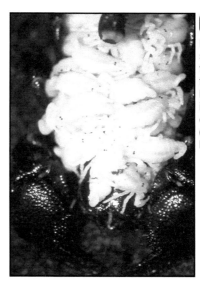

21.3

Newly emerged scorpions ride on their mother's back for several months before becoming independent and dispersing.
(© Zoological Medicine Ltd.)

Handling and restraint

Handling and restraint needs to be gentle in order not to damage delicate invertebrates and also not to allow specimens such as tarantulas or scorpions to injure the handler.

Spiders

Many New World theraphosids such as the Mexican redknee and Chilean rose tarantula rely for their primary defence on barbed irritant 'urticating' hairs that are kicked off from their dorsal opisthosoma into the face of potential predators. When handling New World tarantulas, latex gloves are a sensible precaution. A small number of people appear especially sensitive to these irritant hairs and can develop skin rashes or even respiratory distress on exposure. Asian tarantulas and African baboon spiders do not have this defence mechanism, and so will bite much more readily in defence.

Tarantulas may be gently encouraged into the hand with a fine artist's paintbrush. This can also be used to assess the individual's temperament and mood before handling, by gently and repeatedly stroking the first pair of legs. Any aggressive response will indicate that the tarantula is unlikely to tolerate gentle handling attempts.

Tarantulas can also be gently pinned to the substrate by applying finger pressure or using a pencil, over the strong rigid cephalothorax carapace. The tarantula can then safely be grasped and lifted, with the thumb and middle finger between the second and third pairs of legs on either side (Figure 21.4).

Switching off enclosure heating 12 hours before handling may be helpful with some Old World tarantula species, but placing individuals in the refrigerator for 30 minutes, as is sometimes advocated, can result in mortalities.

Trauma is a common cause of captive spider deaths. An awkward drop from as little as 20 cm can rupture the opisthosoma of a large terrestrial tarantula. For this reason tarantulas should always be handled over a table.

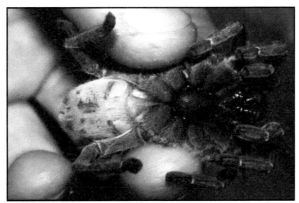

21.4 Safe handling of a *Pterinochilus* tarantula. This is an African species and lacks irritant hairs, so does not necessitate latex gloves. (© Zoological Medicine Ltd.)

Tarantulas laying on their back are normally undergoing ecdysis (Figure 21.5) and should not be handled, as they are susceptible to trauma at this time. Dead spiders are normally found in an upright position with their legs in flexion beneath them, as the legs have flexor muscles only and rely on haemolymph pressure for extension.

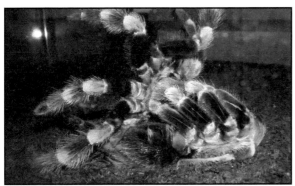

21.5 Tarantulas, such as this Mexican redknee, normally undergo ecdysis on their back, and should not be disturbed or handled during this process. (© Zoological Medicine Ltd.)

Scorpions
Safe handling of imperial scorpions is accomplished by grasping the tail dorsoventrally with padded forceps (Figure 21.6); they cannot twist the distal tail to sting to the side. Some other more venomous scorpion species have a more muscular tail, which may be grasped laterally at the distal third with padded forceps.

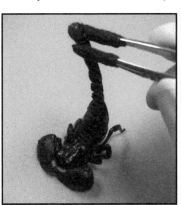

21.6 Handling an imperial scorpion using padded forceps to grasp the tail. (© Zoological Medicine Ltd.)

Diagnostic approach
If individuals are kept in small enclosures these should ideally be brought into the veterinary surgery. The water bowl can be emptied prior to transportation to prevent spillage.

History
A thorough history – with emphasis on husbandry – is essential, as the majority of health problems encountered in pet invertebrates will be husbandry-related. Behavioural changes can be an important indicator of some conditions. Tarantula keepers often notice Panagrolaimidae-infected tarantulas (see later) first by the distinctive behavioural changes they demonstrate, such as anorexia and reluctance to move, and either an abnormally huddled posture or standing on 'tip toes'.

Clinical examination
A macroscopic visual examination can be aided by the use of a low magnification stereomicroscope. Flattening arthropods such as scorpions with clear plastic sheeting on to a plate of glass, or simply placing the specimen in a clear-walled container, will allow gross visual examination.

Imaging

Radiography
Radiography is of very limited value in invertebrates such as arthropods; their cuticle consists of proteins, and very little soft tissue differentiation is evident even in large specimens. Cuttlefish are an exception: traumatic fractures of the cuttlebone and resorption lesions associated with bacterial infections may be visualized radiographically. Radiography can also be useful in shelled molluscs, such as GAL snails, to evaluate severe shell cracks after trauma and to help plan repairs to provide adequate stabilization.

Ultrasonography
Ultrasonography can be useful, especially in GAL snails (Figure 21.7). A small amount of water is all that is needed, as the copious mucus secreted by the gastropod foot is a perfect natural coupling gel. Snails are less likely to retract when water is used, rather

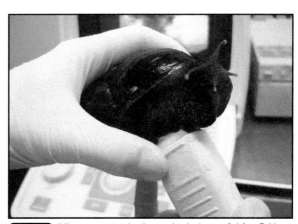

21.7 Ultrasonography is particularly useful for GAL snails. (© Zoological Medicine Ltd.)

than normal ultrasound gels which appear to irritate some specimens. Small 7.5–10 MHz curvilinear probes will give good definition, and structures such as the oral radula, pharynx and cranial digestive tract, as well as developed eggs, are relatively easily visualized. Ultrasonography can also be useful in determining the origin and thus prognosis of a prolapse (see later). Doppler ultrasonography has been reported to be useful in auscultating and monitoring heart rate in GAL snails (Rees Davies *et al.*, 2000). Its most useful application is in determining if a deeply retracted snail is just in deep aestivation or, in fact, dead.

Some arthropods such as tarantulas do not have discrete visceral organs that are amenable to ultrasound examination. Ultrasonography has, however, been used to screen tarantulas for the presence of large endoparasitic acrocercid larvae in the opisthosoma (Johnson-Delaney, 2006). Unfortunately, while individuals could be identified, attempts at treatment by aspiration of the parasite have been unsuccessful and resulted in the spider's death.

Endoscopy

Endoscopy is a useful diagnostic modality in invertebrates, as it provides magnification of these small patients. Endoscopic evaluation of oral discharges in tarantulas can allow differentiation of microscopic panagrolaimid nematodes from bacterial infection, without the need for microscopy. Endoscopic examination of the lung of pulmonate terrestrial snails via the pneumostome (Figure 21.8) is easy and can help demonstrate to clients that the snails are not infected with *Angiostrongylus cantonensis* or parasitic mites. Prolapses could also be examined, and endoscopy may even be useful in evaluating obstructive egg retention in large insects.

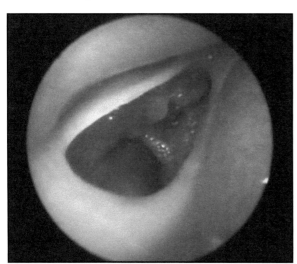

21.8 Endoscopic view of the pulmonary sac via the pneumostome in an East African GAL snail. The pulmonary sac can be examined for nematode or mite infections. (© Zoological Medicine Ltd.)

Microbiology

Bacterial and fungal culture can be performed on samples from lesions, or on oral or anal discharges, but interpretation of the significance of any organisms isolated can be difficult. Some entomopathogens are difficult to culture using standard veterinary techniques. A strong pure culture of a *Bacillus* species, of which there are numerous entomopathogenic and toxin-producing species, is more likely to be significant than a mixed culture. Due to rapid gut breakdown and bacterial invasion after death, culture *post mortem* is often unrewarding.

Faecal examination

Faecal samples may yield protozoans such as Coccidia and gregarines, but many insect species normally harbour a high gregarine parasite load asymptomatically in captivity (Figure 21.9). Similarly, millipedes commonly have a high nematode burden on examination without showing clinical signs; the author has not examined a millipede *post mortem* that has not had numerous gastrointestinal nematodes present.

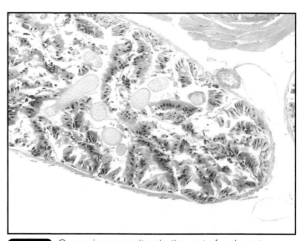

21.9 Gregarine parasites in the gut of a desert locust (*Schistocerca gregaria*). (© Zoological Medicine Ltd.)

Cytology and haematology

Standard stained and unstained cytology can be useful in identifying bacterial, fungal and protozoal infections and lesions, as well as melanization reactions and nodules (Figure 21.10), which are a typical inflammatory response to trauma or infection in insects and many arthropods.

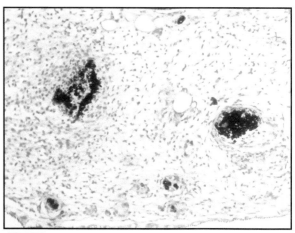

21.10 Many arthropods will react to infections or trauma by forming melanized inflammatory nodules. (© Zoological Medicine Ltd.)

There are some publications on haematology in tarantulas (Figure 21.11) and other invertebrates, but sources often do not agree on nomenclature of cell types, and values vary with life stage and proximity to ecdysis, and also with environmental temperatures, currently precluding any meaningful clinical application.

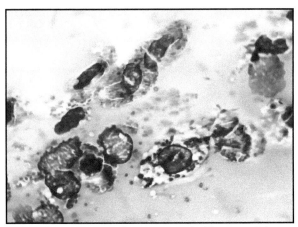

21.11 Blood smear from a tarantula. The green/blue respiratory pigment haemocyanin is contained in crystalline form in special haemocytes (cyanocytes) before being liberated into the haemolymph. Interpretation of invertebrate haematology is still in its infancy. (© Zoological Medicine Ltd.)

Necropsy

In a group invertebrate disease problem, the diagnostic approach usually relies on post-mortem examination and sampling. As gut breakdown and translocation of bacteria occur rapidly, even starting before death, it is better to take samples from live specimens than to use dead individuals.

Simple dissection of viscera immediately following euthanasia and wet mounting between slides (Figure 21.12) can demonstrate infections such as tracheal mites (*Acarapis woodi*) in honeybees which are visible in the respiratory tracheoles, or viral destruction of adipose bodies in Lepidoptera.

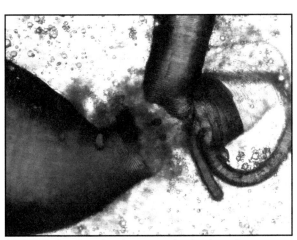

21.12 Section of an insect tracheole viewed microscopically. Such preparations can be examined for evidence of mites, eggs or inflammatory melanization reactions. (© Zoological Medicine Ltd.)

Common conditions

Only a small number of conditions in the most common pet invertebrate species can be briefly covered here; for more detailed information the reader is referred to Lewbart (2006).

Hair loss in tarantulas

As noted above, many New World species of terrestrial tarantula have urticating hairs on the dorsal and caudal aspects of their opisthosoma which they will kick off with their hind legs in the face of predators, or when disturbed. Loss of these hairs in captivity, resulting in an obvious bald patch (Figure 21.13), often indicates environmental stress, such as excessive handling or viewers repeatedly disturbing the spider by tapping on the glass. The hairs will not regrow, but once a new moult occurs the spider will have a new appearance, complete with its full complement of hairs. The condition does not need treatment, but stress should be addressed where needed. Asian tarantulas and African species do not have these irritant hairs, and hence do not develop alopecia. Skin scrapes should not be performed on tarantulas with alopecia as the dorsal opisthosoma overlying the heart, which is typically bald, is thin and can be easily ruptured, leading to fatalities.

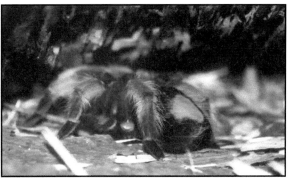

21.13 A bald patch is clearly visible on the dorsal opisthosoma of this Mexican redknee tarantula, presumed due to stress from viewers constantly banging on the glass of its enclosure. (© Zoological Medicine Ltd.)

Endoparasites

There are a large number of endoparasites, such as acrocercid spider-fly larvae and mermithid nematodes in tarantulas, that may be present in asymptomatic wild-caught individuals for months or even years. There is no treatment for these fatal infections, but the emerging parasites usually pose little threat to other captive invertebrates outside their normal geographical range.

Myriapods commonly carry a high load of mixed nematodes in the digestive tract asymptomatically, and these do not require treatment.

Although there is much written about zoonotic *Angiostrongylus cantonensis* nematode infections in GAL snails, this has only been seen in wild snails, and not in the UK. Snails are infected through rat faeces; a person would need to eat an infected GAL snail raw to contract the disease. Endoscopy of the pulmonary sac (see Figure 21.10) may be helpful in demonstrating infection.

Saprophytic soil nematodes (and mites) may be found in the substrate and are not a concern, but often indicate a need to clean the enclosure.

Oral nematodes of tarantulas

Panagrolaimid nematodes appear to be an important emerging problem in captive pet and zoo tarantulas, which has been reported in the UK, several European countries, the USA and Canada. The infection manifests initially with anorexia and lethargy, which progresses to a huddled posture. Death occurs after several weeks. A thick white discharge between the mouth and chelicerae may be noted. This appears at first to be fluid macroscopically, but under endoscopic or microscopic magnification can be seen to consist of a mass of microscopic motile nematodes (Figure 21.14). The diagnosis can be confirmed by visualizing the small, highly motile nematodes (< 0.5–3 mm in length) in a sample of saline flushed over the mouthparts. The nematodes appear to have a symbiotic relationship with bacteria, which cause tissue necrosis on which the nematodes feed. While the mode of transmission is unknown, humpbacked flies (Phoridae) have been suggested as possible vectors, and infections have spread between separate containers in a room. Recent work has also suggested that these nematodes may be related to those of beetles, and this has raised the possibility of mealworm beetles (*Tenebrio molitor*) acting as vectors.

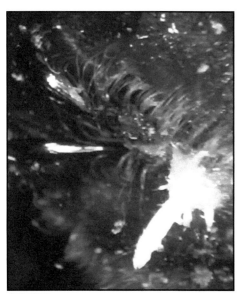

21.14 Panagrolaimid nematodes forming a white fluid-like mass under magnification on the mouthparts of a Goliath birdeater. (© Zoological Medicine Ltd.)

All treatment attempts with different benzimidazole and avermectin anthelminthics, and with antimicrobials for the associated bacteria, have so far been unsuccessful at even prolonging survival time. An important consideration is that related nematode species have been demonstrated to cause a potentially fatal zoonosis of deep anaerobic wounds, with no effective treatment currently available. Since large specimens of *Theraphosa blondi* can have fangs in excess of 3 cm, secondary infection of bite wounds is possible. Due to the possible risk, lack of treatment options, and potential spread in a collection, minimal handling and euthanasia of all affected spiders is currently strongly recommended. There is ongoing research and these guidelines may change within the next few years as more is learnt about these nematodes.

Mites

Mites are a frequently reported problem in captive terrestrial invertebrates (Figure 21.15). Many are saprophytic, rather than parasitic or host-specific. Microscopy can sometimes be helpful, as mites without piercing mouthparts are not parasitic, but this is not always clear. Saprophytic mites are commonly encountered in high-humidity enclosures, or where hygiene is poor. Saprophytic mites can occasionally cause irritation and can cause hermit crabs to abandon their shell. Wood chip and bark substrates are more likely to harbour mites. Some host-specific mites are not particularly harmful, such as *Gromphadorholaelaps schaeferi,* a mite specific to Madagascan hissing cockroaches that feeds off food around the mouthparts.

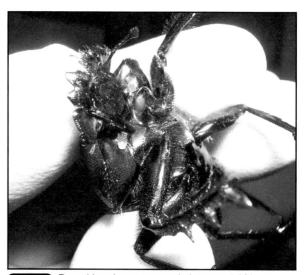

21.15 Parasitic mites on a newly imported African dung beetle. (© Zoological Medicine Ltd.)

Other mites are clearly pathogenic, such as *Varroa destructor* in European honeybees, which also acts as a viral vector and causes colony die-offs. Tracheal mites in a variety of insects may also cause decreased survival and fecundity, even if mortalities are not obvious. Many hobbyists routinely microwave non-flammable substrates in order to prevent mite outbreaks. A commercially available predatory mite, *Hypoaspis miles,* that is sold to control fungus gnats and pest thrips has also been used successfully in large collections of tarantulas; they appear to control the mites in the enclosure without irritating the spider.

Numerous other methods have been described, depending on the affected species, including: removing all substrates; removing visible mites with petroleum jelly/ultrasound gel on a cotton bud or fine artist's paintbrush; mite removal with sticky tape; and applying a 1:200 dilution of ivermectin with a fine artist's paintbrush. New arrivals should always be quarantined in separate rooms to an invertebrate collection for 30 days, and enclosures can be encircled with double-sided sticky tape to catch any mites leaving the enclosure.

Fungal infections

Two basic types of fungal infection are seen in captive arthropods. The first is most commonly seen in individual pets and manifests as visible fungal growth on the exoskeleton while the individual is still alive. The majority of these are opportunistic infections, often due to poor environmental hygiene, and respond well and rapidly to topical treatment with weak povidone–iodine.

The second type of infection demonstrates visible fungal growth only after an individual's death, and usually indicates an entomopathogenic fungus. These commonly invade the coelom, multiplying with no external signs until the animal's death, when external fruiting bodies rapidly emerge and produce spores. These infections are very difficult to manage in collections once spores have contaminated a room. In severe cases, destocking for several months and fumigation may be needed before keeping can recommence. In some cases affected individuals may show colour changes or behavioural abnormalities shortly before death, but often there are no ante-mortem clinical signs.

Hermit crabs out of shell

It is not normal to find land hermit crabs out of their shell. There can be numerous causes, which include: severe systemic illness; enclosure temperatures that are too warm; stress; stealing of the shell by another hermit crab (extra shells of a variety of sizes should be available in the enclosure); ecdysis, very occasionally; and irritants, such as mites. Shells can be removed and boiled to kill mites. If sufficient shells are not available, plastic containers such as film canisters may be useful as temporary 'pseudoshells'.

Poisoning

Most modern dedicated agricultural pesticides are rapid-acting and non-cumulative, and are an uncommon source of intoxication in pets, but it may occur if treated vegetables are fed to herbivorous species. Commercial flea and tick treatments, household sprays, and fumigation of nearby properties are more problematical. Some species, such as phasmids, appear very sensitive to even household aerosols. Arthropods, particularly tarantulas, appear to be sensitive to fipronil toxicity due to its residual nature; this is another reason for veterinary surgeons to use latex gloves when handling patients. Care should be taken when using containers previously used for snakes that fipronil was not used to treat snake mites; treated enclosures have killed spiders several months later, despite being washed. Signs of intoxication can include anorexia and decreased mobility, or incoordination and twitching, depending on the compound. Some other compounds appear

less harmful than would be supposed: the author has used 1:200 dilutions of ivermectin topically on large scorpions and tarantulas to treat mites without any apparent ill effects.

Prolapses

Prolapses are not uncommonly seen in GAL snails. When the bursa copulatrix or dart apparatus prolapses, it may be replaced with a lubricated probe or moist cotton bud, and there is a good prognosis. Digestive tract prolapses usually indicate severe systemic disease and are invariably fatal.

Trauma and dehydration

Trauma (see Wound repair, below) and resultant dehydration (see Rehydration, below) are common problems in pet invertebrates.

Dysecdysis

Dysecdysis is a common problem in arthropods, particularly tarantulas, in captivity. Good nutritional status and hydration are important in preventing dysecdysis. Misting during the actual ecdysis is often not particularly helpful, as the arthropod cuticle is relatively water-resistant and the surface tension of water prevents it entering the narrow space between the new and old cuticle. Adding a surfactant such as household detergent can be useful, but care must then be taken not to apply this in the vicinity of the book lungs (or spiracles in insects) to avoid asphyxiation. Dysecdysis is relatively uncommon in adult scorpions, but a form can occur in newly emerged scorpions when embryonic membranes are desiccated and become trapped. Moistening for several minutes on wet tissue paper, followed by careful removal of the membranes with a cotton bud, can be performed.

It is essential to avoid the temptation to interfere or try to assist during ecdysis. The new cuticle is soft and fragile to allow body expansion to occur; sclerization takes place over the first few hours to days. In contrast, the old cuticle is hardened and strong, and attempting to remove this usually results in dismembering the patient by tearing the new fragile cuticle. Even if several limbs are trapped or distorted, it is best to wait 12–36 hours until the new cuticle has hardened before attempting to trim retained cuticle away with fine scissors, attempting gentle removal with surfactants, or inducing autotomy of affected limbs (see Autotomy, below). Many tarantulas will autotomize limbs safely during this period (see Figure 21.20); it is still advisable to apply cyanoacrylate adhesive to the site to prevent haemolymph leakage.

Egg binding

Egg binding is occasionally seen in females. If it is a recurrent problem in a collection, it is possible that there may be an environmental problem such as lack of suitable or sufficiently deep ovipositing substrate, or insufficient humidity. Careful removal of the obstructed ootheca (capsule containing the eggs) is possible in affected large individuals such as cockroaches (Figure 21.16).

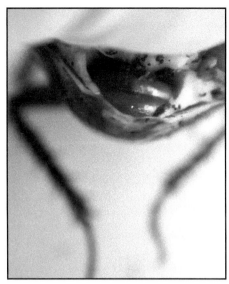
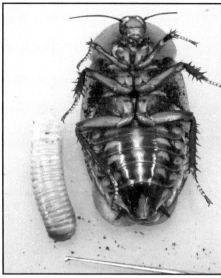

21.16 This false death's head cockroach (*Blaberus discoidalis*) suffered dystocia because the ovipositing substrate was too shallow. The large ootheca was removed manually to relieve the obstruction. (© Zoological Medicine Ltd.)

Notifiable Diseases

Veterinary surgeons dealing with honeybees (*Apis mellifera*) should be aware that, at time of going to press, there are currently three Notifiable Diseases in the European Union according to EC Directive 92/65/EEC. These are:

- American foulbrood (Figure 21.17a), a bacterial disease caused by *Paenibacillus larvae* var. *larvae*
- The small hive beetle (*Aethina turnida*), an African species, now problematic in the USA, Canada and Australia

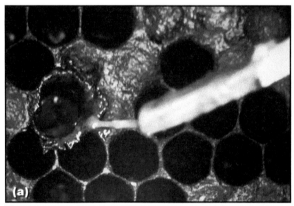
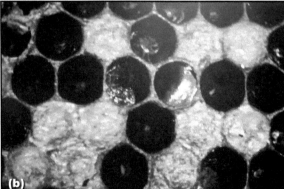

21.17 **(a)** The pathognomic ropey thread seen in American foulbrood in the European honey bee. **(b)** European foulbrood leaves a dry scale in the cell. (Courtesy of DL Williams.)

- *Tropilaelaps* spp. mites, originating from the Asian giant honeybee (*Apis dosata*).

The United Kingdom includes one further Notifiable Disease:

- European foulbrood (Figure 21.17b), a bacterial disease caused by *Melissococcus plutonius*. Lightly infected hives may be treatable with oxytetracycline administered by licensed inspectors.

While *Varroa destructor* mites are the most economically important health problem of honeybees, since their recognition in the UK in 1992 they have become endemic and so are no longer notifiable. The parasite originates from Asia, where it naturally occurs on the Asian honeybee *Apis cerana*. The mite feeds on adult European honeybees and brood, causing weakness, as well as acting as a vector for viruses such as deformed wing virus (DWV). Infested colonies eventually die out if not treated. Further difficulty in control has arisen with the recognition of pyrethroid-resistant mite strains in the UK since 2001.

In the UK, the National Bee Unit offers diagnostic testing of these as well as other common bee diseases, such as the protozoan *Nosema apis*, the amoeba *Malpighamoeba mellificae*, viral sacbrood, and fungal chalkbrood (*Ascosphaera apis*). The unit also offers treatment advice, and further offers testing and monitoring of suspected incidents of pesticide intoxication of bees with the Wildlife Incident Unit.

The Office International des Epizooties (OIE) lists *Varroa destructor* and tracheal mites (*Acarapis woodi*) of bees as Notifiable, along with several diseases of crustaceans and molluscs of commercial concern.

Supportive care

Supportive care in pet invertebrates usually consists of correcting underlying environmental problems, particularly temperature and humidity, and the correction of fluid deficits.

Drug administration

Therapeutic usage of medications in pet invertebrates is anecdotal at present. Veterinary surgeons are referred to Lewbart (2006) for further information.

Rehydration

Snails

If dehydrated or kept under dry conditions GAL snails will retract and seal themselves into their shell and aestivate; this can last for several months. It can be difficult to tell whether a snail is dead or simply deeply retracted and aestivating; this can usually be accomplished using a small-headed pulse Doppler probe to auscultate vascular flow (see Figure 21.19). Rehydration is accomplished by placing the snail in a shallow tray of warm water, which in emerged snails should not cover the pneumostome entrance to the lung just beneath the lip of the shell. Water appears to be more effective than 0.9% physiological saline, due to the increased osmotic gradient.

Arthropods

Severely dehydrated spiders are unable to move, as extension of appendages is dependent on haemolymph pressure. The easiest treatment in most cases is to place the cephalothorax of the spider in a very shallow dish of water. Care must be taken not to submerge the book lungs on the ventral opisthosoma. Most spiders will rehydrate over a few hours. In more severe cases, intrahaemolymph injections of sterile isotonic fluids may be performed using a 30-gauge insulin needle and syringe, into the dorsal midline of the opisthosoma, where the heart lies (Figure 21.18). Tarantulas have a closed arterial and open venous system, and fluids will be effective even if the heart is missed. As the cuticle is inflexible, it is advisable to seal all needle puncture sites with tissue adhesive.

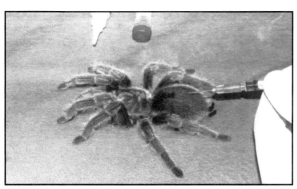

21.18 Fluids may be administered into (or haemolymph sampled from) the heart, which lies in the dorsal midline of the opisthosoma in tarantulas. Needle puncture sites should be sealed with cyanoacrylate adhesive to prevent haemolymph leakage. (© Zoological Medicine Ltd.)

Scorpions can similarly be injected via the soft pleurite membranes between the hard dorsal and ventral plate-like tergites. O'Brien (2008) recommends using sterile water rather than saline in phasmids as their haemolymph contains little sodium.

If treating arthropods for dehydration secondary to suspected trauma or haemolymph loss, it is advisable to keep individuals on paper towels for 48 hours instead of the normal substrate to detect any signs of continued leakage. Haemolymph is pale and often difficult to see otherwise.

Anaesthesia and analgesia

O'Brien (2008) provides a detailed review of anaesthesia in invertebrates, including aquatic species.

Snails

Practical anaesthesia of some gastropods, such as GAL snails, appears to be difficult. In contrast to arthropods, which appear resistant to volatile anaesthetics, pulmonate terrestrial snails appear very sensitive, and the author has inadvertently killed GAL snails with what would be normal volatile anaesthetic concentrations in other species. Girdlestone et al. (1989) found effective dose 50 (ED_{50}) concentrations for reversible anaesthesia, judged on loss of whole body withdrawal reflex, to be only 0.83% v/v halothane, and 1.09% v/v isoflurane. Sodium pentobarbital baths were found to provide insufficient anaesthesia by Joosse and Lever (1959). Zachariah and Mitchell (2009) recommend shallow tricaine methane sulphonate (MS-222) at 100 mg/l, but Joosse and Lever (1959) found this method caused mortalities. If using a bath for terrestrial gastropods such as GAL snails, the bath should be sufficiently shallow so as not to cover the pneumostome (opening to the lungs), found just beneath the shell rim in the mantle.

A relatively reliable and safe method for inducing surgical depth anaesthesia across numerous different pulmonate snail species has been described by Mutani (1982). Snails were placed in shallow baths of 0.08% sodium pentobarbital at 27°C for 30 minutes, followed by a shallow bath of both 0.08% sodium pentobarbital and 0.3% MS-222, with complete surgical depth anaesthesia occurring within 20 minutes. Revival occurred within 60 minutes of being placed in normal water. While this technique may or may not be practical in a veterinary clinical setting, anaesthesia of pet snails should be regarded as higher risk than that of arthropods, and this information conveyed to owners when consent is sought. Anaesthetic depth is judged on foot and whole body withdrawal reflexes, and it is possible to monitor heart rate by means of a Doppler ultrasonography probe (Figure 21.19).

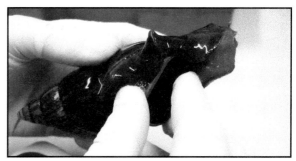

21.19 Doppler ultrasonography can be used to auscultate vascular flow and monitor anaesthesia in gastropods, as well as differentiating aestivating from dead individuals. (© Zoological Medicine Ltd.)

Arthropods

Most common pet arthropods, such as tarantulas, scorpions and insects, can be safely anaesthetized with 4–6% isoflurane concentrations. This may be performed in a double anaesthetic chamber to prevent the patient escaping up the tubing (Figure 21.20). Anaesthesia is judged on loss of righting reflex. Induction can be slow, taking up to 20 minutes in tarantulas, which predominately use anaerobic muscle activity and rely on passive diffusion of gas via the book lungs. Induction is more rapid in insects, which contain spiracles and a tracheolar respiratory system.

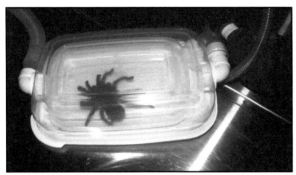

21.20 A double anaesthetic chamber prevents the patient escaping up one of the tubes. This tarantula is demonstrating the loss of righting reflex. (© Zoological Medicine Ltd.)

Crustaceans are problematical to anaesthetize. Crustacean neurotransmission depends on peptides and hydroxytryptamine glutamate, in addition to more orthodox neurotransmitters, and their response to anaesthetic agents can vary in comparison with other species. Injections of anaesthetic drugs such as ketamine, lidocaine and xylazine via the arthrodial limb joint membranes has been described (Lewbart, 2006) but may result in limbs being autotomized. MS-222 is not particularly effective in many crustaceans. Clove oil has been used in some aquatic crustaceans, but induction can take over an hour and concentrations recommended vary widely, from 0.03 to 1 ml/l. Halothane was effective in anaesthetizing freshwater crayfish in under 15 minutes using concentrations of 0.5% v/v (Ingle, 1995).

Analgesia

Currently, it is unknown how invertebrates interpret noxious stimuli, which in vertebrates would be perceived as pain. Appropriate anaesthesia should prevent any response to noxious stimuli and therefore meet the requirements for analgesia in invertebrates. While hypothermia is sometimes used to facilitate handling, this is believed to cause immobilization rather than any loss of sensation and is therefore not considered humane anaesthesia. Some invertebrates are particularly sensitive to rapid temperature changes and 'cold stress'.

Common surgical procedures

It comes as a surprise to many veterinary surgeons that surgical procedures are indeed possible in invertebrates.

Limb amputation

Limb amputation is fairly easily accomplished in most arthropods, and may be needed in cases of trauma where there is uncontrolled haemolymph loss. The arthropod cuticle is brittle and not easily sectioned without fragmenting, so incisions should be made in the joint membranes. Wounds or stumps of amputated limbs should be sealed with tissue adhesives; it is best to apply this in several individual layers. Care should be taken around the base of appendages not to glue other limbs, or seal spiracles or book lung openings, and especially in the proximity of the tiny oral cavity in tarantulas and the surrounding filtering hairs, blockage of which will result in inability to suck up liquid food.

Autotomy

Tarantulas and other spiders are able to perform limb autotomy (Figure 21.21). This evolved to allow animals to discard a badly damaged limb, escape if trapped by dysecdysis, or survive an unsuccessful mating attempt.

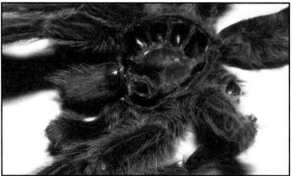

21.21 This shed tarantula cuticle contains a trapped limb that the spider had autotomized. (© Zoological Medicine Ltd.)

Autotomy can be induced by firmly grasping the femur segment of the limb. Grasping more distal limb segments does not usually lead to the spider autotomizing its leg. Autotomy is a voluntary act and cannot be performed with the spider anaesthetized. The usual autotomy site is between the coxa and the trochanter. The pedipalps may also be autotomized, but this may affect feeding. The spider may shed the limb itself, by rapidly jerking the coxa dorsally while the grasped femur retains its position, but usually the veterinary surgeon needs to snap the femur rapidly upwards. The coxal apodeme fractures and the joint membrane ruptures dorsally under the tension. Only the gracilis muscle traverses the autotomy site, inserting on the trochanter. This generally detaches easily, and retracts into the coxa. The remaining muscles insert on thickenings of the joint capsule (sclerites), and contraction of these function to pull the wound edges closed, limiting haemolymph loss. It is strongly advised to apply cyanoacrylate adhesive after any autotomy, as there is a risk of haemorrhage starting at a later point, and spiders have been lost up to a month later from this. The limb will usually regenerate during the next ecdysis, and will return to normal size and appearance within 2–3 ecdyses. Foelix (1996) reported a specimen where all the legs and pedipalps were automomized, which was then hand-fed until the next ecdysis, when all the appendages regenerated.

Wound repair

Molluscs
Radiography can help in determining the extent of shell damage. Shell repair in gastropod snails is performed by cleaning and apposing fragments, and covering the cracks with micropore tape followed by an epoxy resin repair (Lewbart and Christian, 2003). Tissue adhesives are not suitable, as they tend to seep into cracks, acting as a foreign body and preventing healing from occurring.

Integument wounds in cephalopods have been reported to heal well with standard monofilament absorbable sutures (Boyle, 1991).

Arthropods
While Johnson-Delaney (2000) has reported the use of sutures in tarantulas, the author performed an experimental study with different suture materials in Chilean rose tarantulas (Pizzi and Ezendam, 2005) and found the opisthosoma cuticle to have no practical suture-holding ability whatsoever. Sutures simply tore through the cuticle, resulting in larger wounds and the tarantulas' death. The author has found tissue adhesives or commercial cyanoacrylate 'superglue' to be the best trauma repair method in arthropods such as spiders. Large or lacerated wounds in the tarantula opisthosoma have been repaired using a small patch of micropore tape covered with several layers of tissue adhesive, and these have healed by the following ecdysis. The same technique has been successful in scorpion dorsal mesosoma or metasoma wounds. When using cyanoacrylate, several layers should be applied and allowed to dry to build a sturdy repair. Commercial 'superglue' gels do not appear to be usable.

Euthanasia

Invertebrates are not covered by animal welfare legislation in most countries. An exception is the UK Animal (Scientific Procedures) Act 1986 which, through the 1993 amendment, includes a single invertebrate species, *Octopus vulgaris*.

Euthanasia should always aim to be as humane as possible; otherwise there is little sense in a pet invertebrate owner approaching a veterinary surgeon. The method of euthanasia is also determined by what the cadavers will be needed for. Some owners may want the cadaver for display (e.g. large tarantulas), while in other cases post-mortem histology or bacteriology may be desired.

Euthanasia is usually practically performed by using anaesthetic agents, followed by pithing, immersion in a fixative (e.g. alcohol or formalin), or freezing.

While conscious immersion in alcohol is commonly used by entomologists in the field, in the author's experience some small spiderlings and insects will demonstrate frantic activity for over 5 minutes, and this method is hence not recommended unless animals are first anaesthetized. It is strongly recommended that crustaceans are pithed during euthanasia.

References and further reading

Boyle PR (1991) *The Care and Management of Cephalopods in the Laboratory.* UFAW, Potters Bar

Cooper JE (1987) A veterinary approach to spiders. *Journal of Small Animal Practice* **28**, 229–239

Foelix RF (1996) *The Biology of Spiders, 2nd edn.* Harvard University Press, Cambridge, MA

Frye FL (1992) *Captive Invertebrates: A Guide to their Biology and Husbandry.* Krieger, Malabar, FL

Girdlestone D, Cruikshank SG and Winlow W (1989) The actions of the volatile general anaesthetics on withdrawal responses of the pond snail *Lymnaea stagnalis. Comparative Biochemistry and Physiology* C **92**, 39–43

Ingle RW (1995) *The UFAW Handbook on the Care and Management of Decapod Crustaceans in Captivity.* UFAW, Potters Bar

Johnson-Delaney C (2000) *Exotic Companion Medicine Handbook for Veterinarians.* Zoological Education Network, Lake Worth, FL

Johnson-Delaney CA (2006) Use of ultrasonography in diagnosis of parasitism in goliath bird eater tarantulas (*Theraphosa blondi*). *British Veterinary Zoological Society Proceedings*, pp. 102

Joosse J and Lever J (1959) Techniques for narcotisation and operation for experiments with *Lymnaea stagnalis* (Gastropoda Pulmonata). Proceedings, *Koninklijke Nederlandse Akademie van Wetenschappen, Amsterdam*, **2**, 145–149

Lacey L (1997) *Manual of Techniques in Insect Pathology.* Academic Press, San Diego

Lewbart G (2006) *Invertebrate Medicine.* Blackwell Publishing, Ames, IA

Lewbart G and Christian L (2003) Repair of a fractured shell in an apple snail. *Exotic DVM* **5**(2), 8–9

Mutani A (1982) A technique for anaesthetising pulmonate snails of medical and veterinary importance. *Zeitschrift für Parasitenkunde* **68**, 117–119

O'Brien M (2008) Invertebrate anaesthesia. In: *Anaesthesia of Exotic Pets*, ed. LA Longley, pp.279–295. Saunders–Elsevier, St. Louis

Pizzi R (2002) Induction of autotomy in Theraphosidae spiders as a surgical technique. *Veterinary Invertebrate Society Newsletter* **2**(18), 2–6

Pizzi R (2008) Disease management in ex-situ invertebrate conservation programs. In: *Zoo and Wild Animal Medicine: Current Therapy*, ed. M Fowler and E Miller, pp. 88–96. Saunders–Elsevier, St. Louis

Pizzi R, Carta L and George S (2003) Oral nematode infection of tarantulas. *Veterinary Record*, **152**, 695

Pizzi R and Ezendam T (2005) Spiders and sutures: or how to make wounds a whole lot worse. *Veterinary Invertebrate Society Newsletter* **2** (21), 18–20

Rees Davies R, Chitty JR and Saunders R (2000) Cardiovascular monitoring of an *Achatina* snail using a Doppler ultrasound unit. *Proceedings, British Veterinary Zoological Society* p.101

Reichling SWB and Tabaka C (2001) A technique for individually identifying tarantulas using passive integrated transponders. *Journal of Arachnology* **29**, 117–118

Schultz SA and Schultz MJ (1996) *A Mechanical Mom for Tarantulas.* American Tarantula Society, Carlsbad, NM

Schultz SA and Schultz MJ (1998) The Tarantula Keeper's Guide. *Barron, Hauppauge, NY*

Smith M, Goodrum L *et al.* (2008) The importance of hive health in apiculture from a veterinary perspective. *UK Vet* **13**(8), 65–69

Tanada Y and Kaya HK (1993) *Insect Pathology.* Academic Press, San Diego

Williams D (2002) Invertebrates. In: *BSAVA Manual of Exotic Pets, 4th edn*, ed. A Meredith and S Redrobe, pp. 26–33. BSAVA Publications, Gloucester

Zachariah T and Mitchell MA (2009) Invertebrates. In: *Manual of Exotic Pet Practice*, ed. MA Mitchell and T Tully, pp. 11–38. Saunders–Elsevier, St. Louis

22

British and European Union legislation

Peter Scott

Introduction

There are some clear categories of legislation which apply to exotic pets. It is not within the scope of this chapter to cover all aspects of the legislation in any depth but the major pieces are indicated here. These cover:

- Import/export
- Sale
- Keeping, pets, performance and zoos
- Health (including zoonotic diseases)
- Medicines
- General.

An important area to consider is the interaction between veterinary surgeons and the public. If clients will not consult a veterinary surgeon because they feel that they will be reported to the authorities when an illegality is suspected, it may not be in the best interests of the animal. Unless a particular legal requirement to report acquired knowledge is placed on veterinary surgeons by legislation, then breaking client confidentiality and trust should only be considered after discussion with the Royal College of Veterinary Surgeons (RCVS). Veterinary surgeons should certainly be able to guide clients towards their basic legal obligations with regard to their pets.

Import and export

Import and export legislation is partially wrapped up with the sale and keeping of some species, but the primary legislation to be aware of is that covered by CITES.

Endangered species legislation

The 'Washington' Convention on International Trade in Endangered Species of Wild Fauna and Flora, more commonly known as CITES, aims to protect certain plants and animals by regulating and monitoring their international trade to prevent it reaching unsustainable levels. The Convention came into force in 1975, and the UK became a Party in 1976. There are now over 150 Parties. The CITES Secretariat is administered by the United Nations Environment Programme (UNEP).

The species covered by CITES are listed in three Appendices, according to the degree of protection they need:

- *Appendix I*: includes species threatened with extinction. Trade in specimens of these species is permitted only in exceptional circumstances
- *Appendix II*: includes species not necessarily threatened with extinction, but in which trade must be controlled in order to avoid utilization incompatible with their survival
- *Appendix III*: includes species that are protected in at least one country, which has asked other CITES Parties for assistance in controlling the trade.

A specimen of a CITES-listed species may be imported into or exported (or re-exported) from a State Party to the Convention only if the appropriate certification has been obtained beforehand and presented for clearance at the port of entry or exit. There is some variation in the requirements from one country to another and it is *always* necessary to check on the national laws.

Wildlife trade regulations

European Union

CITES has been implemented in the EU since 1984 through a number of Regulations.

Council Regulation (EC) No. 338/97: deals with the protection of species of wild fauna and flora by regulating the trade in these species.

Commission Regulation (EC) No. 1808/2001 (this replaced Commission Regulation (EC) No. 939/37): these set out the rules for the import, export and re-export of the species to which they apply. The regulation of trade is based on a system of permits and certificates that may only be issued when certain conditions are met.

In the EU the CITES Appendices (1, 2 and 3) are replaced by Annexes (A, B and C) to EC Regulation 338/97. This may appear confusing but the lists can differ a little. The system allows for tighter controls within Europe than perhaps are operated elsewhere, so whilst operating CITES as a basis, the EU may upgrade the level of 'supervision' given to a species. Current species lists are held by the UNEP World Conservation Monitoring Centre and can be viewed on their website.

- *Annex A*: includes all species listed in *Appendix I* of CITES, plus certain other species included because they look the same, need a similar level of protection, or to secure the effective protection of rare taxa within the same genus.
- *Annex B*: includes all the remaining species listed in *Appendix II* of CITES, plus certain other species included on a 'lookalike' basis, or because the level of trade may not be compatible with the survival of the species or local populations, or because they pose an ecological threat to indigenous species.
- *Annex C*: includes all the remaining species listed in *Appendix III* of CITES.
- *Annex D*: includes those non-CITES species not listed in *Annexes A* and *C*, which are imported into the Community in such numbers as to warrant monitoring.

Aside from trade restrictions (see below) CITES also requires that anyone breeding or displaying for commercial gain any species listed in Appendix I requires a licence under Article 10, referred to as a 'specimen-specific' licence. Sale of a listed animal requires an Article 10 certificate. Zoos with many such animals usually apply for Article 60 certificates, which are collection-specific, and act as a blanket licence for all of the animals and plants they hold.

United Kingdom
The Department for Environment, Food and Rural Affairs (Defra) Animal Health is now the UK CITES Management Authority and is responsible for ensuring that the Convention is implemented in the UK. Its role includes enforcement and issuing permits and certificates for the import and export, or commercial use of, CITES specimens. Applications for CITES permits are referred to a designated CITES Scientific Authority for advice on the conservation status of the species concerned.

Control of Trade in Endangered Species (Enforcement) Regulations 1997 (COTES): principally enforces the CITES legislation in the UK.

Customs and Excise Management Act 1979

It was widely felt by conservation groups that the weak powers of the COTES legislation accounted for the relatively few prosecutions under it, and this resulted in harsher penalties being introduced in 2003. There are provisions within COTES for power of entry and provision for offences by corporate bodies. Prosecutions may also involve the Customs and Excise Management Act 1979 for import offences, which has more substantial penalties.

Importing into the United Kingdom:

Directive 92/65 EEC (the 'Balai' Directive): covers importation from within the EU.

Commission Decision 2000/666/EC: covers importation from countries outside the EU.

Importation from the EU requires an official export health certificate. Importation from 'Third Countries' (outside the EU) requires a general licence and must comply with the conditions laid down in Commission Decision 2000/666/EC, which currently requires imports only from countries which are members of OIE. Exports are dealt with in a similar fashion. Certification of animals for import and/or export is complex and requires consultation every time with Defra Animal Health.

Practical pointers regarding importing and exporting animals

- Determine the species: this sounds easier than it may be, but could be crucially important in moving an animal from one country to another.
- Check current lists and requirements as these change fairly frequently.

For the owner:

- Defra Animal Health should be contacted regarding any CITES requirements.
- If appropriate for exportation, certificates should be obtained and submitted to the destination country for their CITES team to approve importation (failure to do so could lead to confiscation of the animal).
- For importation, a submission to Defra Animal Health for CITES approval should be made. If approved, an import certificate will then be issued.

For the veterinary surgeon:

- Advise the owner to clarify the situation regarding importing or exporting an animal with Defra Animal Health.

Commercial importation
This is a complex business involving a number of steps, encompassing both CITES and health controls. Many changes have taken place over recent years and more are under way, so it is always advisable to clarify the position with Defra Animal Health.

Veterinary surgeons should be aware that CITES rules are implemented differently in different parts of the world. Performing animals cause special problems where they may be imported into a country for a particular job, which may be for a matter of days or on a contract for several years. If the stay is long-term but ownership is not changing, it may be necessary for the animal to travel back to its country of origin simply for renewal of paperwork.

Diagnostic samples
It is important to note that currently CITES rules apply to all tissues from CITES specimens, including samples taken for diagnostic purposes. The Global Wildlife Division of Defra Animal Health should be contacted and appropriate paperwork obtained prior to sending samples outside the EU.

Sale

Pet Animals Act 1951

Pet Animals Act 1951 (Amendment) Act 1982

See also specific comments regarding the sale of threatened species under CITES, and of European species under the Wildlife and Countryside Act 1981.

British Veterinary Association (BVA) and local authority consultative groups have guidelines for inspection under the Pet Animals Act, which specifies housing dimensions and standards for shops. Considerations during an inspection should cover the basic 'Five Freedoms' (see below).

However, this legislation is likely to be repealed soon and covered within secondary legislation under the Animal Welfare Act 2006. Inspection may well be moved into an industry-regulated scheme monitored by United Kingdom Accreditation Service (UKAS).

Keeping, pets, performance and zoos

Animal Welfare Act 2006

Animal Health and Welfare (Scotland) Act 2006

The Animal Welfare Act 2006 applies to all vertebrate animals designated under the Act as 'protected' or 'for which a person is responsible'.

- An animal is a 'protected animal' if it is of a kind which is commonly domesticated in the British Isles (whether or not under the control of humans).
- An animal is a 'protected animal' if it is under the control of humans, whether on a permanent or temporary basis; or it is not living in a wild state.
- A person 'responsible for an animal' is the person responsible for an animal whether on a permanent or temporary basis and includes being in charge of it. A person who owns an animal is always regarded as being the person who is responsible for it.

A person commits an offence if they do not take such steps as are reasonable in all circumstances to ensure that the needs of an animal for which they are responsible are met to the extent required by good practice. For the purposes of this Act, an animal's needs shall be taken to include:

- Its need for a suitable environment
- Its need for a suitable diet
- Its need to be able to exhibit normal behaviour patterns
- Any need it has to be housed with, or apart from, other animals
- Its need to be protected from pain, suffering, injury and disease.

The appropriate national authority may issue, and may from time to time revise, codes of practice for the purpose of providing practical guidance in respect of any provision made by or under this Act. In England, where the Secretary of State proposes to issue (or revise) a code of practice under Section 14, they must:

- Prepare a draft of the code (or revised code)
- Consult appropriate persons appearing to represent any interests concerned about the draft
- Consider any representations made by the consulted persons.

At the time of writing the codes of practice are just beginning to appear, but it is unlikely that official Defra Animal Health codes of practice will exist for any 'exotic pets' other than monkeys and rabbits. However, the various strategy groups established by the England Implementation Group are developing authoritative strategies in all sectors and further developing Good Practice Guidelines from which care sheets can be derived.

In addition, Section 8 of the Animal Welfare Act 2006 creates a new concept and an offence if a person fails to take steps to meet the needs of an animal. This is a really difficult concept and one which is likely to be difficult to establish clearly when an offence is or is not being committed. The real problem is that it is an offence to not take steps to meet an animal's welfare needs.

Wildlife and Countryside Act 1981

The Wildlife and Countryside Act 1981 creates many powers to regulate the taking of listed species from the wild, sale and possession, prohibiting injuring or release without a licence. For example, there are complex rules regarding the ringing of raptors and the registration and sale of UK-bred passerines; this area is currently under review.

Dangerous Wild Animals Act 1976

Dangerous Wild Animals Act 1976 (Modification) (No. 2) Order 2007

Under the Dangerous Wild Animals Act 1976 owners and potential owners of certain species are required to obtain licences from the local authority to keep the animals. It incorporates a requirement for inspection of premises to ensure welfare and safety. This legislation had laudable aims but poor compliance, and a major review was undertaken in 2001.

Greenwood *et al.* (2001) carried out a study into the Dangerous Wild Animals Act 1976 on behalf of Defra Animal Health, and following lengthy consultation a second Modification Order was produced. The Dangerous Wild Animals Act 1976 (Modification) (No.2) Order 2007 revisited and reduced the list of species included. The list is now felt to be more 'meaningful', listing species which are genuinely dangerous and which should be in controlled ownership. A summary of the animals covered by the Dangerous Wild Animals Act 1976 is given in Figure 22.1. Zoos, circuses and pet shops are exempt from the Dangerous Wild Animals Act.

Mammals
Aardvarks Apes Badgers (except Eurasian) Bears including pandas Bovids (except domestic buffalo, cattle, goats and sheep) Camels Caribou (except domestic reindeer) Cats (black-footed, domestic, kodkod, rusty-spotted; except bay, Geoffroy, little-spotted, Pallas, sand and wild) Civets (African, large-spotted, Indian, Malay) Elephants Fishers Fossas Giant anteater Giraffes Hippopotamus including pygmy Horses including zebras (except donkey and domestic) Hyaenas (except aardwolf) Kangaroos (Eastern grey, red, wallaroo, Western grey) Lemurs (except woolly, bamboo and gentle) Monkeys (New World) (except night (owl), squirrel and titi) Monkeys (Old World) Moose Okapi Otters (except European) Peccaries Pigs (Old World: wild boar, warthog) Ratel Rhinoceros Seals (except common and grey) Tapirs Tasmanian devil Tayra Walrus Wild dogs (except foxes, raccoon dogs and domestic dog (not dingo)) Wolves Wolverine Also included: any mammalian hybrids with at least one parent of a dangerous wild animal included on the list and any animals of which at least one parent is such a hybrid. This does not apply to the cat hybrids (see the Modification Order 2007 for further information)
Birds
Cassowary Ostrich
Reptiles
Alligators Burrowing asps Caimans Some Colubridae (e.g. Amazon false viper, Argentine black-headed, boomslang, Peruvian racer, rear-fanged venomous snakes (African vine, Montpelier), red-necked keelback, South American green racer, yamakagashi Crocodiles All Elapidae Gharials including false gharials Sea snakes All Viperidae
Invertebrates
Scorpions (buthid, Middle Eastern thin-tailed) Spiders (brown recluse, Sydney funnel web, violin, wandering, widow)

22.1 Summary of animals covered by the Dangerous Wild Animals Act 1976.

Performing Animals (Regulation) Act 1925
Performing Animals Rules 1968

The Performing Animals (Regulation) Act 1925 and the Performing Animals Rules 1968 require any person who exhibits or trains any performing (vertebrate) animal to be registered with a local authority. The term 'exhibit' is defined as 'exhibit at any entertainment to which the public are admitted, whether on payment of money or otherwise…' and to 'train' means 'train for the purpose of any such exhibition'.

This provision applies to circuses and also to other situations, such as cabarets, film-making and plays, that involve animal performances and there is no exemption for excluding zoos. The definitions in the Act also appear to cover some of the training and performance with animals that takes place in zoos. However, it might be expected that training that is carried out to assist in the routine management of an animal (and not intended as preparation for performance) would not involve registration.

Controls for 'exotic' performing animals are likely in the future, possibly in the form of industry-generated Good Practice Guidelines and/or within Zoo Licensing legislation.

The Zoo Licensing Act 1981 (Amendment) (England and Wales) Regulations 2002
The Zoo Licensing Act 1981 (Amendment) (Wales) Regulations 2003
The Zoo Licensing Act 1981 (Amendment) (Scotland) Regulations 2003
The Zoo Licensing Regulations (Northern Ireland) 2003
EC Zoos Directive (1999/22/EC)
Secretary of State's Standards for Modern Zoo Practice

The Zoo Licensing Act 1981 (Amendment) (England and Wales) Regulations 2002 includes all places where animals not normally domesticated in the UK are displayed to the public for 7 days or more per year, whether a charge is made or not. This can range from a conventional zoo to a council operated park with aviaries. This Act is primarily concerned with public safety, although animal welfare issues are also covered. The recent Amendments to the Act comply with EC Zoos Directive (1999/22/EC) to provide for good standards of animal care, and to set the framework for the participation of zoos in conservation, research and education.

The Secretary of State's Standards for Modern Zoo Practice are the standards to which zoos and public aquaria must operate. The general standards are based around the 'Five Freedoms' and are presented as five principles:

- Provision of food and water: requiring attention to nutritional content, method of presentation and natural behaviour of the animal or bird

- Provision of a suitable environment: consistent with species requirements (spatial requirement, appropriate 3D environment)
- Provision of animal healthcare: to protect the animal from injury and disease
- Provision of an opportunity to express most normal behaviour: taking into account enrichment and husbandry guidelines
- Provision of protection from fear and distress: including group composition, sex ratios and stocking levels.

These principles provide a good structure for assessing any animal accommodation. The current standards are available from Defra Animal Health.

Health

Health and Safety at Work etc. Act 1974

Control of Substances Hazardous to Health (COSHH) Regulations 1988

Public Health (Control of Disease) Act 1984

Public Health (Infectious Diseases) Regulations 1988

The legal aspects of zoonotic diseases are important. The Health and Safety at Work etc. Act 1974, and the Control of Substances Hazardous to Health (COSHH) Regulations 1988 both apply here. Civil law relating to negligence also has a bearing with regard to clients and veterinary staff who may become infected or injured (Animals Act 1971, see below). COSHH sheets are now required to be prepared for zoonotic diseases.

Control of hazardous substances

The Control of Substances Hazardous to Health (COSHH) Regulations 1988 apply to biological agents and there is a Biological Agents Approved Code of Practice (ACOP) in addition to the general COSHH requirements. Biological agents are classified into Groups 1–4, with Group 1 being the least dangerous and Group 4 the most dangerous.

A suitable and sufficient risk assessment (Figure 22.2) must be carried out for any work activity involving the deliberate use of biological agents (e.g. research, medical care) or for any circumstances where exposure is incidental to the activity (e.g. veterinary work, farm work). The risk assessment should cover the agents (form, effects, hazard groups), the likelihood of exposure and disease, the possibility of substitution with a less hazardous agent, control measures, monitoring and health surveillance.

Detailed guidance is available on appropriate control measures, especially for intentional work with biological agents. The Health and Safety Executive (HSE) must be notified of the use, storage or consignment of biological agents. Protective clothing and equipment should not become a means of transmitting agents. Monitoring of exposure should be carried out if a suitable technique is available. Information should be

Identify all the hazards: those aspects of work that have the potential to cause harm	Substances Equipment Work processes Work organization Biological agents
Identify any specific regulations that must be complied with	
Assess all the risks: the likelihood that the harm will occur from the hazards identified	Be systematic in approach
Ensure that all aspects of the work activity are considered	Waiting room Consulting room Laboratory Operating theatre and preparation room Kennels/hospital facilities
Address what actually happens in the workplace, not what the staff handbook or practice manual says should happen	
Ensure that everyone who might be affected is considered	Veterinary staff (veterinary surgeons, veterinary nurses, kennel staff) Office staff Night cleaners Maintenance staff Visitors
Identify groups of workers particularly at risk	Young workers Inexperienced workers Lone workers Workers with disabilities Pregnant workers
Take account of existing preventive or precautionary measures and whether they are working properly	Isolation Effects to treatment Disinfection Air flow

22.2 Risk assessment.

provided to employees in writing, particularly when dealing with highly infective agents.

Public health

Other legislation relevant to zoonotic diseases includes:

- Public Health (Control of Disease) Act 1984: this is regarded as the key piece of legislation covering communicable diseases and gives various powers to the medical authorities
- Public Health (Infectious Diseases) Regulations 1988: this is the key legislation listing notifiable diseases in humans and updating controls. It includes rabies, tuberculosis, leptospirosis and anthrax.

Psittacosis

Psittacosis (chlamydiosis/chlamydophilosis/ornithosis) is perhaps the most significant zoonotic disease associated with birds. It should be recognized that people have died following becoming infected from their birds. At the same time it is a popular diagnosis (or misdiagnosis) in humans following disclosure that they have a pet bird.

Psittacosis or Ornithosis Order 1953

Diseases of Animals Act 1950

Diseases of Animals (Extension of Definition of Poultry) Order 1953

The Psittacosis or Ornithosis Order 1953 extends the definition of the expression 'disease' for the purposes of the Diseases of Animals Act 1950 to include 'psittacosis' or 'ornithosis'. The Order also provides for the detention and isolation of birds affected, or suspected of being affected, with this disease, and for the cleansing and disinfection of premises and utensils for such birds. The Order, together with the Diseases of Animals (Extension of Definition of Poultry) Order 1953, also enables the power of compulsory slaughter to be used, at the Government Minister's discretion, in respect of poultry affected with, or in any way exposed to, psittacosis/ornithosis. This Regulation brings 'parrots' within the definition of poultry.

Zoonoses Order 1989

Animal Health Act 1981

The Zoonoses Order 1989, made under the Animal Health Act 1981, designates organisms of the genus *Salmonella* and the genus *Brucella* as zoonoses, enabling powers (including those relating to the slaughter of poultry) under the Animal Health Act 1981 to be used to reduce any risk to human health from these organisms. Under this Order the term 'poultry' has been extended to include birds of any species. The Order provides for the imposition of control measures, including quarantine, movement restrictions, cleansing and disinfection.

Diseases of Animals (Seizure) Order 1993

This Order lists psittacosis (ornithosis) amongst the diseases to which it applies and essentially provides for the collection of samples, which can then be tested to exclude Newcastle disease and avian influenza.

- An inspector or veterinary inspector shall have power to seize anything (other than a live animal) whether animate or inanimate, by or by means of which it appears to them that a disease to which Section 35(1) of the Animal Health Act 1981 applies might be carried or transmitted.
- An inspector or veterinary inspector exercising powers under this Order shall dispose of the thing seized by destruction, burial, treatment or such other method of disposal as they think expedient to prevent the spread of disease.

Treatment and control

Various treatment regimes have been suggested for psittacosis, although doxycycline (Ornicure) is the only authorized drug for use in UK. The owner of the bird(s) must be advised about the zoonotic risks and about the difficulty of guaranteeing a complete clearance of organisms. Compulsory slaughter of psittacines has

never been carried out on the grounds of psittacosis infection. A number of veterinary surgeons have recommended this as a course of action but it is not required in the UK, and indeed is not widely considered necessary and may lead to claims for compensation.

Despite all of this psittacosis in humans is not currently a notifiable disease in the UK. For a time, to gather information, it was made notifiable in three local authorities (Cambridge City, South Cambridgeshire and East Cambridgeshire).

Diseases of Poultry (England) Order 2003

This Order makes avian influenza and Newcastle disease notifiable in any species of bird.

Fish

Aquatic Animal Health Directive 2006/88/EC

New legislation regarding fish and fish health is in the process of passing through consultation. The important legislation is the transposition of the Aquatic Animal Health directive 2006/88/EC into national legislation. Secondly, for unclear reasons secondary standards to assist the Environment Agency in dealing with novel parasites in fish being moved around the country are being introduced via the Marine Bill.

Medicines

Veterinary Surgeons Act 1966

Veterinary Surgeons Act 1966 (Schedule 3 Amendment) Order 1988

Medicines Act 1968

For the purposes of the Veterinary Surgeons Act 1966 the definition of 'animals' includes birds and reptiles but not fish. Pressure at the time that the Act went through the House of Lords resulted in fish being removed, despite strenuous efforts to have them included. The legal status of the exclusion is unclear since mammals are not specifically included either. However, treatment is still controlled by The Medicines Act 1968.

The RCVS has held in the past that it is the responsibility of veterinary surgeons to provide emergency first aid for all species and to ensure that the client can reach more experienced help where required. The veterinary surgeon should personally make contact with another colleague who can deal with the case. In circumstances where no practice in the area has the necessary expertise, the RCVS makes it clear that the practice which received the case initially must take all reasonable steps to obtain assistance so that the public (and the animals) are not denied help.

The Veterinary Surgeons Act 1966 (Schedule 3 Amendment) Order 1988 changes the type of treatment which can be carried out on animals (as covered by the 1966 Act) by the owner. It therefore makes no reference to fish.

Medicines (restrictions on the administration of veterinary medicinal products) Regulations 1994 (SI 1994/2987) as amended by SI 199712884 (Amelia 8)

These Regulations establish in UK law the prescribing cascade, and the requirements for minimum withdrawal periods and for record keeping by veterinary surgeons adopted by the EC in 1990. These requirements were incorporated in the Code of Practice for the Prescribing of Medicinal Products by Veterinary Surgeons introduced by the BVA in 1991 and, subsequently, in the RCVS Guide to Professional Conduct.

In summary, when no authorized veterinary medicinal product exists for a condition in a particular species, and in order to avoid causing unacceptable suffering, veterinary surgeons exercising their clinical judgement may prescribe drugs for one or a small number of animals under their care in accordance with the following sequence:

1. A veterinary medicine authorized in the UK for use in another animal species or for a different condition in the same species.
2. If there is no such medicine, use either:
   (a) A medicine authorized in the UK for human use
   (b) A veterinary medicine from another Member State or country outside the EU in accordance with an import certificate from the Veterinary Medicines Directorate (VMD).
3. If there is no such medicine, a medicine prepared extemporaneously by a veterinary surgeon, pharmacist or a person holding an appropriate manufacturer's authorization.

There are additional requirements for treating food-producing animals: drugs must be authorized for use in food animals, otherwise the treated animal (or eggs) should not be eaten.

General

Abandonment of Animals Act 1960

Protection of Animals Act 1911

The Abandonment of Animals Act 1960 makes it an offence of cruelty under the Protection of Animals Act 1911 to abandon an animal without reasonable excuse in circumstances likely to cause it suffering. For example, prosecutions have been sought in regard of pet cockatiels released when an owner moved house.

Animals (Scientific Procedures) Act 1986

The Animals (Scientific Procedures) Act 1986 as amended states that regulated procedures causing pain, distress or lasting harm in live vertebrate animals and the octopus must be authorized. Researchers and premises must also be authorized. This Act applies to zoos and fieldwork. It does not apply to procedures which are recognized veterinary, agricultural and animal husbandry practices. Most behavioural observation is not covered by the Act.

Animals Act 1971

This Act makes provision with respect to civil liability for damage done by animals. It places liability on the keeper, who at the time may not be the owner.

References and further reading

Cooper ME (1987) *An introduction to Animal Law.* Academic Press, London

Greenwood AG, Cusdin PA and Radford M (2001) *Defra Research Contract: CR0246. Effectiveness Study of the Dangerous Wild Animals Act 1976*

Health and Safety Executive (HSE) (2000) *Common Zoonoses in Agriculture.* HSE Books, London

Roberts V and Scott-Park F (2008) *BSAVA Manual of Farm Pets.* BSAVA Publications, Gloucester

Useful websites

The Department for Environment, Food and Rural Affairs (Defra) Animal Health: www.defra.gov.uk/animalhealth/cites

Health and Safety Executive (HSE): www.hse.gov.uk

Health Protection Agency: www.hpa.org.uk

The ICUN Red List of Threatened Species: www.iucnredlist.org

Joint Nature Conservation Committee (JNCC): www.jncc.gov.uk

United Nations Environment Programme (UNEP) World Conservation Monitoring Centre: www.unep-wcmc.org

Veterinary Medicines Directorate: www.gov.uk/vmd

23

North American legislation

Cathy Johnson-Delaney

Introduction

Veterinary surgeons within the United States (US) must be familiar with local, state, federal and international regulations pertaining to the exotic pet trade, zoological and wildlife species. This includes transportation, sale, animal husbandry, agricultural impact and public health implications, in addition to the legalities of private and public ownership of exotic species. Canadian veterinary surgeons have a smaller number of regulations and agencies that apply to exotic pets and wildlife. Both countries accept international policy concerning animals set by the 'Washington' Convention on International Trade in Endangered Species of Wild Fauna and Flora (CITES) (see Chapter 22).

Air transportation of live animals

Major airlines in both the US and Canada are members of the International Air Transportation Association (IATA), which was established to standardize air transport policies and sets humane guidelines for shipping animals. The Live Animal Regulations were developed to ensure the safety and welfare of all species of animal during air transportation. More than 230 airlines comply with these regulations, which are endorsed by CITES. IATA sets the standard for animal shipping crate design, size and material to ensure safe accommodation for the animal and safety for the airlines. In the US these crate standards are accepted as meeting or exceeding the transportation requirements of the Animal Welfare Act 1966.

United States

Several different federal government departments and agencies are involved with exotic animals and wildlife.

- The United States Department of Agriculture (USDA) includes the Animal and Plant Health Inspection Service (APHIS). The mission of APHIS is to promote the health and well being of US citizens and export customers through administration of federal laws and regulations (in cooperation with state governments), which pertain to animal and plant health, quarantine, humane treatment of animals, and the control and eradication of pests and disease.

- The Animal Health (AH, formerly Veterinary Services) Division of APHIS controls quarantine, importation of agricultural animals and birds, and interstate transportation. The AH Division also oversees the National Veterinary Services Laboratory in Iowa, as well as programmes such as brucellosis eradication and bovine spongiform encephalopathy surveillance.
- The Animal Care (AC) Division of APHIS is responsible for enforcement of the Animal Welfare Act 1966.
- The United States Department of the Interior (USDOI) includes the Fish and Wildlife Service (FWS). The FWS is responsible for enforcing US and international wildlife protection laws including:
  - CITES
  - Endangered Species Act 1973
  - Lacey Act 1900
  - Bald Eagle Protection Act 1940
  - Wild Bird Conservation Act 1992
  - Feather Import Quota: Tariff Classification Act 1930
  - Migratory Bird Treaty Act 1918
  - African Elephant Conservation Act 1989.
  The FSW is also responsible for permitting owning, selling and/or transporting captive-bred wildlife.
- The United States Department of Commerce (USDOC) includes the National Marine Fisheries Service (NMFS). The NMFS in conjunction with the FWS is responsible for the enforcement of the Marine Mammal Protection Act 1972 and the Endangered Species Act 1973 as it pertains to cetaceans and pinnipeds. The NMFS is also responsible for administering the Fur Seal Act 1966, which prohibits the taking of northern fur seals as well as the sale, importation, transportation and possession of northern fur seals or their parts.
- The United States Department of Health and Human Services (USDHH) oversees the Centers for Disease Control and Prevention (CDC).
- The CDC's office of Global Migration and Quarantine enforces the Public Health Service Act 1946.

Figure 23.1 provides a summary of US regulations and the animals to which they apply.

Animals	Regulations
Artiodactyla (even-toed ungulates)	Animal Welfare Act 1966 (AWA); CITES; Endangered Species Act 1973 (ESA); Lacey Act 1900 (LA); United States Department of Agriculture (USDA) quarantine and importation regulations (except hippopotamuses)
Carnivora (carnivores)	AWA; CITES; ESA; LA (including injurious animal regulations, LA-INJ); Marine Mammal Protection Act 1972 (MMPA; e.g. polar bears, sea otters)
Cetacea (whales, dolphins, porpoises)	AWA; CITES; ESA; LA; MMPA
Chiroptera (bats)	AWA; CITES; ESA; LA; LA-INJ; Public Health Service Act 1946 (PHSA)
Dermoptera (flying lemurs)	AWA; LA
Eagles	Bald and golden: Bald Eagle Protection Act 1940 (BEPA); ESA
Edentata (anteaters, sloths, armadillos)	AWA; ESA; CITES; LA
Hyracoidea (hyrax)	AWA; LA
Insectivora	AWA; CITES; ESA; LA
Lagomorpha (hares, rabbits, pikas)	AWA; CITES; ESA; LA; LA-INJ (European rabbit)
Mandarin duck	Feathers only: Feather Import Quota (FIQ): Tariff Classification Act 1930
Marsupialia (marsupials)	AWA; CITES; ESA; LA
Migratory birds	Migratory Bird Treaty Act 1918 (MBTA); CITES; ESA
Monotremata (platypus, echidnas)	AWA; CITES; LA
Perissodactyla (odd-toed ungulates)	AWA; CITES; ESA; LA; USDA quarantine and importation regulations (not rhinoceroses)
Pheasants (5 species)	Feathers only: FIQ
Pholidota (pangolins)	AWA; CITES; ESA; LA
Pinnipedia (seals and sea lions)	AWA; CITES; ESA; MMPA; Fur Seal Act 1966 (FSA) (northern fur seal only, which is exempt from the MMPA)
Primata (primates)	AWA; CITES; ESA; LA; PHSA
Proboscidea (elephants)	AWA; CITES; ESA; LA
Psittaciformes (parrots)	Non-US: Wild Bird Conservation Act 1992 (WBCA); CITES; ESA; PHSA; USDA quarantine and importation regulations
Ratites (ostriches, emus, rheas, cassowaries)	Eggs and chicks only: USDA quarantine and importation regulations; CITES; ESA; PHSA
Rodentia (rodents)	AWA (except domestic rats, mice); CITES; LA; LA-INJ; PHSA
Scandentia (tree shrews)	AWA; CITES; ESA; LA
Sirenia (manatees, dugongs)	AWA; CITES; ESA; LA; MMPA
Testudinata (turtles and tortoises)	PHSA; CITES; ESA (does not include leather back turtles or marine chelonians)
Tubulidentata (aardvarks)	AWA; CITES; LA

23.1 US regulations and the animals to which they apply.

Quarantine, import and export regulations

Animal quarantine, import and export regulations are administered by the AH Division of APHIS. The regulations apply to all avian species, members of the order Artiodactyla (except hippopotamuses) and members of the order Perissodactyla. The USDA should be contacted for specific requirements prior to the import or export of any animal. In addition, prior to export, the country of receipt should also be consulted for requirements.

Health certificates

Animals transported across state lines are required by the AH Division of APHIS to have a certificate issued by a USDA accredited licensed veterinary surgeon, certifying that the animal is free from infectious disease, including rabies. Most states have adapted the federal form (record of acquisition, disposition or transport of animals) for domestic animals, but for non-domestic species the federal form is required. The veterinary surgeon is responsible for submitting a copy of the certificate to the state of origin's state veterinary office.

Birds

Birds imported for pet or zoological display must be accompanied by an import permit issued in advance of the shipment in compliance with the Wild Bird Conservation Act 1992 and CITES. A health certificate issued by a government veterinary surgeon of the exporting country is required. Birds are inspected by a USDA veterinary surgeon at the designated port of entry, and are then quarantined for 30 days in a USDA approved facility (privately owned or government operated) at the port of entry.

All birds are screened for Newcastle disease and fed an antibiotic diet to suppress *Chlamydophila psittaci*. Birds imported as pets are quarantined at the owner's expense. Birds imported from Canada that have been in the owner's possession for at least 90 days prior to importation, and pass a health inspection at a designated Canadian border port, are not required to undergo quarantine.

In 1989 importation of ratites (cassowaries, emus, ostriches and rheas) was prohibited due to exotic ectoparasite arthropod infestation of ostriches arriving from Africa and Europe. In 1990 the ruling was modified to permit restricted entry of certified parasite-free chicks and hatching eggs.

Ungulates

A permit is required to import ruminants (including cervids), swine and horses from certain countries into the US. Elephants, hippopotamuses, rhinoceroses and tapirs must be treated for ticks.

Animal Welfare Act 1966

The Animal Welfare Act became law in 1966 and has been amended several times. The intent was to ensure humane treatment of warm-blooded animals used for exhibition, research or as pets. The Animal Welfare Act 1966 excludes birds, rats and mice. It is administered by the AC Division of APHIS, which issues registrations to animal breeders/dealers (including pet stores that sell non-human primates and other exotic small mammals such as sugar gliders or hedgehogs), transporters, exhibitors (zoos, collections open to the public, circuses, entertainment animals) and research facilities. The requirements for animal care as set down in the Act must be met or exceeded before registration is issued. In this context, exhibitors also includes aquariums that show mammals. Private zoos, collections and 'sanctuaries' are exempt unless they sell, trade or transport animals across state lines. Many exhibitors request inspection and registration to gain legitimacy for their programmes.

The regulations cover humane health and husbandry standards (feeding, water quality, ambient temperature, space and furnishings, handling, transportation, detailed facility structure and veterinary care) along with requirements for environmental enrichment and promotion of psychological well being. The Animal Welfare Act 1966 requires that institutions conducting animal research have a review committee (Institutional Animal Care and Use Committee, IACUC) as well as documentation of all activities conducted under the Act.

Bald Eagle Protection Act 1940

The Bald Eagle Protection Act was enacted in 1940 and has been amended several times. It prohibits the taking, possession or transportation of bald eagles (*Haliaeetus leucocephalus*) or golden eagles (*Aquila chrysaetos*) or their parts, nests or eggs without a permit. Sale, exportation and importation is also prohibited. This Act is administered by the FWS. Permits may be granted for scientific, exhibition or Native American religious purposes, or as part of depredation control. At the time of writing, the Act is being reviewed due to the population recovery of the two species.

Endangered Species Act 1973

The Endangered Species Act was enacted in 1973 and continues to be challenged and amended. It is intended to prevent the decline of wild animals and plants by prohibiting or restricting import, export, possession or commerce of critical species.

- Species in danger of extinction are listed as 'Endangered'.
- Species likely to become endangered are listed as 'Threatened'.

The two lists include wildlife and plants both native and foreign. If a species recovers, it may have its status changed or be removed from the list completely. For example, the bald eagle (*Haliaeetus leucocephalus*) was listed as endangered in 1973, and removed from the list in 2007 as the population had rebounded and was deemed stable.

The addition of species to the lists can be initiated by private individuals, the Secretary of the Interior or the Secretary of Commerce through the NMFS. The procedure is complex and requires scientific proof of population decline. A critical habitat for the proposed species must be designated within 1 year of the listing. All proposals must be published in the Federal Register and are open to public comment.

Permits for prohibited activities (e.g. scientific research, propagation programmes, zoological, horticultural or botanical exhibition) may be granted by the FWS. Captive-bred wildlife registration regulation of the Endangered Species Act became effective in 1979. This decreases the permit requirements for captive-born exotic, endangered or threatened species when prohibited activities enhance the propagation or survival of the species. 'Enhancing the propagation or survival of the species' includes activities that are shown not to be detrimental to the survival of wild or captive populations of the affected species. It provides for:

*   Healthcare
*   Management of populations (by culling, contraception, euthanasia, grouping or handling) to control of survivorship and reproduction, using similar practices of animal husbandry employed to maintain captive populations that are self-sustaining and possess as much genetic vitality as possible
*   Accumulation and holding of living wildlife that are not immediately needed or suitable for propagation or scientific purposes
*   Transfer of wildlife between individuals to relieve crowding or other problems that hinder the propagation or survival of the captive population at the location from which the wildlife would be removed
*   Exhibition of living wildlife in a manner designed to educate the public about the ecological role and conservation needs of the affected species.

Individuals, wildlife and zoological facilities are eligible to apply for captive-bred wildlife registration.

Wild Bird Conservation Act 1992

The Wild Bird Conservation Act 1992 established a new federal system to limit or prohibit importation of exotic bird species. It imposed an immediate moratorium on certain exotic bird species identified by CITES, and provided the procedure for the Secretary of the Interior to suspend trade in any CITES-listed bird species and remove trade suspensions on other species. The Act directed the Secretary of the Interior to publish in the Federal Register the list of exotic bird species for which trade was allowed, and provided procedures for determining such species. The Act provided criteria to determine whether exotic bird breeding facilities in other nations 'qualified' to export species to the US.

The Wild Bird Conservation Act 1992 allows for the periodic review of trade in non-CITES species, and authorizes the Secretary of the Interior to impose emergency moratoria or quotas if necessary for species conservation. The Act also directs the Secretary of the Interior to request information from exporting nations on their conservation programmes

for wild birds. It also designates purposes for which the Secretary of the Interior can issue permits (i.e. exemptions) for the importation of exotic birds. In addition, the Act has established guidelines for civil and criminal penalties for violations of the law, as well as enforcement guidelines and funding. It established an Exotic Bird Conservation Fund and directs the Secretary of the Interior to select, for assistance, projects in countries of wild bird origin. The Act also requires review of additional wild bird conservation programmes.

Feather Import Quota: Tariff Classification Act 1930

This Act, administered by the FWS, sets limits on the importation of skins and feathers from six bird species (it does not apply to live birds):

*   Blue-eared pheasant (*Crossoptilon auritum*)
*   Gold pheasant (*Chrysolophus pictus*)
*   Lady Amherst pheasant (*Chrysolophus amherstiae*)
*   Reeves pheasant (*Surmaticus reevesii*)
*   Silver pheasant (*Lophura nycthemera*)
*   Mandarin duck (*Aix galericulata*).

Lacey Act 1900

The Lacey Act was originally passed in 1900 and has been amended several times. It includes provisions that prohibit the importation, transportation or acquisition of any wildlife or their eggs, designated as injurious (LA-INJ) to the environment, to people, or to wild or agricultural animals and plants, into the US without a permit. The Act also makes it illegal to ship injurious wildlife across state lines. Species considered to be injurious include those of the genus *Pteropus, Atilax, Cynictis, Helogale, Herpestes, Ichneumia, Mungos, Suricata, Oryctolagus* or *Cuon*. The Act also prohibits the transportation in interstate or foreign commerce of wildlife taken, transported, possessed or sold in violation of any state or foreign law, international treaty, US regulation or Native American tribal law. The Act is enforced by the FWS and assists foreign countries and individual states to enforce their wildlife conservation laws.

Migratory Bird Treaty Act 1918

The Migratory Bird Treaty Act was passed in 1918 and implements treaties between Great Britain, Canada, Mexico, Japan, the former Union of Soviet Socialist Republics (USSR) and the US to protect migratory birds. It makes it illegal to take, possess, buy or sell a listed species. Permits for banding, marking, scientific collection, depredation control, taxidermy, waterfowl sale and disposal, falconry, and special purposes may be granted by the FWS. Sport hunting of certain migratory game birds is permitted in accordance with federal hunting regulations. Public, scientific and educational institutions are exempt from the Act but are required to maintain records on acquisition and disposition of listed species.

Public Health Service Act 1946

The Public Health Service Act 1946 was introduced to prevent the spread of communicable diseases by certain imported animals and applies to psittacine birds, turtles, tortoises and terrapins including their eggs (non-marine species), non-human primates, and domestic cats and dogs. Non-human primate importers must meet the requirements of CITES, the Endangered Species Act 1973 and the Animal Welfare Act 1966.

At the time of writing, the Act prohibits importation of more than six viable turtle eggs of a live turtle with a carapace length of ≤10 cm without a permit. A permit is not required for turtles with a carapace length >10 cm or for those marine species belonging to the families *Dermochelidae* and *Chelonidae*. The intent is to ensure that only individuals who have demonstrated that turtles will be isolated or confined in appropriate holding facilities to prevent human infection from *Salmonella* are granted permits. The regulation concerning the 10 cm turtle carapace rule is being debated as vendors of turtles are trying to prove that they can breed, distribute and maintain *Salmonella*-free turtles and tortoises for the pet trade.

The Act also requires that transportation of psittacine birds across state lines must be accompanied by a permit issued by the state health department in the receiving state, if such a permit is required by the state. In addition, transportation of psittacine birds can be restricted by order of the US Surgeon General in areas that have been declared to be infected with psittacosis (*Chlamydophila psittaci*).

Canada

Canada has far fewer regulations concerning exotic pets, zoological species and wildlife than the US.

Environment Canada

Canada Wildlife Act 1973
Migratory Bird Conservation Act 1994
Wild Animal and Plant Protection and
Regulation of International and
Interprovincial Trade Act (WAPPRIITA) 1992
Environmental (Species and Public Protection)
Amendment Act 2008
Environmental Management Act 2004

The primary regulation is the Canada Wildlife Act 1973, enforced under Environment Canada. This Act specifies the creation, management and protection of wildlife areas (designated National Wildlife Areas). Environment Canada also enforces the Migratory Bird Conservation Act 1994, which protects and conserves migratory birds and their habitats. The Wild Animal and Plant Protection and Regulation of International and Interprovincial Trade Act (WAPPRIITA) protects Canadian and foreign animals and plant species from illegal trade. It also protects Canada's ecosystems from introduction of harmful species and allows for measures necessary for efficient enforcement of CITES.

Under WAPPRIITA is the Species at Risk Assessment (SARA) provision. This provision allows for the protection and recovery of endangered or threatened plant and animal species, and for a list of these species to be generated. It also provides the framework to allow the different governments in Canada, organizations and individuals to work together to implement the regulations and decisions pertaining to the provision. In addition, SARA also establishes penalties for committing offences under WAPPRIITA. The Committee for the Status of Endangered Wildlife Species in Canada (COSEWIC) continually reviews the status of wildlife species in relation to the provision, and the Habitat Stewardship Program provides information concerning the regulations and decisions to the public.

At present, there are few laws in Canada that prevent the ownership, sale or trade of exotic animals. In 2008 British Columbia passed the Environmental (Species and Public Protection) Amendment Act (which amends the Canada Wildlife Act 1973 and the Environmental Management Act 2004). The Environmental (Species and Public Protection) Amendment Act 2008 fills regulatory gaps for managing and regulating ownership of alien species within the province. The Act also has the authority to address possession, breeding, release, trafficking, shipping or transportation of alien species, including tigers, venomous snakes and other animals which are potentially harmful to the public and/or native wildlife. The Act can also set penalties for offences. Under the Environmental (Species and Public Protection) Amendment Act 2008, the Minister can prohibit or regulate keeping of a listed alien species, making it an offence to acquire, possess or sell a listed species unless authorized within the regulation.

The Environmental (Species and Public Protection) Amendment Act 2008 is being considered as the first step in setting standards for exotic animal ownership, care, trade and transport. In March of 2009 new regulations under the Canada Wildlife Act 1973 were enacted. The new regulations prohibit the breeding, acquisition, selling or possessing of any listed exotic animal. Accredited zoos, research and educational facilities will be required to apply for permits from the Ministry of Environment for each animal. The film industry will also be regulated and required to obtain permits for temporarily bringing in any listed animal. A full list of controlled alien/exotic species and the requirements and restrictions under the new regulations are available from the Ministry of Environment.

Canadian Food Inspection Agency

Health of Animals Act 1990

The Animal Health Imports division of the Canadian Food Inspection Agency (CFIA) is responsible for the Health of Animals Act 1990 and regulations concerning pet importation. Requirements for importation of pet species are available from the CFIA website. The categories are listed as:

- Amphibians, reptiles and birds from the US
- Cats, dogs, fish, foxes, skunks and birds from other countries
- Ferrets (from the US), guinea pigs, gerbils, mice, rats, chinchillas, hamsters and other pet rodents
- Horses (from the US), pet rabbits, pet primates, scorpions or spiders.

Animals from countries other than the US have different requirements. For example, a pet ferret from the US does not require an importation permit but does require a vaccination certification for rabies within 1 year. If the ferret is under 3 months of age, no certificate or vaccination is needed.

References and further reading

Vehrs KL (1996) Appendix 3: Summary of United States wildlife regulations applicable to zoos. In: *Wild Mammals in Captivity Principles and Techniques*, ed. DG Kleiman *et al.*, pp. 593–599. University of Chicago Press, Illinois

Wells-Mikota SK (1993) Wildlife laws, regulations and policies. In: *Zoo and Wild Animal Medicine: Current Therapy 3*, ed. ME Fowler, pp. 3–10. WB Saunders, Philadelphia

Useful websites

Animal and Plant Health Inspection Service (APHIS)
www.aphis.usda.gov

Canadian Food Inspection Agency (CFIA)
www.inspection.gc.ca

Canadian Wildlife Service (CWS)
www.cws-scf.ec.gc.ca

Centers for Disease Control and Prevention (CDC)
www.cdc.gov

Fish and Wildlife Service (FWS)
www.fws.gov

International Air Transportation Association (IATA)
www.iata.org

List of birds protected under the Migratory Bird Treaty Act 1918
www.fws.gov/migratorybirds

Ministry of Environment
www.env.gov.bc.ca/fw/wildlifeactreview/cas

Conversion tables

Biochemistry

	SI unit	Conversion	Non-SI unit
Alanine aminotransferase	IU / l	x 1	IU / l
Albumin	g / l	x 0.1	g / dl
Alkaline phosphatase	IU / l	x 1	IU / l
Aspartate aminotransferase	IU / l	x 1	IU / l
Bilirubin	μmol / l	x 0.0584	mg / dl
Calcium	mmol / l	x 4	mg / dl
Carbon dioxide (total)	mmol / l	x 1	mEq / l
Cholesterol	mmol / l	x 38.61	mg / dl
Chloride	mmol / l	x 1	mEq / l
Cortisol	nmol / l	x 0.362	ng / ml
Creatine kinase	IU / l	x 1	IU / l
Creatinine	μmol / l	x 0.0113	mg / dl
Glucose	mmol / l	x 18.02	mg / dl
Insulin	pmol / l	x 0.1394	μIU / ml
Iron	μmol / l	x 5.587	μg / dl
Magnesium	mmol / l	x 2	mEq / l
Phosphorus	mmol / l	x 3.1	mg / dl
Potassium	mmol / l	x 1	mEq / l
Sodium	mmol / l	x 1	mEq / l
Total protein	g / l	x 0.1	g / dl
Thyroxine (T4) (free)	pmol / l	x 0.0775	ng / dl
Thyroxine (T4) (total)	nmol / l	x 0.0775	μg / dl
Tri-iodothyronine (T3)	nmol / l	x 65.1	ng / dl
Triglycerides	mmol / l	x 88.5	mg / dl
Urea	mmol / l	x 2.8	mg of urea nitrogen / dl

Temperature

	SI unit	Conversion	Conventional unit
	°C	(x 9/5) + 32	°F

Haematology

	SI unit	Conversion	Non-SI unit
Red blood cell count	10^{12} / l	x 1	10^6 / μl
Haemoglobin	g / l	x 0.1	g / dl
MCH	pg / cell	x 1	pg / cell
MCHC	g / l	x 0.1	g / dl
MCV	fl	x 1	$μm^3$
Platelet count	10^9 / l	x 1	10^3 / μl
White blood cell count	10^9 / l	x 1	10^3 / μl

Hypodermic needles

	Metric	Non-metric
External diameter	0.8 mm	21 G
	0.6 mm	23 G
	0.5 mm	25 G
	0.4 mm	27 G
Needle length	12 mm	$^1/_2$ inch
	16 mm	$^5/_8$ inch
	25 mm	1 inch
	30 mm	$1^1/_4$ inch
	40 mm	$1^1/_2$ inch

Suture material sizes

Metric	USP
0.1	11/0
0.2	10/0
0.3	9/0
0.4	8/0
0.5	7/0
0.7	6/0
1	5/0
1.5	4/0
2	3/0
3	2/0
3.5	0
4	1
5	2
6	3

Index

Index

Index

Index

Index

BSAVA Manuals

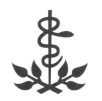

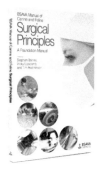
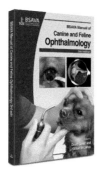
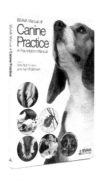
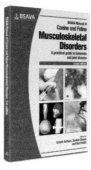
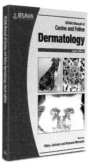
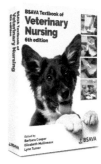

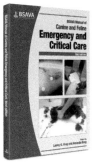
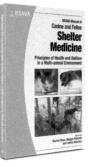
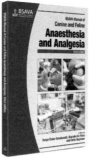
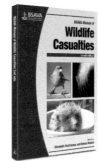
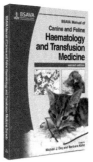
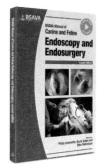

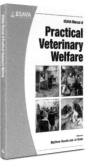
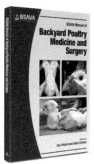
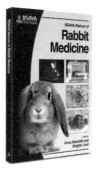
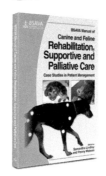
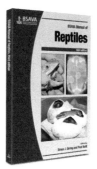
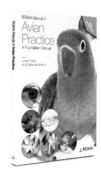

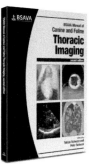
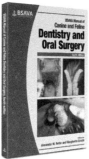
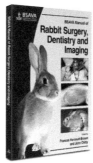
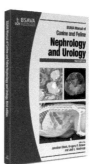
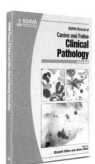

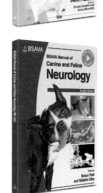
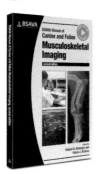
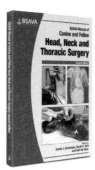
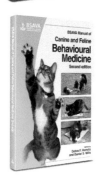
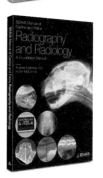

Tel: 01452 726700   Fax: 01452 726701

Email: administration@bsava.com   Web: www.bsava.com

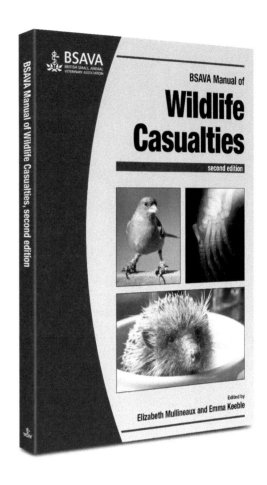